Oral Healthcare and Technologies:

Breakthroughs in Research and Practice

Information Resources Management Association
USA

IGI GLOBAL
DISSEMINATOR OF KNOWLEDGE

www.igi-global.com

Published in the United States of America by
IGI Global
Medical Information Science Reference (an imprint of IGI Global)
701 E. Chocolate Avenue
Hershey PA, USA 17033
Tel: 717-533-8845
Fax: 717-533-8661
E-mail: cust@igi-global.com
Web site: http://www.igi-global.com

Library of Congress Cataloging-in-Publication Data

Names: Information Resources Management Association, editor.
Title: Oral healthcare and technologies : breakthroughs in research and practice / Information Resources Management Association, editor.
Description: Hershey, PA : Medical Information Science Reference, [2017] | Includes bibliographical references.
Identifiers: LCCN 2016046529| ISBN 9781522519034 (hardcover) | ISBN 9781522519041 (ebook)
Subjects: | MESH: Dental Health Services | Oral Health | Biomedical Technology
Classification: LCC RK52 | NLM WU 29 | DDC 362.1976--dc23 LC record available at https://lccn.loc.gov/2016046529

British Cataloguing in Publication Data
A Cataloguing in Publication record for this book is available from the British Library.

List of Contributors

Table of Contents

Preface

The constantly changing landscape surrounding modern oral healthcare makes it challenging for experts and practitioners to stay informed of the field's most up-to-date research. That is why IGI Global is pleased to offer this single-volume comprehensive reference collection that will empower students, researchers, and academicians with a strong understanding of these critical issues by providing both broad and detailed perspectives on cutting-edge theories and developments. This compilation is designed to act as a single reference source on conceptual, methodological, and technical aspects, as well as to provide insight into emerging trends and future opportunities within the discipline.

Oral Healthcare and Technologies: Breakthroughs in Research and Practice is organized into three sections that provide comprehensive coverage of important topics. The sections are:

1. Clinical Applications.
2. Diagnostics and Imaging.
3. Education, Literacy, and Health Services.

The following paragraphs provide a summary of what to expect from this invaluable reference source:

Section 1, "Clinical Applications," open this extensive reference source by highlighting the latest trends and clinical uses of oral healthcare research. Through perspectives on computerized analysis, tissue engineering, and nanoparticles, this section demonstrates valuable clinical applications in the dental industry. The presented research facilitates a better understanding of how emerging technologies enhance healthcare.

Section 2, "Diagnostics and Imaging," includes chapters on novel innovations for dental image processing methods and perspectives on diagnosis techniques. Including discussions on X-ray images, muscle pain disorders, and splint therapy, this section highlights the changing landscape of image analysis and diagnostics in dental medicine. These inclusive perspectives contribute to the available knowledge on the implementation of technological tools in medical settings.

Section 3, "Education, Literacy, and Health Services," presents coverage on the benefits and methods of disseminating medical knowledge and research to the public. Through innovative discussions on social networking, teleconsultations, and healthcare delivery, this section contains pivotal information on the value of proper health literacy. The presented research assists in advancing current practices in public health education.

Although the primary organization of the contents in this work is based on its three sections, offering a progression of coverage of the important concepts, methodologies, technologies, applications, social issues, and emerging trends, the reader can also identify specific contents by utilizing the extensive indexing system listed at the end.

As a comprehensive collection of research on the latest findings related to *Oral Healthcare and Technologies: Breakthroughs in Research and Practice,* this publication provides researchers, practitioners, and all audiences with a complete understanding of the development of applications and concepts surrounding these critical issues.

Section 1
Clinical Applications

Chapter 1
Digital Occlusal Force Distribution Patterns (DOFDPs): Theory and Clinical Consequences

Robert C. Supple, DMD
Private Practice, USA

ABSTRACT

This chapter describes the many clinical applications of Digital Occlusal Force Distribution Patterns (DOFDPs) recorded with the T-Scan Computerized Occlusal Analysis system. Movements made by the Center of Force trajectory as force travels around the dental arches during the occlusion and disocclusion creates these patterns. The repetitive occlusal contact data points locate the force distribution received when teeth occlude against each other. These force distribution patterns correlate to intraoral compromised dental anatomy found in radiographs, photographs, and during the clinical examination of teeth and their supporting tissues. Moreover, they directly influence the envelope of motion, the envelope of function, and head and neck posture. This chapter illustrates with clinical examples the correlation between Stomatognathic System structural damage and repeating patterns of abnormal occlusal force distribution. The T-Scan technology isolates these damaging regions of excess microtraumatic occlusal force, absent of clinician subjectivity, thereby helping clinicians make an accurate, organized, and documented occlusal diagnosis.

INTRODUCTION

Technological Innovation and Dental Medicine

New paradigms brought on by technological advances offer fresh perspectives and solutions to old problems. As an example, the Hubble telescope is a technological advance that changed humanity's perception of the universe (Figure 1). Concepts evolve over years or decades, and sometimes over centuries. Technology can validate concepts developed by master teachers of the past, not by seeking to change the definition or the parameters of a concept, but rather to provide undeniable proof of a concept's inherent soundness.

DOI: 10.4018/978-1-5225-1903-4.ch001

Figure 1. T-Scan Sensor technology and Hubble Telescope were both major innovations in their respective disciplines, because they made visible what was previously invisible

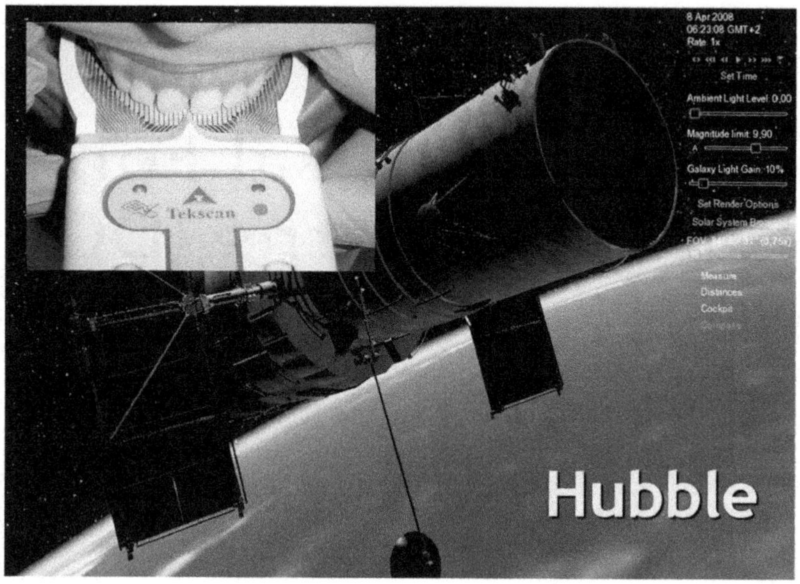

The science of occlusion has developed using traditional, accepted definitions (contained within the Glossary of Prosthodontic Terms) as a method of standardizing the interpretation of concepts related to the Stomatognathic system. Traditional occlusion is the study of spatial relationships that uses non-digital tools, such as stone casts, facebow transfers, and articulators, to assess these spatial relationships. Modern dental technologies, such as digital photography and radiology, enhance the diagnosis made with traditional, non-digital methods, which then further develop the science.

Digital applications will continue to grow as dental professionals keep finding ways of incorporating technology into the diagnosis and treatment of many dental conditions. Implementation must be simple, make sense to patients, and motivate them to seek comprehensive treatment. Digital data should also be affordable, productive, organized, and practical for clinicians to employ. Currently, digital technologies assist during diagnosis, treatment sequencing, and treatment. They also electronically document, educate, and monitor patient progress. Specialized software applications can image, design, and fabricate restorations while facilitating future diagnostic and treatment innovations. In Dental Medicine's digital evolution, computer-based applications are becoming instruments of change. Ultimately, economic benefits that provide a win-win situation for both patients and practitioners will transform evolution into revolution, providing Dental Medicine with new and innovative solutions.

In the oral cavity, articulating paper is the "Standard of measurement" used by every dentist worldwide, to "measure" and analyze occlusal contact pressure. Interestingly, articulating paper does not actually measure occlusal force or occlusal contact pressure (Carey et. al., 2007; Saad, et. al., 2008; Qadeer et. al., 2012), but is widely believed (surprisingly) to be able to do that by its appearance characteristics. Presently, no published study shows articulating paper markings can measure occlusal force.

Alternatively, the T-Scan system's recording sensor (HD Sensor, Tekscan Inc., S. Boston, MA, USA) transcends the analog generation of occlusal tools by acquiring differing relative occlusal contact force levels from all contacting teeth, thereby removing the occlusal contact force, pressure, and timing information from within the oral cavity, and displaying it on a computer monitor for instantaneous clinician viewing and analysis. In the same way that telescopes and microscopes opened our eyes to objects that had never been seen before to produce new theories that challenged our imaginations, the T-Scan technology opens new perspectives and possibilities for occlusal research, while offering occlusal solutions for every clinician who marks occlusal contacts with articulating paper, and then chooses the contacts for treatment by subjectively interpreting the marking's appearance (Kerstein & Radke, 2013).

Today's reality for diagnosing and improving the Standard of patient care, is correctly oriented and sized data images that are viewable in multiple dimensions. Diagnostic relative occlusal force scans record high-quality data measurements which are then archived in clinical records. With the T-Scan technology (Version 8, Tekscan Inc., S. Boston, MA, USA), form, function, and anatomy in motion can be imaged in a video format that explores the possibilities of advancing occlusal knowledge, while achieving healthy, efficient, occlusal function for patients.

Relative Occlusal Force Measurement is an Advance in Dental Occlusion

Experience and clinical observation teach that an occlusion can adapt and change. Measuring the force of an occlusal contact that has been generated by the envelope of function over time, illustrates where, when, why, and how adaptation to the applied force within the Stomatognathic system has occurred. The resultant occlusal force patterns tell the story about the occlusion's past, dictates treatment in the present, and predicts the survivability of the occlusion going forward into the future. Digital force recordings are simple to take, require less than a minute to complete, do not emit radiation, and require as little as 100 KB of storage to maintain.

Qualitative interpretation of articulating paper ink marks made by the clinician has been the accepted Standard of Care. Dentists use articulating ink to mark the occlusal contacts in vertical and horizontal directions, but the real question for clinicians to consider is, "what do the colored marks truly describe?" Current research is showing clearly that paper markings do not correlate to force levels (Carey et. al, 2007; Saad et. al., 2008; Qadeer et. al., 2012), which is contrary to what has been advocated and widely accepted for a very long time. Moreover, this method has recently come under scientific scrutiny as being highly inaccurate (Kerstein & Radke, 2013). A Subjective Interpretation study performed with 295 practicing dentists reported that older, more experienced practitioners demonstrated no better skills at choosing forceful occlusal contacts than did younger, less experienced clinicians. More importantly, the study showed that when dentists observe articulating paper markings to choose high and low force occlusal contacts, they will choose incorrect contacts 88% of the time, when basing their contact selections on the appearance characteristics of the paper markings (Kerstein & Radke, 2013).

As an alternative to the subjective interpretation of articulating paper markings, digital force scans can clarify which colored articulating paper markings are the truly problematic contacts, by grading the occlusal contacts to 256 differing levels of relative occlusal force. This method objectively determines the contacts that are time-premature, or possess occlusal force excess.

In the past, the art and science of measuring oral articulations and cycles of repetitive occlusal contact depended solely on the skill and knowledge of clinicians who interpreted what the colored ink that was transferred onto the occlusal surfaces of teeth, meant clinically. A digital force pattern added onto an articulating paper marking's appearance will either validate the original diagnosis, or offer an alternative thought process because of the clinical visualization of the additional relative occlusal force data. Articulating paper has value in marking the occlusal contacts, but computer generated occlusal force measurements divide and organize the differing contact points into accurate, meaningful information that is not available to the clinician who solely relies on traditional ink markings. Digitally, the occlusal contact forces are represented to the clinician by colored pixels and columns that form the building blocks of a 3-Dimensional occlusal force video, which greatly improves the study of a patient's occlusion.

T-Scan I

Computerized occlusal analysis was introduced in April 1987 by a group of engineers led by Dr. William Maness (Maness, 1987; Maness, Benjamin, Podoloff, Bobick, & Golden, 1987; Maness & Podoloff, 1989). The T-Scan I technology (Tekscan Inc., S. Boston, MA, USA) created a new paradigm in the measurement of occlusal contacts by introducing empirical evidence recorded with a sensor that was designed and fabricated to collect occlusal force data electronically. The first generation of scans quantified and qualified articulating paper marks, illustrated the engagement of the mandible going into and out of maximum intercuspation (MIP), and captured the duration of posterior teeth engagement during excursive function (Kerstein & Wright, 1991). The recorded data was displayed for playback and analysis in two and three dimensions with frame-by-frame graphical video animations. The fourth occlusal dimension, visible for the first time in the history of Dental Medicine, was occlusal contact "time durations."

Maness, the creator of the T-Scan I System, predicted that force scans would uncover the mysteries of occlusal diagnosis, and provide for therapies that traditional articulating paper markings had not yet solved (Maness, 1987). He pointed out that this technology had applications in occlusal adjustment procedures, TMJ disease, restorative dentistry, periodontics, and orthodontics. It also offered promise in analyzing the functional health of the muscles of mastication, by using occlusal contact pattern reproducibility and total time-duration of closure from first occlusal contact through into habitual occlusion, as a measure of occlusal health (Maness, 1987).

Digital force scans opened the doors of Dental Medicine to a new frontier in occlusion, because it allowed clinicians to see what was invisible to the naked eye, and to discover a level of occlusal reality that was not suspected to exist. This new digital force measurement technology made it possible for clinicians to expertly detect, assess, and target excess occlusal contact force, completely absent of clinical subjectivity. The concepts that emerged using the T-Scan I generated new occlusal applications and a level of occlusal precision and control that did not exist prior to its invention.

However, any new technology needs to enlist early adopters to cross the chasm of resistance, and produce platforms that validate the technology's accuracy, reliability, and usefulness, while creating excitement about the product's possible clinical applications. As with all things computer, there existed (and still exists today) a new-user learning curve that must be mastered to reach clinical implementation competency (see chapter 4 for a detailed explanation of the user skills required to attain T-Scan mastery). Clinicians and educators who presently want to learn to use the T-Scan technology, would greatly benefit from taking advantage of the experience of the early adopters who have significantly reduced the learning curve for the later adopters.

Today, the ability to measure, change, and monitor the dynamics of the Stomatognathic system using objective occlusal force data is potentially available in every clinical dental space that has a computer.

Because the current version of the T-Scan contains a patient database (T-Scan I did not have a patient database), scans recorded today can readily be compared to future scans of the same patient. This allows the clinician to better understand long-term occlusal diagnostic information about a patient's function over time, and the adaptive process that the teeth and related structures have undergone trying to accommodate the ongoing cycles of occlusal force distribution.

The conclusions reached from analyzing the digital occlusal force distribution data provide knowledge that clinicians can use to produce educated treatment results. This new occlusal force information has created new questions from patients, allowed for the development of new occlusal theories, changed concepts that have been espoused in older philosophies, and created opportunities for performing meaningful occlusal research.

This chapter represents the initial attempt by the author to publish these observed (for the past 15 years) clinical relationships between recorded patterns of unbalanced occlusal force distribution and structural changes in the teeth, the periodontium, and the structures of the Temporomandibular joint complex. These patterns of force distribution that occur during maxillomandibular engagement are recorded in a digital format, and provide improved diagnostic insight into the functional dynamics of the Stomatognathic system, in comparison to traditional, non-digital, and subjectively interpreted, occlusal indicators. The T-Scan's 2 and 3-Dimensional objective force measurements bring articulating paper markings into the digital age of Dental Medicine.

Digital Occlusal Force Measurement as Part of a Comprehensive Patient Exam

The diagnosis made from a comprehensive oral health assessment is usually multifactorial. Three components of a comprehensive oral exam are diagnosing how teeth occlude, how healthy is the supportive anatomy, and how efficient is a patient's ability to function. Alternatively, subjective ink mark interpretation limits the profession's ability to translate ink markings into meaningful force information. Recorded occlusal force data studied over time can be obtained from any patient, and can be taken at any age in their occlusion's evolution. The ultimate goal should become to turn comprehensive oral exams into clinical opportunities that prevent, or limit pathology from further compromising Stomatognathic system anatomic structures.

Digital occlusal force scans often illustrate violations of sound occlusal force distribution that challenge the anterior and condylar guidance, while exposing the existence and locations of forceful, prolonged, and premature occlusal interferences. This information will likely transform the clinicians' diagnostic skills, and motivate them to update their practice business model, to provide patient's with faster, more accurate, and higher-quality occlusal services.

The addition of the T-Scan computerized occlusal analysis system to the comprehensive examination gives clinicians:

- A *diagnostic* tool capable of predicting impending occlusal force problems that, once isolated, can be prevented with targeted intervention.
- A *precision* tool for identifying problematic occlusal contact points.
- An *orientation* tool that accurately pinpoints areas within the dental arches where the anatomy is stressed by excess occlusal force, and might lead to altered mandibular function.
- A *documentation* tool that collects and stores occlusal force and timing measurements for future comparison.
- An *educational* tool for doctors, staff, and patients.
- A *communication* tool effective at boosting case acceptance by motivating patients to own their occlusal problems that require treatment.

- A *monitoring* tool that measures occlusal force changes over time.
- A *treatment* tool that measures immediate and long-term occlusal intervention results.
- A *practice-enhancement* tool.
- A *digital upgrade* to traditional analog articulating paper Subjective Interpretation.

Digital Occlusion as a New Paradigm

Changing a habits and developing a new paradigm to replace old patterns involves a learning curve. However, the benefit of adopting the T-Scan technology is that there becomes a measured rationale to occlusal diagnosis and treatment. Clinicians have developed their own philosophy of occlusion based on pattern recognition and past clinical experience. Anatomic structural changes like wear facets, muscular pain, abfraction formation, or periodontal pockets absent of plaque, are diagnostic clues for the clinician that the occlusion is compromising the structure.

Every patient has a mandibular envelope of motion, an envelope of function, and a repetitive habitual force cycle. *Force cycles* involve the engagement and release of force when the mandible lands in maximum intercuspation (MIP), and then reverses direction away from maximum intercuspation. Proprioception constantly changes in the oral cavity such that the teeth, the CEJ, and the foundation structures incrementally adapt to the repetitive force cycle, over time. A pathologic force cycle causes structural damage, whereas a physiologic force cycle will be preservational of the system's structures.

The future of occlusal analysis will be to capture occlusal force information accurately, and to diagnose the change as physiologic or as pathologic. The challenge going forward will be to understand in a digital format, the dynamic relationship between occlusal force application during the processes of occluding and disoccluding.

The differences between using analog articulating paper from the past, and using today's digital occlusal technology are outlined in Table 1.

Clinical Uses of Force Scans

There are a variety of clinical uses that digital occlusal force scans offer daily occlusal practice. They are:

- To accurately visualize occlusal contact force content, time of occurrence, location, and intensity, outside of the oral cavity for improved diagnostic visualization.
- To record in real-time, functional force movies that measure the occlusion and disocclusion contacts in different posture orientations.
- To create, analyze, and archive force scans for future occlusal history referencing.
- To measure occlusal contact forces in an entire arch so that all forceful contact points can be properly identified. This method eliminates false positive paper markings and saliva concerns, while measuring the effect that combined occlusal materials contribute to the occlusal function.
- To increase the diagnostic accuracy and precision of any articulating paper mark, and to better identify where microtrauma and occlusal interferences may cause structural damage.
- To isolate the intensity, direction, and sequence of force as it occurs on any tooth, groups of teeth, or over an entire arch.
- To combine the findings of a force scan with other digital diagnostic technologies to better understand occlusal function.

Table 1. Comparison of measuring occlusal contacts with Articulating Paper vs. T-Scan technology

Measuring Envelope of Function Occlusal Contacts with Analog vs. Digital Tools		
Occlusal Force Data Characteristics and Measurements	**Analog (Articulating Paper)**	**Digital (T-Scan)**
Location of contact	✓	✓
Intensity of contact		✓
Plane(s) of contact / frame(s) of analysis*	1	100-300*
Sequence of contacts		✓
Shape of a full arch of contacts	Possibly	✓
Repeating contact patterns		✓
Force transfer movement in any direction	Possibly	✓
Occlusion timing (duration of contact)		✓
Disclusion timing (release of contact)		✓
Premature contact identification	Possibly	✓
Accurate recording in a wet field		✓
Contact not influenced by occlusal materials		✓
Immediate dynamic playback in 2 and 3 Dimensions		✓
Instantaneous, real-time display of an entire arch that is visible to patient on a monitor		✓
Envelope of function movies		✓
Recording of a CO movie (habitual force pattern)		✓
Recording of CR movie (skeletal force pattern)		✓
Storage and retrieval of pre, mid, and post treatment measurements		✓
Capable of interfacing with other digital diagnostic technologies		Absolutely

* Articulating paper shows a single static image of contacts while the T-Scan plays back multiple frames of occlusal engagement in 0.01 second long intervals, or.003 second-long intervals in Turbo-mode

- To aid in the development of a treatment sequence.
- To establish a quality control standard for occlusal management and the balancing of the Stomatognathic system, that will help prevent adaptation from exceeding physiologic limits.
- To increase co-discovery and patient acceptance through education and recognition.
- To advance the future clinical care of the human occlusion with a "measure, predict, and prevent" model.
- To advance concepts, techniques, applications, and knowledge in the diagnosis and treatment of occlusal problems digitally and biometrically, rather than observationally and subjectively.

FORCE CYCLE DEVELOPMENT AND FORCE SCANS ANALYSIS

Introduction to Point, Line, Frame, and Pattern

This section of the chapter illustrates how the T-Scan technology enhances the information that articulating paper marks have been previously thought to provide. As was previously stated, modern studies show that paper markings do not illustrate force content in any reliable way. Alternatively, force scans record and quantify occlusal forces as they are transferred onto occluding teeth, in a measurably repeatable way (Kerstein, Lowe, Harty, & Radke, 2006; Koos, et. al., 2010). Therefore, a new T-Scan user must grasp the inherent differences between articulating paper ink markings, and real-time occlusal force movies that are displayed in two and three dimensions. A force movie reports on every occlusal contact which can be reviewed for analysis, one frame at a time, forwards, backwards, or in super slow motion, comparable to how instant replay describes sports on television.

Initially, the amount of acquired occlusal force data may appear as overwhelming to a new T-Scan user. Therefore training and frequent clinical practice are both required to expand a new user's T-Scan implementation knowledge. A single frame of T-Scan data can appear somewhat similar to articulating paper marks, which can make the data somewhat easier for a new user to understand and interpret. However, each T-Scan recording displays all recorded contacts throughout the arch, whereas articulating paper often marks only a few teeth unilaterally, or regionally. Additionally, the digital force data is unaffected by saliva or the differing occlusal dental materials, which often hinders the clinician from visualizing the paper contact markings.

To simplify undergoing the paradigm shift required to recognize and employ digital occlusal data, the contact information can be analyzed with four T-Scan software features (Table 2):

- **Points:** Point data illustrates where the primary contact locations exist, and visualizes their relative force intensity.
- **Lines:** Center of Force trajectory lines that extend from one contact point to another define the primary direction of force transfer across and within the arches.
- **Frames:** In function, the mandibular plane engages the maxilla, stops in MIP, and releases from occlusal contact, thereby producing a force cycle that lasts approximately one second in duration. The T-Scan's 0.003-0.01-second-long force movie frames describe each force cycle in small time increments, that illustrate in great detail the occlusal contact order and the differing contact force intensities, and how they sequentially occurred in real-time.
- **Patterns:** Force patterns illustrate the cyclic and repetitive application of force distributed over the contacting teeth. As force cycles change over time, the envelope of function and the envelope of motion can change as well.

Table 2. Summary of the occlusal information described by Points, Lines, Frames, and Patterns

	Points	Lines	Frames	Patterns
Force Location	✓	✓	✓	✓
Force Intensity	✓	✓	✓	✓
Force Order	✓	✓	✓	✓
Timing/Sequencing	✓	✓	✓	✓
Occlusal Interference	✓	✓	✓	✓
MIP	✓	✓	✓	✓
Force Direction		✓	✓	✓
Force Distribution		✓	✓	✓
Envelope of Function			✓	✓

Frame-by-frame data playback aids in the determination of what a single forceful contact point can structurally influence. By combining the displayed excess force locations with the time of their occurrence in the closing contact sequence, the clinician is better able to answer the questions:

- *Where is excess force located?* The location of a high intensity contact that persists for a prolonged period of engagement and release, denotes an interference that puts the surrounding anatomy at potential structural risk.
- *What is at risk structurally?* A high-intensity, long duration contact, as well as a cluster of excessively forceful contacts, requires the involved anatomy to adapt and accommodate the force content of the contact(s). Over time, this structural adaptation could damage the involved anatomy because the absorption of the force by the muscles, the teeth, the cementoenamel junction (CEJ), and the condyle-disc assemblies, requires the system to absorb the force in order to minimize the effects of the excessively forceful contacts on functional equilibrium.
- *How to use?* Force scans find and describe interference locations that prevent functional balance between the mandible and the maxilla. Therefore, using this computer-isolated excess force detection methodology, assists the clinician in locating interferences which often result from an unbalanced skeletal plane of occlusion, and those that are formed from either poorly aligned natural teeth or prosthetic replacements. These detected regions of force excess may be a single contact, a single tooth in total, or on groups of teeth. Additionally, when considering occlusal intervention, the force scan guides the clinician when performing any mitigating treatment.
- *Why intervene?* The envelope of force and envelope of function should remain balanced as patients age in order to maintain a physiologic healthy occlusion. When the force envelope is unbalanced, the function and the system are induced to adapt, and may become pathologic. Motion at odds with structural design is at best adaptive, and at worst, destructive.
- *When to assess?* A force scan of MIP can be taken at any age, at any time, and whenever excessive force might be thought to be a contributing factor to structural breakdown. Therefore, any exam can be an opportunity to take a force distribution measurement. Hygiene recall, new patient exams, and emergency assessments, all are potential opportunities to teach both patients and clinicians about the quality of the force distribution and its management while the patient ages over the course of time.

Points: Intensity of Contact Force

In Dental Medicine, "points" and diagnosis are often related. Clinicians use an explorer point to find tactile irregularities in teeth and restorations, periodontal probes are used to quantify degrees of epithelial attachment breakdown, fingers palpate Temporomandibular joint ligaments, assess fremitus teeth, isolate muscle trigger points, and articulating paper is used to mark points of occlusal contact.

A "contact" is the state of physical touching. A recorded contact is used to visualize force and timing information, which brings life and meaning to traditional paper ink marks. All questions regarding the intensity of small dots, the force content of large marks, the contact locations, and the sequence, are answered with a properly recorded force scan. The "guess factor" or the Subjective Interpretation of what a clinician might think an articulating mark means is eliminated, while experience using digital occlusal force data teaches confidence and improved clinical judgment.

Applying simple concepts to the recorded T-Scan data is a strategy for the new user to learn successful T-Scan data analysis skills. Begin by observing the 2-Dimensional "Point View" (Figure 5, bottom pane), which displays and quantifies every loaded, square-shaped sensor sensel. In the 2-Dimensional "Point View," the T-Scan data resembles traditional articulating paper dots.

The 2-Dimensional Point View" illustrates:

- The varying intensity of the differing occlusal contacts;
- Any changes in contact position due to force movement across the surface of the contacting teeth;
- The contact timing sequence and contact order;
- The distribution of force as the mandible engages the maxilla and then releases.

Point contact data locates the contacts within the arch and registers their intensity using sensels embedded in a Mylar matrix. Each T-Scan sensor has 400 sensels per square inch (Figure 2). Sensels are like pixels that can detect 256 varying levels of occlusal contact force intensity.

Points can appear and then disappear as opposing teeth make and then break contact. The varying levels of contact intensity are displayed in a graded color-coded format based upon the activated sensel's electronic Digital Output (*DO*). Each loaded sensel illustrates the physical interaction that occurs when mandibular teeth engage the maxillary teeth, which transfers force onto the *plane of occlusion*. Every contact in the arch is organized and displayed in the order it occurred during the movement (Figure 2). The character of a point contact, including a cluster of point contacts (Figure 3), is critical to the amount of destruction a contact or a group of contacts can cause over a period of time. Points that receive chronically higher occlusal force levels over time should be considered microtraumatic to the anatomy involved. As such, *Points* are a collection of diagnostic data that predict the location of structural microtrauma that can induce system structural adaptation.

Contacts can be functional or parafunctional over the life of a single tooth, as well as to the system that surrounds it. A parafunctional interference is a violation of motion and of function that is not in harmony with the occlusal design. Non-working cusps are much more susceptible to fractures (Bader, Shugars, & Sturdevant, 2004). Unbalanced microtrauma produces extra stress and a vector of force that is not in harmony with the long axis of the involved tooth, or with the design of the system as a whole. Teeth are designed to receive force along their long axis to best dissipate the contact energy. As such, over the long-term, a parafunctional interference that is in contact from the beginning of a force cycle,

Figure 2. The left pane shows a T-Scan sensor schematic design. The middle pane shows displayed T-Scan point contact data with the COF trajectory superimposed. The right pane illustrates a single sensel (outlined) within the grid of many sensels, embedded in the Mylar sensor matrix.

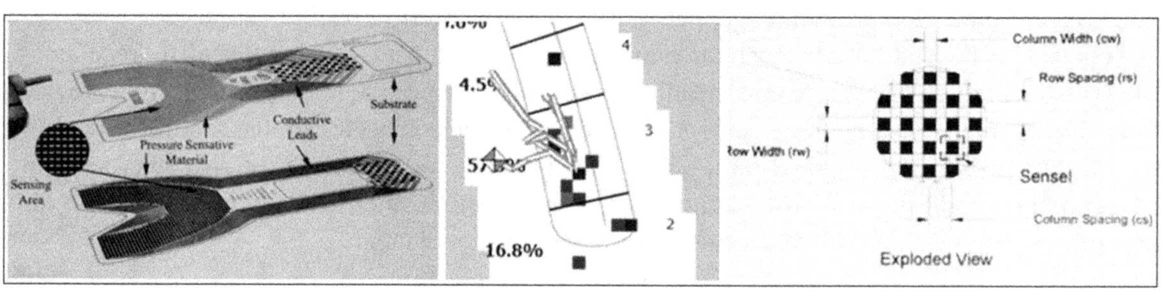

Figure 3. The distribution of 2-Dimensional point contacts (left pane) and the 3-Dimensional columnar presentation (right pane) of those same 2-Dimensional point contacts, with both views displayed at MIP. Tooth #18 contacts tooth #15 with higher force compared to all other contact areas as the patient occludes into MIP. The overall force balance is good (the COF is centered), with the exception of one contact point that can causes microtrauma to the distobuccal cusp of tooth #15.

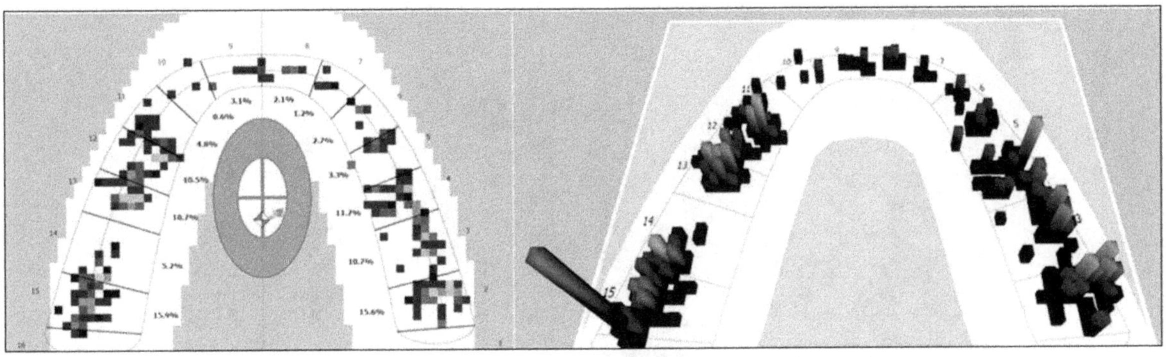

and remains in contact until the mandible separates from the maxilla to release the applied force, will likely erode the integrity of the surrounding anatomy. Prolonged intensity creates resistance, interference, or microtrauma, all of which impedes the system's balance.

Most force scans often have a large amount of dark blue sensel activation that defines areas of minimal or light force, which spread out across the sensor surface (Figure 3). The T-Scan since version I, has repeatedly demonstrated that large articulating paper markings may or may not register intense or high force areas. In addition, not all points that register high intensity are pathologic. Higher force contacts that register as red or pink in color require further investigation as to their location, time of occurrence during the sequence of the force cycle, and the duration of time within the cycle the high force remains present. A red or pink contact that initially appears near the end the force cycle (above 90% of Total Force near MIP) will never be as damaging as one that appears early in the force cycle (for example, at 25% of Total Force), and then maintains that high level of contact force within that cycle until MIP is reached, well past 90% of Total Force.

A basic and simple application to record, is to instruct patients to close down on a sensor and squeeze their teeth together in the same manner they would when dentists use articulating paper (Figure 3).

Defining Cluster Points

Cluster point contacts are collected groups of contact points that appear early in closure (occlusion) and leave late in release (disocclusion) (Figure 4). These clusters are often primary closure *occlusal interferences*, which can also be present during excursive movements. Note in Figure 4, that when the patient slides in all directions, the articulating paper leaves ink within the visible wear facets suggestive of a group function occlusal scheme. Clusters of heavy, prolonged force usually indicate a strong occlusal interference. The mesial marginal ridge of tooth #15 and the distobuccal incline of tooth #14 are the first points of contact when the mandible is gently directed into the maxillary plane of occlusion.

Figure 4. An example of Cluster Points. The left pane shows teeth #11 to #15 marked with blue articulating paper. Tooth #15 receives the strongest grouping of occlusal interferences noted in the T-Scan data, which is not accurately demonstrated by the articulating paper mark distribution. The dominance of this posterior left cluster prevents the entire system from achieving balance.

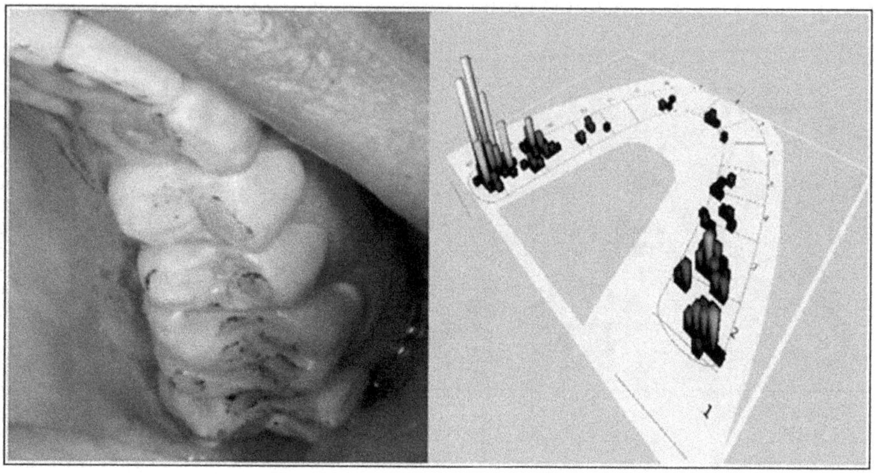

Points Outline the Entire Dental Arch

Point data can affect a single tooth (see Figure 6a), but point data as a system provides insight into the diagnosis of the mandible's favored pathway of function. Asking a patient to "tap-tap" on a recording sensor is similar to the common technique of marking contacts with articulating paper. However, it differs in that the T-Scan displays and illustrates where in the arch specific teeth touch forcefully, because the Point contact display outlines the entire dental arch around all of the recorded occlusal contacts. Figure 5 shows the recorded force pattern made following two "taps" on the sensor. The entire distribution of all points that occurred into MIP is displayed for analysis, with the COF target and the COF trajectory superimposed over the target. Point contacts repeat their sequence and distribution when the mandible engages the maxilla. Repeating points define force cycles which direct the envelope of function into and away from contacts that interfere with a balanced occlusion.

Points of Microtrauma Can Promote Pathology

Forceful point contact can raise concerns about potentially compromised clinical anatomy that may be present in one contact area, or over an entire arch. Measuring the force in the area of concern often leads to a diagnosis that will direct the clinician to investigate that area for structural damage. Intense points that arrive early and leave late in the force cycle often lead to the visualization of the system's weakest link. Over time, these pathologic forceful point contacts will eventually destroy the anatomy in question and/or alter the proprioception of the system. Problematic point contact can also be matched to radiographs, photographs, or clinical observation of structure compromise during examinations, all of which aid the clinician in arriving at a more informed diagnosis. Digitally recorded occlusal contact point data does not replace articulating paper (because the T-Scan sensor does not "mark" the involved teeth), but this data does define, clarify, and organize problematic contact points for analysis by the clinician.

Figure 5. This recorded force pattern was made following two "taps" on a T-Scan sensor. All point contacts that occurred on the way into MIP are displayed around the arch. Note that the left side point distribution is different from that of the right side. The gray Center of Force target (COF) and the red COF trajectory lines illustrate the history of where the total force summation was located in previously recorded "tapping" movements. The left and the right sides of the arch have an equal amount of points in contact, but the points on the left side are twice as intense.

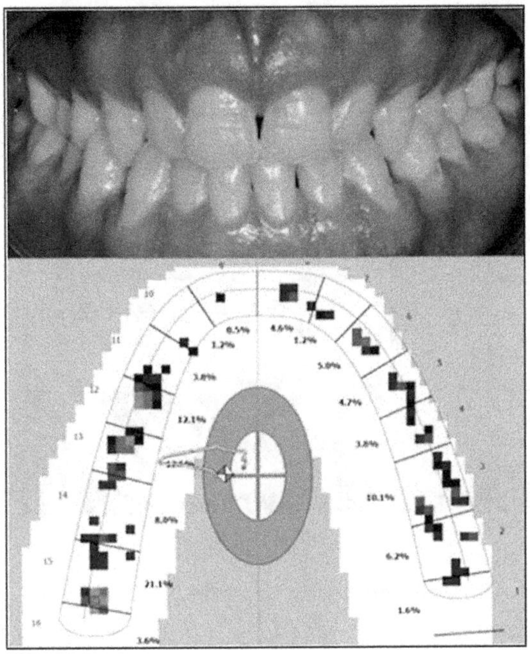

Figures 6a and 6b demonstrate how a longstanding, forceful occlusal interference caused microtrauma that weakened the surface tooth structure, thereby allowing bacteria to populate in the resultant enamel defect and cause decay (Figure 6a). This was the patient's first required restoration since having sealants placed at age 12. The patient presented not reporting tooth discomfort, but with a chief complaint of right Temporomandibular joint pain, with an early "click" present upon opening and during the left lateral excursion. The patient also complained of experiencing right temporal headaches. These symptoms indicated that a diagnostic force scan should be recorded. The extreme point contact force present on tooth #31 matched the location of the enamel micro fracture, and the resultant caries (Figure 6b).

To summarize, the following factors should be considered important when analyzing contact *Point* data:

- Points illustrate a patient's occlusal contacts at the beginning, middle, and end of a recorded force cycle.
- A point indicates that a single sensel was triggered by the demonstrable force contained within an occlusal contact.
- Points organize contacts by tooth surface location, by position within the arch, and by varying occlusal force intensity.
- Contact intensity can be viewed in 3-Dimensions using a measured range of colored columns, and can be organized in 2-Dimensions by relative occlusal force percentages per tooth.

- Points can be individually isolated or form clusters, indicating that greater occlusal contact area is under excessive load. The clinician can review the timing, coordination, and duration of every point contact by playing back the force scan and observing the 3-Dimensional columnar animation.
- Playing back force movies in slow motion quickly teaches the clinician how point distribution patterns influence the mandible's path of closure (*occlusion*).
- Force point data is component information of Lines, Frames, and Patterns that occur within the envelope of function.

Figure 6a. Decay was removed from a 22-year old patient in the exact location where a high intensity contact on tooth #31 existed (Figure 6b). Microtrauma over time from the prolonged and intense contact point, fatigued and weakened the enamel allowing bacteria to create decay.

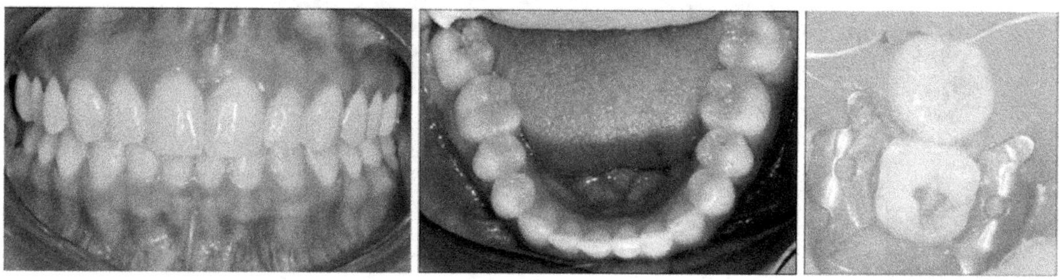

Figure 6b. Tooth #31 was then restored and adjusted to lessen the applied occlusal force, such that the right TM joint felt better to the patient and lessened its "click." Six weeks following the restoration and this minimal occlusal correction, the right temporal headaches abated and no clicking was present in any mandibular movement.

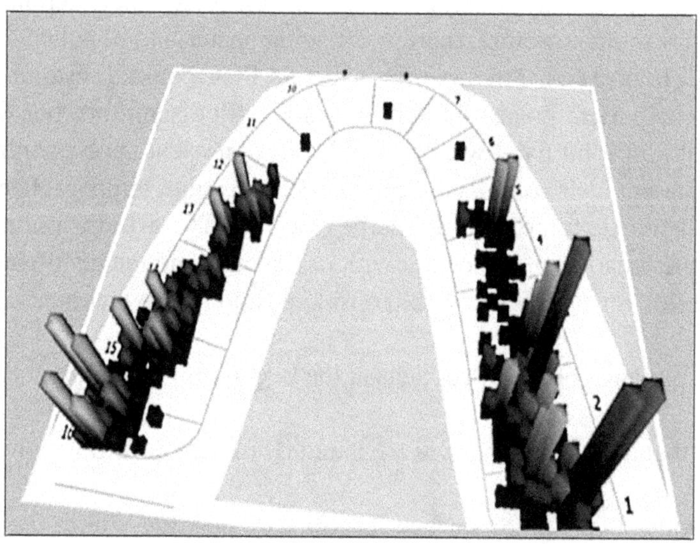

Lines Indicate the Direction of Force Transfer

During a mandibular closure into full contact when occlusal force compression, intercuspation, and decompression transpire on the teeth sequentially, the Center of Force trajectory (COF) creates "red and white lines" that track where the COF icon travels around the 2-Dimensional ForceView window, in response to the changing total force summation. The trajectory lines describe the changing history of total force summation, which is positionally determined by the closure contact sequence, and the sequential contact force intensity changes that occur around the dental arch. As contact forces evolve on individual teeth in sequence during mandibular compression, the force summation moves toward higher contact force concentrations and away from lesser force concentrations. This process of force concentration reverses when the mandible moves away from MIP, and teeth sequentially disengage. The force summation's positional changes are illustrated in the 2D ForceView window, by a red and white diamond-shaped icon followed by its red-colored line trailer. Each leg of the trajectory line represents 0.003 second-long segments (in Turbo Mode recording), or 0.01 second-long segments (in non-Turbo Mode recording).

The differing positions the COF marker assumes during the entire process of intercuspation results in line formation. The shorter lines are in length, the less are the number of individual legs that constitute the COF trajectory line. The more centered along the midline of the 2-Dimensional ForceView the COF trajectory lines travel, the more balanced are the occlusal forces between the right and left halves of the dental arch, all through the closure and release contact sequence.

When the mandible moves and the dentition engages, the digital force lines locate the origin of the occlusal force, and track its progress from the earliest contact points through to its final destination when the COF icon stops moving at MIP. These force lines significantly increase the occlusal diagnostic capability of the clinician, because the lines confirm the locations of the primary occlusal contacts that are controlling, guiding, or steering the force summation's directional movement. Lines change direction because the force concentration changes as more and more teeth make occlusal contact. Trajectory lines diagnose in real time, the force transfer from one location to another, and can be analyzed either one frame at a time (in slow motion), or in continuous movie playback.

In order to generate trajectory line data, position a patient's head upright to record the mandible's habitual sequence of force contact distribution (Figure 5). Patients should be instructed to "tap" their teeth together two or three times in succession, with the recording sensor properly interposed between the arches. The software then produces a moving line that will indicate the direction of force movement during the closure sequence, where the number of contact locations and points displayed at the beginning of a line and the numbers of contact points present at the end of a line, will be different. In addition, the combined force percentages at the beginning of a line will be different from the percentages of high force located at the end of most lines.

Many lines may appear similar, but the force summation is unique to each individual. The timing and the location of the higher intensity contact points, both play roles in the pathway traveled by the trajectory line. The type, style, speed, and characteristics of lines diagnose the challenges that the mandible must navigate as teeth engage during repeated "tapping" closures. Line recordings, which develop different characteristics and configurations when observed in the 2-Dimensional ForceView window are showcased in Figures 7- 15, where differing "tap-tap-tap" mandibular closures were recorded.

Some observable trajectory line characteristics are that:

- Lines organize points (Figure 7).
- Lines can repeat (Figure 8).
- Lines can be curved, angled, or irregular in shape (Figure 9).
- Lines can be long and straight (Figure 10).
- Lines can describe the presence of a closure occlusal interference (Figure 11).
- Lines can illustrate a first contact on a habitual closure arc, followed by a squeeze into MIP (Figure 12).
- Lines can be v-shaped, demonstrating both engagement (occlude) and release (disocclude) (Figure 13).
- Lines can describe left (and right) lateral excursions (Figure 14).
- Lines can describe a protrusive excursion (Figure 15).

Lines may move posteriorly into the back of the arch (Figures 8 and 9) or move sideways across the arch (Figures 10- 13). The majority of lines move from light to heavy force before stopping (Figures 7- 12) and move within a specific area of the arch. For example, in Figure 7, the lines are located in the posterior right area of the arch. Figure 11 illustrates lines located in the middle right area of the arch. Figure 18 shows two lines that travel into the center of the arch.

Figure 13 is different. In this example, the line movement starts on the right side of the arch but stops in the COF target center (occluding force), and then changes direction as the force gradually releases upon opening. The occluding lines (anterior right side to the middle) and the disoccluding lines (middle

Figure 7. Lines organize contact points in the 2-Dimensional ForceView window. Here, the patient closed on a sensor to establish a baseline, then "tapped" his teeth together three times, resulting in three lines formed by the movement of the COF marker. Only four contact locations occurred in MIP due to this patient presenting with an anterior open occlusion. The lines moved from right to left as the sequential intensity changed from light to heavy force. The location of all the force transfer is in the posterior right segment of the arch. The lines repeat and isolate to the arch locations indicating which teeth are dominating the force transfer.

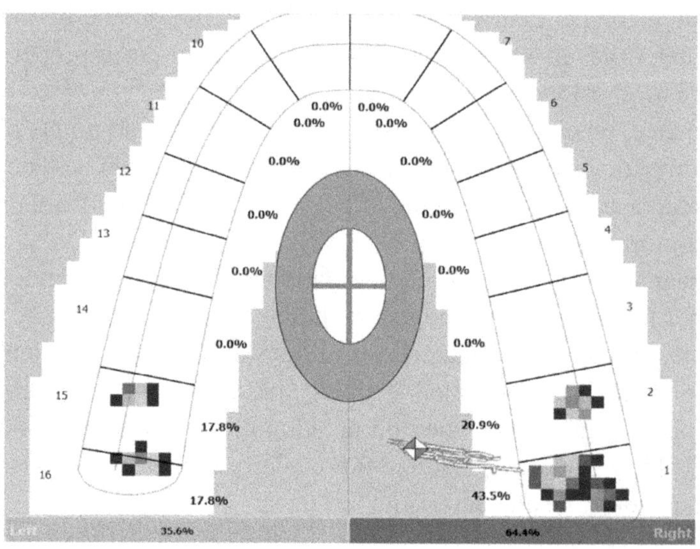

Figure 8. An example of repeating lines where a "tap-tap" pattern shows that the anterior teeth engage first, and then the occlusal force is directed in a posterior left direction as the occlusion reaches MIP. The lines then repeat for a second time. The two individual red trajectory lines are crooked, but show the same movement and the same characteristic pattern. Each "tap" line starts in the gray COF zone and moves from right to left and posteriorly, as the teeth engage, release, and repeat during the second "tap" onto the sensor.

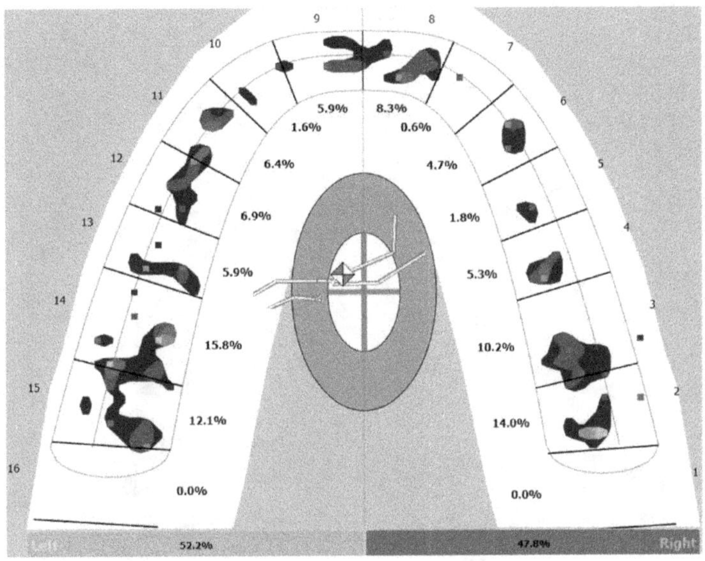

Figure 9. There are two sets of lines in this example. The first "tap" recorded only the front teeth indicating that the pathway of closure had resistance in the anterior region, which is often an indication that the envelope of function is limited by the anterior arch arrangement. The second "tap" line (in the center) is an example of a jammed, compressed, or wiggly line, which indicates a stressed squeeze into MIP. Here the force travels from the anterior right to the middle left. The line changes direction often as more contacts sequentially influence the force to move posteriorly. Every bend in the line results from a slight occlusal contact force change within the arch, which influences and directs where the COF icon moves next.

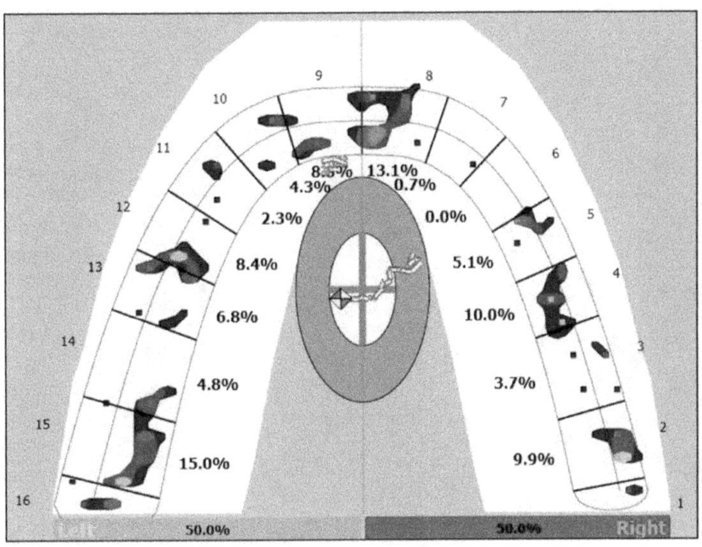

Figure 10. An example of multiple long, straight, repeating lines, which indicate that the teeth on the left and right are occluding nearly simultaneously. Unlike the trajectory lines in Figure 9, these lines do not wedge because the force transfer is released rapidly. The force intensity and shape of the arch on the right side is different from those on the left, but the total force within the arch is balanced at the maximum force frame. These lines are very straight, indicating that a short time frame (0.02 - 0.04 second) has passed during force transfer from closing to opening.

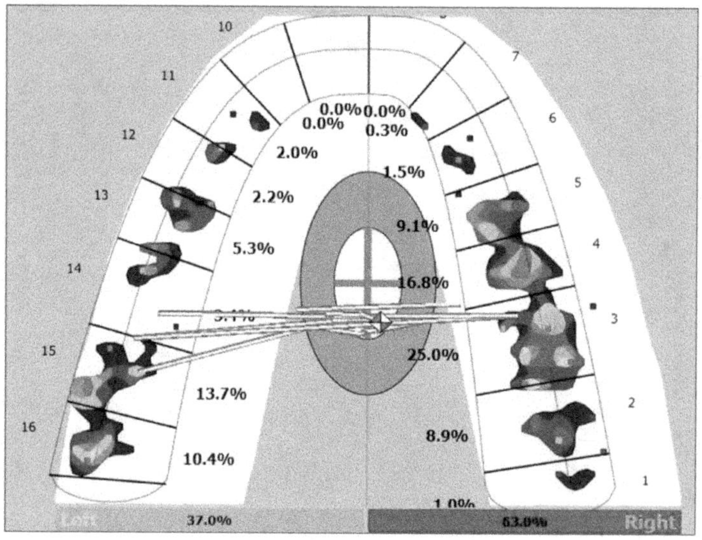

Figure 11. An example of lines that describe the presence of an occlusal interference comprised of cluster points. Here, a few lines start in the posterior right quadrant where teeth #3 and #4 receive 47.9% of the total force. Microtrauma over time may lead to pathology in this region of the arch. The lines commence where the occlusal interference rises forcefully in advance of the left side teeth contacting. The COF trajectory moves towards the left side but stops right of the white portion of the COF target, never crossing the midline. The posterior right teeth within this closure sequence initiate and dominate all other occlusal contact engagements in and out of MIP.

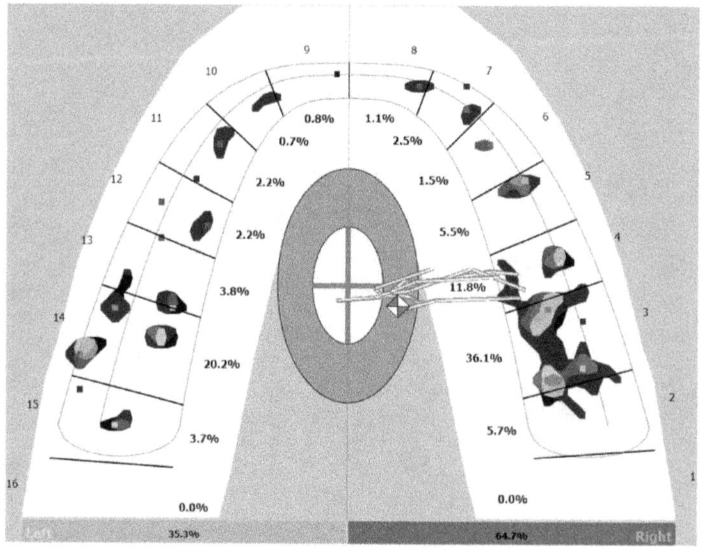

Figure 12. An example of a Bimanual Manipulation technique (Dawson, 2007) closure line pattern. This pattern is dominated by the occlusal interference present on teeth #2 and #31. Note that the start of the line stagnates during the Bimanual Manipulation (the red circle of lines) in the right posterior quadrant, because there is a prolonged force buildup that occurs as the first right posterior teeth occlude when the condyles are manipulated on the Centric Relation arc of closure. Then the line moves towards the COF target as the patient leaves the Centric Relation manipulated position, and self-slides on a habitual arc to finally squeeze into MIP.

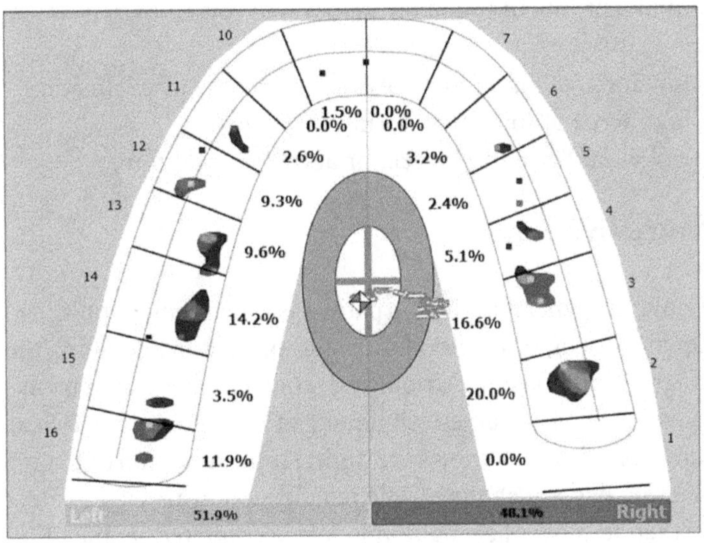

Figure 13. An example of v-shaped lines. Here, a patient self-closes into MIP with the right anterior region contacting slightly before the teeth on the left side. This frame indicates that at 94.16% of Total Force, the force summation is centered when most of the teeth are in contact. When the patient begins to disocclude, the force leaves towards the left side. The short nature of these lines indicates that there is rapid and balanced contact timing in and out of MIP. The lines on the right side of the midline represent occlude and present with different character and direction than the lines on the left side of the midline, which represent disocclude.

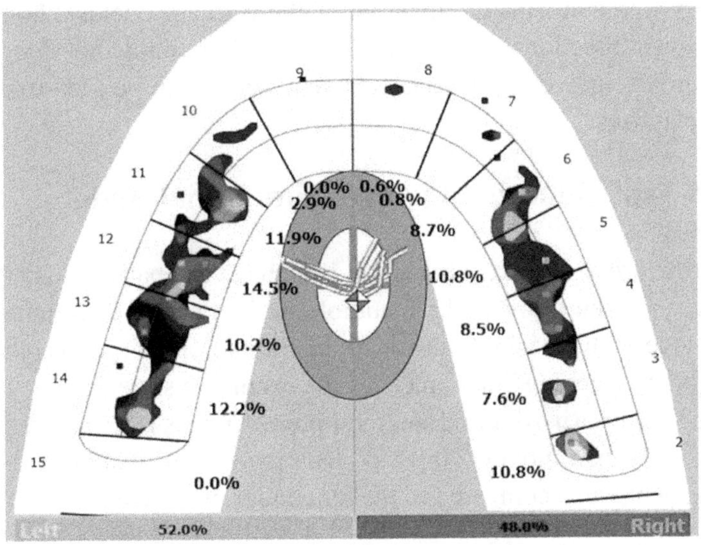

to anterior left) are equal in length and mirror each other. Lines that demonstrate disclusion indicate that an occlusion has the potential to release force out of heavy contact, thus minimizing the effects of isolated areas of microtrauma. Figure 13 is an example of balanced and centered force distribution (*occlusion* and *disocclusion*) into and out of MIP.

Lastly, it has been the author's observation that most trajectory lines (over 70%) move from the right arch half to the left arch half. Future research will be required to isolate why force movement does not appear to commence equally between the left and right directions.

There are three essential facts about line interpretation to remember:

- Lines move from low force to high force during the process of occlusion.
- Lines move from high force to low force during disocclusion.
- Lines stop movement at 100% of total force, or at 0.00% total force.

Left, Right, and Protrusive Lines

In traditional analog articulating paper markings, a patient is asked to close the mandible until the dentition engages, and to "tap" up and down, or to slide left, right, or forward, to allow the clinician to visualize contact locations and lines of ink transfer. Articulated stone casts can also be used to visualize closure and lateral excursive movements. The same technique can be used with a T-Scan sensor to record and analyze excursive movements. Figure 14 shows the digital representation of the information traditionally obtained with the articulating paper technique. The patient was instructed to close into the sensor so all teeth intercuspated, and then to move their mandible left, as directed by the clinician.

The trajectory line illustrates a force transfer that starts at the base of the COF target where the maximum number of contacts occurred, and then moves left, to stop at the final single canine-to-canine contact point. All contacting teeth involved in the slide are recorded in sequence and may be reviewed and analyzed in super slow motion to verify the nature of the excursive contact pattern. The displayed frame shows only the end of the excursion, but the trajectory line describes the entire force movement to the left as the excursion evolved.

The playback of an excursive movie displays information that traditional articulating paper cannot provide. All the teeth in the arch that are responsible for the left lateral movement are recorded in sequence. The trajectory line confirms the location of the primary occlusal contacts that control and steer the force summation's directional movement. The line direction is not direct from MIP to canine disocclusion, as there are excursive interferences present which can be identified when analyzing the movie in slow motion playback.

Combining a "Tap-Tap" Recording with a Directional Slide

The digital method for recording an excursive slide is to have the patient start the slide from a static (usually MIP) position, and then to move the mandible in the desired direction (Figure 14). Combining the "tap-tap" technique with a desired movement or slide in one direction, changes the line pattern generated resultant from the "tapping" that precedes the excursive slide.

The line representing the protrusive movement in Figure 15 does not start from a stopped MIP position (as in Figure 14), but from a moving "tap-tap" location. In this example, the distobuccal cusp of tooth #14 is out of alignment when compared to the remainder of the teeth in the arch, such that it is the

Figure 14. An illustration of the last frame recorded of a patient moving their mandible in a habitual left lateral excursive movement. This is an example of a curved line that began when all teeth were intercuspated in MIP, after which the patient slid their mandible to the left. The final contact point was located on the canine cusp tip that received 100% of the total force, because it was the only remaining point of contact.

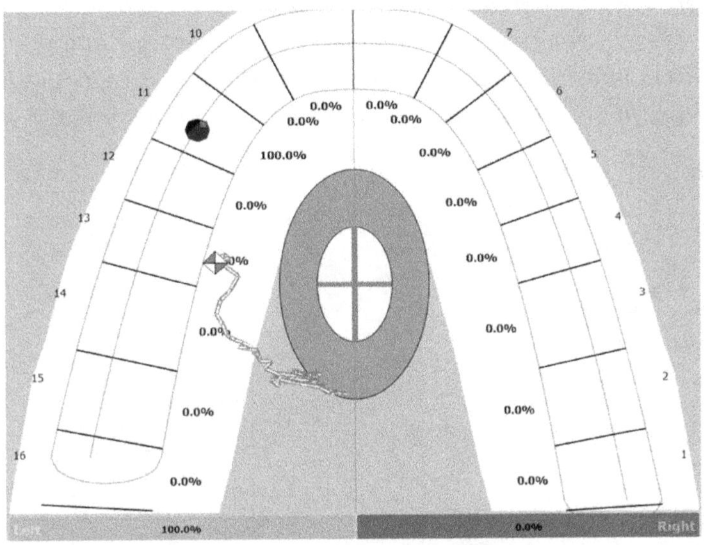

primary occlusal interference in the left lateral and protrusive movements made out of the MIP position. The data obtained from a protrusive or lateral excursive slide recording made after the patient "taps" can easily be correlated to clinical photographs and articulated stone casts for diagnosis.

Lines Define Occlusal Force Summation Direction and Character

In summary, the *COF trajectory lines* have the following force descriptive attributes:

- The sequential contact order in which multiple point contacts occur during a mandibular closure defines how the COF trajectory moves (historically) through the arches. This movement is what creates the trajectory line path.
- The location and direction that a line takes from beginning to end, indicates how the occlusal force summation is being transferred. This can be observed to some degree, with articulated stone casts and photographs for additional clinical confirmation.
- Lines can be curved, angled, and/or change direction, as the force summation of all sequentially contacting teeth drives the occlusal force summation to make directional changes.
- Non-linear and jagged lines show force level changes from one point contact to another, or from one group of contact points to another.
- Lines can be manipulated and controlled by the clinician through targeted occlusal adjustments made to the involved "time-early" or "force-excessive" occlusal contacts.
- Lines describe the direction of force summation movement, and define the shape and character of Digital Occlusal Force Distribution Patterns resultant from repetitive force transfer cycles.

Figure 15. "Tap-tap and slide forward" is a technique that combines the repeated "tapping" of the teeth with a protrusive excursion. The left upper pane shows a patient who "tapped" on a sensor a few times before the mandible moved protrusively without discluding all the posterior teeth. The top right pane shows a later sequence within the protrusive movement, when the force line moves anteriorly, indicating that the left side of the arch controls the protrusive movement. The lower left photograph shows the habitual closure position. The lower right photograph shows the hanging distobuccal cusp of tooth #14 (see black arrow in lower right pane), which is an occlusal interference that prevents a balanced force transfer from one mandibular position to another. The distobuccal cusp of tooth #14 directs the excessive left side "tapping" closure force, and controls the early portion of the protrusive movement.

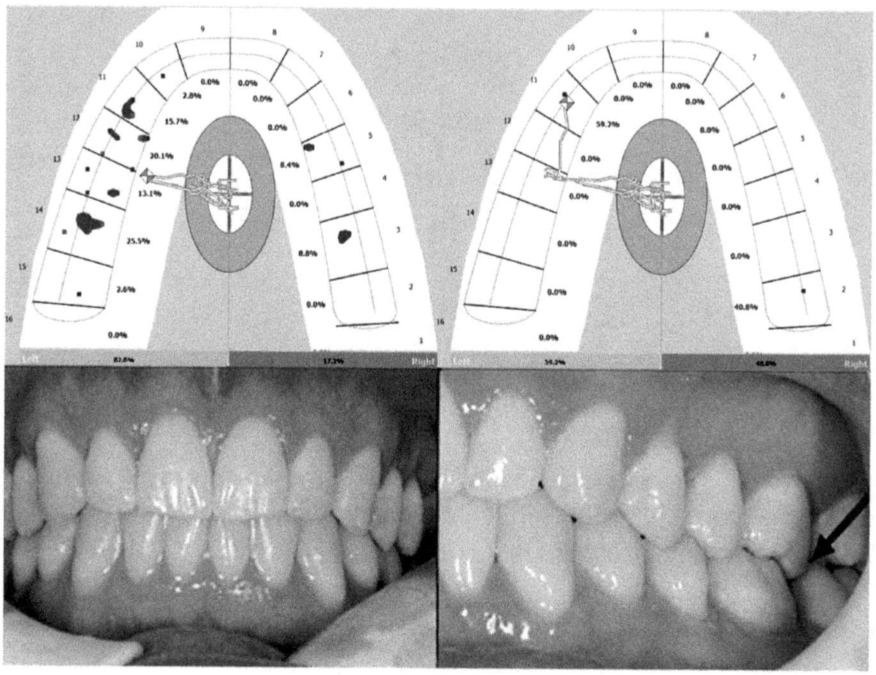

Theoretical Planes of Occlusion

Customarily, a *plane* is defined as a flat, two-dimensional surface (Wikipedia, 2013). However, the plane of occlusion is not flat, and the Glossary of Prosthodontic Terms defines it as the average plane established by the incisal and occlusal surfaces of the teeth. Generally, it is not a plane but represents the planar mean of the curvature of these surfaces (Academy of Prosthodontics, 2005). Similar to the idea that COF trajectory lines may not always be straight, the plane of occlusion is actually a uniquely formed 3-Dimensional space that accepts the mandibular teeth as they engage the maxillary teeth. Force engagement encounters both resistance and release during an envelope of function movement.

A *force cycle* will outline in successive force movie frames the boundaries of engagement into and out of the plane of occlusion (Figure 16), and map the force summation from the first point of contact all the way into MIP. Then, throughout the movement of opening, the sequence of contact reverses until the last point of contact disappears at the end of disocclusion, when the mandible push-off completely disengages the maxilla. It has been stated that the repetitious movements of the mandible determine the envelope of function, which does have favored pathways of function (Dawson, 2007). Consequently, it has been suggested that when teeth interfere with these favored paths, there will be deformation or dysfunction such that the weakest link will exhibit structural damage (Dawson, 2007). Recorded force distribution cycles expose the mandibular challenge faced in achieving a balanced landing, and unimpeded take-off from MIP.

The maxillary plane of occlusion is a stationary platform which the mandible contacts and leaves during the recording of a force cycle. Every recorded force frame describes a fractional time increment of the mandible's forceful engagement with, or release from, the stationary maxilla. These scans make diagnostic predictions of whether there exists asymmetric force transmission between the maxillary and mandibular occlusal planes. The clinician will require the additional information obtained from a face bow transfer, articulated diagnostic casts, and clinical photographs, to better visualize the source of the violation that produces non-ideal maxillary and mandibular occlusal contact interactions. In this way, matching DOFDPs to mounted models, digital radiographs, and photographs, illustrates to the clinician how the mandible navigates in and out of interocclusal contact.

Once the mandible reaches the border position of *occlude*, and begins to leave MIP, the opening movement force data alerts the clinician to a very important occlusal concept. Does the heavy force reduce and release, or is the envelope of disocclusion trapped by microtraumatic force? Unbalanced *occlusal planes* often trap force and promote dysfunction.

Lastly, it is important to note that the condylar position, the anterior guidance, the posterior guidance, the envelope of motion, the envelope of function, and the cranial posture patterns, are all variables that influence the mandibular closure movement in and out of the maxillary occlusal plane (See Figure 37).

Occlusal Interference and Clinical Planes of Occlusion

The T-Scan's 2-Dimensional planar data allows the clinician to measure the orientation of the applied occlusal force within the arch, and track it into, onto, and out of the maxillary occlusal plane. If the

Figure 16. The blue outline above the teeth graphically represents the three-dimensional boundaries established when unbalanced occlusal force is delivered to a non-uniform occlusal plane.

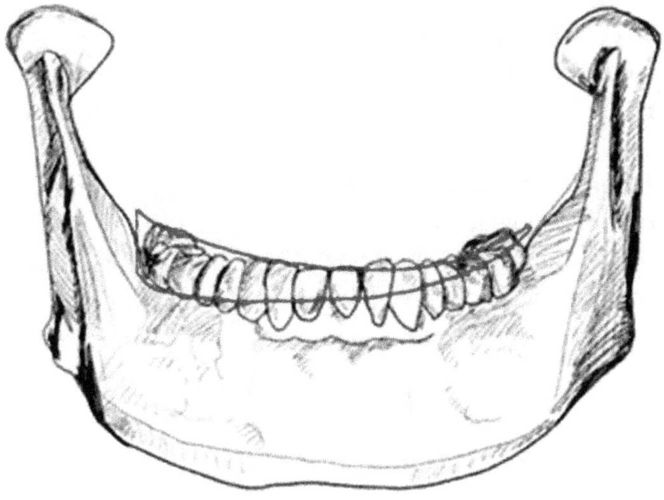

occlusal forces are unbalanced, the plane of occlusion will likely be asymmetric in one of three planes (transverse, sagittal, and horizontal). Additionally, the chiropractic pitch, yaw, and roll vectors can also be affected by the shape of the arch, the anterior-posterior axis (the curve of Spee), and the mediolateral axis (the curve of Wilson) (Carlson, 2003).

By age 15, the force distribution on the posterior and anterior sections alerts the clinician to the presence of an occlusal interference in the mandible's preferred pathway to MIP. The posterior segments must be efficient on the working side and in harmony with the non-working side.

The adjective "anterior" means "placed near or toward the front." The word "anterior" in reference to the occlusion can also mean "anterior to the condyles." The term anterior guidance can be somewhat confusing. Any tooth in front of the condyles necessarily includes all the posterior teeth. Therefore, it is possible for a posterior tooth to control the mandible's anterior guidance into and out of MIP. The reality is that Dental Medicine has only one definition for a posterior or anterior tooth that alters the favored pathway of the mandible. The term *interference* is used to describe any deflection or limitation to a preferred movement of the mandible.

The first tooth that touches and provides anterior proprioceptive control over the mandibular movement has been defined as the *anterior control*. What follow is a series of contacts anterior to the condyles that guide the mandibular teeth into the upper occlusal table and the upper occlusal plane. If a molar is the first tooth to make contact, then that posterior tooth controls the maxillomandibular interocclusal interaction, and interferes with the effectiveness of the anterior guidance and the condylar guidance.

Definitions

- **Posterior Guidance:** Does not have a definition in the Glossary of Prosthodontic Terms. Dental Medicine has termed posterior teeth that occlude prematurely an *occlusal interference*, but the term is vague and calls for a more complete definition.

Dental Medicine has historically used other definitions to provide an understanding of how the posterior teeth should fit, guide, and articulate:

- **Interference (1783) :** Any tooth contact that interferes with or hinders harmonious mandibular movement.
- **Occlusal Interference:** Any tooth contact that inhibits the remaining occluding surfaces from achieving stable and harmonious contacts.
- **Occlusal Prematurity:** Any contact of opposing teeth that occurs before the planned timing of the intercuspation.
- **Deflective Occlusal Contact (Also Known as Prematurity):** Contact that displaces a tooth and diverts the mandible from its intended movement.
- **Deflection (1605) :** A continuing eccentric displacement of the mandibular midline's incisal path, that is symptomatic of a restriction in normal mandibular movement.
- **Occlusal Plane:** The average plane established by the incisal edges and occlusal surfaces of the teeth.

The Anteroposterior Curve: The Theoretical Curve of Spee

The Curve of Spee has been defined as the anatomic curve established by the occlusal alignment of the teeth when projected onto the median plane, beginning with the cusp tip of the mandibular canine and following the buccal cusp tips of the premolar and molar teeth, continuing through the anterior border of the mandibular ramus, that ends at the anterior most portion of the mandibular condyle (von Spee, 1890).

The curve of Spee is an anatomic 3-Dimensional shape that describes a symmetrical *mandibular* plane in the anteoposterior axis. Figure 17 shows a mandibular arch that matches the definition of a symmetrical curve of Spee. However, the plane of occlusion is a static 3-Dimensional shape found in the maxillary arch. The ideal anteroposterior plane of the mandible may or may not be in harmony with the anteroposterior plane of occlusion of the maxilla.

The Buccolingual Arch Shape (the Theoretical Curve of Monson)

The theoretical curve of Monson is where each cusp and incisal edge touches or conforms to a segment of the surface of a sphere, that is 8 inches in diameter, with its center in the region of the Glabella (Academy of Prosthodontics, 2005). A 3-Dimensional sphere, where the posterior occlusal contours in all three planes (horizontal, vertical, and transverse) are in harmony, represents an ideal curve of Monson.

The shape of the maxillary arch and vault of the palate are diagnostic indicators found in patients with upper airway resistance. At a young age, the myofunctional habits of the tongue and swallow reflex help define the shape and width of the palate, which in turn defines the buccolingual dimension of the plane of occlusion. Diagnostic intraoral signs of the skeletal and neuromuscular status of the oral cavity include tongue size, vaulted palate, narrow maxillary and mandibular arches, and an unbalanced posterior occlusal plane (Figure 18). A narrow adult arch limits, constricts, or modifies lateral mandibular movements, and promotes excessive posterior occlusal force distribution patterns. Often, a narrow maxillary arch on one side is the cause of a unilateral crossbite.

Figure 17. An example of an asymmetrical maxillary occlusal plane and a mandibular arch with a symmetrical curve of Spee. The anteroposterior plane of the mandibular arch does not engage the plane of occlusion with balanced posterior force, because the posterior right maxilla is asymmetric in shape and position. A force scan recording of MIP will diagnose the primary points of interference that prevent synergy between the two arch shapes.

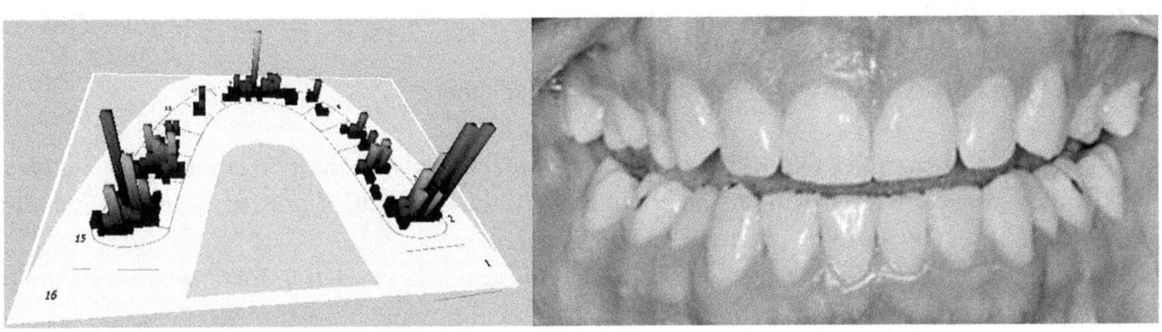

Figure 18. The width of the mandibular and the maxillary arches is narrow in the buccolingual dimension. A narrow upper arch coupled with a tongue thrust will result in a skeletal growth pattern that can lead to the formation of an anterior open occlusion. The 3-Dimensional posterior force distribution illustrates the location of the primary occlusal interference (teeth #s2 and 31).

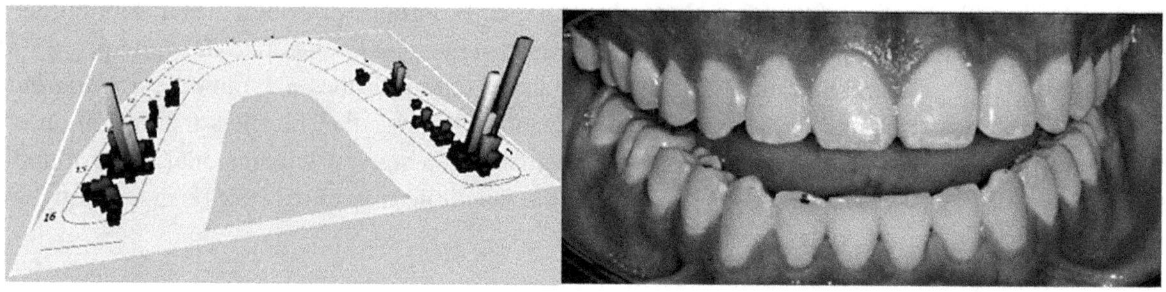

The Mediolateral Curve (The Theoretical Curve of Wilson)

Theory suggests that occlusal planes should be spherical in nature, such that the curvature of the cusps when projected on the frontal plane should result in the concave curvature of the mandibular with a convex curve in the maxillary arch (Wilson, 1911). Further suggested descriptions of these frontal curves indicated that an equal lingual inclination of the right and left molars should make the tips of the corresponding cross-aligned cusps be aligned along the circumferences of a circle. Additionally, the transverse cuspal curvature of the maxillary teeth is affected by the equal buccal inclinations of their long axes. The curve of Wilson is characterized by the buccal cusps of the lower posterior teeth being higher than the lingual cusps, and vice versa of the posterior teeth in the upper arch (Wilson, 1911).

The ideal curve of Wilson presumes that the mandibular arch and the maxillary arch match each other geometrically, which they seldom do (Figure 19). The mandibular concave plane should fit symmetrically into the maxillary convex plane, with all contacting teeth aligned axially. In Figure 20, the mandibular arch and the plane of the mandibular teeth have symmetrical curves of Wilson and Spee. However, the maxillary plane of occlusion does not conform to the mandibular curve of Wilson.

Figure 20 illustrates that despite the poor tooth interdigitation in the anterior right quadrant, and the non-ideal shapes of the maxillary arch, the anteroposterior curve and the mediolateral curve, the overall occlusal force summation of the system demonstrates balance. The extraction of tooth #18 helped to center the force distribution in MIP. The maxillary arch is narrow and both the curve of Wilson and the curve of Spee are less than ideal.

In theory, these three clinical asymmetric planes should not form a physiologic occlusal design, but when combined with the occlusal contact distribution and the individual varying tooth contact intensities, the COF icon centers.

In review, a summary of the above *Frame* section details that:

- Frames build force cycles that start with the first contact, evolve as more teeth intercuspate on the way into complete intercuspation, and continue until the last contact releases when the mandible is opened vertically, or moves laterally in an excursion.
- Within a force cycle, the sequence of contact points and their relative force content define the individual frames that describe force distribution in real-time.

Figure 19. An example of an ideal mandibular plane that must enter into and exit from, a less than ideal maxillary plane of occlusion. The mandibular curve of Wilson does not match the maxillary one, resulting in an unbalanced force cycle. Note how the lingual inclination of the posterior teeth locates significant occlusal force on the second molars. Also, note how the uneven mandibular anterior incisal edges have worn the corresponding maxillary anterior incisal edges when the patient slides protrusively.

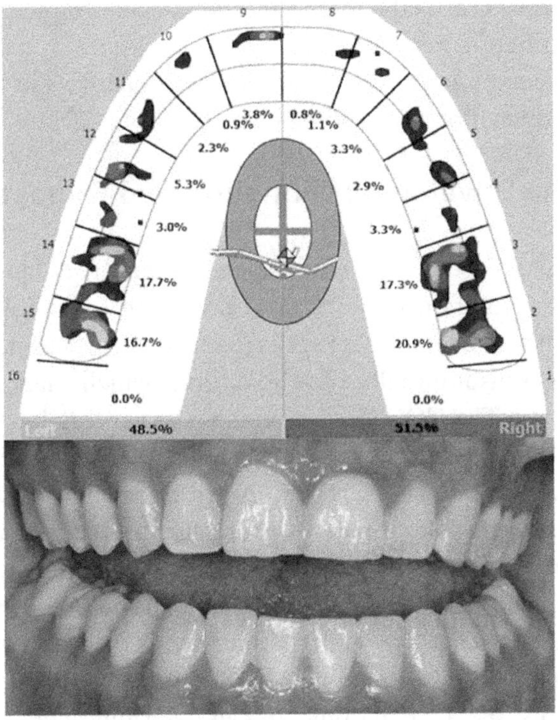

Figure 20. The COF alignment is centered in MIP despite the anatomic curves being non-ideal. The upper arch is narrow and both the curve of Spee and the curve of Wilson are asymmetrical. Yet, the patient presented with a centered COF. The force distribution on the left side of the arch is very different from the force distribution on the right side, but they offset each other resulting in overall balance.

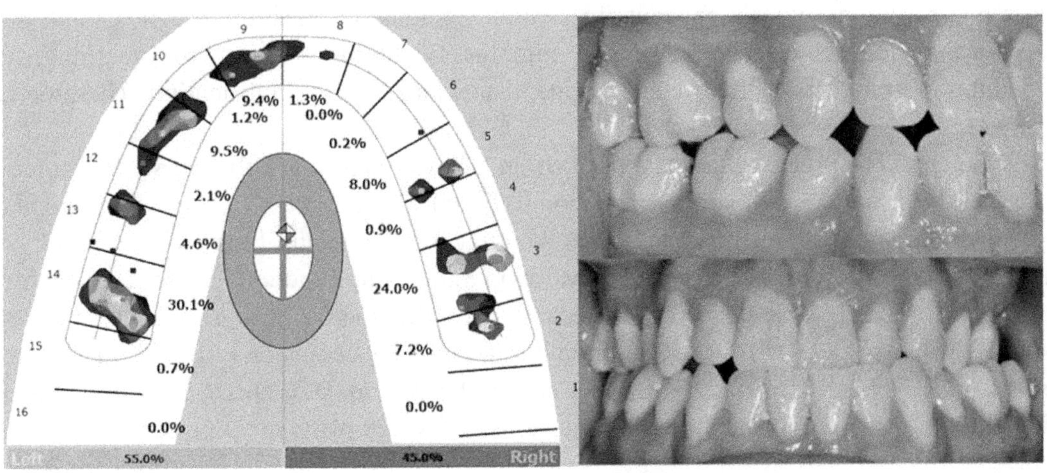

- The direction and the duration of force transferred in a force cycle are critical to the future prognosis of an overloaded tooth, teeth, dental implant, or the structures that support them.
- Quality force cycles present with minimal occlusal interference, and demonstrate good anterior guidance. The applied force enters and exits the dentition quickly and with minimal resistance.
- Frame data is the foundation from which a clinician can understand the character and quality of the differing force patterns described later in this chapter (see Habitual Force Distribution Pattern and Skeletal Force Distribution Pattern).
- Head posture will influence the arc of closure and can change the force distribution, and thus change the character and location of the force cycle (Carlson, 2003).

Patterns: Measuring the Envelope of Function and Repeating Force Cycles

The envelope of function produces contact and release patterns that are unique to an individual, representing a signature of the muscularly-ingrained interaction between the mandible and the maxilla. The word "signature" describes a patient's unique muscle engram pattern. A repeating force pattern develops when a patient "taps" on a recording sensor initially with light force, which changes into maximum force, and then lessens to a releasing force. The COF icon summates the varying intensities of the occlusal force cycle and moves around the 2-Dimensional ForceView, while the actual occlusal force travels into and out of repeating intercuspations. A Digital Occlusal Force Distribution Pattern (DOFDP) is a diagnostic force map that shows how occlusal force cycles repetetively engage the occlusal surfaces of contacting teeth.

It should be noted that force cycles can both be functional and dysfunctional. As such, the structural adaptation to the repeating functional or dysfunctional applied force will influence the Temporomandibular joints, the masticatory muscles, the teeth, the airway, the skeletal posture, and the periodontal tissues that supports the teeth. The result may be physiologic, pathologic, or both over the life of an occlusion. Using force patterns, the T-Scan clinician can determine how dysfunctional force patterns created damage in structures that did not adapt well to the cyclical force application. The T-Scan can also monitor the occlusal treatment undertaken to correct the destructive force distribution, and stop the ongoing structural maladaptation.

Envelope of Function

Function is one of the more basic concepts in Dental Medicine because the diagnosis and treatment must work for the patient to be accepting of the outcome. Function must work for breathing, swallowing, mastication, posture, comfort, efficiency, appearance, and TM joint lubrication. Therefore, it must be operational.

The oral function is a process that must perform in sickness and in health, every day. It requires the oral cavity and the structures that support function to literally 'grind it out.' Success, for a dentist who is diagnosing and treating a patient's mandibular position and the occlusal landing, is to seek harmony and balance for both in action. The ultimate question in diagnosing function is "are all the components working in a healthy and stable condition?" Because everything and everyone adapt and change over time, a sound clinical strategy to restore functional harmony to the occlusion is to minimize excess force locations that will cyclically stress the structures and/or the system. DOFDPs simply alert the clinician where the mandible is going to encounter resistance to its favored pathway of closure.

It is important to note that the entire process of occluding and disoccluding while "tapping" on a sensor is accomplished in fractions of seconds. DOFDPs are a diagnostic tool that connects the mandible to the cranium using force transfer as a measurement. The recordings are done for the purpose of understanding how the mandible and the dentition are engaging the maxillary occlusal plane. The orientation of the entire mandible, including the condyles, is determined by proprioception and engrained into functional patterns over time. Force is transferred when the mandible stops and force transfer can be measured from the first contact made to the final stop position (MIP). DOFDPs record an objective measurement using force transfer as a diagnostic parameter to better understand the challenge the mandible encounters when seeking a centered pathway of function. Harmony in function minimizes dysfunction and promotes longevity, which is every patient's primary goal.

The data does not tell the clinician how the mandible functions, but the patterns do provide valuable insight into whether the mandible is able to function in an efficient manner. A balanced landing (occlude) of the mandibular dentition or prosthetics is preferred, because the force distribution can be spread out, shared, and dissipated efficiently. An unbalanced landing (interference to *occlude*) will alter the mandible's orientation and require the dentition or the prosthetics to absorb and distribute the force in a less than efficient manner.

The mastication of food is a process different from the one in involved in occluding because the bolus limits tooth-to-tooth contact. However, the envelope of motion and the envelope of function are repeatable muscle engrams dictated by the sensory receptors of the Temporomandibular joints and the periodontal ligaments. The force directed into and out of the dentition and/or prosthetics during mastication varies depending on the consistency of what is being chewed. In addition, the intensity and duration of the force required are predicated on the efficiency of the system. Prolonged function, such as the simple repetitive process of chewing gum, may be easy for one person and impossible for another. Every patient's diet is unique but the quality and efficiency of function is directly dependent on the patient's ability to chew.

In *Principles of Esthetic Integration,* which was translated at the turn of the 20th century, the author suggested that Dental Medicine make a philosophical transition to integrate dental restorations where form follows function, such that establishing that dynamic equilibrium should be the goal of a soundly functioning occlusion (Rufenacht, 2000). Human adaptation to form and function will likely find its own biologically acceptable dynamic equilibrium over time. The process of understanding occlusal disease causation (diagnosis) and achieving dynamic equilibrium (treatment) is a clinician's lifetime endeavor, with the ultimate goal of creating function without friction for every patient's occlusion.

The Clinical Technique of Recording Digital Occlusal Force Distribution Patterns (DOFDPs) Using the T-Scan Occlusal Analysis System

A Habitual Force Distribution Pattern (HFDP) is recorded with a patient sitting upright in the dental chair, in a similar position to that of eating. The T-Scan sensor is then inserted intraorally with the T-Scan sensor support resting between the maxillary central incisors' facial embrasure, with the sensor held away from, but parallel to the maxillary occlusal plane. The *record button* on the recording handle is then activated, after which the patient is asked to first swallow and squeeze through the sensor into firm intercuspation, then to open and to "tap" firmly onto the sensor 3 or 4 times in succession, before finally re-squeezing into a second firm intercuspation.

Each recorded "tap" captures a force sequence, such that the patients will better load the teeth and the Temporomandibular joints with each successive "tap." The summary of all the "taps" creates a pattern that defines the force distribution of a patient's occlusion. The squeeze at the end of recordings illustrates the force distribution of complete habitual intercuspation. Because of the swallowing, repetitive "tapping," and finally squeezing into MIP, a HFDP movie is routinely recorded over a 5-7 second-long time frame.

Incremental playback allows the clinician to view a typical force pattern at differing stages of evolution, where changes in the COF icon position illustrate how the force is transferred onto all contacting teeth (Figures 21- 24).

Figure 21. A typical force pattern at 25% of complete closure. The COF icon is located in the posterior right quadrant with widespread low occlusal contact forces visible.

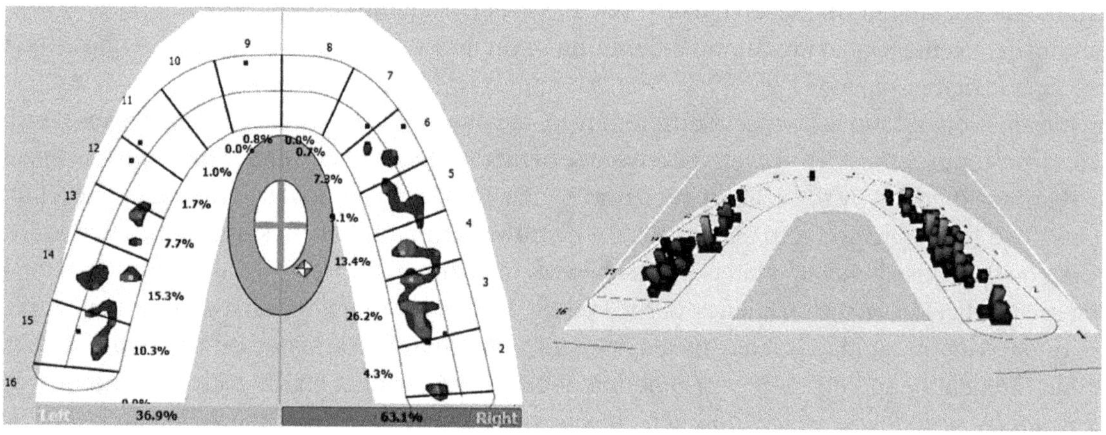

Figure 22. The same force pattern at 50% of complete closure. The COF icon has moved across the midline to the left posterior quadrant as teeth #14 and #15 rise in force, while the right side maintains low occlusal forces.

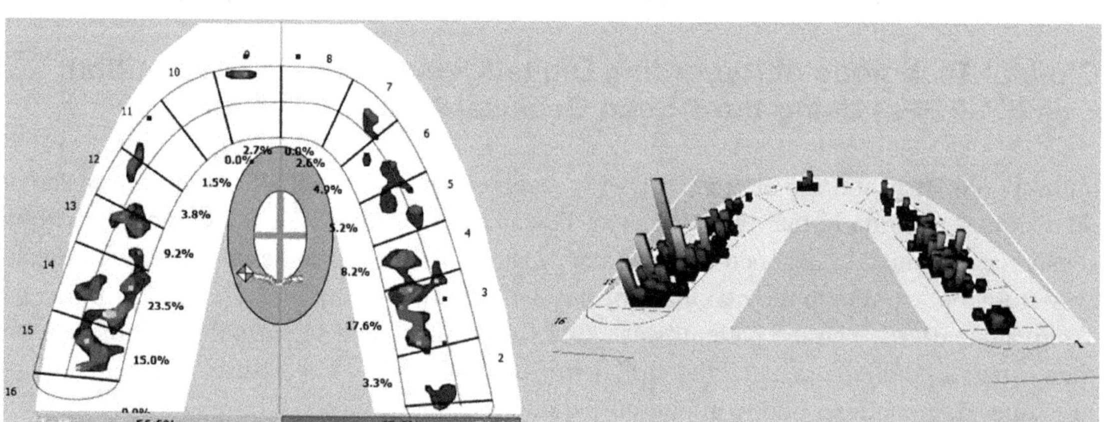

Figure 23. After the second "tap" of the cycle, the patient has released from MIP causing forces to drop to 44% of total force. The first "tap" force lines start to repeat with the second "tap" forming the pattern's shape. The second force cycle is complete when the mandible releases from the maxillary occlusal plane to 0.00% force. The third force cycle begins when the first occluding contact point initiates the identical sequence of repeating contacts.

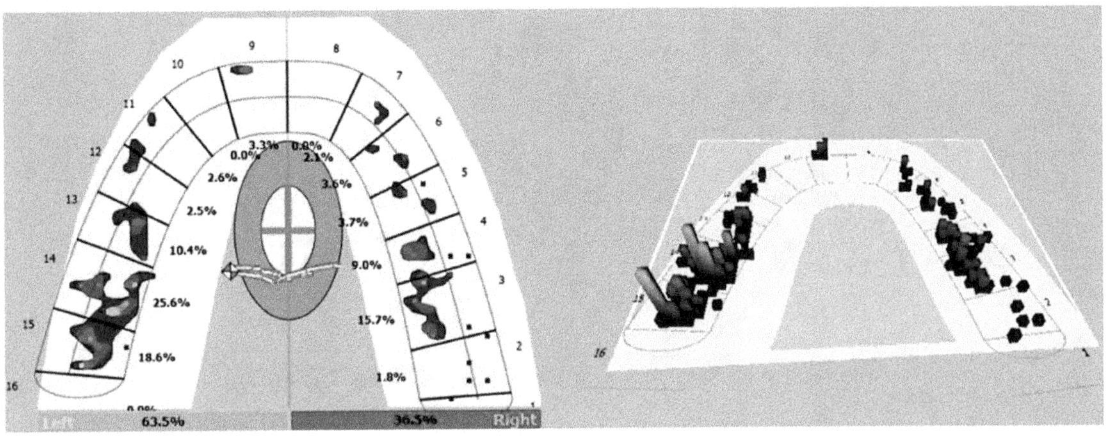

Figure 24. The final frame of a completed force pattern when the force distribution is recorded at 100% of closure (occlude). The patient re-squeezed into complete intercuspation following four "taps" that resulted in four recorded force cycles.

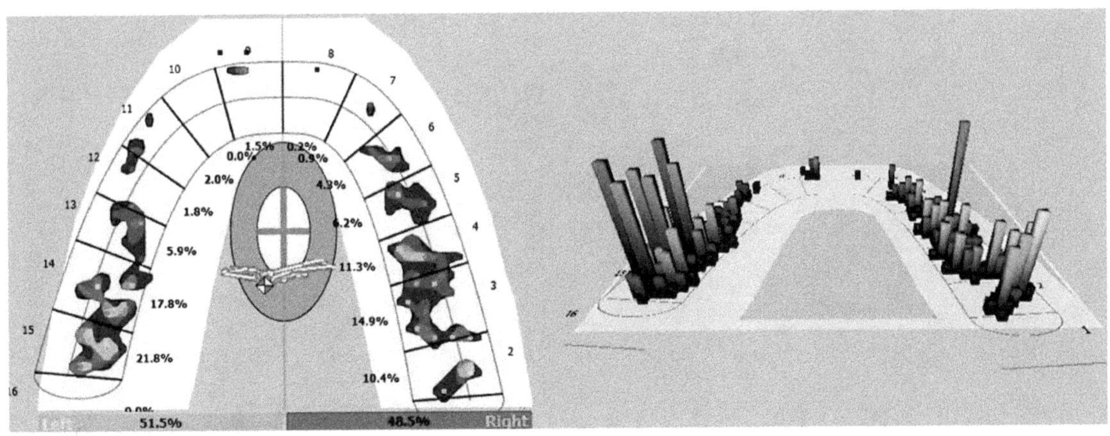

The Diagnostic Visualization of Pattern Characteristics

Habitual Force Distribution Patterns show the direction, the sequence, the intensity, and the repetition of occlusal force that isolates to different positions within the dental arch. It has been the author's observation that there are six different, but consistently observed, occlusal force patterns that will be discussed in significant detail later in this chapter (Figures 25 - 30, and 44 - 49).

The differing patterns can reveal how an occlusion will age, which teeth are involved in guidance, and how the occlusal force is absorbed by the supportive structures. Over the lifespan of a dentition, many factors may accelerate the anatomical changes observed in the TM joints, the muscles, the teeth,

Figure 25. Force cycle pattern #1: Distal posterior, either left or right

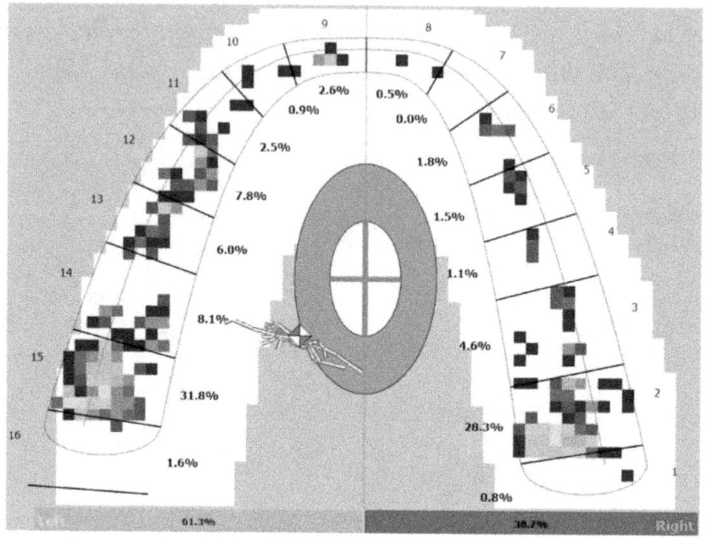

Figure 26. Force cycle pattern #2: Middle posterior, either left or right

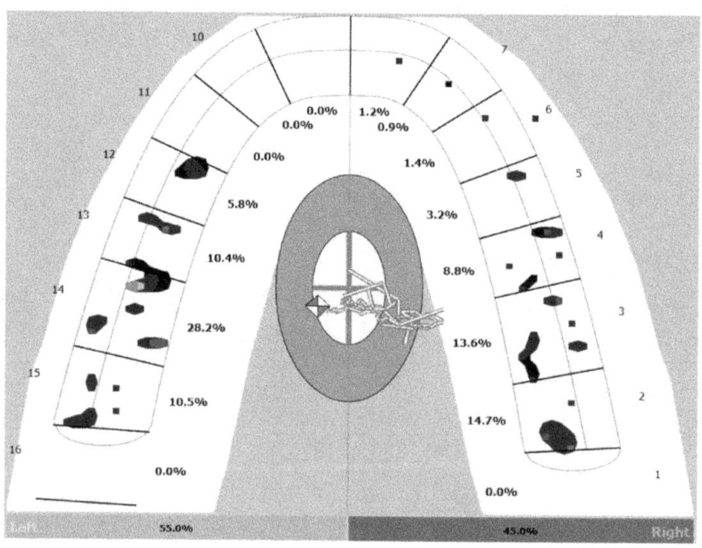

the gingival tissues, the bones, and the neck posture. However, repeated and aberrant occlusal force distribution will be a significant contributory factor to accelerating structural breakdown.

In an ideal occlusion, the condylar guidance and the anterior guidance should be independent of each other. Both guidance systems are in functional harmony with the envelope of function contacts, when the two systems are not codependent on each other (Dawson, 2007). Occlusal interference makes either the condyles or the anterior teeth functionally dependent on the other, producing dysfunctional patterns of force. A dysfunctional relationship begins when a person's anatomical structure ages faster than its ability to adapt, remodel, or repair. An occlusal force that interferes with a braced centric closure, or is

Figure 27. Force cycle pattern #3: Anterior dominant

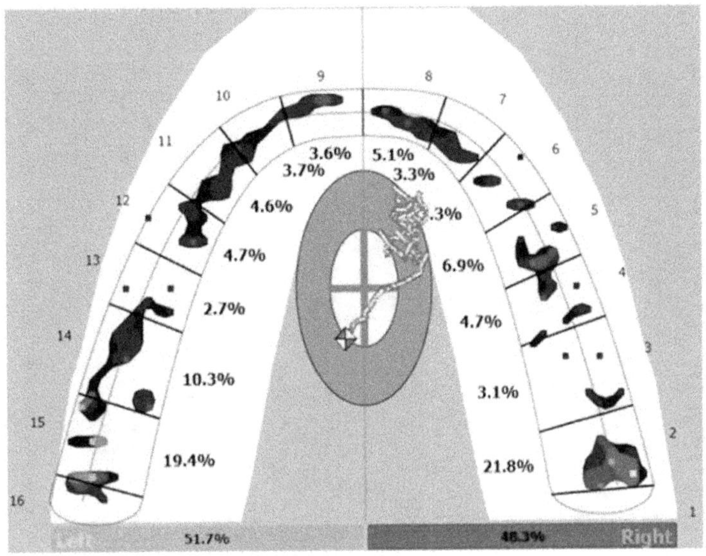

Figure 28. Force cycle pattern #4: Centered within the Center of Force target

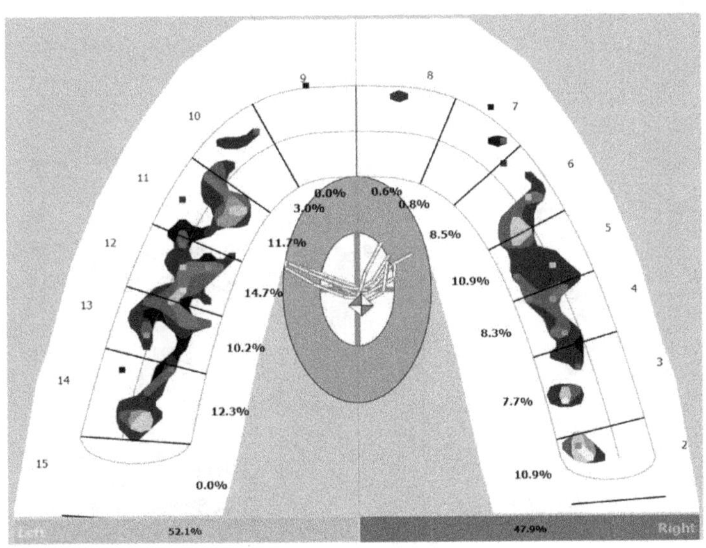

present during eccentric mandibular movements, can alter the articular disc's lateral pole position on the condyle. While some patients can continuously adapt physiologically and not demonstrate structural breakdown or clinical symptoms, others will be unable to.

In summary, *Digital Occlusal Force Distribution Patterns*:

- Result from recorded repetitive force cycles. There patterns describe how force is transferred to the occlusal surfaces of functional tooth contacts.

Figure 29. Force cycle pattern #5: Anterior open occlusion, posteriorly dominated

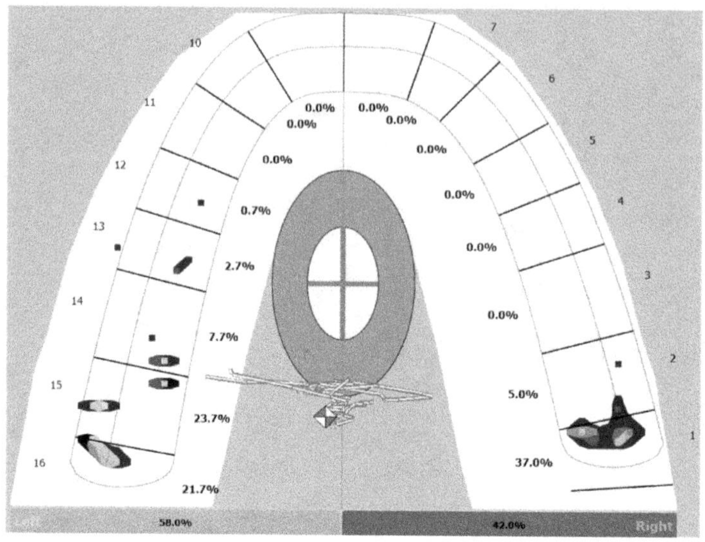

Figure 30. Force cycle pattern #6: Anteroposterior or posteroanterior, either along or across the arch

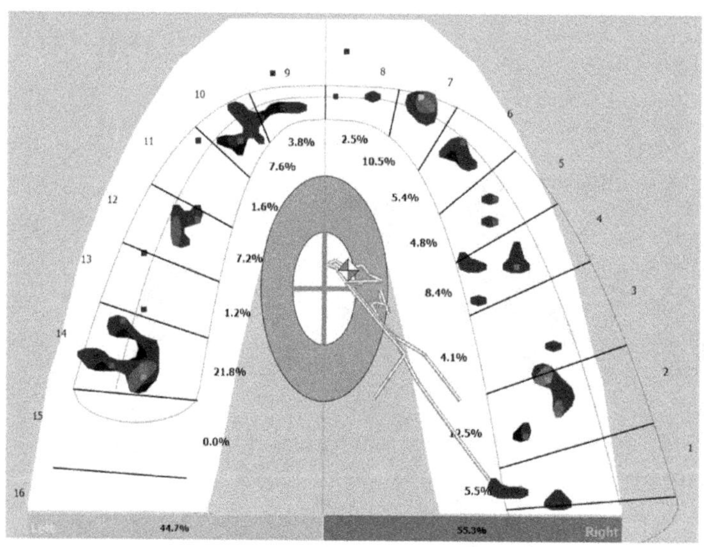

- Can be followed over time and be compared to previous ones, to observe changes to the force distribution across the lifespan of an occlusion.
- Can be isolated in one of six different arch locations.
- Are strongly influenced by head posture, and will change orientation when the head is in a vertical or a horizontal position.
- Connect the condylar guidance and the anterior guidance to compromised structural anatomy.
- Can be analyzed to observe where isolated locations of intense excessive occlusal force exist, which place the involved occlusal surfaces at risk.

PATTERN SPECIFICS

Posture and DOFDPs

The relationship between muscle triggers in the head, neck, shoulders and Digital Occlusal Force Distribution Patterns have been studied by this author for the past 15 years. What has been observed over that time span, is that force distribution patterns change whenever posture is altered or stressed due to injury or trauma. The recorded force distribution patterns of patients who benefit from physical therapy, massage therapy, chiropractic care, personal training, yoga or other forms of structural alignment, change as symptoms subside and as trigger zones are neutralized. Splint therapy, occlusal therapy, TMD therapy, and restorative treatment will also change the DOFDPs, and can potentially improve head and neck posture. If confirmed by further research, these considerations can improve our understanding and treatment of muscular-skeletal conditions that are associated with Temporomandibular joint disorders, occlusal changes, and tooth loss (Cuccia & Caradonna, 2009).

There are many available treatments for Temporomandibular disorders that do not involve direct treatment of the teeth. Postural adaptation of the cranium will influence the way teeth seat into each other, which is reflected in the noticeable differences of recorded force patterns when the head position is altered, such as when the head is positioned forward of the spine when sitting, or when the patient is laid supine. Gravity adds to the head postural change (Novak, 2006), which indirectly influences the mandibular and occipital condylar positioning such that the closure arc of the mandible is greatly influenced.

Digital Occlusal Force Distribution Patterns capture the process of teeth occluding in different head postures, or when the mandible is manipulated into position by a clinician. Each posture provides a unique occlusal force recording. The variations of the repetitious movements of the mandible can be minimized and studied by recording DOFDPs in different diagnostic postures. The author uses four different postural positions to diagnose, study, and explain the effects of microtraumatic force on an occlusion. Each force pattern is named for the postural information it provides:

- **The Habitual Force Distribution Pattern (HFDP):** The HFDP illustrates a patient's habitual occlusal force distribution as contact is transferred from the mandible to the maxilla in an upright seated position, similar to the one adopted while eating (Figure 31).
- **The Skeletal Force Distribution Pattern (SFDP):** The SFDP illustrates a patient's occlusal force distribution when a patient experiences reduced cervical muscular tension. This state is induced by having the patient recline, and then an assistant applies a moderate amount of downward pressure to the front of the patient's shoulders, which stretches the shoulders backwards to help immobilize the cervical muscles, the infrahyoid muscles, and the digastric muscles. Isolating the head, neck, and shoulders prior to taking the scan will produce a condensed, more direct, and less adaptive mandibular closure into and out of *occlude,* which generally results in a more retruded force pattern than does the HFDP (Figure 32).
- **The Manipulated Force Distribution Pattern (MFDP):** The MFDP illustrates a patient's occlusal force distribution when the mandible is manipulated into Centric Relation, prior to a force cycle recording where the clinician restricts the condylar movement to control the arc of closure. The most common manipulated position is achieved using Bimanual Manipulation (Dawson, 1983), during which the condyles are gently seated along the Centric Relation arc of closure. The

purpose of manipulating the mandible is to provide a controlled skeletal-condylar relationship into and out of Centric Relation occlusal contact (Figure 34).

- **The Vertical Force Distribution Pattern (VFDP):** A VFDP illustrates a patient's occlusal force distribution when a patient is standing. Leg length, hip position, and upper body alignment can influence head, neck, and mandibular position. The information examines the influence of posture and body positioning on the occlusal force distribution (Figure 35).

Recording a Habitual Force Distribution Pattern (HFDP)

Instruct the patient to sit in the dental chair, in a position similar to one adopted while eating and chewing.

- Insert the sensor in the patient's mouth, and position the sensor support between the maxillary central incisors with the sensor parallel to the maxillary occlusal plane.
- While observing the T-Scan recording desktop, depress the *record button* on top of the recording handle to initiate a 5 - 7 second-long force recording.
- Ask the patient to swallow and then to squeeze into the sensor by clenching the teeth together firmly to set a baseline mandibular position similar to MIP.
- Ask the patient to "tap" the teeth firmly onto the sensor three or four times in succession and finally, ask the patient to squeeze the teeth together in order to complete the recording.

Recording a Skeletal Force Distribution Pattern (SFDP)

Recording a Skeletal Force Distribution Pattern (SFDP) requires two staff members working together to capture the occlusal force data.

Figure 31. The left pane shows the proper head position, T-Scan recording handle position, and sensor position parallel to the maxillary occlusal plane, used to record the HFDP movie (displayed in the right pane). The resultant COF pattern is centered near the middle of the arches with reasonable bilateral force equality. The HFDP scan diagnoses the mandible's preferred force pathway as it enters and exits the upper plane of occlusion.

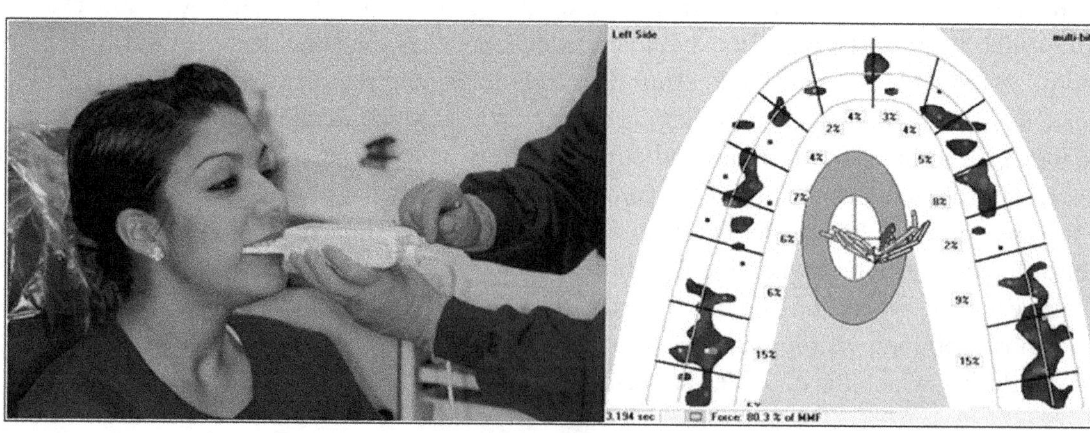

- Place the patient in a supine position in the dental chair. Have an assistant apply a moderate amount of downward pressure to the front of the patient's shoulders using a neck support, while asking the patient to take a deep breath and to exhale slowly (Figure 32). This will pull the patient's shoulders back helping to immobilize the cervical muscles, the infrahyoid muscles, and the digastric muscles. Pre-stretching the shoulders back using a karate belt before recording will aid the patient in attaining the proper shoulder position (Figure 33).
- While observing the T-Scan recording desktop, depress the *record button* on top of the recording handle to initiate a 5 - 7 second-long force recording.
- Ask the patient to swallow and then squeeze into the sensor by clenching the teeth together firmly to establish a baseline MIP.
- Then ask the patient to tap the teeth firmly onto the sensor three or four times in succession and finally, to squeeze the teeth together to complete the recording.

A small support or rolled towel can be placed under the patient's neck to help relax cervical muscles and prevent overstretching. Before recording a skeletal force distribution pattern (SFDP) in a dental chair, a useful stretch relieves muscle tension that can influence the position of the mandible's pathway to closure. Patients can incorporate this stretch at home on a daily or on a periodic basis. Start by wrapping the belt around the mid-back and under the armpits. Each end of the belt is then laid over the front of the shoulder and crossed around the back (Figure 33). The ends of the belt are held in the hands, which are then extended downwards to pull and stretch the shoulders up and back.

The skeletal force distribution pattern (SFDP) takes into account variations of the postural adaptation of the atlanto-occipital joint. The position of the atlas fossa in the cranial base is slightly posterior, medial, and inferior to the glenoid fossa. Stabilizing the cranium in a supine position minimizes the postural adaptation of the atlas, and provides a fixed head and neck position to measure the mandible's pathway

Figure 32. The properly reclined head position and shoulder restriction when recording an SFDP. Note that the T-Scan recording handle and sensor are positioned parallel to the maxillary occlusal plane. The patient swallows and squeezes into the sensor three or four times in succession, and then clenches the teeth together firmly. In this head position the mandible's pathway can change the force engagement pattern since the SFDP is generally posterior and lateral compared to the HFDP recorded from the same patient. Also note how the yellow arch shape outline is slightly different from that in Figure 31.

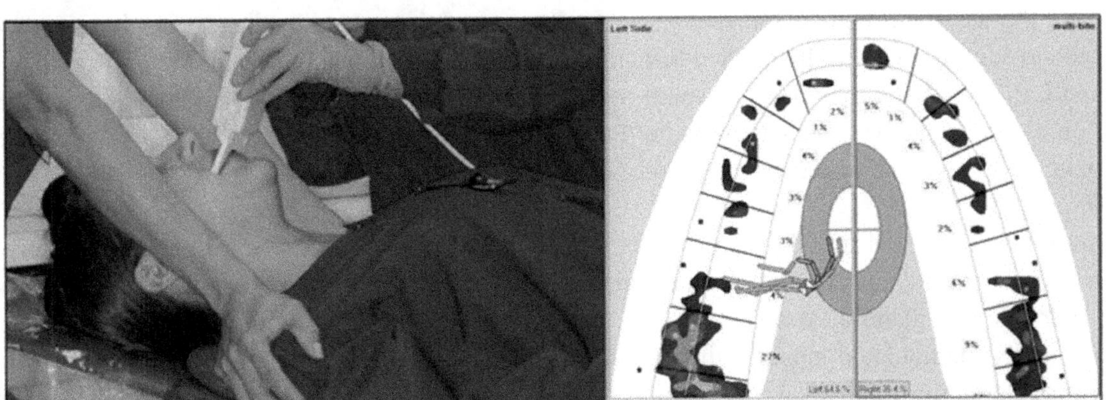

Figure 33. The karate belt stretch opens up the shoulders before recording a SFDP. It improves posture and assists the dentist in locating occlusal resistance to a balanced mandibular engagement.

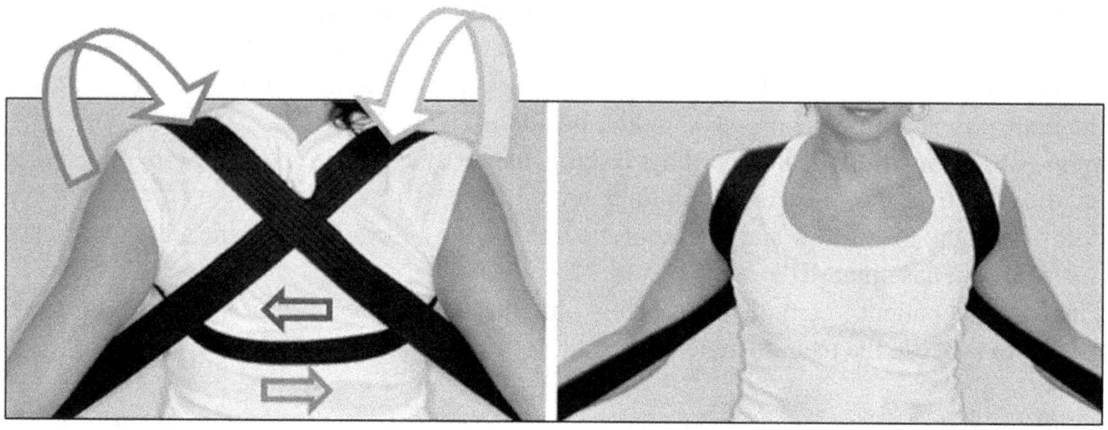

into the occlusal plane. Experience has taught the author that equilibration procedures performed using the skeletal and manipulated patterns reduce the number of teeth that require adjustment because the primary occlusal interference (*the anterior control*) is identified and corrected. Eliminating the strongest and the most aggressive occlusal interference first begins the process of restoring equilibrium to a system. A safe and effective strategy in the treatment of the Stomatognathic system is to adjust minimally for maximally improved occlusal results.

Recording a Manipulated Force Distribution Pattern (MFDP)

Any manipulation directed by the operator will provide force transfer information in the desired regulated position. Manipulating the mandible to isolate one or both condyles into a seated position limits condylar mobility, and produces unique force distribution patterns.

- To record a CR to MIP slide, have the patient recline in the same supine position used in the SFDP recording, and then have the chairside assistant insert the sensor in the patient's mouth parallel to the occlusal plane (vertically).
- While holding the patient's mandible (Figure 34) and observing the T-Scan recording desktop, have the assistant depress the *record button* on top of the recording handle, to initiate a 5 - 7 second-long force recording. Then bimanually manipulate the patient's mandible into the sensor and CR, by initiating a guided closure until the initial CR point of contact registers on the T-Scan ForceView windows. The patient is held there momentarily by the clinician, after which the patient self-closes and squeezes into maximum intercuspation.

From the manipulated first point of contact in CR, it is also possible to record lateral excursive and protrusive movements, or repeated patient "self-tapping" closure movements, while both condyles are gently braced in the glenoid fossae.

Bimanually manipulated closures that are controlled by the clinician identify the primary anterior (to the condyle) controlling interocclusal contacts that can influence the position of the condyles during unguided, habitual function. This is because all points of contact into MIP are activated when the patient squeezes from the CR contact into MIP. This application enhances the diagnostic value of bimanually manipulated articulating paper slide markings, by both qualifying the definitive location, and quantifying the force characteristics of the CR contact.

Recording a Vertical Force Distribution Pattern (VFDP)

- Have the patient stand upright with feet shoulder width apart, eyes looking straight ahead, parallel to the floor (Figure 35).
- Insert the sensor in the patient's mouth parallel to the maxillary occlusal plane.
- While observing the T-Scan recording desktop, depress the *record button* on top of the recording handle to initiate a 5 - 7 second-long force recording.
- Ask the patient to swallow and to squeeze into the sensor by clenching the teeth together firmly to establish a baseline MIP starting position.
- Then ask the patient to "tap" the teeth firmly onto the sensor three or four times in succession and finally, ask the patient to squeeze the teeth together in order to complete the recording.

Standing patterns, when compared to HFDPs, SFDPs, and MFDPs generally display less teeth contacting, and consequently less force intensity on the occlusion.

In addition to T-Scan sensors, Tekscan also manufactures the MatScan technology (MatScan, Tekscan, Inc. S. Boston, MA, USA), which provides dynamic and static foot pressure distribution measurements. Standing foot pressure distribution can be correlated in real time to both electromyographic activity and occlusal force (right pane). The right pane of Figure 35 illustrates demonstrates the possibilities of integrating digital data from differing sources, to better understand postural functional adaptation.

Figure 34. Using Bimanual Manipulation, a guided closure is initiated until the patient makes the initial point of contact registered by the sensor in CR, after which the patient self-squeezes into maximum intercuspation. This manipulated force pattern registered mostly blue to light green force levels because Bimanual Manipulation is a low-force generating movement.

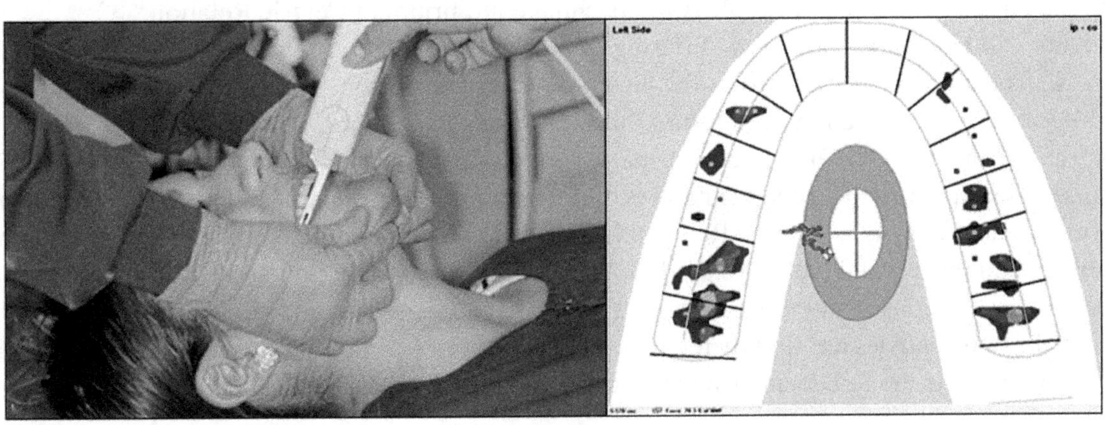

Figure 35. With the patient standing upright, feet shoulder-width apart, looking straight ahead, the patient swallows, squeezes into intercuspation, and "taps" the teeth firmly through the sensor three or four times in succession. The displayed force pattern (middle pane) represents the mandible's engagement into MIP while standing.

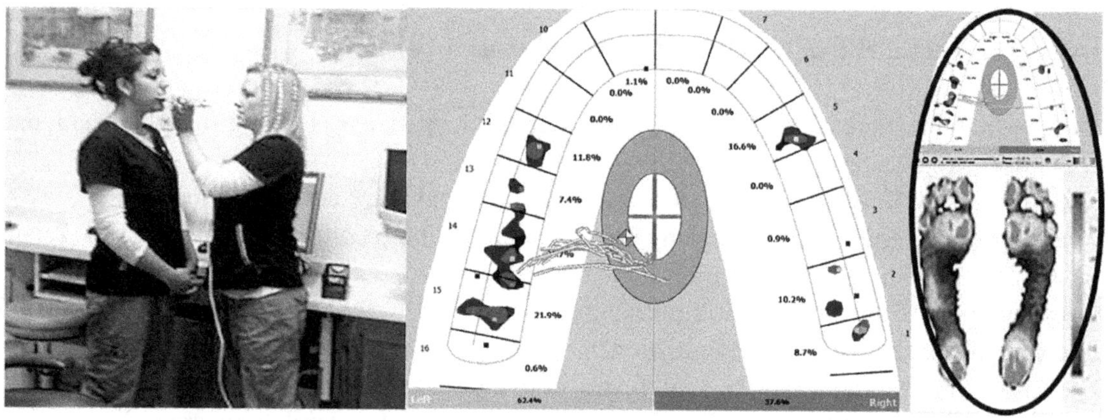

HFDP, SFDP, and MFDP

The three force distribution patterns recorded with patients in a dental chair when either sitting or supine (HFDP, SFDP, and MFDP), can all be used to identify the first points of contact when the mandible engages the maxilla, which provides resistance to a mandible's pathway toward equilibrium in the various postural positions. In some patients, all these force distribution patterns are similar in arch location and trajectory. In other patients, the arc of mandibular closure produces a different force distribution pattern (Figures 31, 32, and 34) that can be diagnostic of the relationship between forward head posture, condylar position, and occlusal force engagement.

Figure 36 is an example of three force distribution movies taken on the same patient using three different positions for the two condyles. In the HFDP, the condyles are free to adapt within the envelope of motion and the envelope of function. The SFDP diminishes the forward movement of the two condyles by immobilizing the head thus measuring a different mandibular pathway. An MFDP is designed to measure the first anterior control contact when the mandible is maintained in a Centric Relation condylar position. The condyles and the head posture are restricted in a MFDP to diagnose the primary force interference that prevents the mandible from reaching equilibrium in Centric Relation.

Patients will generally exhibit two differing digital force patterns; one that is *habitual* and one that is *skeletal*. The habitual pattern favors the "teeth together" occlusion, while the skeletal pattern is so named because it records an arc of closure that minimizes head, neck, and condylar adaptation. The author uses the habitual (HFDP) pattern to assess a post-adapted occlusal condition, the skeletal (SFDP) pattern to reflect a pre-adapted condylar and occlusal condition, and the manipulated (MFDP) pattern to identify the actual site of the Centric Relation interference. When the HFDP and the SFDP are similar, the habitual and the skeletal pathways produce similar envelopes of motion and envelopes of function.

The primary difference between the occlusion in the habitual position and in skeletal position is that in the latter, the two condyles are slightly restricted in the glenoid fossae, thus changing the arc of closure. When the HFDP and the SFDP are different (Figure 36 compared to Figures 43 and 44), it indicates the

Figure 36. Differing patterns recorded from the same patient sitting, supine, and supine with a controlled mandible closure. Primary resistance to a balanced force distribution is located by identifying the Centric Relation 1st point of contact (MFDP), the skeletal envelope of function (SFDP), and an adapted envelope of function (HFDP).

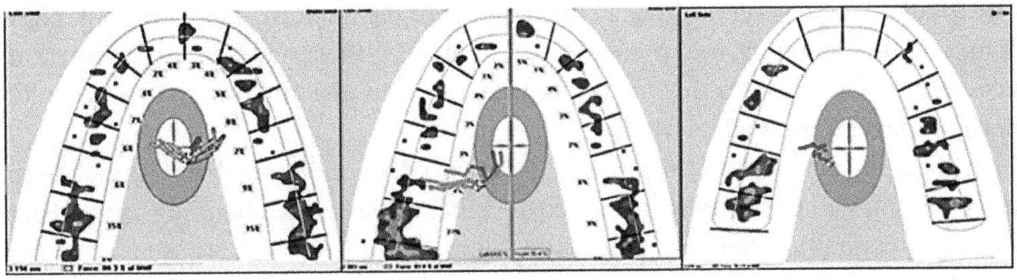

HFDP	SFDP	MFDP
Reveals the adapted pathway of the mandible's engagement into, onto, and out of the upper occlusal plane while the patient is sitting.	Reveals the favored mandibular pathway when the patient is in a supine position with the neck supported and the shoulders held back securely.	Bypasses the adapted pathway engram using a bimanual technique while the patient is in a supine position to reveal the first points of contact named the **anterior controls**.

degree to which the occlusion has had to adapt in order to function around the primary force resistance that prevents bilateral balance. When the COF trajectory icons in the HFDP, the SFDP, and the MFDP match closely near the center of the target area, the mandible is best positioned for minimal occlusal interference in both the envelope of motion and the envelope of function.

When HFDP ≠ SFDP or MFDP

The HFDP is an adapted closure pattern different from the SFDP in most patients. The SFDP that is recorded in a supine position usually is found posterior and lateral compared to the adapted or habitual arc of closure that is recorded in a sitting position. The orientation of each condyle (Figure 40) in the glenoid fossae is therefore slightly different. In Figure 36, the true primary interference found in both the SFDP and the MFDP scans, is located in the left posterior area (#15 - #18). This contact is the *anterior control* that prevents a balanced bilateral engagement of contacts. The SFDP and the MFDP are better indicators of the true site of resistance to the mandible's pathway because they limit adaptive movement of the condyles. All three patterns should be recorded before and after treatment to document changes.

When HFDP = SFDP = MFDP

When all three patterns are similar, adaptation to the mandible's preferred pathway is minimal, and the first points of contact match location or are very similar, in all three scans. This offers triple confirmation of the location of the interference using objective data that validates a consistent mandibular engagement position with respect to the applied force distribution onto the occlusion. This favorable distribution results in a bilaterally balanced occlusal design indicated by the COF icon resting in the elliptical gray and white zone when the patient squeezes into MIP (see Figure 38).

Patterns and Structure Constantly Change

To *occlude* means to come together, where the occlusion facilitates the gathering of contacts when closure of the mandible into the maxillary arch ensues. The resultant occlusal force of each contact when received by the plane of occlusion is either in harmony with the anatomy and free from interference, or not in harmony with the anatomy, and presents interferences either to the arc of closure and/or during excursive movements. Those forces that are not in harmony with the anatomy will accelerate the necessary force-dissipation structural adaptation.

Moreover, a changing envelope of motion and envelope of function coupled with a changing occlusal contact landing pattern, will continually influence how the teeth react to changing applied occlusal force levels. Structural and systemic changes occur daily, monthly, and yearly, because the mandible is often in function during sleep, while chewing, swallowing, and while engaging in any habit which involves the teeth and/or dental prostheses. "Ideal" occlusions generally have good force distribution patterns (Figure 38), but even the most beautiful natural and/or reconstructed occlusions age and adapt. Microtrauma and friction inhibit and/or prevent harmonious functional adaptation (see Figure 39).

Many factors accelerate change to the involved oral structures and functional patterns of the mandible (see below). Some are acute problems like an infection, but most structural changes result from chronic dysfunction and take years to develop. Individual genetics, dental care, and patient education allow many humans to maintain healthier teeth, gingiva, and bones throughout their lifetime. However, each decade of life increasingly challenges the teeth, gingiva, and Temporomandibular joints with the force the muscles generate during long-term occlusal function. The repetitive microtrauma from teeth landing on each other with varying force concentrations and for varying contact durations will change how the *occlusion* functions. Simply stated, the more teeth are together, the more likely that applied occlusal force will alter the proprioception that directs the structural support system to adapt to the force, inducing changes throughout life.

Functional and structural factors that influence and change *force distribution patterns* are:

- The alignment, position, quality, and resistance of the teeth and supportive bone.
- Congenitally missing or any extracted tooth/teeth.
- Orthodontic treatment, endodontic treatment, occlusal adjustment procedures, and restorative treatment that alters occlusal contact.
- Carious lesions (occlusal, proximal, and root surface) and other structural pathologies.
- Adaptation to normal function, parafunction, or dysfunction.
- Periodontal, foundational, and environmental disease.
- Cementoenamel junction adaptation to applied occlusal force (abfraction formation and periodontal recession).
- Wear facets, stress fractures, and variations of the occlusal anatomy of the teeth and/or prosthetic replacements.
- Corrective surgery, oral or periodontal.
- The quality of dental care rendered (materials, timing, and technique).
- Patient diet, nutrition, heredity, and the quality of home care.
- Tongue and airway function from birth, throughout life.
- Head and neck posture during sleep, at work, at play, and at rest.

- Any systemic change that affects the homeostasis of the oral anatomy, such as hormonal changes from pregnancy, or chronic medication use from ongoing disease, dry mouth, diabetes, etc.
- Splint therapy, chiropractic treatment, and physical or massage therapy that can alter the mandible-to-cranium spatial relationship.

Digital occlusal force contact measurements greatly improve the occlusal diagnostic process, as well as, through computer-guided occlusal intervention, increase the longevity of structural components that, if left untreated, create microtrauma and accelerate the adaptive processes. Resistance to the mandible's favored pathways will likely lead to long-term structural compromise and pathway alteration. Altered pathways trigger adaptation and ultimately result in pathology to the system and to structure.

Occlusal splints can minimize the structural damage and promote functional harmony. Occlusal splint therapy is the art and science of establishing neuromuscular harmony in the masticatory system by creating a mechanical disadvantage for parafunctional forces (Dylina, 2001). Splints have traditionally been used to separate the structural integration of the mandible and the maxilla. The purpose of a splint is to position the mandible against the cranium in a different location from the habitual closure position. In addition, the proprioception of the sensory receptors of the periodontal ligaments and the Temporomandibular joints will be altered with a splint in place. The different materials and designs of the splint have the ability to change the mandible's pathway, the position of both condyles, and the reflex engrams of the masticatory muscles. In this way, a splint allows the clinician to observe changes between the habitual position and the splint-modified closure position for both diagnostic and therapeutic purposes. In some patients, a simple therapeutic splint has the potential to improve the quality of their daily life, as has been documented in the case of headache, TMD, and sleep apnea sufferers (Dylina, 2001).

Chronic microtrauma necessitates correction, such that a poor force distribution can be changed by one or more intervention procedures. Treatments can change force distribution and can potentially transform pathologic adaptation variations into a consistent physiologic arc of closure. A primary goal in occlusal treatment is to achieve functional harmony between the anatomy and the Stomatognathic system. In this way, a clinician can alter, adjust, or completely change how the force is distributed into and out of the plane of occlusion. Good clinical judgment and objective data can improve the prognosis and longevity of the treatment provided.

A clinician may choose to alter a poorly distributed force pattern by any number of methods:

- Monitor the occlusion as it adapts naturally.
- Make a postural change (physical therapy, etc.).
- Employ splint therapy.
- Equilibrate the dentition.
- Restore the dentition, as needed.
- Rebuild entire arch(es).
- Move the teeth orthodontically.
- Realign the arches with Orthognathic surgery.

Treatment options depend on a clinician's objectives. Altering a single tooth may or may not have an effect on the force distribution of the system. The alteration of multiple teeth in a short period of time greatly increases the possibility that the contact force engagement will change throughout the arch. Orthodontics, a full arch reconstruction, or a new denture will completely alter contact force distribution and vary in mandibular engagement within the Stomatognathic system. Digital contact measurement taken before and after treatment can guide the intervention, and document the improvements made to the involved structures.

The Diagnostic Value of Digital Occlusal Force Distribution Patterns

The sensory receptors of the TM joints, periodontal ligaments, and the muscles provide a constant feedback mechanism that controls the forces against the teeth. Factors such as the growth of the facial bones, the force of muscle contractions during mastication, and the natural tendency of the teeth to drift are probably all far more important in maintaining occlusal homeostasis, than is the oft-mentioned anatomy (Enlow, 1990).

The engram (the masticatory "muscle memory") has been shown to be a conditioned reflex whose muscle conditioning lasts less than two minutes, which is far shorter than previously thought. This reflex, reinforced and stored in the masticatory muscles with every swallow, adjusts masticatory muscle activity to guide the lower arch unerringly into its intercuspated position (ICP). These muscle adjustments compensate for the continually changing internal and external factors that affect the mandible's entry into the ICP (Lerman, 2011).

One thing that has been stated as appearing certain, is that the repetitive movements of the mandible that determine the envelope of function are far more complex, and far more influenced by exquisitely sensitive sensory systems, than can be explained by simplistic explanations. However, clinical observation is too consistent to be ignored. The mandible does have favored pathways of function, and if teeth interfere with these favored paths, there will be a price to pay in deformation or dysfunction. The weakest link will be the prime focus of the damage (Dawson, 2007).

Force cycle recordings that create DOFDPs and measure the mandible's engagement are influenced by:

- The position of head and neck (SFDP).
- The condylar orientation (MFDP).
- The anterior orientation (HFDP).
- The posterior plane of occlusion (SFDP).

The orientation of the mandible's pathway, the position of the two condyles, the anterior controls, and the posterior plane of occlusion determine guidance, control, and contact for the mandible to *occlude* and *disocclude* in a cyclical, repeatable pattern (Figure 37).

Figure 38 describes a patient with excellent anatomical architecture and a healthy occlusion, where the occlusion does not violate any of the four occlusal imperatives, presented in Figure 37. The HFDP is well-balanced, with the occluding and disoccluding lines lying close to the center of the COF target. The alignment of the teeth, coupled with a slightly posteriorly centered COF icon position, is diagnostic of preservational force dissipation, rather than of destructive force application. The anterior segment is tightly coupled (with minimal fremitus on #8 only), and the posterior plane of occlusion is symmetrical in both design and in the balance of force. Only the posterior left maxillary plane, the lack of contact of teeth #11 to #22, and fremitus detected on tooth #8, prevent this patient from having the elusive, "perfect occlusion."

Figure 39 shows a maladaptive HFDP. The COF trajectory icon (the upper pane) indicates that excessive anterior contact forces are present. The poor alignment of the posterior teeth, the bilaterally uneven

Figure 37. Each force distribution pattern has the potential to verify four variables that influence mandibular engagement of the favored pathway. Destruction occurs when the condylar orientation (the "back end"), the anterior orientation (the "front" end), and the posterior plane of occlusion (transverse or "side to side") are functionally codependent, and work against each other during the mandible's engagement with the maxilla.

The condylar orientation	The anterior orientation	The posterior plane orientation	The mandibular pathway

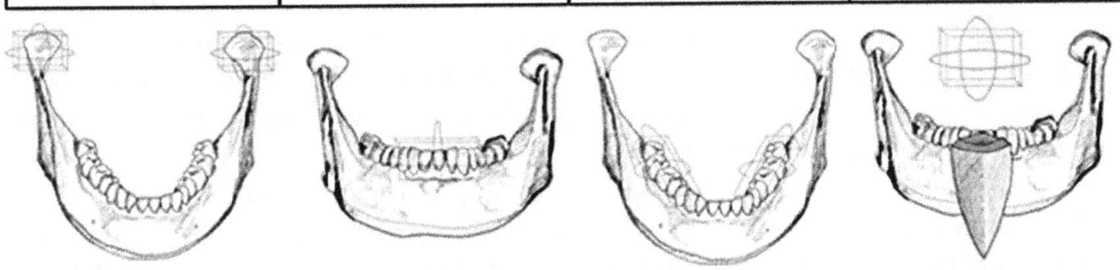

is the first determinant of occlusion	is the second determinant of occlusion	ideally should not interfere with the two determinants	is defined by the envelope of motion and the envelope of function

Figure 38. A functionally harmonious HFDP that is well-balanced, with the occluding and disoccluding lines being close to the center of the COF target.

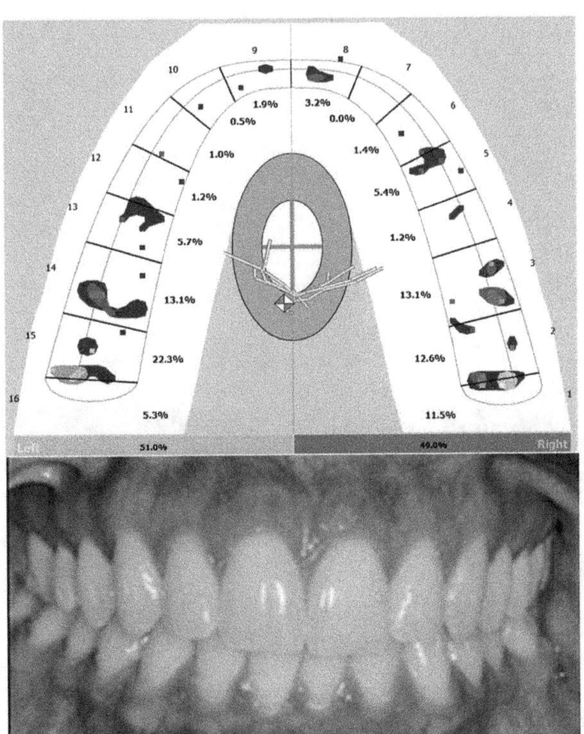

occlusal plane, and the adaptive condylar orientation all contributed to the dysfunction of the anterior anatomy. The anterior position of the force summation (COF) diagnoses destructive force dissipation within this dentition. This excessive anterior force was present years before the tooth structure changed into its present condition. As demonstrated by the force distribution pattern, this occlusion violates all four imperatives of harmonious function, free from codependent adaptation.

Most patterns demonstrate both functional and dysfunctional elements. Patterns are generally dictated by the involved dental anatomy and the repetitive function of the masticatory apparatus over a patient's lifetime. Many HFDPs are present years before they cause any damage, making the patterns an excellent diagnostic tool that allows a clinician to slow down or prevent the consequences that repetitive habitual stress will force on the muscles, the ligaments, the TM joints, the teeth, or the supportive alveolar bone. DOFDPs enable a "predict and prevent" model of patient care, as they identify occlusal interferences long before the eventual destruction manifests itself.

It has been the author's experience that force cycles that are isolated within a region of the dental arch will have identical characteristics and cause similar symptoms in patients whose force cycles occur in the same region. Lines and patterns that behave similarly from one patient to the next often result in similar positive or negative, intra or extraoral structural changes.

Figure 39. A maladapted HFDP in which excessive anterior contact forces are present, illustrated by the origin of the COF trajectory lines

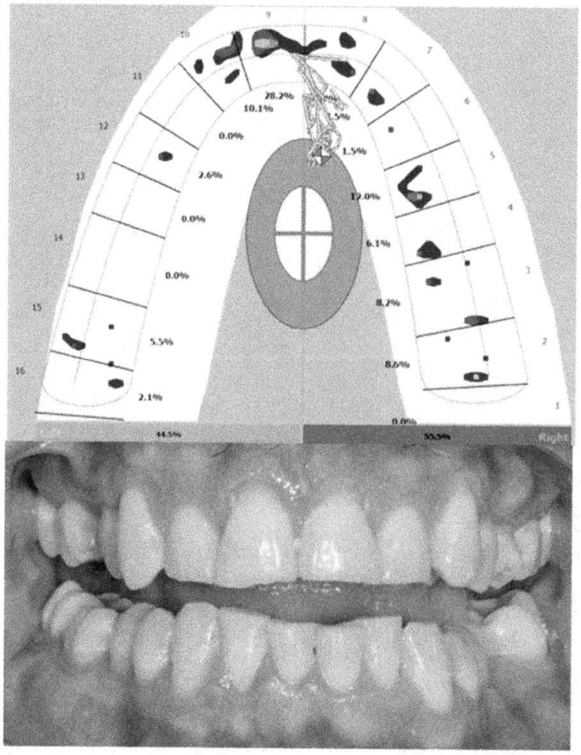

The Condylar Orientation Is the First Determinant of Occlusion

The goal in treating all patients is to give them the functional freedom that comes with a healthy occlusion. A violation of, or validation of the *first and/or second determinant(s) of occlusion* (Dawson, 2007) can be documented with an objective force cycle measurement. The condylar path dictates how the back end of the mandible moves. That is the *first determinant of occlusion* (Figure 40) (Dawson, 2007). The "back end" refers to the alignment of the TM joints with the posterior dentition behind the canines. An ideal arrangement would be two healthy condyles with good range of motion, in harmony, with minimal occlusal interference. The second determinant is the anterior orientation, which dictates how the "front end" of the mandible moves. Ideally, both the back half and the front half of the arch should work together harmoniously along with a stable and consistent arc of mandibular closure. The posterior planes of occlusion often determine the character of the mandible's behavior in function or in dysfunction because they are rarely symmetrical in all three dimensions.

Dual condylar orientation accurately describes condylar function, because each condyle must first function by itself, and then function in harmony with the other condyle. Each condyle influences its counterpart during growth and function. Condylar skeletal orientation over a lifetime of mandibular motion is critical to the stability of the mandible's favored pathways at rest, in function, and during sleep. If one condyle is asked to function in a less than ideal position, then the ipsilateral condyle may consequently be required to change its orientation within the glenoid fossa, which will ultimately alter the mandible's preferred pathway. Ideally, each condyle/fossa unit should act independently from the other and function in an efficient, healthy position by itself, while in harmony with the other. Condyles

Figure 40. Every patient has two Temporomandibular joints and one occlusion. Each condyle head (known as the "ball") should physiologically rest and function within the glenoid fossa (the "socket"). The orientation icons illustrate, in 3-Dimensions, the mandible's dual-hinged position within the glenoid fossae. These icons suggest that each condyle has the possibility of finding an adapted position within the glenoid fossa in any mandibular movement, over time.

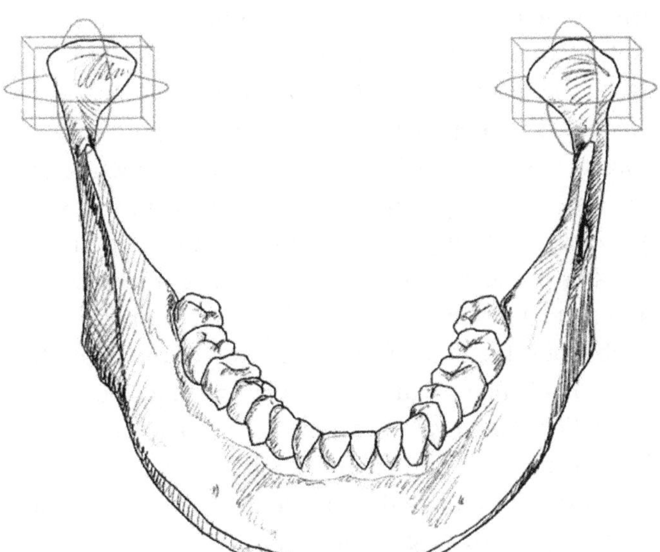

that do not function in perfect harmony at rest or in function, either by themselves or in combination with the counterpart condyle, must adapt structurally over time. Adaptation may be physiologic, pathologic, or both to the TM joints and to the Stomatognathic system.

Condyles that are properly located spatially within the glenoid fossa at rest and in function, are assumed to be in the center or in the *centric* position. The word *centric* in Dental Medicine always refers to the condyles. Ideally, the two glenoid fossae should be mirror images of each other in shape, size, and volume. However, if the two temporal bones are not mirror images of each other, the two condyle heads will adapt differently to their respective glenoid fossa contours. Different socket shapes and positions will affect condylar orientation, thus making the TM joints functionally codependent on each other, thereby altering both the occlusal force distribution, and the mandible's pathway in motion and in function.

As an adjective used in Dental Medicine, the term *centric* can be confusing to the reader because it is often combined with other words which have different meanings. *Centric Relation*, *Centric Occlusion*, *Long Centric*, *Habitual Centric*, and *Myocentric,* are all terms used in Dental Medicine to describe differing anatomic occlusal concepts that are describing differing mandibular positions.

Because the condyles are attached to the posterior portion of the mandible, and because the mandible is a single bone, it then is a physical fact that the adapted position of the condyles in the fossae will be influenced by the occlusion of the teeth, and vice versa. The occluding teeth may or may not create an ideal condyle-to-fossa relationship because the contact of the teeth may direct the condylar anatomy into a muscularly-braced, rather than a ligamentally-braced position. Many patients adapt to such a condition and live with it for years without structural damage, but many do not.

Motion at odds with design is at best inefficient, and at worst, destructive. This occurs when the envelope of motion is not in harmony with the envelope of function. The cause and effect relationship of condylar orientation can be minor, or catastrophic to one or both condyles, to a single tooth or to the entire system. Both adaptation and destruction of tissue result when structure and movement cannot coexist in functional harmony.

The Anterior Orientation Is the Second Determinant of Occlusion

The diagnosis and treatment of the anterior orientation requires an understanding of the integration of morphology, biology, esthetics, and function (Rufenacht, 2000). The Stomatognathic system seeks to establish equilibrium between the head, the condyle, the neck, and the occlusal posture. The anterior orientation is an excellent diagnostic component of the mandible's preferred pathway (Figure 41). Force distribution patterns recorded at any age, provide objective data as to when and where the anterior teeth are opposing resistance to the mandible's preferred pathway of closure, or when and where any tooth or teeth anterior to the condyles are preventing a friction-free mandibular closure pathway.

One of the primary functions of the anterior teeth is to protect the back teeth from excursive movement occlusal surface frictional interactions. However, if the posterior teeth and the condylar orientation are not in harmony with each other, then the anterior pathway of the mandible will be altered, and the structure of the anterior teeth will change. Both the condylar guidance posteriorly, and the anterior guidance should determine the functional pathways of the mandible. The *second determinant of occlusion* is controlled by the teeth, where the anterior guidance determines how the front end of the mandible moves (Dawson, 2007). It is also important to realize that an occlusal plane is only acceptable if it permits the anterior guidance to disclude the posterior teeth effectively and rapidly.

Figure 41. The anterior orientation must function in harmony with the teeth, the pathway of the mandibular movement, and the condylar orientation. The anterior region consists of the maxillary and mandibular canines, lateral incisors, and central incisors. The orientation icon suggests that the anterior segment of the mandible will seek an adapted position within the upper anterior teeth during mandibular movements.

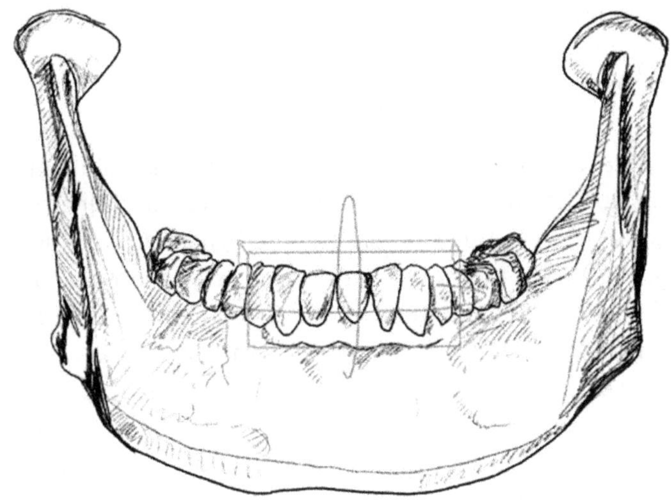

The diagnostic determinants of the anterior orientation are:

- **Anterior Guidance:** The influence of the contacting surfaces of anterior teeth on tooth-limiting mandibular movements.
- **Canine Guidance (Also Named Canine-Protected Articulation):** A form of a mutually-protected articulation in which the vertical and horizontal overlaps of the canine teeth disengage the posterior teeth in mandibular excursive movements.
- **Incisal Guidance:** The influence of the contacting surfaces of the mandibular and maxillary anterior teeth on mandibular movements.
- **Occlusal Plane:** The average plane established by the anterior incisal edges and occlusal surfaces of the posterior teeth.
- **Head, Neck, and Condyle Orientation:** The influence of posture on mandibular movements.

The anterior teeth are only one of the segments establishing the position for the anterior orientation. The myriad of systems posterior to the canines and incisors must also be in balance for the anterior orientation to be in harmony with the Stomatognathic system. In dental occlusion, guidance describes how the mandible is guided into the maxilla for both occlusal function and swallowing. The anterior teeth primarily direct the horizontal movement of the mandible in and out of intercuspation, while the posterior teeth direct the vertical movement of the condyle/disc assemblies into the glenoid fossa of the Temporomandibular joints.

The presence of wear facets on the lingual and incisal surfaces of the upper anterior teeth and lower facial and incisal edges, often indicate resistance to the engrained adaptive patterns of mandibular motion and to the mandible's preferred pathway. The anterior, canine, and incisal guidance systems are all factors that influence the envelope of function and the anterior orientation of the mandible. To achieve equilibrium in the anterior segment, the orientation of the head and neck, the condyles, and the posterior dentition must also be in harmony. The two force patterns described in Figures 50 and 51 illustrate two different anterior guidance patterns; one that is preservational and one that is destructive. These two different mandible-to-cranium pathways result in different adaptive responses of the anterior teeth, and will dissimilarly affect the longevity of the occlusion and of the system.

The Posterior Plane Orientation

The term *occlusal interference* refers to interference to comfortable mandibular function (Dawson, 1989). The occlusal interference is not determined by occlusal contacts alone, but also involves the anatomy of the Temporomandibular joints, the limiting influence of the ligaments, and the shape and orientation of the occlusal plane (Storey, 1979). The ideal occlusal plane is only theoretical because all patients have a unique 3-Dimensional orientation of their natural or prosthetic teeth within the supportive bone, which may or may not be ideal in shape and/or quality. The clinician must understand that the shape of the bone determines the position of the dentition. An interference to a balanced mandibular pathway is often caused by the position a tooth assumes within the bone and within the arch. The *occlusal table*, which is the functional portion of the occlusal surface of the posterior teeth (Academy of Prosthodontics, 2005), is where the interferences appear when resultant from poor tooth position within the arch.

Occlusal disharmony is a phenomenon in which contacts of opposing occlusal surfaces are not in harmony with other tooth contacts, and/or the anatomic and physiologic components of the craniomandibular complex. A DOFDP can be diagnostic for occlusal disharmony present on the occlusal table, by alerting the clinician to exactly which tooth, teeth, or prosthetic replacement(s), is the cause of the interference. It is important to note that asymmetric arch foundations may still demonstrate a balanced DOFDP, if the dentition and/or prosthetics have been corrected to compensate for the skeletal asymmetry.

The two posterior occlusal planes are a 3-Dimensional representation of what controls the vertical and transverse force that occurs during mandibular engagement with the maxilla. To prevent functional codependency, microtrauma, interference, and occlusal deflection, each plane must meet the conditions of the first and second determinants of occlusion (Figure 42). In theory during function, the x-y-z axes of the occlusal plane (the transverse, sagittal, and horizontal posterior planes) of the static upper arch should match the mandibular posterior spatial orientation.

The Mandible's Pathway

Mandibular position, like a number of other automatic somatic activities, is largely reflexively controlled, even though it can be altered voluntarily. Reflex engrams guide the mandible in its favored pathways, and DOFDPs provide objective data on the structural obstacles that divert, limit, and/or prevent the mandible from using its natural preferred pathway of least resistance to and from *occlude* (Figure 43). In function, the force recorded (within the *red* zone) influences how the patient, through proprioception, orients the mandible in space (*blue*) on the way into occlusal contact. Alternatively, after the process of occlusion completes and stops at maximum intercuspation (MIP), it is followed by the mandible disoccluding, when it reverses course and moves back into the envelope of motion.

The receptors of the Temporomandibular capsular area appear to be far more important in the control and guidance of mandibular function and position than it has previously been thought. Much of our knowledge of mandibular position and its regulation have been derived from studies of adults. It may

Figure 42. The orientation icons suggest that there are two posterior segments, both of which will seek an adaptive position in mandibular movements, over time. The two posterior segments are independent of each other in some functional patterns of engagement, but each alone can be very dependent on the ipsilateral side within most mandibular positions. This is one valid reason for measuring all the contacts within the entire arch together at one time, resultant from any functional mandibular movement.

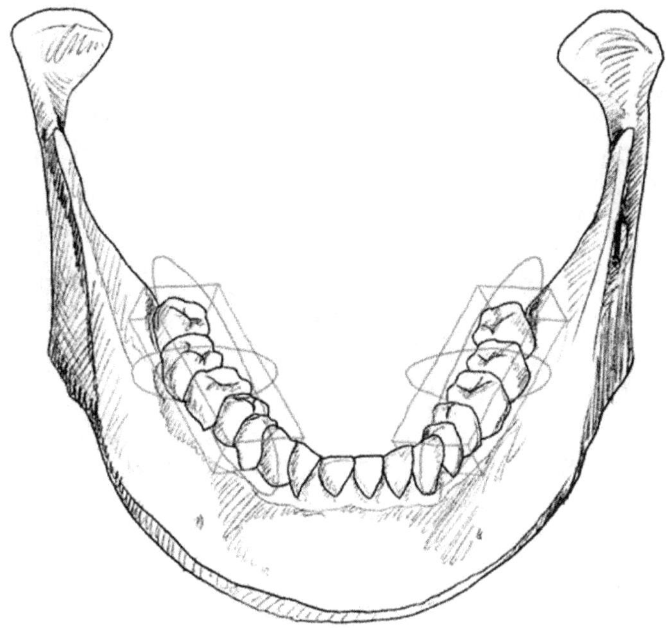

be hazardous to casually transfer these concepts to the growing child, despite that the concepts may be correct for older persons. According to one author, knowledge about many aspects of developmental mandibular neurophysiology has been considered to be incomplete (Enlow, 1990).

The entire context of occlusal harmony is based on the precise relationship of the teeth and how the mandible moves in function versus parafunction. The starting point for understanding the envelope of function is to first understand the envelope of motion (Dawson, 2007). Figure 43 illustrates the concept that only the mandible moves. The two condyles are allowed to work separately within the envelope of motion but become codependent in the envelope of function.

When the teeth are apart, the mandible in space is controlled by the integrated Stomatognathic system which, through its development, assimilates an integrative neurologic process that dictates the motor behavior of the neuromusculature and the Temporomandibular joints. Movement engrams in the envelope of motion set up the approach and landing of the mandible into maximum intercuspation, the ultimate "stopped" position. Instantaneously, the direction reverses as the process of disclusion starts. The "push off" to release the engagement of contact is often times the most aggressive display of force intensity observed in a force cycle. The reason is that in many occlusions, the force transfer to get into MIP is quick and easily accomplished by the patient. However, the force transfer to exit MIP is difficult because occlusal surface friction prolongs the tooth separation while raising the contact force intensity. This force intensity results in prolonged microtrauma that can deform the involved specific local structure and induce dysfunction to the overall system.

Figure 43. The graphic located between the condyles is an orientation icon used to illustrate the 3-Dimensional movement of the mandible's pathway into, onto, and out of MIP. An extension of Posselt's diagram is overlaying the mandible in space, illustrating its range of motion in all three planes. The three-dimensional spatial orientation of the mandible to the maxilla influences the envelope of motion (blue) to seek equilibrium within functional border positions (red).

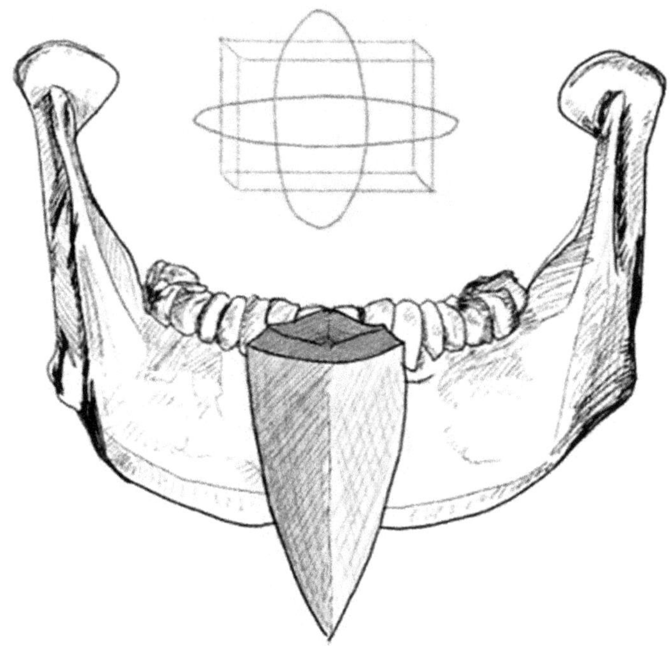

Dental and skeletal asymmetries that develop from myofunctional habits during growth produce adaptations which will limit the range of motion, and create a unique Posselt's envelope. The awareness of the mandible in space during swallowing, breathing, sleeping, and mastication will define a truly individualized envelope of motion. As such, the neuromuscular function of mandibular movement and the functional anatomy of the two TM joints will adapt in structure and shape. Pathologic TM joints create poor condylar orientation and repetitive condylar motion patterns, will alter the DOFDPs over time. Conversely, any prolonged intense force that is either located or distributed throughout the dental arch can change both of the condyles' orientation within the glenoid fossae.

Detailed Analysis of Arch Position and Digital Occlusal Force Distribution Pattern Locations

Force cycle engagement is present in every occlusion. Force pattern recordings document how force is transferred during an entire occlusal cycle: occlusion, MIP, and disocclusion. The diagnostic patterns show direction, sequence, intensity, and repetition of force. Some patterns dominate the anterior teeth while others are located more posteriorly. Some remain in small, isolated locations and others include a contact point from every tooth or prosthetic replacement in the arch. Most patterns favor one side of the arch, indicating that a balanced bilateral occlusion is not very common.

Each pattern has a growth and development phase, an airway and posture phase, an oral health phase, and a treatment history phase, as an occlusion ages. As such, every individual has a unique pattern that can change over time; slowly for some, and quickly for others. Understanding pattern behavior and why patterns change is essential to the diagnosis, treatment, and maintenance of an occlusion.

Digital Occlusal Force Patterns occur in one of six arch locations (Figures 44 - 49; and Figures 25 - 30):

- **Force Cycle Pattern #1:** Distal posterior, favoring either the right or left arch-half (Figure 44).
- **Force Cycle Pattern #2:** Middle posterior, favoring either the right or left arch-half (Figure 45).
- **Force Cycle Pattern #3:** Anterior force with minimal or no posterior contact (Figure 46).
- **Force Cycle Pattern #4:** Centered within the Center of Force (COF) target (Figure 47).
- **Force Cycle Pattern #5:** Posterior force with no anterior coupling (Figure 48).
- **Force Cycle Pattern #6:** Anterior initially, then moving posteriorly, or posterior initially then moving anteriorly, either along or across the arch (Figure 49).

Force Cycle Pattern #1: The Distal Posterior, Either Right or Left Pattern

Figures 50 - 52 detail force cycle pattern #1. Figure 50 illustrates the first "tap" that begins to form a distal left posterior force distribution pattern. The COF trajectory line represents the initial COF pathway made from the first points of contact to MIP, that can diagnose the presence of repetitive microtraumatic posterior force distribution as the patient re-occludes during the repeated "tapping". The anterior teeth make no contact, which lessens the protection of the posterior teeth in function. The red COF line moves from posterior left horizontally to the right, indicating that the left molars occlude before the right teeth do. Each "tap" will reproduce a similar line in the same location in the arch as the force contact points

Figure 44. Force cycle pattern #1: Distal posterior (left or right). The force cycle is limited to a few molars that control the entire occlusion, preventing even contact distribution in both the vertical and horizontal movements. This is a clear violation of the first determinant that can stress the condylar orientation in every mandibular position.

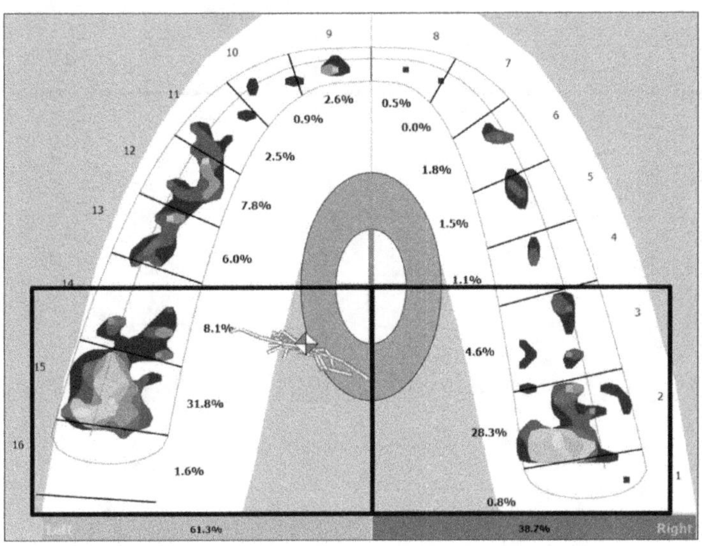

Figure 45. Force cycle pattern #2: Middle posterior (right or left). This force cycle shows limited amounts of anterior guidance in horizontal movements, with extra vertical force concentrated on one side of the arch, both of which can alter the envelope of function. Transverse force may or may not be an issue depending on the degree of skeletal asymmetry present.

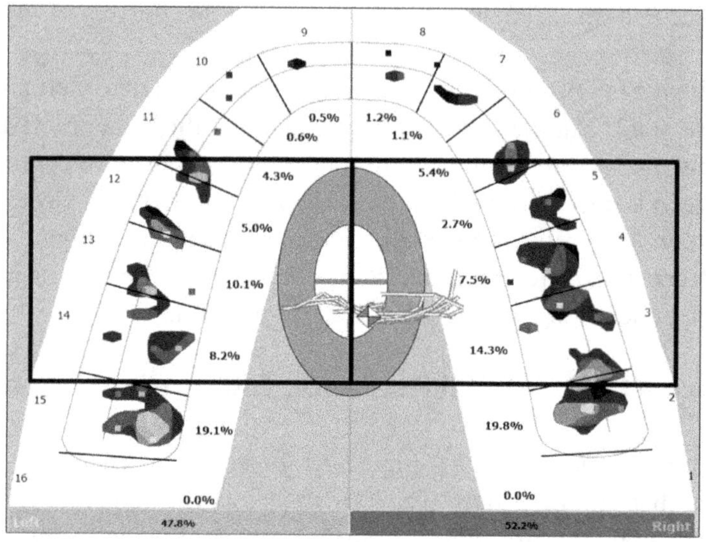

Figure 46. Force cycle pattern #3: Anteriorly dominated. Lack of posterior vertical force can destroy the anatomy in the anterior segment. The teeth, a prosthesis, and the supporting foundation structures can be stressed, forced to adapt, and age quickly. Force distribution exclusive to the anterior region occurs because of missing posterior teeth, or from a lack of vertical stops.

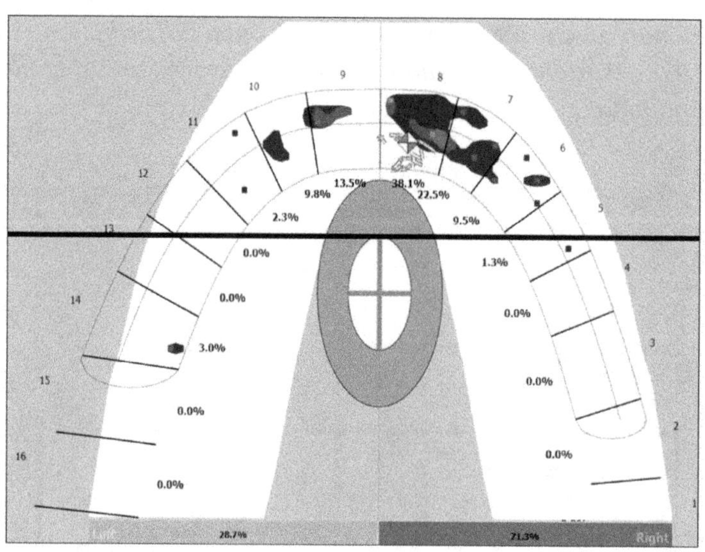

Figure 47. Force cycle pattern #4: Centered within the Center of Force target. Very few occlusions distribute force equally within the posterior occlusal plane during both the occluding and disoccluding envelopes of movement. The anterior orientation and the condylar orientation are either independent of each other, or are equally codependent when a force pattern is visibly centered in function, sleep, and rest.

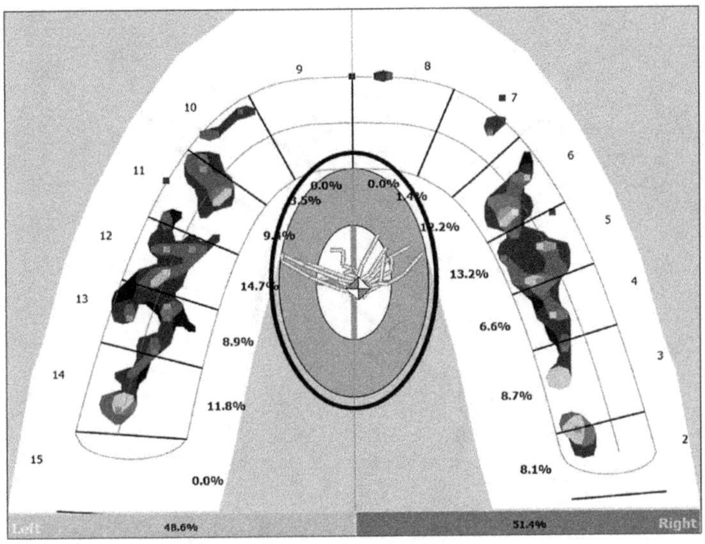

Figure 48. Force cycle pattern #5: Posterior dominant with an anterior open occlusion. The open anterior bite is generally a pathologic occlusion. It has the potential to become physiologic if the tongue and cervical posture balance out the excessive posterior vertical force cycle.

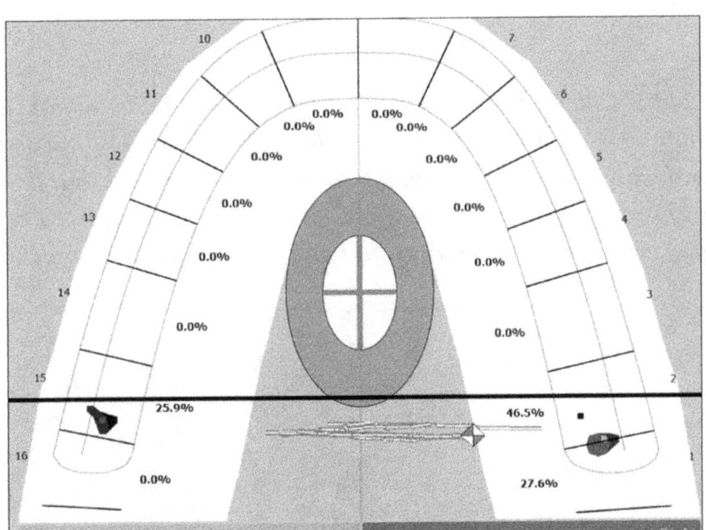

Figure 49. Force cycle pattern #6: Moves either anteroposteriorly or posteroanteriorly, along or across the arch. This is a potentially damaging force cycle pattern because the anterior and the posterior teeth work against each other in every functional position. Thick anterior crowns and wide posterior bridges often contribute to this unfavorable force distribution pattern.

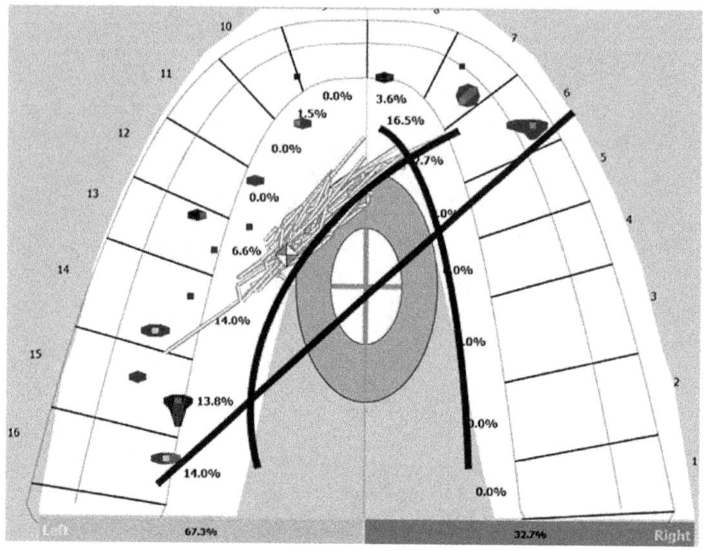

repeat the identical contact pattern. The left side hits first and the right side directs the movement as the microtraumatic cycle repeats itself with each subsequent "tap" until the pattern is completed (Figure 51). This example of a young occlusion illustrates how the recorded force data instructs the clinician where to find the occlusal interferences.

Figure 50. An example of the first line of the pattern displayed where the molars are controlling all the contacts is the very beginning of a force cycle that will develop as a dominating distal left posterior force pattern. The red COF trajectory line moves from left to right which means that the left molars touch first followed by the later right tooth contacts in just five frames (0.15 seconds). The arrows correlate the clinical articulating paper marks of the contacts that are prevent an easy entry into MIP.

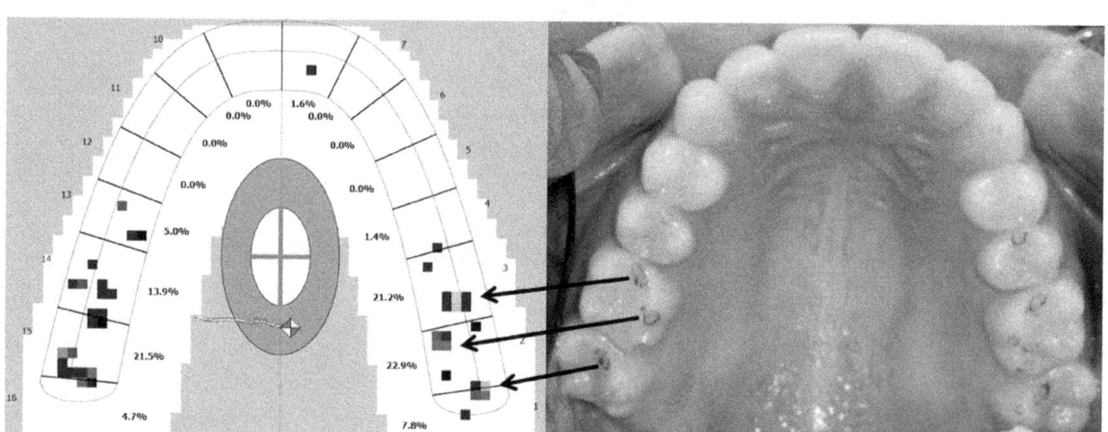

Figure 51. The completed Habitual Force Distribution Pattern (HFDP) (from Figure 50), which repeats exactly the same tooth sequence when the patient "tapped" five times. Most of the force dominates the posterior left quadrant and does not allow the mandible to enter the maxillary occlusal plane without resistance from the primary interference to the mandible's favored pathway. The condylar position, the cervical posture, and the muscles of mastication are codependent in function because of poor anterior guidance and an unbalanced, unilateral posterior force distribution.

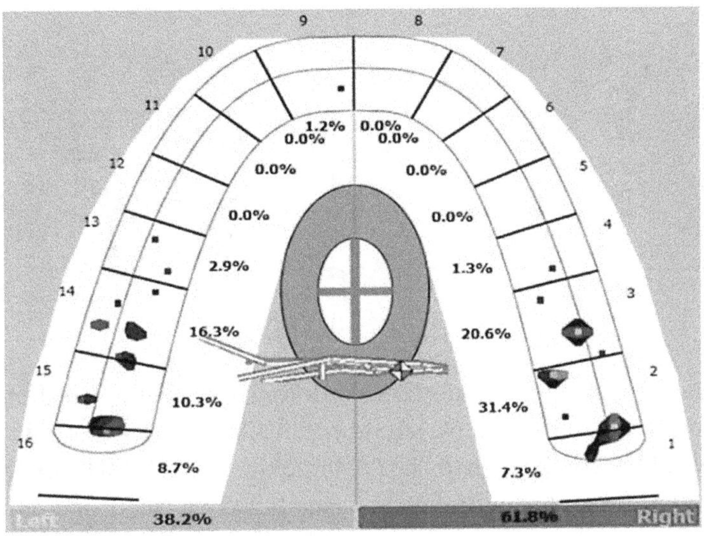

Pattern #1 Characteristics

- **Head and Neck Posture:** A cervical trigger point at the base of the skull is often present on the side where the posterior force dominates. All muscles of mastication are codependent often producing unilateral temporal headaches, when stressed.
- **Condylar Orientation:**The lateral pole of the more forceful side can be tender as the condyle is positioned forward and slightly medial on the side where the force is heavy. The opposing condyle is often positioned up and backward.
- **Anterior Orientation:** The anterior orientation does not protect the posterior teeth due to the lack of canine or premolar contact.
- **Posterior Plane of Occlusion:** Without canine protection, there is occlusal interference in every plane of mandibular function. High intensity unilateral transverse force can accelerate both structural and systemic pathology.
- **Mandibular Pathway:** The mandible's pathway to engage a balanced plane of occlusion encounters interference from the back of the arch. The result is an adaptation or compensation of the envelope of motion. Heavy regional force also alters the envelope of function and directs the mandible's favored pathway around the excessive posterior force, making a balanced closure into intercuspation difficult to achieve.

Clinical Observations: Experience from scanning all patients over the past decade indicates that thirty percent (30%) of habitual force cycle patterns (HFDPs) and fifty percent (50%) of skeletal force cycle

Figure 52. Three examples of distal posterior force patterns that demonstrate where the mandible's envelope of function encounters occlusal interference. The left pane shows a pixilated force scan demonstrating that most of the force distribution is located in the posterior left quadrant. The middle pane is a good example of a skeletal force pattern that demonstrates isolated force distribution only in the posterior right quadrant. The right pane shows an HFDP where the COF lines trace occlude and disocclude, even though the force concentration of the intercuspation is located in the posterior left portion quadrant.

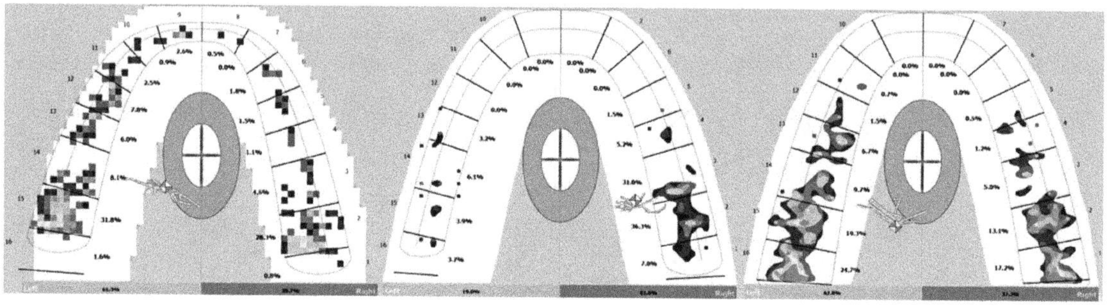

patterns (SFDPs) fall into this category. A posteriorly dominated envelope of function violates the first determinant of occlusion. The result is often a strong cervical muscle trigger point and tenderness when palpating the lateral pole of the condyle, on the heavy force side. Patients who experience muscle tension headaches who positively respond to splint therapy, usually have a No. 1 or a No. 2 pattern.

Force Cycle Pattern #2: The Middle Posterior Pattern, Either on the Left or Right Arch-Half

Figures 53 and 54 detail force cycle pattern #2. The patient shown in Figure 53 initially loads force near the arch middle. However, after a few additional "taps," the force moves over towards the posterior right teeth. The change from a centered habitual pattern to a posteriorly oriented pattern results from the condyles changing position and seating more fully as the patient "taps" the teeth together a few more times in succession. In turn, with more "taps," the force builds on the right occlusal interferences more so than on the left teeth. In this HFDP (left pane of Figure 53), the first premolars contact when the mandible is "tapping" and squeezing into MIP at 100% force. However, the upper left pane photograph shows a different occlusion, where the first premolars do not make contact.

Force Cycle Pattern #2 Characteristics

- **Head and Neck Posture:** Cervical, temporal, and lateral pterygoid muscles on the more forceful side are forced to adapt. Unilateral temporal headaches are common with this pattern.
- **Condylar Orientation:** Lateral ligaments supporting the articular disc on the more forceful side have to adapt because of excessive occlusal interference. These patients often complain of TMJ pain.
- **Anterior Orientation:** The anterior teeth do not adequately protect the posterior segment (left or right), when one side is overloaded compared to the other.

Figure 53. A posterior right HFDP, which resulted from the condyles seating more fully, and forces increased on the right posterior teeth as the patient repeatedly "tapped" his teeth together. The anterior open skeletal occlusion concentrated the occlusal forces posteriorly and to the right side. The upper right photograph shows the mandible in a Centric Relation occlusal position, but the HFDP shows canine contact when the patient completes the pattern by squeezing into MIP. Tooth #28 shown in the lower right pane has an ink mark on its distal-occlusal surface. However, the photograph in the upper right pane shows that tooth #28 does not make any occlusal contact. In this example, the patient's habitual occlusion differs from his skeletal occlusion.

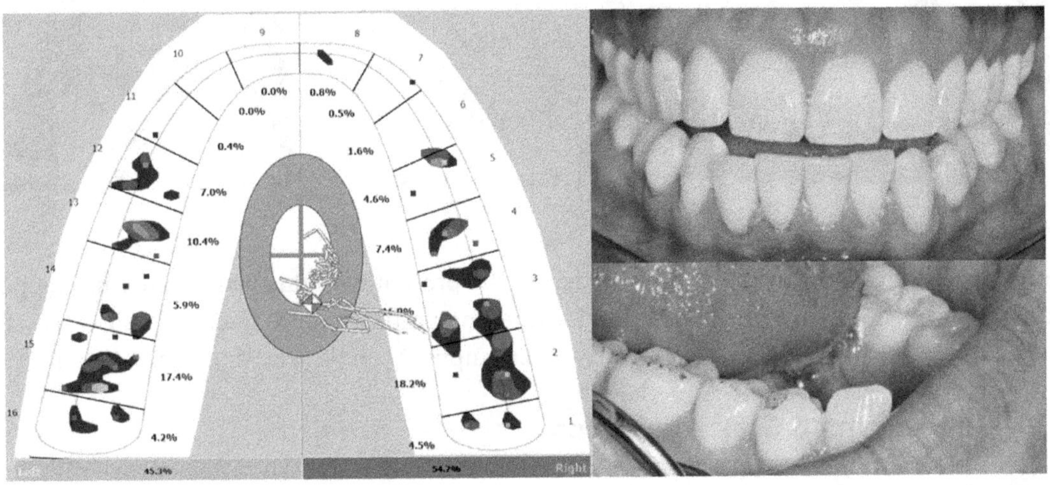

- **Posterior Plane of Occlusion:** Without anterior protection, an occlusal interference is likely present during closure. A narrow maxillary arch is often associated with a dominant lateral force distribution.
- **Mandibular Pathway:** Mandibular motion is altered because the mandible cannot readily engage the maxilla due to occlusal interference and a unilateral force imbalance. Heavy regional force constrains the envelope of function causing the mandible to adapt around, into, or behind the excessive posterior force. This makes closure into balanced intercuspation difficult to achieve. These patients often complain of Cervical Dentin Hypersensitivity.

Clinical Observations: The posterior force alignment affects the anatomy through forced adaptation. Headaches, TMJ strain, sore ligaments, and cervical muscle triggers can be experienced on the same side as the dominating occlusal force. CEJ adaptation within the periodontium and in the cervical regions of teeth is also commonly seen with this pattern. Over the years, it has been observed by the author that twenty-five percent (25%) of patients present with a Pattern #2 force distribution.

Force Cycle Pattern #3: The Anterior Dominant Pattern

Figures 55 and 56 detail force cycle pattern #3. Figure 55 is an example of a deep overbite patient presenting with excessive anterior force and minimal posterior contact. Note how the first five "taps" are concentrated between teeth #s5 and 8, before the COF icon moves left posteriorly when the patient squeezes into MIP. In this example, the front teeth control the mandible's closure and receive excessive

Figure 54. Three middle posterior force patterns, two with a left dominant distribution of force contact (outside panes), and one with a right dominant force distribution (middle pane). Note that the COF icon rests close to the border of the target's white zone as the mandible seeks equilibrium when the patient squeezes into MIP. However, the repeating "tap-taps" show force distribution that is dominated by a lateral interference preventing simultaneous bilateral closure.

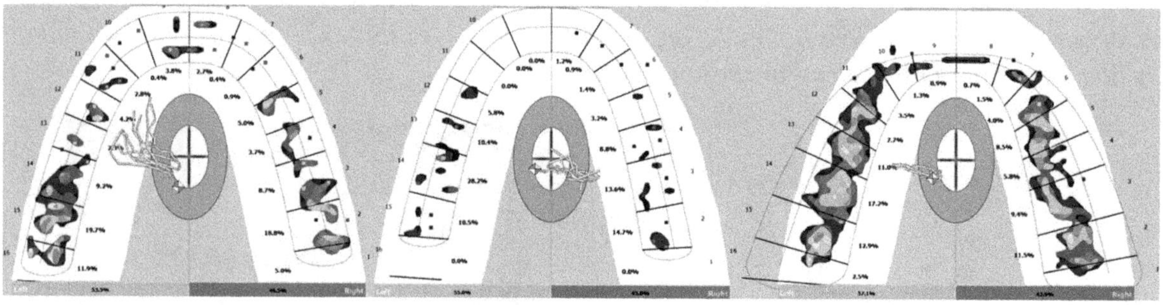

force with every occlusal engagement. Most patients who present with this pattern are missing posterior teeth. A maxillary denture opposing a mandibular free-end partial denture (Kennedy Class I) will often present with this pattern. The lack of posterior vertical support can destroy the anterior teeth over time.

Force Cycle Pattern #3 Characteristics

- **Head and Neck Posture:** Cervical strain and temporal headaches are common when the anterior segment forces the mandible backwards, and jams the condyles in a posterior position within the glenoid fossa. Figure 55 is a good example of posterior condylar displacement.

Figure 55. Here is an example of a deep overbite patient presenting with excessive anterior force and minimal posterior contact. The first five "taps" are concentrated right-anteriorly before the COF moves left posteriorly at MIP. The front teeth control the mandible's closure and receive excessive force with every envelope of function engagement. The lack of posterior vertical stops combined with the deep overbite can force the condyles posteriorly, exacerbating pain in the ears.

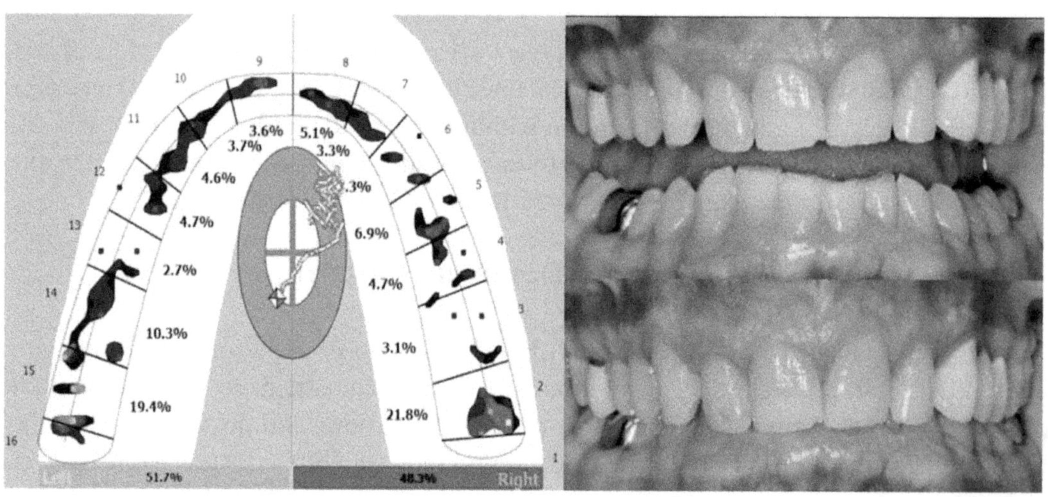

- **Condylar Orientation:** The lack of significant posterior occlusal support in some patients allows the condyles to find the center of the glenoid. In other cases, the condyles are forced backwards because of restriction within the envelopes of motion and function.
- **Anterior Orientation:** The anterior segment is dominating the occlusal function in every mandibular movement causing either excessive wear, increased mobility, or damage to the anterior tooth structure.
- **Posterior Plane of Occlusion:** Most anterior force pattern patients have no occlusal interferences present because either the posterior teeth are missing, or the posterior vertical stops are not readily engaged.
- **Mandibular Pathway:** Mandibular motion is dominated by anteriorly-controlled occlusal function. The anterior segment assumes most of the force which promotes incisal edge wear, increased CEJ stress, and soft tissue recession. Occlusions without posterior support in MIP can be very destructive of the anterior anatomy.

Clinical Observations: The extra force on the anterior segment can have an effect similar to that of a deprogramming splint. No posterior contact implies that there is no occlusal interference, so the condyles seat firmly in the glenoid fossae minimizing muscle triggers on the neck and around the TM joints. The lack of posterior contact will accelerate anterior wear, or force the mandible into a retruded position in MIP. Retruded mandibular pathways can create muscle pain and limit the envelope of motion. One must better balance the anterior guidance with the condylar guidance when posterior vertical stops are absent.

Force Cycle Pattern #4: The Centered-Within-the-COF-Target Pattern

Figures 57 and 58 detail force cycle pattern #4. This centered force pattern lies in the ideal position with respect to a positive force distribution and ideal occlusal force characteristics. It is extremely rare to keep a lifelong perfect occlusion/disocclusion pattern, or occlusion with a balanced MIP landing. Young patients who present with balanced occlusion and centered HFDPs and SFDPs are more common, but as an adult, they will generally change into a posteriorly dominated force pattern. The majority of adult

Figure 56. Three anterior dominant force patterns, where the COF trajectory lines stay anterior to the final COF location, indicating that the anterior force concentration begins on the anterior teeth, and is more substantive than on the posterior occlusal contacts. Force can be directed posteriorly with each successive "tap" as illustrated in the left pane, or across the anterior teeth as shown in the other two panes.

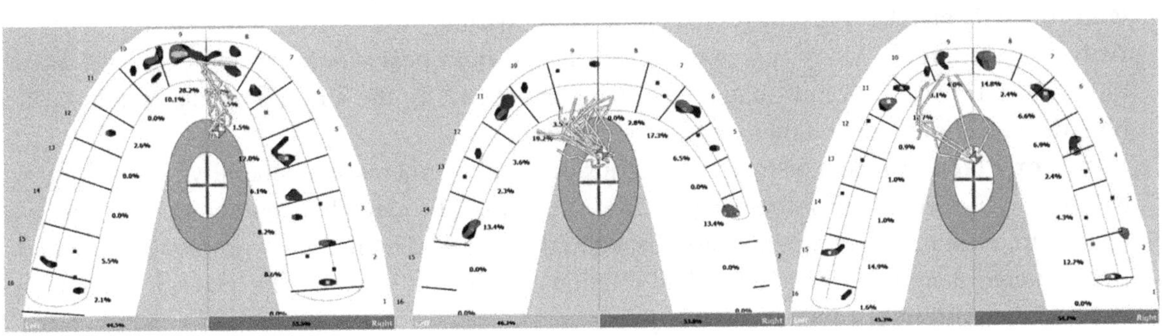

Figure 57. This example of a centered pattern contains an unbalanced posterior force distribution. Opposing teeth #s14 and 19 receive 27.7% of the total occlusal force while the implant crown in the #20 site is not loaded. A centered force pattern can result when excessive force concentration exists in a small region of the arch (teeth #s14 and 19), that is offset and equaled by most or all of the teeth on the opposite arch half. The natural dentition in the photographs is worn both anteriorly and posteriorly, yet the adapted occlusion has produced a centered force distribution pattern.

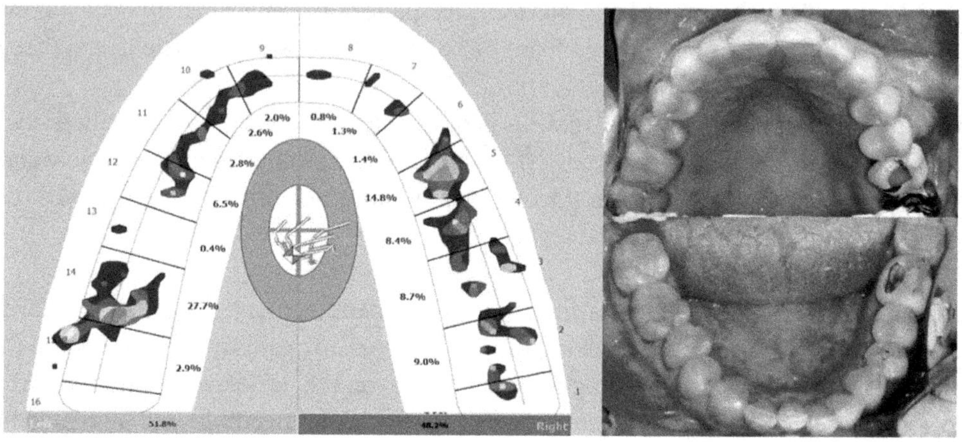

centered patterns either result from excellent dental treatment, a worn dentition, or an adapted mandibular pathway that is seeking equilibrium.

Figure 57 is an example of a centered force pattern where excessive force concentration in a small region of the arch is offset and equaled by the many teeth that have worn down through years of function. An implant crown on tooth #20 receives 0.4% total force while the root-canalled and crowned teeth #s14 and 19 receive 27.7% of the total occlusal force. The force pattern is centered, but the force distribution is not balanced on either side of the arch. Most centered patterns observed in a middle-aged adult are the result of “retrofit” dental procedures and adapted oral anatomy.

Force Cycle Pattern #4 Characteristics

- **Head and Neck Posture:** A mandible in harmony with the cranium during function can only help idealize the position of the occipital condyles.
- **Condylar Orientation:** This type of HFDP and SFDP pattern is usually indicative of good condylar health and range of motion. However, patients with an adaptive centered pattern can present with stressed condyles and a restricted envelope of motion.
- **Anterior Guidance:** Many centered patterns reveal both posterior wear and excessive anterior tooth wear. However, in most patients with a centered COF, the anterior guidance is protecting both the posterior teeth and the condylar orientation.
- **Posterior Plane of Occlusion:** The posterior occlusal segments are generally in harmony with each other, especially when the occlusal force mapping of the teeth is symmetrical in shape and demonstrates similar contact intensity throughout the arch. The potential problem with an adaptive centered pattern is the codependent relationship of posture, condylar position, and anterior wear on the posterior occlusion.

Figure 58. Three centered-within-the-COF-target force patterns; two with definitive anterior contact (outside panes). and one with slight anterior occlusal contact and significant bilateral posterior occlusal contact force (middle pane). Note that the COF icon rests within the COF target, but not always in the exact middle.

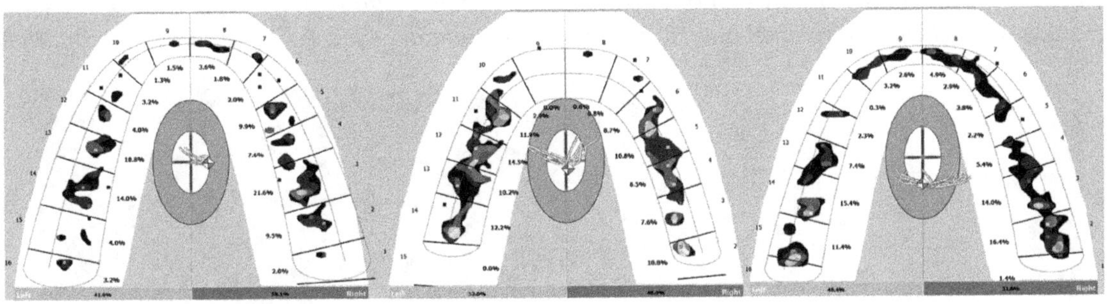

- **Mandibular Pathway:** Most patients with a centered HFDP and/or SFDP demonstrate unrestricted envelopes of motion. The envelope of function distributes force bilaterally in patients with a balanced and centered HFDP and/or SFDP.

Clinical Observations: The natural aging process creates multiple effects that result from this pattern. The mandible will seek equilibrium over time and may present with a centered pattern HFDP, even if some or all of the oral anatomy is stressed from isolated areas of excessive force concentration. It should be noted that a centered HFDP does not mean there will also be a centered SFDP, because posture of the head and neck can cause the COF icon to move out of the COF target. The "ideal" center of force distribution is rare in that only 20% of patients (mostly young) have been observed by the author to present with a centered pattern. These patients that do have a centered pattern are often able to maintain a healthy occlusion that demonstrates minimal structural adaptation.

Force Cycle Pattern #5: The Anterior Open Occlusion Pattern

Figures 59 - 61 detail force cycle pattern #5. Figure 59 illustrates the growth pattern of a natural anterior open occlusion. Myofunctionally, the anterior control in the open occlusion patient can be the tongue, which fills the open anterior space to skeletally interfere with the both the development of the arches and the anterior tooth intercuspation. In function, the anterior segment cannot protect the posterior teeth, while the unbalanced posterior excessive force concentration alters the condylar position, thereby inducing structural adaptation of the disc assembly. This can lead to the development of detectable joint vibrations.

Every anterior deprogramming splint has the possibility of changing the pathway of the mandible because the condyle position in the glenoid fossa is altered when the posterior teeth are separated. As is evidenced in Figure 60, an occlusal change can occur when using an NTI appliance that decreases the frequency and intensity of headaches. DOFDPs can document the "before" and "after" force profile of any occlusal splint that alters the position of the mandible relative to the maxilla.

Figure 59. A natural anterior open occlusion where the arches are narrow, the palate is vaulted, and the limited tongue space prevents the anterior teeth from coupling. The tongue fills the open anterior space to skeletally interfere with both the development of the arches and the anterior tooth intercuspation. Only the posterior teeth generate occlusal force. Without anterior protection, the excessive force concentration on the left alters the condylar position. The T-Scan data could be interpreted as a distal posterior pattern #1 but the natural anterior open occlusion makes it a #5 skeletal occlusal pattern.

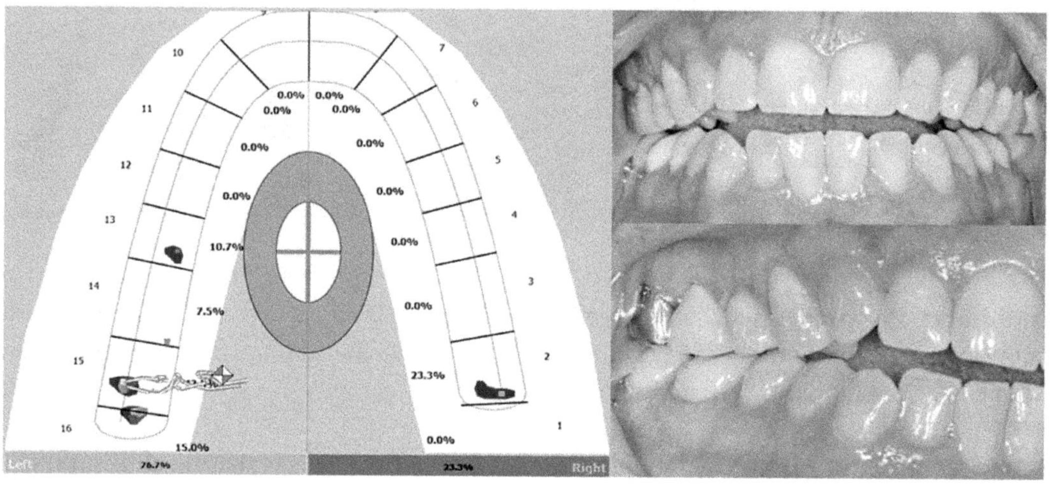

Figure 60. This is an example of a patient who has two bites. The top right photograph shows the habitual occlusion in the "teeth together" position. The force scan on the left is the HFDP of the occlusion seen in the upper right photograph. The lower right photograph shows the occlusal position of the mandible when in the seated condylar position. The T-Scan illustrates the force distribution of the habitual occlusion when the majority of teeth are in contact. However, the skeletal force pattern (SFDP) would appear very different because only the two second molars would be in contact. This would suggest the possibility of this patient exhibiting a skeletal asymmetry.

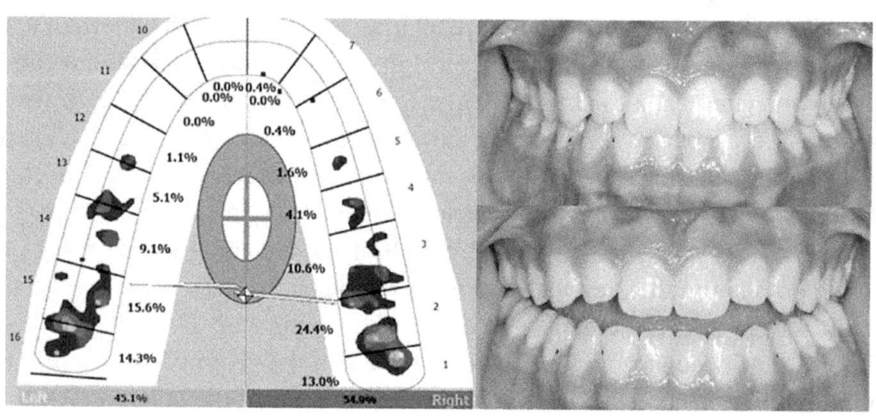

Force Cycle Pattern #5 Characteristics

- **Head and Neck Posture:** This pattern always presents a skeletal concern. Chronic forward head posture creates cervical stress, and limits the lateral movement of the atlas.
- **Condylar Orientation:** The force on both condyle heads is directed upward and backward. During growth, early myofunctional habits can create asymmetries between the glenoid fossa, the condyles, the ramus height, and the maxillomandibular orientation.
- **Anterior Guidance:** The only anterior control is exerted by the tongue, which occurs at rest and during swallowing. Its presence within the open occlusion space prevents tooth eruption.
- **Posterior Plane of Occlusion:** Dominated by the second molars in every movement. The shape of the mandibular angle is obtuse which prevents contact of the anterior teeth.
- **Mandibular Pathway:** Patients mostly exhibit vertical mandibular motion. Lateral movements of the mandible are limited because of the bilateral posterior group function and lack of anterior guidance. The neck posture can limit and narrow Posselt's envelope. Some patients function asymptomatically despite the lack of anterior occlusal contact, but many open occlusion patients suffer significant myogenous symptomatology.

Clinical Observations: These patients are very prone to migraine-type headaches, cervical stress, and non-physiologic adaptive condylar structural changes. Patients often have prior ear, nose, and throat conditions, can exhibit myofunctional tongue habits, and demonstrate forward head posture. Only a few teeth receive force during function and the anterior control is always a posterior tooth, when the tongue is not positioned over the teeth.

Force Cycle Pattern #6: The Anteroposterior or Posteroanterior Pattern

Figures 62 and 63 detail force cycle pattern #6. An anteroposterior pattern behaves like the anterior dominated force pattern. Alternatively, the posteroanterior pattern behaves like a posterior dominated force pattern. Figure 62 is an example of a middle-aged patient's posteroanterior pattern. During the closure into intercuspation, the COF starts in the posterior right quadrant and moves anteriorly when the mandible is squeezed into MIP. This mandibular pathway has to wedge into the plane occlusion because all of the dental restorations do not provide a balanced force landing.

Figure 61. Three anterior open occlusion patterns. Note the far posterior position of the COF in all patterns, and the horizontal nature of the force transmission exhibited in the trajectory lines.

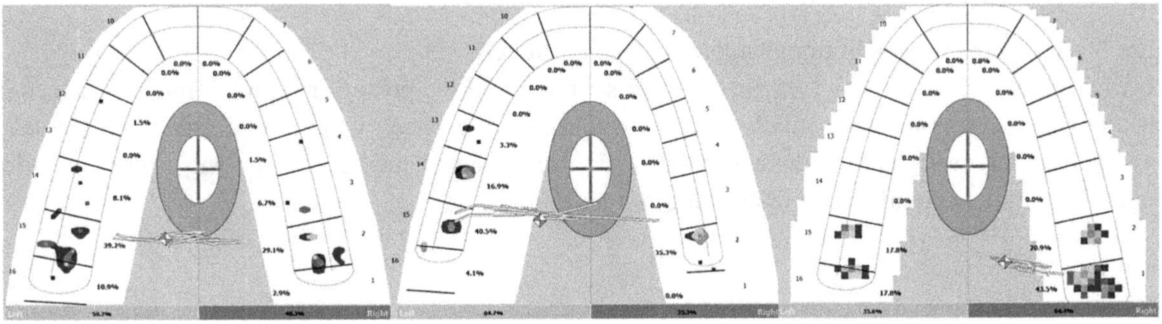

Figure 62. A posteroanterior pattern where the closure COF begins in the posterior right quadrant because an early contact present on tooth #3's, gold crown. The COF later moves left-anteriorly, away from the interference on tooth #3,when the anterior teeth and the left side Nesbit partial denture begins to make occlusal contact. Note that the denture tooth #13 has been worn out of contact, as it receives only 1.2% of the total force. Alternatively, its neighboring natural tooth #14, comprises nearly half the force percentage of the left side (21.0% of the 44.7% total left side occlusal force).

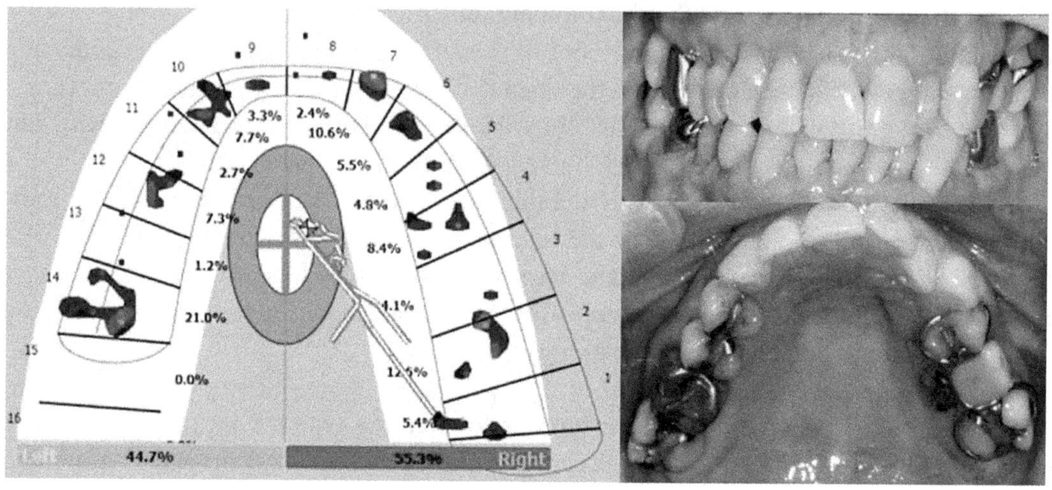

Force Cycle Pattern #6 Characteristics

- **Head and Neck Posture:** The Temporomandibular condyles and the occipital condyles will change position over the years to accommodate the anteroposterior or posteroanterior force transmission.
- **Condylar Orientation:** The anteroposterior force can routinely stress the condylar position within the glenoid fossa. Posterior interference prevents the condyles from achieving a fully seated position in function.
- **Anterior Orientation:** With the anteroposterior force transmission, the anterior guidance can show signs of stress because the posterior occlusal support is somewhat compromised.
- **Posterior Plane of Occlusion:** The posteroanterior force produces long-term stress, in and around the posterior teeth because those teeth are constantly early in the closure contact cycle.
- **Mandibular Pathway:** Often the patient will attempt to adapt forward, to escape a posterior occlusal interference, only to run into an anterior one, or vice-versa. Many of these patients exhibit tight muscles, tender condyles, and off-centered head posture.

Figure 63 illustrates three additional anteroposterior patterns.

Clinical Observations: Any time the anterior segment and the posterior segment must work against each other, one component will likely lose, depending on the zone of force predominance. However, many equilibrated cases have a centered pattern (Figure 63, left pane), demonstrating a long occluding line into MIP and an equally long disoccluding line out of MIP.

Figure 63. Three anteroposterior patterns. The first two patterns (left and middle panes) exhibit fairly reasonable balance and good COF trajectory and icon positioning. The third pattern (right pane) demonstrates very poor COF trajectory and icon positioning because of a severe occlusal force imbalance present on the left side, between the opposing left canines and the opposing left first molars.

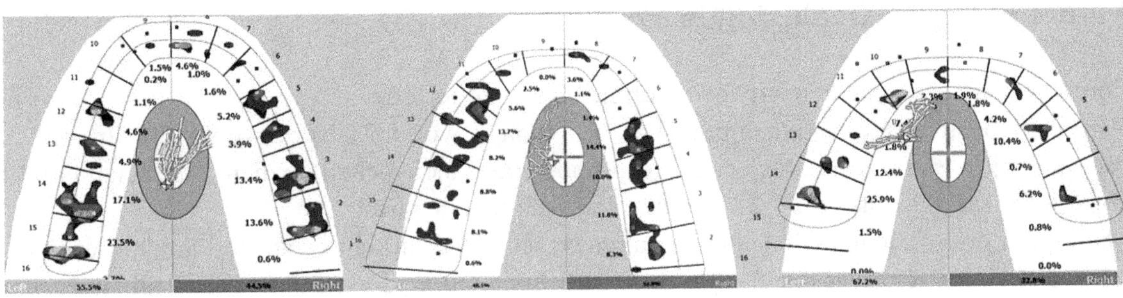

SOLUTIONS AND RECOMMENDATIONS

The Solution is to Measure

A technology that leads to a more accurate diagnosis which is obtained in less clinical time, should become readily accepted by the dental profession. Articulating paper has value but digital occlusal contact force movies measure occlusal forces sequenced in motion, dynamically. The paradigm shift requires the clinician to view the T-Scan recording sensor as "smart" articulating paper that presents to the clinician digital force and time data. Any condyle-directed, muscle-directed, or habitual pathway of occlusal engagement can be recorded as a force cycle. This data offers insights into the occlusal force distribution that cannot be obtained with traditional occlusal indicators. It is therefore essential in the diagnosis and treatment of occlusal dysfunction.

It is highly practical to use the T-Scan technology when educating patients, when making a diagnosis, and when performing occlusal treatment. It is clinically prudent to add the recording of force scans to the customary radiographic and diagnostic procedures performed at the time of a clinical examination. Combining force scan data with clinical photographs that show anatomic occlusal force structural adaptation, such as in abfraction formation, gingival recession, and occlusal wear, often explains why the structural adaptation and/or damage has occurred.

The concept of *Occlusion Confusion* has arisen because there are many different occlusal philosophies advocated, therefore there are many different interpretations of what the word "occlusion" actually describes. Confusion should be of concern to the profession because it indicates that Dental Medicine continues to struggle to uncover the etiologic puzzle of occlusal development, dysfunction, and adaptation.

Clarity to occlusion confusion is available to the clinician who employs the T-Scan technology in daily practice. The digital data helps the clinician to see occlusion as "a simple act or process", where the masticatory muscles transfer energy onto the natural teeth (with or without prosthetic alteration) and their supporting tissues. This energy conduction, which occurs when two objects engage, repeatedly occurs with each swallow and functional mandibular movement the patient makes. Alternately, disocclusion (disclusion) is the separation of the teeth by exiting the intercuspated contact position, which reverses the energy conduction off of the teeth and the supporting structures. Force cycle conduction and release cannot be measured with conventional articulating paper. In fact, the Subjective Interpretation of an articulating paper mark is nothing more than a clinician's guess at its force content (Kerstein & Radke, 2013). Therefore, it is the author's recommendation that occlusal function should be measured with the T-Scan technology to improve the Standard of patient care that the field of Occlusion currently accepts.

The Future of Digital Occlusion is Now

- Computers are available in nearly every clinician's operatories.
- Digital applications (Apps) are commonplace in today's world. They are wholly user-friendly.
- Patients enjoy visual technologies, and can understand their benefits when a clinician employs objective measurements with which to make an accurate diagnosis.
- The digital era of Dental Medicine has already generated an unprecedented amount of data in many differing disciplines that has yet to be fully explored, understood, and clinically integrated.
- Articulating paper has definite value, but it has yet to solve the "occlusion confusion" puzzle.
- T-Scan sensors provide a new paradigm that includes objective force and timing data that describes every contact point, in both sequence and duration.
- The present day T-Scan gives the clinician the capability to measure, record, study, and better treat the effects that poor occlusal force distribution has on both younger and older populations, over the long-term. This insight may help prevent significant adaptive structural breakdown of the differing components of the Stomatognathic system.

FUTURE RESEARCH DIRECTION

Force measurement is a relatively new metric that translates mandibular engagement into objective force and timing data. Using force intensity, duration, and distribution, as metrics to measure the occlusal scheme represents a new paradigm for Dentistry. Force reproduction of the T-Scan system has been shown to be highly reproducible (Kerstein, Lowe, Harty, & Radke, 2006; Koos, Godt, Schille, & Goz, 2010), thereby proving the usefulness of this technology. However, although DOFDPs have been observed over the past 15 years to provide accurate occlusal force data that can be repeatedly evaluated over time, they lack formal research that validates force distribution patterns as a scientifically useful clinical measurement.

Three possible future research directions that could potentially study DOFDP data sets are:

- Growth and development related to the evolution of DOFDPs.
- The relationship between the atlas orthogonal joint and maxilla-to-mandible engagement.
- Headache etiology associated with a "measured", unbalanced occlusion.

Growth, Development, and the Evolution of DOFDPs

Force patterns evolve during the transition from a deciduous to an adult dentition. This evolution has not been studied. Van der Linden stated in 1989 that the occlusal morphology of the posterior teeth is not to achieve better chewing, but instead to secure a positive guiding role in facial growth (Van der Linden, 1989). Because myofunctional habits, airway development, and the directional growth of the cranial base influence the mandible's pathway, a study could be designed to determine if force distribution patterns taken at a young age could predict the symmetry, or lack thereof, of future cranial skeletal growth.

Cranial Posture and Mandibular Engagement

The muscles of mastication act as antagonists to the suprahyoids and infrahyoids, and promote balance for the cranium. If the tension in the muscles of mastication is greater than the tension in the hyoids, then the head will be displaced backward. In the reverse case, the head will posture forward. Moreover, if the tension in the muscles of mastication is unequal from one side of the head to the other, the axis will rotate, while differences in the horizontal level of one condyle to the other may induce the body posture to adapt to properly support the head.

These postural alterations resultant from muscular imbalances can influence the two "bites," each patient can demonstrate (the habitual occlusion, and its skeletal variation). The mandible's skeletal approach (as determined by a SFDP) may be the primary favored pathway for some individuals, whereas the habitual engagement (as determined by an HFDP) may function better for others. A study could compare the HFDP and the SFDP to the orientation of axial complex, to assess whether cranial posture plays a role in the development of occlusal dysfunction. The results of this type of study have potential treatment implications for clinicians who diagnose problems with the atlas orthogonal joint.

DOFDPs and Headaches

The headache associated with Temporomandibular disorders is listed by the International Headache Society under classification 2, as "tension-type headache". This type of headache appears to be linked to parafunctional activity, intermittent TM joint clicking, masticatory muscle tenderness, a reduced envelope of motion, and force cycle patterns demonstrating excessive posterior occlusal force distribution. These observed associations between mandibular function and tension-type headache requires additional research to determine causation. A study could be designed to determine if certain DOFDPs were consistently observed in the tension-type headache patient. The results could potentially elucidate that one or more specific DOFDPs would be a diagnostic predictor of headaches that are causally related to mandibular function.

Should the findings of the above suggested studies prove to be clinically relevant, when combined with the potential results of the many other suggested studies presented in the other chapters contained within this book, they would help usher in an age in Dental Medicine where increased use of digital occlusal technology becomes commonplace.

CONCLUSION

Occlusal concepts rest on architectural and engineering principles, while using articulating paper as the standard to describe the integrated stop position of mandibular engagement lacks any true measurement. All philosophies of occlusion strive to develop a system in which the anatomy of the teeth, the Temporomandibular joints, the neurologic circuitry, the associated ligaments, the masticatory muscles, and the boney arches, all function in health and harmony. These structures are all governed by the proprioceptive receptors within the Stomatognathic system which maintain both homeostasis and function.

As such, adaptation to the applied pressure from occlusal loading influences everything that is biologic within the system.

The idea to record and display occlusal contact force and timing on a video screen in the early 1980s was revolutionary. The development of the T-Scan system back then has made it possible today for every dentist to benefit from learning to use the newest T-Scan version. Modern studies clearly illustrate that the clinical interpretation of ink marking is a highly compromised procedure lacking clinician accuracy, despite the technique being advocated in textbooks, dental schools, and in professional continuing education programs. The quality of a mark is dependent on a dry field, and on the incorrect assumption that natural teeth, gold, non-precious metals, plastic, porcelain, composites, and zirconium will all imprint exactly the same force. Additionally, the dark and wet oral environment makes subjective paper mark interpretation a visually difficult clinical task.

Systems function in a designed way, and yet dysfunction may stress a system in any number of ways. Digital diagnostic procedures are available to oral physicians who wish to provide functional harmony to the Stomatognathic system. Mandibular engagement with the occlusal plane is a repeating event, where problematic occlusal contact may occur during sleep, chewing, swallowing, and exercising. DOFDPs predictably find existing microtrauma. DOFDPs help manage this microtraumic force engagement by providing crucial information to enhance the reliability of the occlusal diagnosis, while also ensuring and monitoring the long-term success of any applied treatments. Despite that some systems will be able to adapt to the repetitive microtrauma, most patients will require help finding functional harmony through improvements that alter any pathologic, repetitive force distribution.

Force scans isolate things that Dental Medicine has not seen before, which have created diagnostic and treatment opportunities that could never be possible with analog articulating paper. Ultimately, the effectiveness of any procedure is only as good as the tools used to measure and verify the results. In this digital era of Dental Medicine, the T-Scan system is a far superior tool for clinicians to employ compared to dental articulating paper. As such, studying Digital Occlusal Force Distribution Patterns (DOFDPs) with the T-Scan technology, offers Dental Medicine a major advance in the quality of occlusal care that is now available to the modern dental patient.

REFERENCES

Academy of Prosthodontics. (2005). The Glossary of Prosthodontic Terms. *The Journal of Prosthetic Dentistry*, *94*(1), 10–92. doi:10.1016/j.prosdent.2005.03.013 PMID:16080238

Bader, J. D., Shugars, D. A., & Sturdevant, J. R. (2004). Consequences of posterior cusp fracture. *General Dentistry*, *52*(2), 128–131. PMID:15101306

Carey, J., Craig, M., Kerstein, R. B., & Radke, J. (2007). Determining a relationship between applied occlusal load and articulation paper mark area. *Open Dentistry Journal*, *1*(1), 1–7. doi:10.2174/1874210600701010001 PMID:19088874

Carlson, J. E. (2003). *Orthocranial Occlusion*. Woodinville, WA: Blue Pine Unlimited.

Cuccia, A., & Caradonna, C. (2009). The relationship between the Stomatognathic system and body posture. *Clinics (Sao Paulo)*, *64*(1), 61–66. doi:10.1590/S1807-59322009000100011 PMID:19142553

Dawson, P. E. (1989). *Evaluation, Diagnosis, and Treatment of Occlusal Problems* (2nd ed.). St. Louis, MO: CV Mosby Co.

Dawson, P. E. (2007). Functional Occlusion: From TMJ to Smile Design. St. Louis, MO: Mosby Elsevier.

Droter, J. R. (2005). An orthopaedic approach to the diagnosis and treatment of disorders of the Temporomandibular joint. *Dentistry Today*, *31*(10), 82–88. PMID:16358802

Dylina, T. J. (2001). A common sense approach to splint therapy. *The Journal of Prosthetic Dentistry*, *86*(5), 539–545. doi:10.1067/mpr.2001.118878 PMID:11725283

Dylina, T. J. (2001). The basics of occlusal splint therapy. *Dentistry Today*, *21*(7), 82–87. PMID:12242839

Enlow, D. H. (1990). Facial Growth (3rd ed.). Philadelphia, PA: W B Saunders Co.

Kerstein, R. B. (1994). Disclusion Time measurement studies: Stability of Disclusion Time. A one-year follow-up study. *The Journal of Prosthetic Dentistry*, *72*(2), 164–168. doi:10.1016/0022-3913(94)90075-2 PMID:7932263

Kerstein, R. B. (2004). Combining technologies: A computerized occlusal analysis system synchronized with a computerized electromyography system. *The Journal of Cranio-Mandibular Practice*, *22*(2), 96–109. doi:10.1179/crn.2004.013 PMID:15134409

Kerstein, R. B. (2010). Reducing chronic masseter and temporalis muscular hyperactivity with computer-guided occlusal adjustments. *Compendium of Continuing Education*, *31*(7), 530–543. PMID:20879206

Kerstein, R. B., Lowe, M., Harty, M., & Radke, J. (2006). A force reproduction analysis of two recording sensors of a computerized occlusal analysis system. *The Journal of Cranio-Mandibular Practice*, *24*(1), 15–24. PMID:16541841

Kerstein, R. B., & Radke, J. (2013). Clinician accuracy when subjectively interpreting articulating paper markings. *The Journal of Craniomandibular & Sleep Practice*, *32*(1), 13–23. PMID:24660642

Kerstein, R. B., & Wright, N. (1991). An electromyographic and computer analysis of patients suffering from chronic myofascial pain-dysfunction syndrome; pre and post-treatment with Immediate Complete Anterior Guidance Development. *The Journal of Prosthetic Dentistry*, *66*(5), 677–686. doi:10.1016/0022-3913(91)90453-4 PMID:1805009

Koos, B., Godt, A., Schille, C., & Göz, G. (2010). Precision of an instrumentation-based method of analyzing occlusion and its resulting distribution of forces in the dental arch. *Journal of Orofacial Orthopedics*, *71*(6), 403–410. doi:10.1007/s00056-010-1023-7 PMID:21082303

Lerman, M. (2011). The muscle engram: The reflex that limits conventional occlusal treatment. *The Journal of Cranio-Mandibular Practice*, *29*(4), 297–303. PMID:22128670

Maness, W. L., Benjamin, M., Podoloff, R., Bobick, A., & Golden, R. F. (1987). Computerized occlusal analysis: A new technology. *The Journal of Practical Dentistry*, *18*(4), 287–292. PMID:3472263

Maness, W. L., & Podoloff, R. (1989). Distribution of occlusal contacts in maximum intercuspation. *The Journal of Prosthetic Dentistry*, *62*(2), 238–242. doi:10.1016/0022-3913(89)90321-1 PMID:2760866

Novak, J. (2006). *Posture, Get it Straight!* (2nd ed.). Andover, MN: Expert Publishing, Inc.

Qadeer, S., Kerstein, R., Kim, R. J., Huh, J. B., & Shin, S. W. (2012). Relationship between articulation paper mark size and percentage of force measured with computerized occlusal analysis. *Journal of Advanced Prosthodontics*, *4*(1), 7–12. doi:10.4047/jap.2012.4.1.7 PMID:22439094

Rufenacht, C. R. (2000). *Principles of Esthetic Integration*. Carol Stream, IL: Quintessence Publishing Co., Inc.

Saad, M. N., Weiner, G., Ehrenberg, D., & Weiner, S. (2008). Effects oflLoad and indicator type upon occlusal contact markings. *Journal of Biomedical Materials Research. Part B, Applied Biomaterials*, *85*(1), 18–22. doi:10.1002/jbm.b.30910 PMID:17618516

Spee, F. G. (1890). Die Verschiebrangsbahn des Unterkiefers am Schadell. *Archiv für Anatomie und Physiologie*, *16*, 285–294.

Storey, A. T. (1979). Controversies related to temporomandibular joint function and dysfunction. In P. Dawson (Ed.), *Evaluation, Diagnosis, and Treatment of Occlusal Problems* (2nd ed., p. 15). St. Louis, MO: The C.V. Mosby Company.

Van der Linden, F. P. G. M. (1986). *Facial Growth and Facial Orthopedics*. Chicago, IL: Quintessence Publishing Co., Ltd.

Plane. (2014). In *Wikipediathe Free Encyclopedia*. Retrieved April 22, 2014, from http://en.wikipedia.org/wiki/Plane

Wilson, G. H. (1911). A Manual of Dental Prosthetics. *The Journal of Prosthetic Dentistry*, *94*(1), 28–29.

ADDITIONAL READING

Carlson, J. E. (2004). *Occlusal Diagnosis*. Wiltshire, UK: Midwest Publications.

Dos Santos, J. Jr. (2007). *Occlusion: Principles & Treatment*. Hanover Park, IL: Quintessence Publishing Co., Inc.

Egoscue, P., & Gittines, R. (1993). *The Egoscue Method of Health Through Motion: Revolutionary Program That Lets You Rediscover the Body's Power to Rejuvenate It*. New York, NY: Harper Collins Publishers, Inc.

Lundeen, H. C., & Gibbs, C. H. (2005). *The Function of Teeth: the Physiology of Mandibular Function Related to Occlusal Form and Esthetics*. Gainesville, FL: L and G Publishers, LLC.

McCoy, G. (2001). *On the Demise of Occlusion*. San Francisco, CA: Self-published.

McCoy, G. (2007). Dental Compression Syndrome and TMD: Examining the Relationship. *Dentistry Today*, *26*(7), 118–123. PMID:17708320

McNeill, C. (Ed.). (1997). *Science and Practice of Occlusion*. Carol Stream, IL: Quintessence Publishing Co., Inc.

Miles, T. S., Nauntofte, B., & Svensson, P. (2004). *Clinical oral physiology*. Copenhagen, DK: Quintessence Publishing Co., Inc.

Racich, M. (2010). *The Basic Rules of Oral Rehabilitation*. Markham, ON: Palmeri Publishing, Inc.

Racich, M. (2012). *The Basic Rules of Occlusion*. Markham, ON: Palmeri Publishing, Inc.

Racich, M. (2013). *The Basic Rules of Facially Generated Treatment Planning*. Markham, ON: Palmeri Publishing, Inc.

Rocabado, M., Johnston, B. E. Jr., & Blakney, M. G. (1982). Physical Therapy and Dentistry: An Overview. *The Journal of Cranio-Mandibular Practice*, *1*, 46–49. PMID:6960091

Sakaguchi, K., Mehta, N. R., Abdallah, E. F., Forgione, A. G., Hirayama, H., Kawasaki, T., & Yokoyama, A. (2007). Examination of the relationship between mandibular position and body posture. *The Journal of Cranio-Mandibular Practice*, *25*(4), 237–249. PMID:17983123

Sperber, G. H. (2001). *Craniofacial Development*. Hamilton, ON: BC Decker, Inc.

KEY TERMS AND DEFINITIONS

Anterior Controls: The first points of contact (tooth, teeth, or prosthetic dentistry) anterior to the condyles when the mandible engages the occlusal plane.

Anterior Orientation (The Second Determinant of Occlusion): The front half of the arch should be free of occlusal interference and function in harmony with the envelope of motion.

Condylar Orientation (The First Determinant of Occlusion): Healthy condylar function and posterior force distribution are balanced vertically, horizontally, and transversely.

Digital Occlusion: The applied concept of using digital technology to diagnose and treat the envelope of motion and the envelope of function.

Equilibrium: The Stomatognathic system seeks equilibrium throughout a lifetime of function. Motion in harmony with design provides the best chance for the system to maintain physiologic function. Maintaining or recreating harmony between motion, function, and design over time, is the ultimate goal when seeking equilibrium for Stomatognathic therapy.

Favored Pathway: The mandible has an engrained anatomic envelope of motion that favors a path of least resistance. An unbalanced force distribution in function alters the system's preferred mandibular pathway. The orientation of the mandible's favored pathway is determined by contributory anatomic factors; the head and neck posture, the condylar position, the posterior occlusal plane, and the anterior occlusal plane.

Force Cycle: The occlusal force transfer from the mandible to the maxilla during the entire occlusion-occlude-disocclusion process, which captures the intensity, direction, and sequence of every occlusal contact, and creates a patient's unique force distribution pattern. It can also be described as the summation of all frames of occlusal force that evolve from the first occlusal contact into MIP, until the last contact out of MIP. A force cycle defines the recorded envelope of force that occurs within the envelope of function.

Measure, Predict, and Prevent: Adult force distribution patterns measure resistance to the mandible's favored pathway within the envelope of function. Elevated and prolonged force intensity often can predict the location of where pathology to the system and to the anatomy, will likely evolve. The concept of prevention is to identify and correct pathologic force before destruction occurs.

Occlusal Interference: In analog dentistry, interference is not defined. In digital dentistry, data defines the intensity, duration, and sequence of every contact point. Cusps and grooves that are not in harmony with an efficient envelope of function can now be identified, studied, and corrected.

Occlusion, Occlude, and Disocclusion: The three phases of a force distribution cycle within the mandible's envelope of function during its engagement (occlusion), at stopping time (occlude), and during its release (disocclusion). Each patient "tap" onto a sensor records all three phases.

Plane of Occlusion: The 3-Dimensional occlusal plane is a wave-like shape that is unique to every individual. Force cycle patterns highlight the mandible's challenge in engaging the maxillary occlusal plane efficiently.

This work was previously published in the Handbook of Research on Computerized Occlusal Analysis Technology Applications in Dental Medicine edited by Robert B. Kerstein, DMD, pages 830-904, copyright year 2015 by Medical Information Science Reference (an imprint of IGI Global).

Chapter 2
Periodontal Treatment and Computerized Occlusal Analysis

Nicolas Cohen, DDS, MS, PhD
Private Practice, France & University of Paris, France

ABSTRACT

This chapter addresses the ongoing controversy regarding occlusion's role in the progression of periodontal disease. Occlusal force has been considered a non-factor in the initiation of periodontal attachment loss. However, the absence of a validated measuring device or quantifying method for analyzing the occlusion has contributed to the confusion that still exists in the scientific community today about the relationship between periodontal disease and occlusion. The development of the T-Scan occlusal measurement technology, which is independent of a clinician's occlusal contact force level subjective assessment, may change the scientific opinion about occlusion's role in periodontal disease. This chapter illustrates how the T-Scan 8 system aids in treating patients who have tissue loss and occlusal issues. Notably, after the major etiologic risk factors of periodontal disease have been controlled, adjusting the occlusion with the T-Scan improves healing outcomes resulting in less inflammation, decreased probing depths, and bone level stability.

INTRODUCTION

The Periodontium is characterized by several tissues:

- Soft tissues such as the keratinized gingiva,
- The free gingiva,
- The periodontal ligament (PDL),
- The hard tissues around the teeth such as bone and cementum.

Periodontal diseases are multifactorial and considered to be of host deficiency origin, which are characterized by the presence of gingival pockets and progressive loss of attachment, with bone resorption occurring around teeth. It is possible to ensure the periodontal health of the patient by keeping these

DOI: 10.4018/978-1-5225-1903-4.ch002

pockets shallow. Clinicians are therefore perpetually faced with the need for probing pocket depths of any detected periodontal pockets.

Clinicians also check for two groups of potential Periodontal disease risk factors, which include:

- Innate human factors (age, sex, ethnicity, genetic predisposition).
- Acquired factors (microbiological factors, smoking, and other systemic disease states).

The link between occlusion and impaired periodontal health has always been a matter of great debate (Green & Levine, 1996). However, occlusion is not generally considered to be a risk factor for periodontal disease, but is rather viewed as an aggravating factor, in the same was as is tobacco use. Despite that in everyday practice, clinicians observe obvious links between occlusion and periodontal parameters, the absence of an "evidence based" occlusal force analysis makes difficult the demonstration of these interrelationships. The T-Scan 8 system (Tekscan, Inc., S. Boston, MA, USA), could help to address unanswered questions. The aim of this chapter is to review how computerized occlusal analysis can be integrated into periodontal practice, and how it can greatly aid the clinician in the treatment of Periodontal Disease.

BACKGROUND

Interrelations between periodontal disease and occlusal forces have been usually defined by the term *Occlusal Trauma*. Stillman was the first to define occlusal trauma, as a traumatic state of the tissues supporting the teeth resulting from the movement of the jaws towards the closed position (Stillman, 1917). In 1978, the World Health Organization (WHO) defined occlusal trauma as a periodontal traumatism caused by stress on the teeth induced directly or indirectly by contacting the teeth present in the other arch (Lindhe, Karring, & Lang, 2008). The American Academy of Periodontology (AAP) defined occlusal trauma as damage to the dental support tissues caused by an excessive occlusal load (Gher, 1996).

There are 2 classifications of periodontal damage resultant from occlusal trauma:

- **Primary:** Primary trauma affects teeth with normal periodontal tissue height (Figure 1).
- **Secondary:** Secondary trauma affects teeth with reduced periodontal tissue height (Figure 2).

With patients who demonstrate the differing periodontal risk factors, secondary occlusal trauma makes treatment more difficult because the compromised teeth are often embedded in a damaged periodontium. When force is applied to the crown of a tooth that has reduced tissue support, the tooth's center of rotation translates more apically, which creates a major lever-arm resultant from the occlusal loading (Figure 2).

Definition of Occlusal Trauma

Occlusal trauma is the term used to describe changes in periodontal state due to the applied force of the masticatory muscles (Sanz, 2005).

When evaluating occlusal trauma on a patient, a number of clinical and radiographic signs and symptoms may be present (Hallmon, 1999; Parameter on occlusal traumatism in patients with chronic periodontitis. American Academy of Periodontology, 2000).

Figure 1. Primary occlusal trauma results from excessive occlusal force with normal support. The center of rotation is near the middle of the tooth.

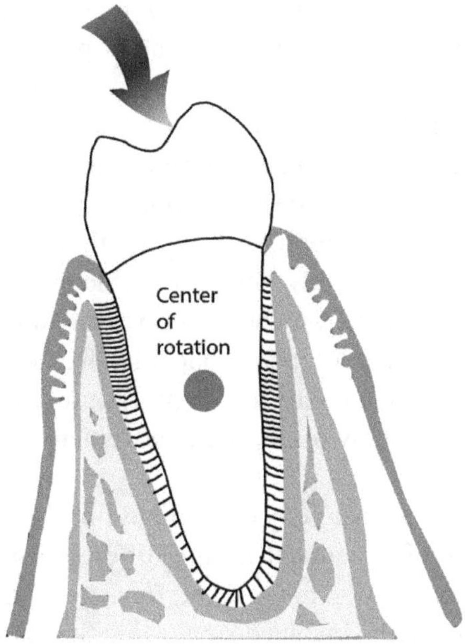

Figure 2. Secondary occlusal trauma results when excessive occlusal force is applied to a tooth with reduced support. The center of rotation moves down into the apical third of the root.

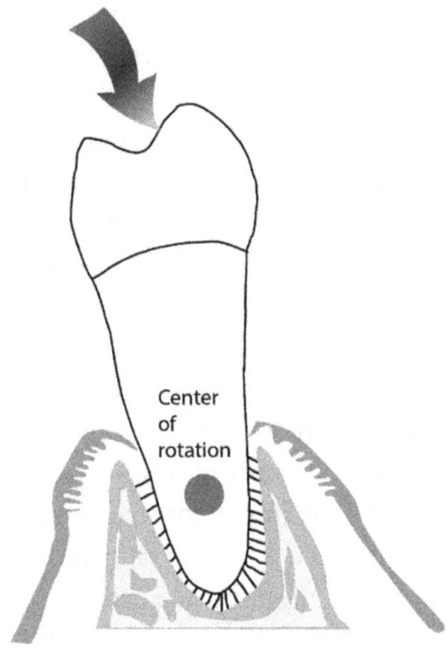

The Clinical Signs and Symptoms of Occlusal Trauma

- Occlusal prematurities and tooth contact discrepancies.
- Pain on percussion.
- Wear faceting.
- Fractured cusps and/or chipped teeth.
- Fremitus.
- Mobility.
- Thermal sensitivity.
- Tooth migration.

Radiographic Findings

- Horizontal and/or vertical alveolar bone loss.
- Widened Periodontal Ligament lamina dura space.
- Root resorption.

Orthodontic Trauma

In orthodontic treatment, tooth movement is created and controlled by the orthodontic appliance (for example, braces), that applies to teeth a particular level of constant force. When a constant force is applied to a tooth, a reaction is observed in the periodontal ligament, which delineates into two zones; a zone of tension, and a zone of pressure. Within the zone of pressure, vascularization and vascular permeability increase, there is thrombosis, and the cells and collagen become disorganized. The osteoclasts are activated to trigger bone resorption, either directly from the resorption bays, or from Howship's lacunae, or indirectly by producing mediators involved in bone resorption. In parallel, the zone of tension induces bony apposition. The entire healing process between the zone of tension and the zone of pressure can take several weeks to pass, after which the ligament and bone show no more signs of resorption, while demonstrating normal tooth mobility and radiographic appearance (Figure 3).

Figures 3a, b, and c illustrate a molar being mesialized and uprighted, which creates a reactive vertical tooth movement. The presence of an antagonist tooth adds a constraint to the uprighting, because the opposing tooth occludes with a significant force that is applied in the opposite direction to the desired vertical extrusive movement. Within the panoramic radiograph (Figure 3d) there is a visible mesial root intra-alveolar radiolucency near the uprighted molar's roots. It extends from the apex up to the furcation. However, after the orthodontic treatment had been completed (Figure 3e), bone apposition has occurred such that the mandibular second molar shows no increased periodontal bone loss than was present prior to orthodontic commencement (Figure 3b). This is an example of how orthodontic movement must be well - controlled, to prevent lasting orthodontic trauma.

Orthodontic treatment constricts movement to a given direction, whereby continuous unidirectional force is applied to a tooth by an orthodontic device. This type of movement is very different from the omni-directional mobility a periodontally compromised tooth may exhibit. Therefore, uncontrolled functional mobility exerts a stronger and more damaging effect on the involved supporting tissues when compared to orthodontically induced mobility, that is somewhat controlled,

Controlled orthodontic movement can be properly described by the term Jiggling:

- **Definition of Jiggling:** Tooth Jiggling results due to an applied constraint that allows for alternating movement only in two opposite direction (buccal-lingual, inciso-gingival, or mesial-distal)

Figure 3a. An intra-oral photograph showing an impacted maxillary canine and a mesially tipped mandibular second molar, prior to orthodontic treatment

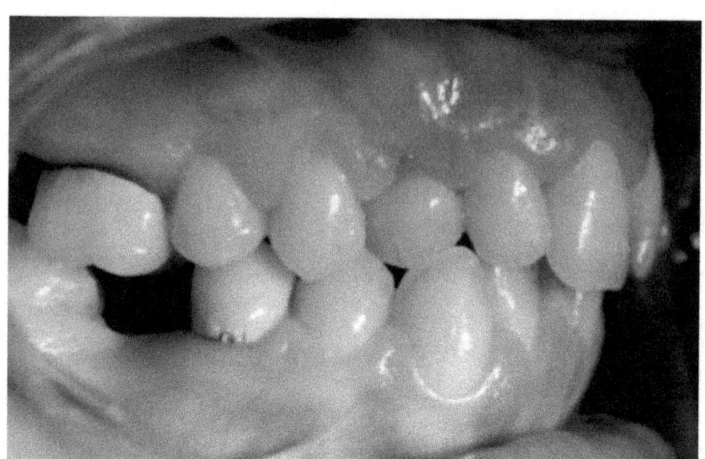

Figure 3b. The pre treatment panoramic radiograph showing the absence of traumatic bone loss, before moving the teeth

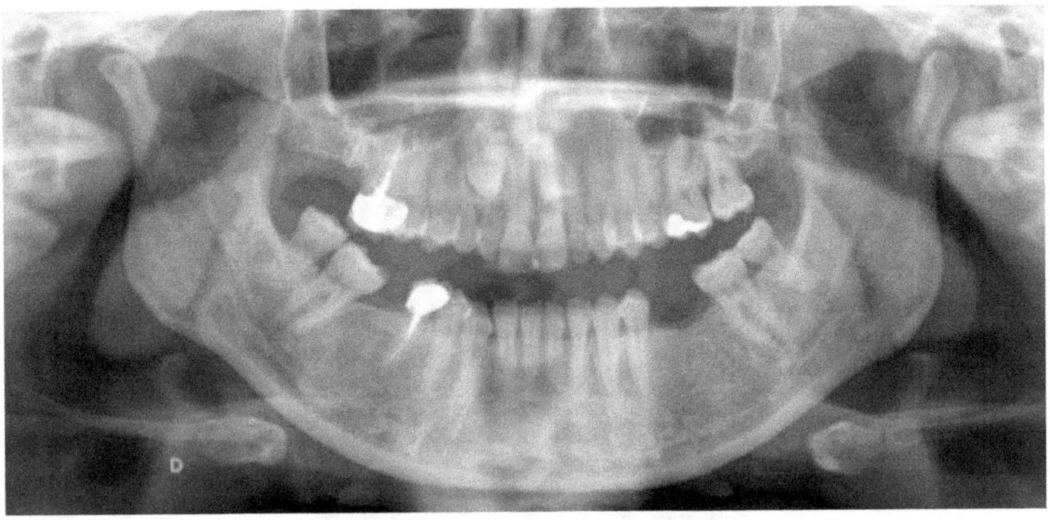

Figure 3c. The progression of orthodontic treatment using traction on the maxillary canine while up-righting the mandibular molar

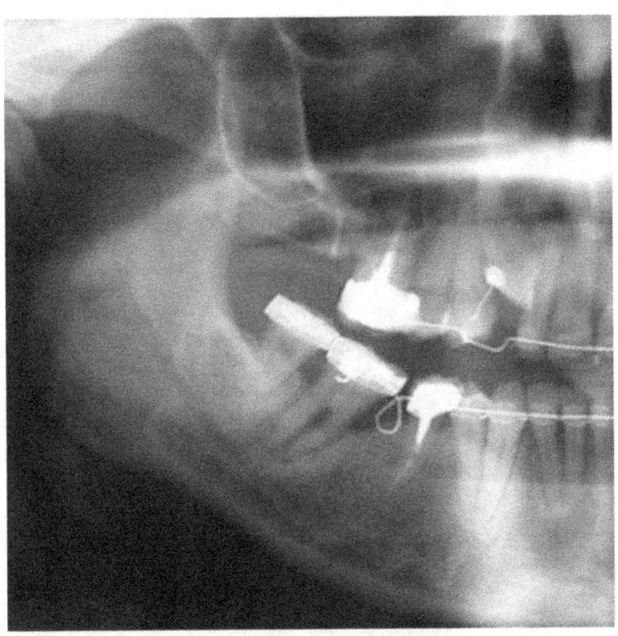

Trauma in Teeth Displaying Periodontal Disease

Many studies that have addressed the occlusion's role in periodontal tissue loss have determined that occlusal trauma does not appear to cause the observed destruction of the dental supporting tissues. However, it has been deemed important to consider occlusion as a potential contributing factor to the

Figure 3d. The mid-orthodontic treatment panoramic radiograph showing the presence of an intra-alveolar radiolucency visible on the mesial aspect of the molar's roots

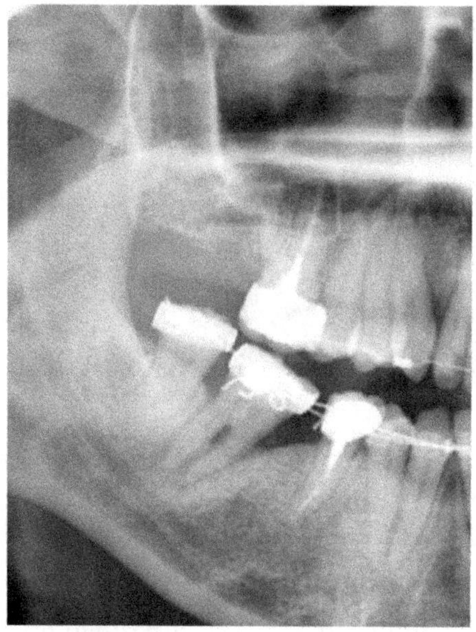

Figure 3e. The post treatment panoramic radiograph after maxillofacial surgery, orthodontic brace removal, and bonded retainers placed intraorally

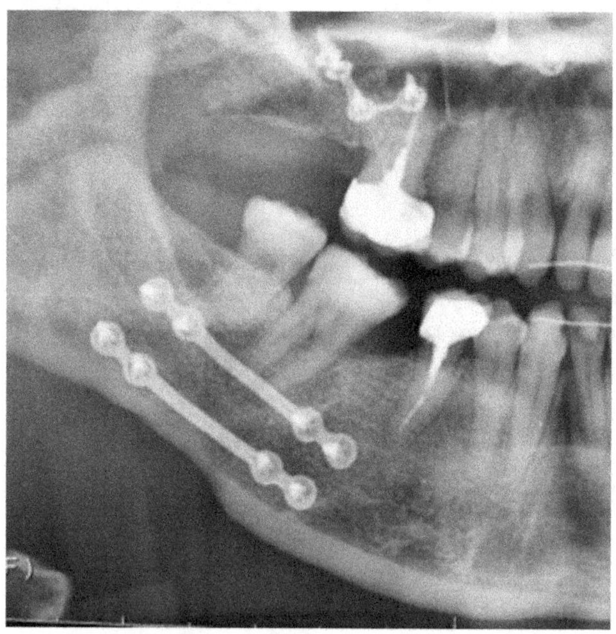

Figure 4. A radiograph that shows the consequences of trauma on a mandibular canine tooth with periodontal disease. The characteristic boney lesion was resultant from a hyperoccluded composite restoration placed on the opposing tooth. Note that the interdental septa is reduced in height.

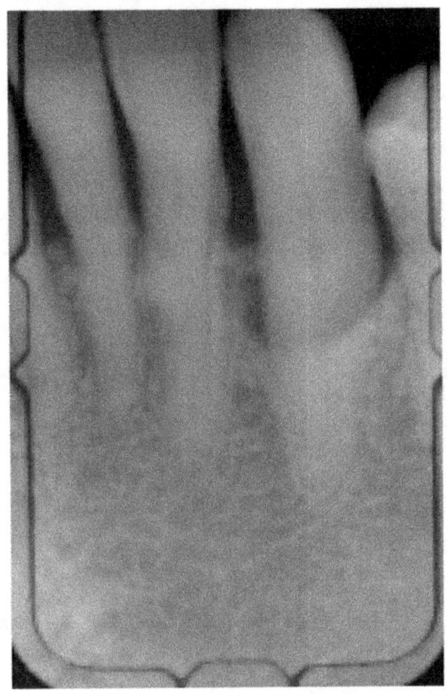

development of periodontal disease. Occlusal trauma is thought to accelerate the process of destruction where teeth may become temporarily or definitively mobile (Lindhe & Svanberg 1974; Nyman, 1978; Meitner, 1975) (Figure 4).

Periodontal Status

Periodontal health is characterized by the presence of bone and soft tissue around the teeth or implants, that exists in a stable state. The nature of the periodontal attachment is essential in assessing health vs. disease, such that and most studies have focused on three attachment parameters (Figure 5):

- The clinical attachment level (CAL).
- The mobility of the tooth.
- The pocket depth (PD).

Different parameters have been used by other clinicians and researchers to evaluate periodontal health. The maintenance of these parameters over the long-term, has been the principal objective of periodontal treatment.

- **ICT:** Inflamed connective tissue.
- **PPD:** Probing pocket depth.
- **PAL:** Periodontal attachment level.

Figure 5. Clinicians routinely use the periodontal probe to evaluate the clinical attachment level (CAL)

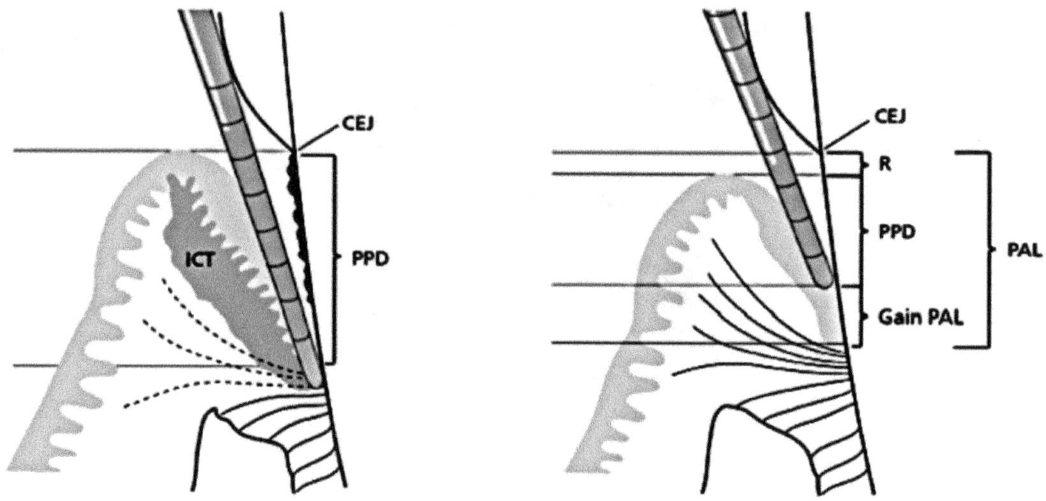

- **CEJ:** Cementoenamel junction.
- **R:** Recession.

The clinical attachment level (CAL) may be assessed with a graduated probe. It is expressed as the distance in millimeters from the CEJ to the bottom of the probable periodontal pocket. In patients who exhibit periodontal disease, there is usually observed widespread pocket depths of > 4 mm.

In recent years, periodontal probing procedures have become somewhat standardized by employing digital measurement when evaluating pocket depths. Most notably, the Florida Probe™ (Florida Probe Corp., Gainsville, FL, USA) has led the way into automated probing (Karpinia, Magnusson, Gibbs, & Yang, 2004). The use of automated probing has been controversial because of the difficulties of consistent clinician pressure calibration. If the clinician applies a high pressure when probing, the probing will be painful for the patient. If the applied pressure is too low, the system can have difficulty evaluating the correct probing depth, especially when infra gingival plaque is present within the pocket (Oringer et. al., 1997). Alternatively, the use of charting software (Florida Probe software version 9, Florida Probe Corp., Gainesville, FL, USA), to record manual probing depths is accurate and effective for the clinician.

There are very few studies that provide high-level evidence illustrating clearly, the effect occlusion has on the development of periodontal disease. Nor are there existing studies that illustrate the outcome benefits of performing occlusal adjustments as part of periodontal treatment (Foz, Artese, Horliana, Pannuti, & Romito, 2012). Generally, clinicians do not systematically carry out occlusal adjustments in every periodontal case, because the occlusion has not been deemed to be an important component of routine periodontal therapy. Occlusion is treated only when the patient experiences discomfort with their occlusal contacts.

Rationale for the Interrelation between Periodontal Disease and Occlusal Factors

Since Karolyi in 1901 first suggested a possible correlation existed between occlusal trauma and "pyorrhea" (Karolyi, 1901), several theories have been described. In the 1930s, Stones claimed that there was a correlation between various aspects of periodontal disease and occlusal problems (Stones, 1938). However, studies on monkeys did not include any controls, and the conclusions drawn were not consistent with the lack of significance of the results. Most of the early publications describing the relationship between occlusion and periodontal disease were based upon clinical observation.

Others studies evaluated tissue samples taken during autopsy, which generated conflicting results regarding occlusion's role in periodontal disease. Weinmann concluded that inflammation progresses along the vessels in the alveolar bone, and that this inflammation was not correlated with occlusal contact (Orban & Weinmann, 1933; Weinmann, 1941). It was not until cadaver studies were performed, in which a rigorous analysis of the potential role of occlusion being a factor influencing the development of periodontal disease, that occlusion was deemed a possible component (Glickman, 1967; Waerhaug, 1979). Glickman observed that teeth subject to strong occlusal constraints displayed greater periodontal tissue loss than teeth with no occlusal constraints. By contrast, Waerhaug, in a study of very similar samples, observed no correlation existed between the loss of marginal tissues around the teeth and the presence of occlusal trauma.

The gold standard for any human study is a randomized-blinded-controlled clinical trial (RCT). Unfortunately, in 1996, the World Workshop in Periodontics declared that it was not ethically justifiable to carry out studies on occlusal trauma without performing both real and mock occlusal adjustments (Gher, 1996). This statement made it impossible to study a correlation between occlusal forces and periodontal disease using an RCT design.

Animal Studies

A number of animal studies using squirrel monkeys (Kantor, Polson, & Zander, 1976; Polson, 1974; Polson, Kennedy, & Zander, 1972, 1974; Polson, Meitner, & Zander, 1976) and beagle dogs (Ericsson & Lindhe, 1977, 1982; Lindhe & Ericsson, 1976, 1982; Lindhe & Svanberg, 1974), evaluated the effect of excessive occlusal force on induced periodontitis. In the squirrel monkeys a mesio-distal compression force that was comparable to an orthodontic force was employed, whereas in the beagle dogs a buccolingual force was applied using a high occlusal contact. Both groups investigated the presence of excessive occlusal forces in the presence and absence of biofilm.

These studies yielded similar results, despite that different animal models and different occlusal forces were used. Excessive occlusal force in the absence of plaque, was found to cause loss of bone density and increased mobility of the affected tooth, but no evidence was found that the occlusal forces alone could cause attachment loss. When the excessive occlusal forces were removed, the loss of bone density reversed. In the presence of biofilm, inflammation of the gingiva and the periodontal supporting structures was observed, and when excessive occlusal forces and plaque were together, more bone density was lost in both animal models. Additionally, in the beagle dog model there was evidence of attachment loss when plaque and excessive occlusal forces were present together (Ericsson & Lindhe, 1977, 1982; Lindhe & Ericsson, 1976, 1982; Lindhe & Svanberg, 1974). However, those results were not observed in the squirrel monkey model (Kantor, Polson, & Zander, 1976; Polson, 1974; Polson, Kennedy, & Zander, 1972, 1974; Polson, Meitner, & Zander, 1976). Both studies agreed that the removal of plaque and the control of inflammation would stop the progression of periodontal disease whether or not excessive occlusal forces were present.

Although these two animal model study series attempted to evaluate the relationship of occlusal forces and biofilm, no specific force levels and force mapping data was gathered from the created occlusal study conditions. "Excessive" load was created empirically by modeling trauma that was far from the reality of occlusal contact physiology. Both studies concluded that there was no evidence indicating that excessive occlusal force alone will cause loss of attachment. Lastly, it is important to understand that even though these studies are very interesting, no animal model demonstrates naturally developing periodontal disease that is consistent with human periodontal disease.

Biologic Pathway

Trauma from occlusion is considered to create a disturbance of tissue homeostasis, where the excessive force induced on teeth mechanically stresses the cells living within the tissues. A tissue reaction then activates a host response which induces many cytokine inflammatory mediators (that are organized within the Cytokine Network) to participate in the disruption of periodontal stability, by activating osteoclastogenesis and inhibiting bone formation. Receptor activator of the nuclear factor kappa B ligand (known as RANKL) occurs, which is an important component in osteoclast cell differentiation, activation, maturation, and survival.

Some researchers have investigated the distribution of RANKL-expressing cells in rat periodontium during lipopolysaccharide-induced inflammation, with or without occlusal trauma (Yoshinaga, Ukai, Abe, & Hara, 2007). Their results demonstrated that RANKL expression on endothelial cells, inflammatory cells, and PDL cells, was involved in inflammatory bone resorption, whereby the expression was enhanced by traumatic occlusion. It has been suggested that RANKL expression in these cells is closely involved with an increase in osteoclasts that are induced by the occlusal trauma (Yoshinaga et. al., 2007).

Osteopontin is an extracellular matrix protein known to be important in cellular attachment, that is produced under mechanical loading. Osteopontin is thought to induce osteoclasts to migrate to resorption sites, where the osteopontin then interacts with CD-44 (a cell-surface glycoprotein) to bind hyaluronic acid, type I collagen, and fibronectin. RANKL has been shown *in vitro* to aid in the constitutive induction of intra-cellular osteopontin. However, no correlation between RANKL distribution and osteopontin production in osteoclasts has been found (Kaku, Uoshima, Yamashita, & Miura, 2005).

Human Cadaver Studies

Glickman's Analysis

- **Glickman's Concept:** Glickman defended the possibility that occlusion was a factor capable of modifying periodontal disease that was induced by plaque. Teeth that had been subject to occlusal trauma seemed to have a disease progression that was different from that of teeth without occlusal trauma. Glickman thus described two zones (Glickman, 1967) (Figure 6):
    - A zone of irritation.
    - A zone of co-destruction.

Figure 6. A schematic drawing of the zone of irritation and the zone of co-destruction, as described by Glickman. The inflammatory lesion in the zone of irritation can propagate into the alveolar bone, while in teeth that are subjected to occlusal trauma, the inflammatory infiltrate can spread directly into the periodontal ligament. Adapted from Carranza, F.A., Jr. (1987). Glickman's Periodontology, Philadelphia, W.B. Saunders, Co., pp. 285, Figure 19-10.

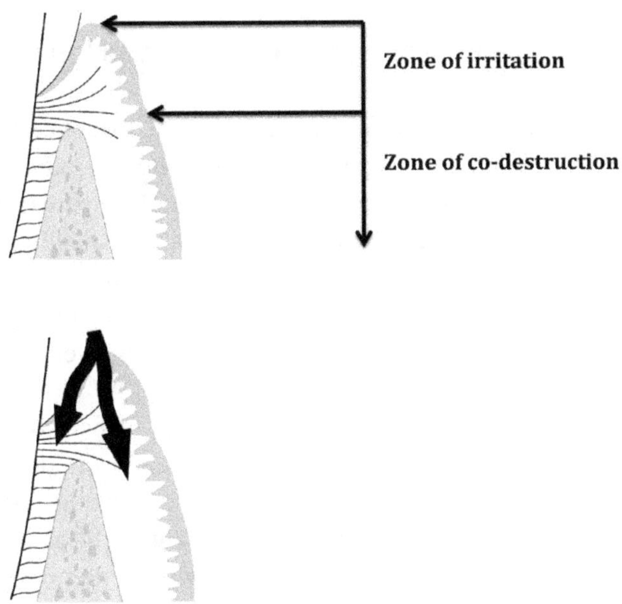

By studying cadaver samples, Glickman determined that the zone of irritation was not susceptible to occlusal problems, because it consisted of mucous tissues. Any inflammation in this zone was thus, dependent purely on the presence of bacterial plaque, where forces applied in the zone of irritation appeared to be dissipated solely within the mucosa. By contrast, the zone of co-destruction was composed of the periodontal ligament and the periodontal bone, which are both susceptible to occlusal trauma. In the zone of co-destruction, applied forces were thought to lead to the development of angular boney lesions. Glickman concluded that there was a causal relationship between occlusal trauma and the presence of angular boney lesions.

Waerhaug's Analysis

- **Waerhaug's Concept:** Waerhaug studied the same type of cadaver samples as Glickman and noted the presence of numerous sites without angular boney lesions that were in the presence of occlusal trauma (Waerhaug, 1979). He thus, refuted Glickman's affirmation concerning a possible causal effect.

These investigations remained controversial for many years, and numerous authors took one side or the other without really providing any high-level scientific evidence to justify their choice.

All the above-mentioned descriptive studies were subject to observer bias. With living patients, the periodontal condition observed is the result of the action of many factors often acting together over many years. Findings from autopsy specimens are even more difficult to interpret because the autopsy sample does not exhibit active human physiology. Often, knowledge of the cadaver's medical history, life habits, and other factors are limited or absent. After death, it is difficult to accurately evaluate the occlusal relationship that existed during life. Moreover, the "occlusal trauma", by definition, depends on masticatory function and muscular force that cannot be evaluated in a cadaver, because the occlusal trauma is not a static phenomenon.

Clinical Studies Involving Occlusal Adjustments and Periodontal Disease

The first clinical studies carried out in 1976, showed healing did not differ between teeth with and without angular lesions, after occlusal adjustment was performed (Rosling, Nyman, Lindhe, & Jern, 1976). In 1980, another study analyzed the healing by differentiating hypermobile teeth from stable teeth. The author concluded that the healing capacities of these two types of teeth were different (Fleszar et. al., 1980).

The effect of occlusal adjustment in the treatment of periodontal disease was studied in 1992. 50 patients were analyzed, of which 22 subjects were treated with occlusal adjustment. Two years after surgery, probing results were better (smaller pockets by 0.5 mm, on average) in the patients who had undergone occlusal adjustment (Burgett et. al., 1992).

The influence of dynamic occlusal interferences on the depth of periodontal pocketing was so ae-valuated in a transverse epidemiological study involving 2,980 subjects that were representative of a Caucasian population (Bernhardt et. al., 2006). Their medical and dental histories, and their different known periodontal risk factors were studied, in addition to present occlusal factors. Interferences on the non-working side were shown to be significantly associated with pocket depth and loss of attachment ($p < 0.0001$). Additionally, there was an increase in pocket depth observed ($p = 0.004$) when a tooth demonstrated both working and non-working side contacts, where the amplitude of the applied forces had some influence on the outcome. These different relationships, even though clearly demonstrated, were not specific, and were considered of little importance compared to the patient's age, history of tobacco use, and the subject's plaque index.

In 2008, a study analyzed the relationship between occlusal force and periodontal healing during the periodontal maintenance phase, three years post treatment. The authors found that a correlation existed between the loss of attachment exceeding 7 mm, and the progression of periodontal the disease despite tissue-based treatment, in the presence of occlusal forces (Takeuchi & Yamamoto, 2008).

In 2009, Nunn and Harrel analyzed occlusal variations and their relationship with periodontal health or disease parameters. Occlusal analysis included the determination of the initial contact, the Cr-CO discrepancy between initial contact in a retruded position (Centric Relation) and contact in maximum intercuspation (Centric Occlusion), the presence of working, balancing, and protrusive contacts in excursive movements. The occlusal analysis was performed by gently manipulating the patient into a retruded position to determine initial (CR) contact. All other contacts were evaluated from the Centric Occlusion (CO) intercuspated maxillomandibular relationship. The occlusal contacts were verified by performing the analyses twice, and confirming occlusal contacts with occlusal marking ribbon. The same examiner performed all examinations. The multiple analyses revealed that the presence of a CR-CO discrepancy and non-working (balancing) contacts, were both associated with deeper probing depths. The data also indicated that posterior protrusive excursive interfering contacts were associated with deeper probing depths (Harrel & Nunn, 2009).

Branschofsky et. al., in 2011, analyzed 288 subjects with chronic periodontitis of varying severities, and 93 healthy subjects, where it was found that secondary trauma from occlusion (premature and balancing side contacts) was frequently seen in periodontally compromised patients. The authors reported that secondary trauma from occlusion was positively correlated with the severity of attachment loss (Branschofsky, Beikler, Schafer, Flemming, & Lang, 2011).

The conclusions that can be drawn from these studies are:

- Occlusal trauma does not initiate gingival inflammation.
- In the absence of inflammation, a traumatogenic occlusion will result in increased mobility, widened PDL, loss of crestal bone height and bone volume, but no attachment loss.
- In the presence of gingival inflammation, excessive jiggling forces do not cause accelerated attachment loss (in squirrel monkeys). Increasing occlusal forces may accelerate attachment loss (in beagle dogs).
- Treating the gingival inflammation in the presence of continuing mobility or jiggling trauma, will result in decreased mobility and increased bone density, but no change in attachment level or the alveolar bone level.
- There is a correlation between occlusal force and degrees of healing during the maintenance phase

Using Computerized Occlusal Analysis during the First Periodontal Appointment

The periodontal examination includes an assessment of the general medical condition, followed by both an extraoral and intraoral analysis. Often, the general medical state of the patient can provide clues to the context of their periodontal disease. Some diseases states like diabetes, have a significant effect on changing periodontal health parameters, as well as on the healing capability of the tissues from rendered treatment (Kardesler, Buduneli, Cetinkalp, & Kinane, 2010).

The extraoral examination is often quite basic, but may reveal the presence of occlusal problems, such as muscle tension and spasm, facial pain, and associated facial asymmetry resultant from skeletal discrepancies.

During the intraoral examination, analyses of the periodontal status involves the recording of the following clinical parameters:

- Hygiene level,
- Periodontal probing depths,
- Bleeding,
- Suppuration,
- Height of the keratinized gingiva,
- Mobility, which is described with mobility classification:
  - Normal mobility.
  - **Grade I:** Slightly more than normal (< 0.2 mm of horizontal movement).
  - **Grade II:** Moderately more than normal (1-2 mm of horizontal movement).
  - **Grade III:** Severe mobility (> 2 mm horizontally, or involving vertical movement).

A summary of the above periodontal parameters is then generated by the companion software at the first periodontal assessment visit, for the purposes of making an accurate periodontal diagnosis (Figure 7).

Figure 7 shows the software charting of a typical periodontal examination. Probing detected areas of recession and furcation involvement on a few teeth. There also was observed the presence of plaque on the lingual surfaces of the lower anterior teeth. When the examination was repeated following treatment during the healing period, the software automatically displays pre and post treatment differences, such has a decrease or an increase of the probing depths.

Occlusal analysis, which is currently done with articulating paper, is often part of the intraoral examination. Articulating paper has several disadvantages for this analysis, including its thickness, the difficulty of marking teeth with ink due to saliva, the impossibility of measuring the timing dynamics of contacts, and the impossibility of measuring occlusal contact force (Carey et. al., 2007; Saad et.al.,, 2008; Qadeer et. al., 2012).

The T-Scan 8 system however, can provide an occlusal analysis that is both faster and more detailed with respect to contact forces, timing, and dynamic movement assessments. Indeed, the identification of interfering contacts is very simple and rapid with this digital technique. For example, by using the T-Scan software feature "Force percentage per tooth" (Figure 8; in the 2 and 3-Dimensional ForceView windows) to correlate individual tooth force percentages with clinically detected mobile teeth, a diagnosis of existing occlusal trauma can be made that is free from clinician subjectivity.

Figure 8a demonstrates a periodontally compromised patient with deep pocketing on teeth #s 14, 15, and 17, as well as teeth #s25, 26, 27 and 28. The pre treatment T-Scan recording showed an extreme force was located on teeth # s25, 26, 27 and 28 (in MIP). The COF icon was located on left side of the arch, revealing a force imbalance existed between the right and left arch halves. Some defibrillation can be noted in the Total Force line within the Force vs. Time Graph, illustrating the patient had muscular difficulty in maintaining force levels while attempting firm intercuspation. Therapeutic occlusal adjustments will be needed before periodontal treatment is instituted, to decrease the impact these occlusal force risk factors may have on lessening periodontal therapy effectiveness.

Nine weeks after T-Scan guided occlusal adjustments were performed, the force mapping is more equalized bilaterally, denoted by the Center of Force being more centered within the arches (Figure 8b). This illustrated the relative force was more equalized between the right and left arch-halves. In addition, the defibrillation disappeared from the Total Force line within the post treatment Force vs. Time graph, indicating the patient no longer exhibited muscular difficulty when maintaining force levels during firm intercuspation.

The CR Prematurity: MIP Slide

The distance that the patient moves between the retruded initial contact (CR prematurity), and the position of maximal tooth contact (Centric Occlusion) is termed the slide between Centric Relation and Centric Occlusion. This slide is often described aside has been termed the CR-CO discrepancy (Celenza, 1984) or the Centric Relation-to-Centric Occlusion slide. This slide is quantified by measuring its length (in mm), in the anterior, vertical, and lateral planes. Following the identification of the initial contact, the clinician can ask the patient to further close their teeth together until maximum intercuspal contact is made. The Centric Occlusion position (known as MIP), is the position that the patient will naturally move to because it is the most comfortable fit of their teeth.

Figure 7. Typical periodontal charting. All clinical parameters are recorded and synthesized into a periodontal chart by the companion software (Florida software version 9, Florida Probe Corporation, Gainesville, FL, USA). Probing depth (6 measurements per site), recession, furcation involvement, mobility, bleeding, suppuration, and quantity of plaque, can all be entered into the patient periodontal chart. Red triangles represent furcation probing.

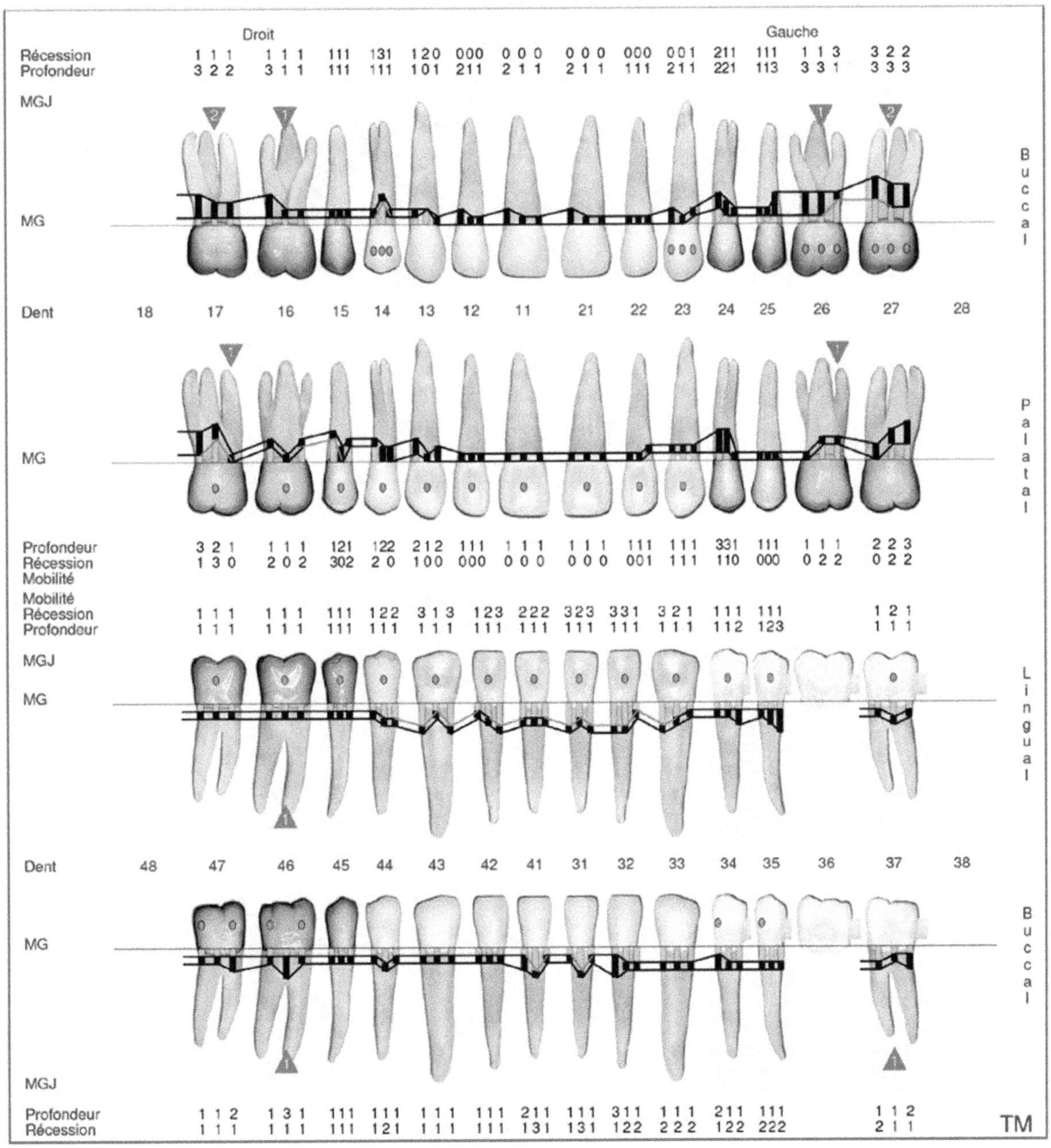

Figure 8a. T-Scan 8 recording of a periodontally compromised patient with excessive force on teeth # s25, 26, 27 and 28 The 2-Dimensional ForceView window shows an occlusal force imbalance was present, described by the left-sided and non-centered position Center of Force (COF) trajectory.

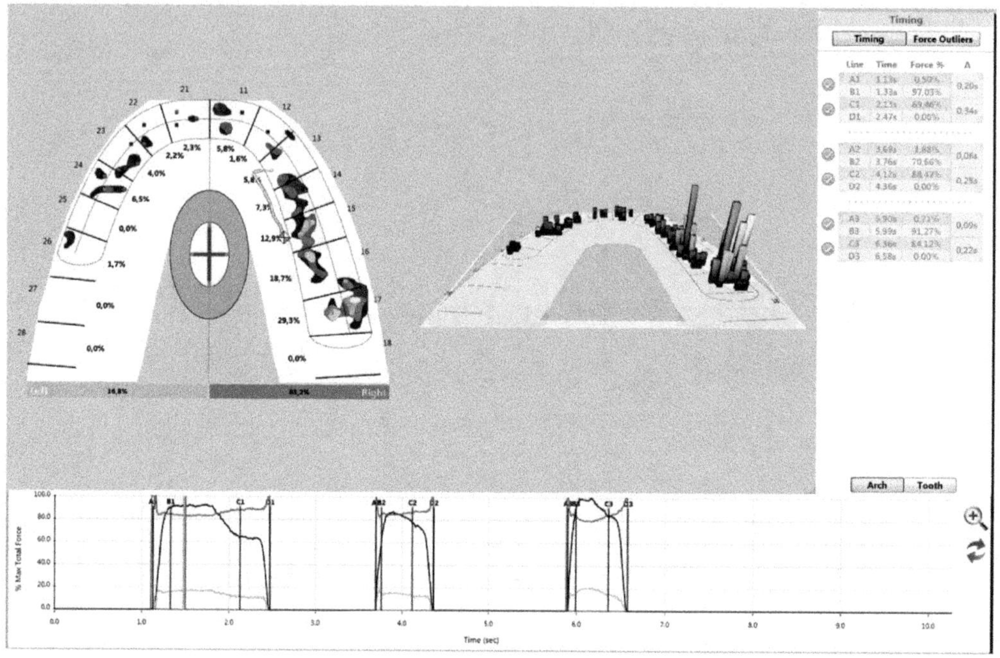

Figure 8b. 9 weeks after T-Scan guided occlusal adjustments were performed, the force mapping was more equalized bilaterally, the Center of Force was more centered, and the pre treatment defibrillation of the Total Force line was absent.

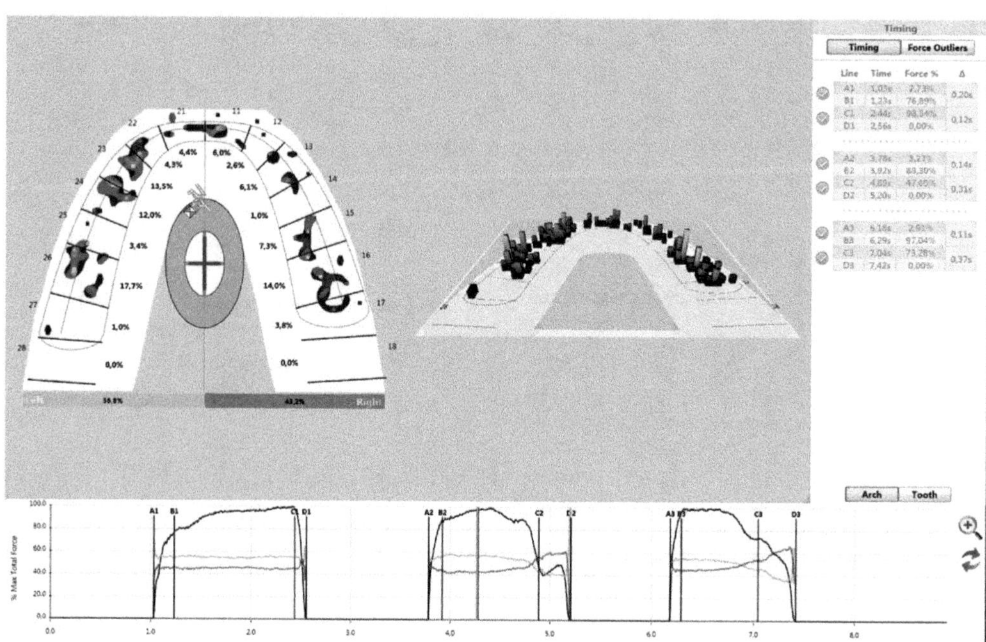

Figures 9a, b, and c, present a patient with significant periodontal disease. The periodontal charting documents deep pockets of 6 to 8 mm, and several mobile teeth. The probing is deepest on teeth #s 2 and 3 for no visibly apparent reason. yet more severe periodontal disease parameters were charted on the right side (Figure 9a). The intraoral photographs reveal the patient had poor oral hygiene, and presented with some areas of tissue recession (Figures 9b, c and d). Figure 9e presents the spider graph as described by Lang and Tonetti (Lang & Tonetti, 1996), which can clarify for the clinician the various periodontal risk factors present. This patient's spider graph indicateas that this patient was at low-risk for additional risk factors contributimg to the periodontal disease state.

Figures 10a shows the pre treatment T-Scan data of the patient shown in Figure 9a - e, who presented with periodontitis. Note the occlusal force overload in the right posterior quadrant, and the severe occlusal force imbalance documented by the very far to the right and non-centered COF trajectory and icon.

Figure 10b illustrates the 1-year post treatment charting, following both periodontal treatment and computer-guided occlusal intervention. There is good tissue healing noted in the follow-up charting, as no more deep pockets were detected with probing (Figure 10b). The periodontal parameters appear to have been stabilized, and the additional risk factors were under control. The 1-year post treatment follow up T-Scan data (Figure 10c) shows there is significantly more occlusal balance with low-force occlusal contacts uniformly distributed on all teeth. Note the COF position was now centered compared to the pre treatment COF position in Figure 10a.

Lateral Interferences and Periodontal Disease

Occlusal interference may occur in protrusion or lateral excursions, and on initial contact in the retruded contact position when the mandible is manipulated into Centric Relation. They may be found on both the working and/or the non-working sides of the dentition. Non-working side contacts have been considered by many authors to be destructive to tooth cusps, their supporting structures, and the musculoskeletal apparatus (Lee, Kwon, Chai, Lucas, Thompson, & Lawn, 2009; Keown, Bush, Ford, Lee, Constantino, & Lawn 2012; Keown, Lee, & Bush, 2012). However, a review article reported that long-term studies performed before 1985, lacked the supporting evidence that removing non-working interferences was beneficial to occlusal function (Bush, 1984). Generally, lateral interferences are still considered to be a controversial subject in correlation to periodontal disease progression, despite that clinicians often observe better stability of periodontal health parameters in patients who present without lateral interferences.

To date, no clear mechanism to explain the pathogenesis of periodontal progression related to occlusal force issues has been established. Nevertheless, Ishigaki et. al. in 2006, used Periotest™ (Periotest classic, Medizintechnik Gulden, Modautal, Germany) to show that occlusal interferences could result in tooth mobility. The authors concluded that chewing movements increased the mobility of specific types of compromised teeth. Alternatively, Kerstein and Radke found that the reduction of Disclusion Times when using the Immediate Complete Anterior Guidance Development (ICAGD) coronoplasty, which is an enameloplasty guided with the T-Scan 8 synchronized with electromyographic recordings, reduced muscular hyperactivity in parallel to the occlusal treatment of lateral interferences (Kerstein & Radke, 2012). One could hypothesize that increased and repeated lateral mechanical stress applied to the periodontal ligament, could be a factor in tissue destruction. Lateral excursive forces are qualitatively different from closure maximum intercuspal forces. Lateral movements with posterior teeth in contact generate shear forces (oblique vector forces in relation to the long axis of the tooth), but centric occlusion forces are more parallel to the long axes of teeth (Rees, 2001).

Figure 9a. Clinical case periodontal charting documenting 6 to 8 mm pocketing with several mobile teeth present

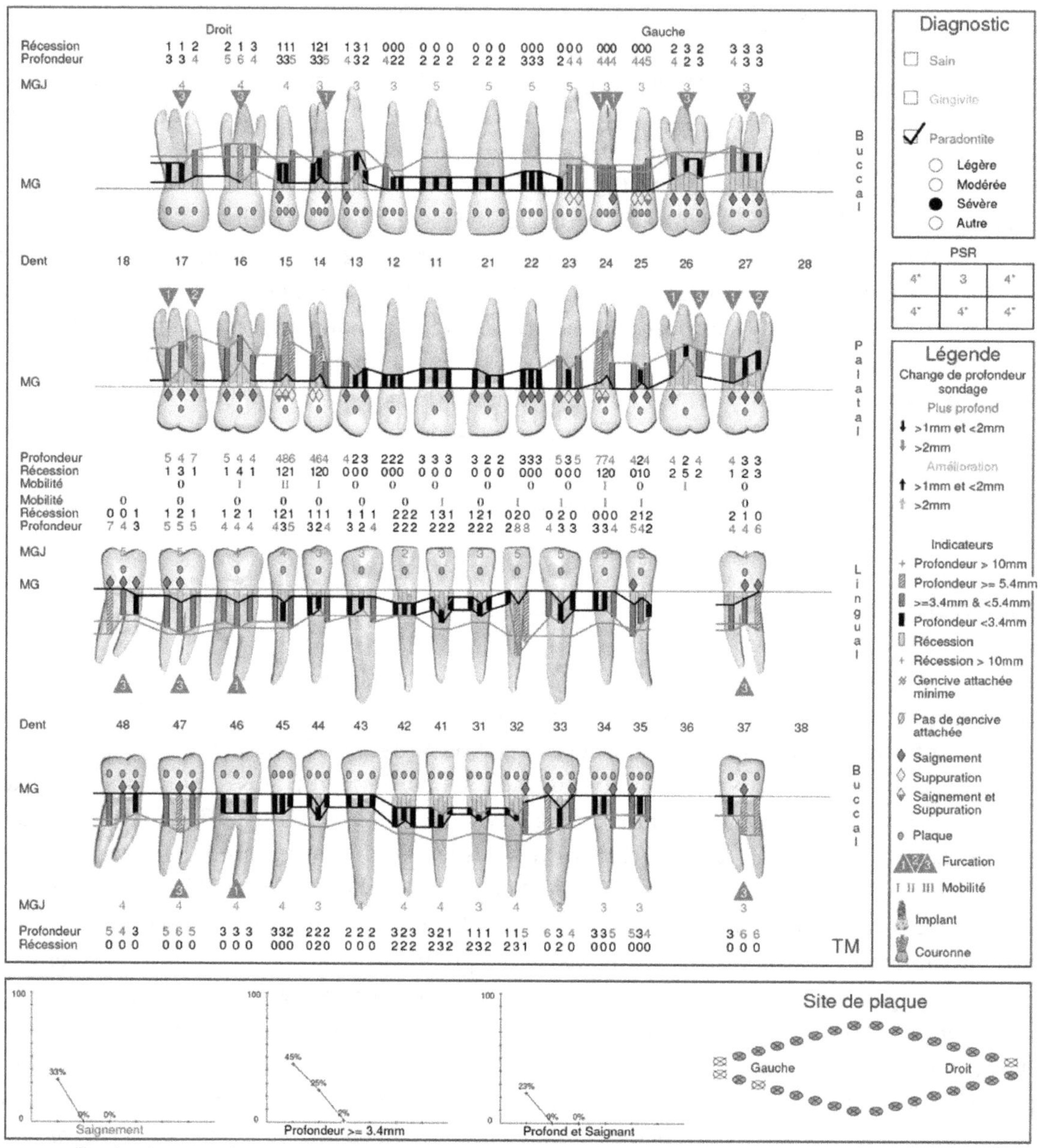

Printed on 21/09/2013 08:33:15 from CABINET2-BUREAU

Because lateral interference mapping was very difficult to obtain prior to the development of T-Scan technology, clinical studies relating periodontal disease progression to differing occlusal parameters was also very difficult to establish. With T-Scan 8 recordings, such data is much more easily obtained and quantified, which could lead to a clearer understanding of how occlusal force and excursive interferences affect periodontal tissue loss.

Figure 9b. Facial view of the patient shown in Figure 9a at initial presentation, with visibly poor hygiene and some gingival recession

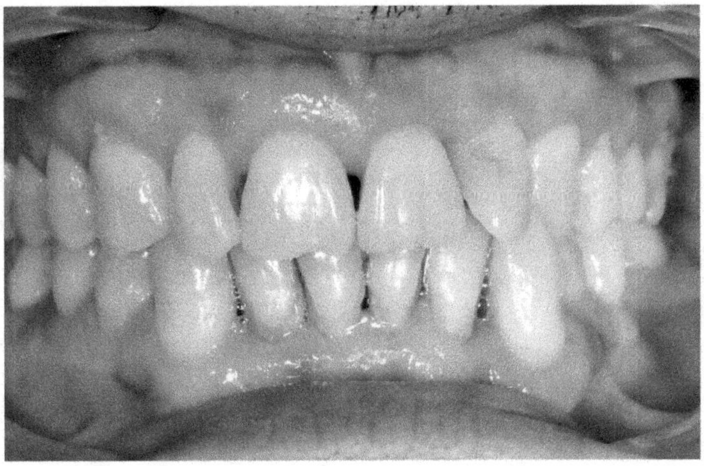

Figure 9c. Left sided view of the patient shown in Figure 9a at initial presentation

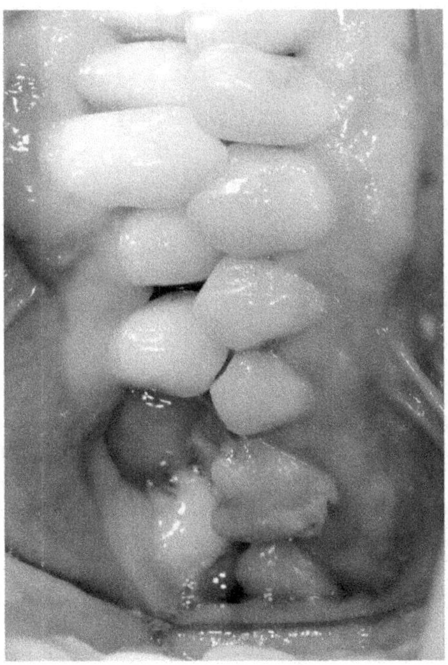

Figure 9d. Right-sided view of the patient shown in Figure 9a at initial presentation

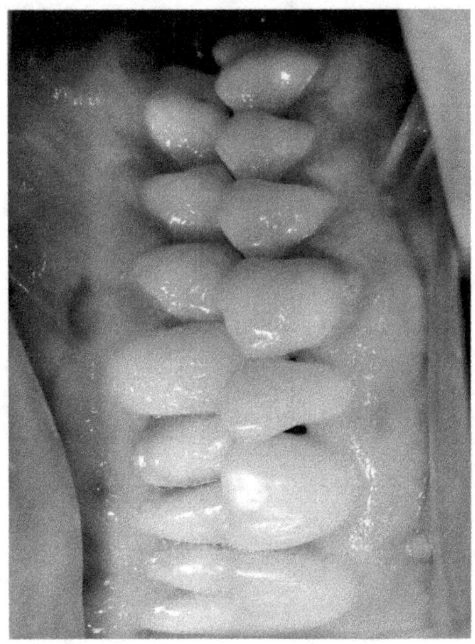

Occlusal Adjustment in Periodontal Treatment

As described earlier, not all studies agree on the existence of a relationship between periodontal treatment and occlusal trauma. However, periodontists routinely include occlusal adjustment in their initial periodontal therapy. Some periodontists carry out this adjustment themselves. Others ask the patient's

Figure 9e. The spider graph determined that this patient was at low-risk for additional periodontal disease contributory factors

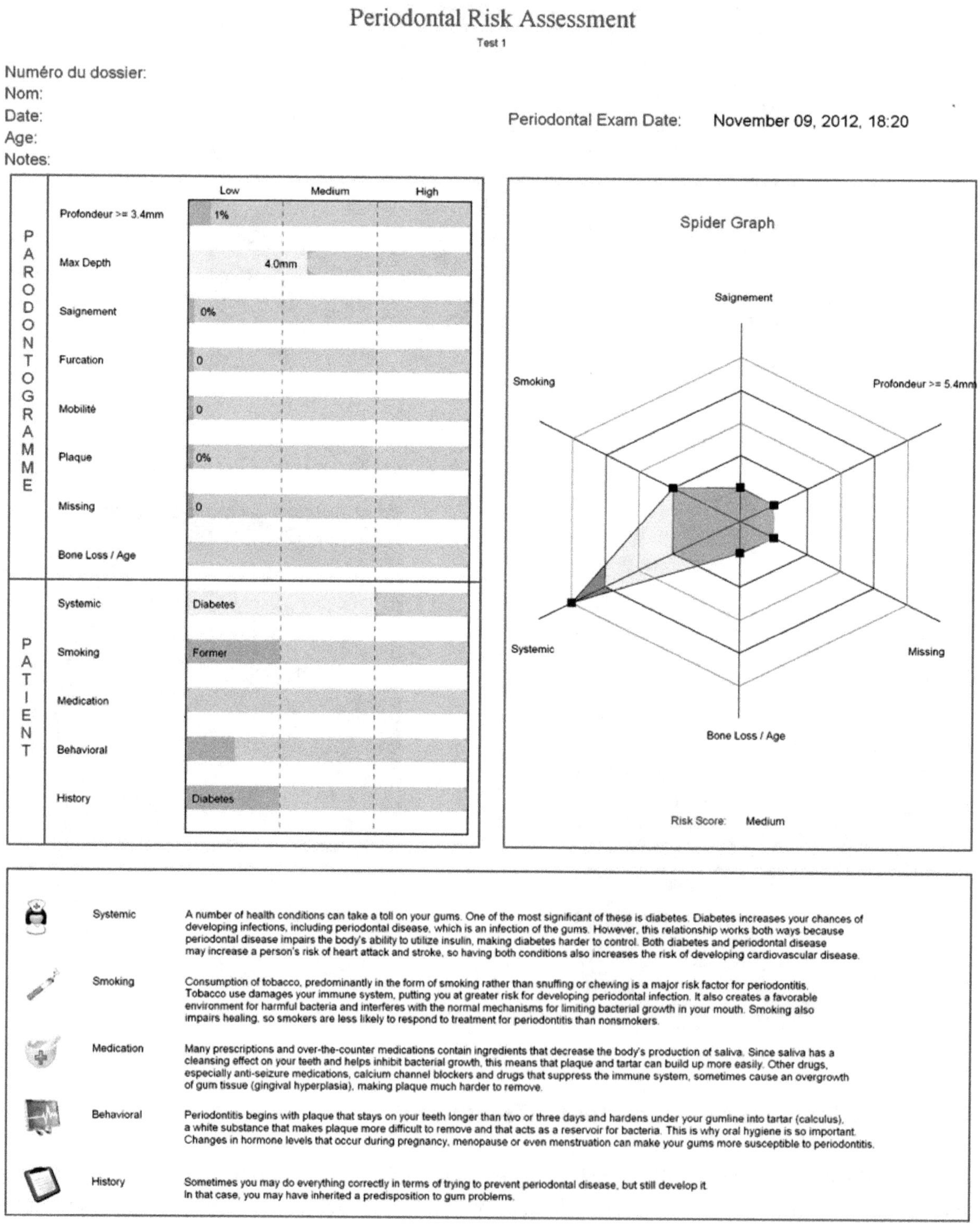

Figure 10a. T-Scan analysis of a patient who presented with periodontitis before any adjustments and periodontal and occlusal treatment had been rendered. A severe occlusal force imbalance existed with COF trajectory and icon very far to the right side of the dental arch.

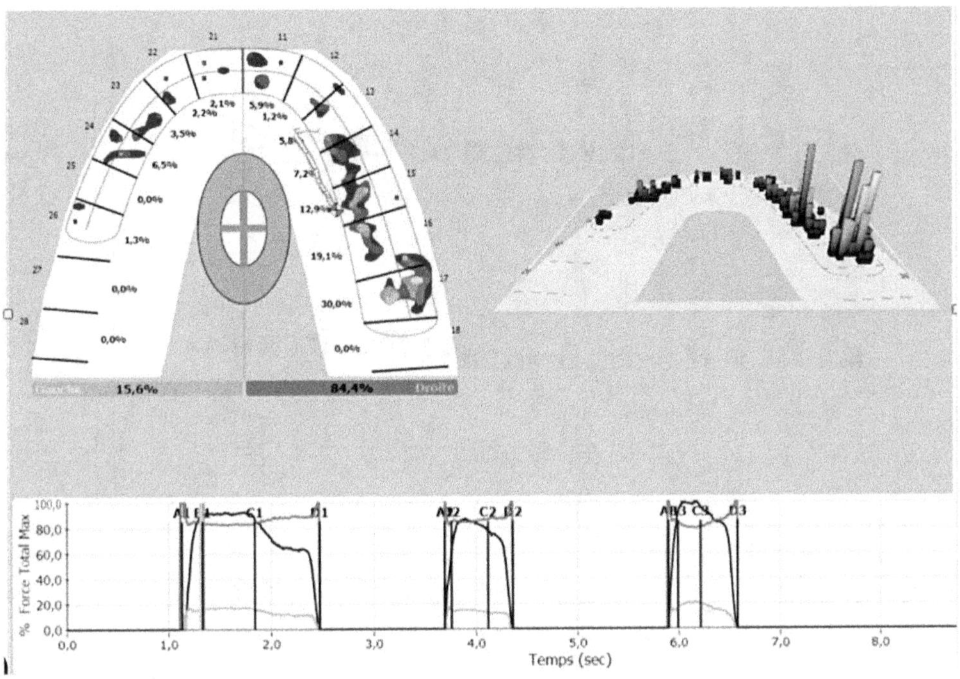

general dentist to perform the procedure. Adjustments are usually carried out before periodontal treatment is initiated, attempting to achieve both a static and a dynamic occlusal force equilibrium. Some authors still advocate occlusal adjustment as an important component of the treatment when trying to regenerate periodontal tissue (Branschofsky et. al., 2011; Harrel & Nunn, 2001; Nunn & Harrel, 2001; Sanz, 2005).

The non-smoking patient illustrated in Figures 11a, b and c, presented with some deep pockets (> 4mm). There was more pronounced periodontal disease detected on the right arch-half, such that the periodontal charting described more right-sided pockets, bleeding, and suppuration. Also, the maxillary incisor's attachment loss was significantly more than that of the mandibular incisors (Figure 11d). All maxillary anterior lingual sulci were widened from the large amount of subgingival brown calculus present, which created significant chronic inflammation and edema of the gingival mucosa. The periodontal charting (Figure 11e) showed the plaque index, the probing depths, the bleeding locations, and the areas of recession the patient presented with.

Of significance, was that this patient demonstrated more than twice the occlusal force concentration on the left arch-half compared to the right arch-half (69.4% left – 30.6% right). This can be seen in Figure 11f, where a pretreatment left-sided COF position was observed within the pretreatment T-Scan data.

Before commencing periodontal treatment, T-Scan 8 computer-guided occlusal adjustments were performed to improve the closure occlusal force balance of the MIP position, and to remove the discrepancy between Centric Relation and Centric Occlusion (Figure 11g). These occlusal corrections homogenized the 3-Dimensional ForceView column heights throughout the arch, and repositioned the Center of Force icon into the middle of the arch halves. These two T-Scan data improvements indicated

Figure 10b. The 1- year post periodontal and occlusal treatment follow-up periodontal charting. There were no more deep pockets detected with probing.

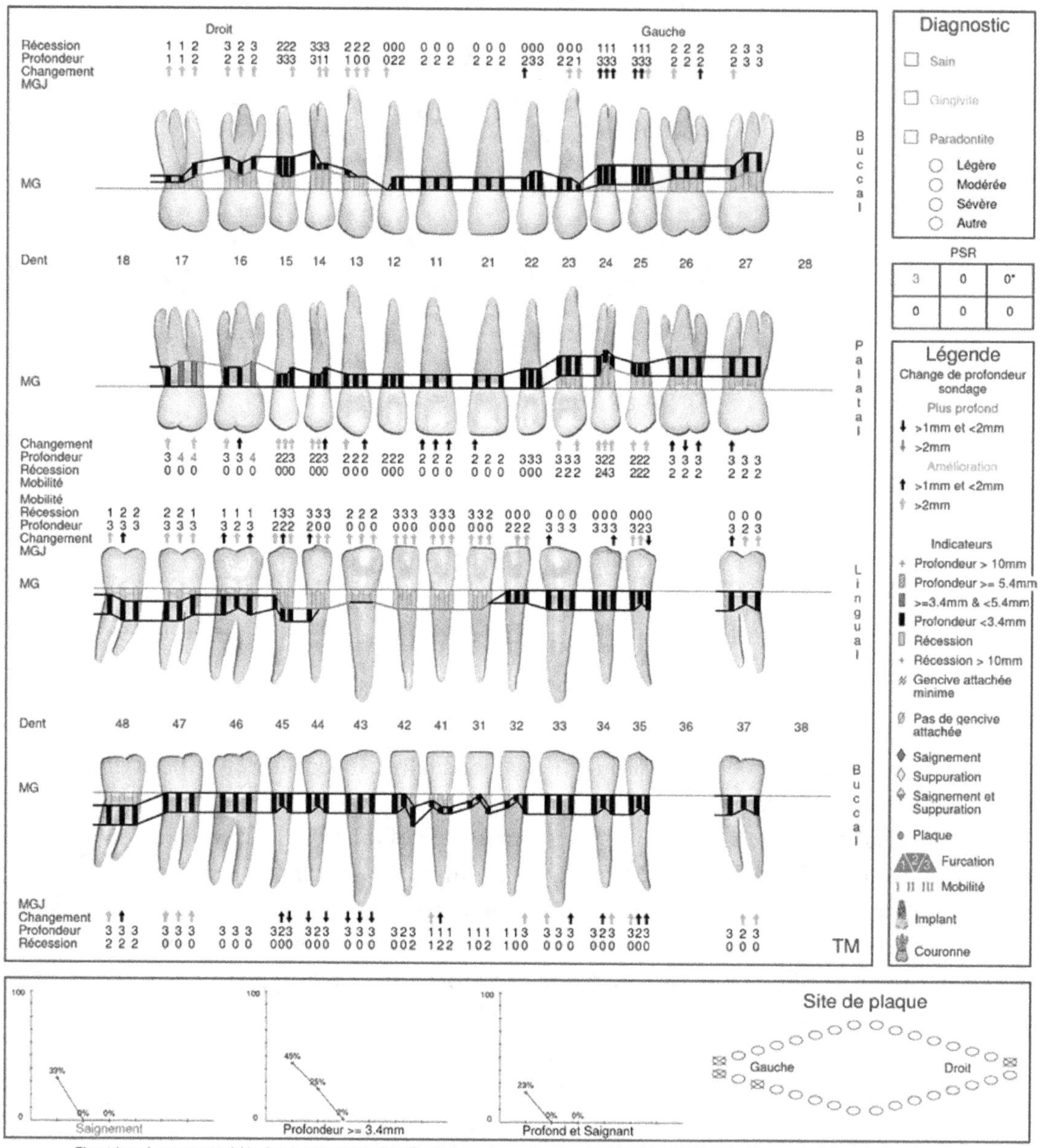

that the performed occlusal adjustments lessened the overall occlusal force imbalance from 69.4% left – 30.6% right (Figure 11f), to 56.6% left – 43.4% (Figure 11g).

The periodontal disease was then addressed using a full-mouth disinfection protocol (Quirynen et. al., 1995). After 1 year, definitive healing was observed, with significant reductions noted in pocket depths, bleeding, and suppuration (Figures 11h - l). 1-year post treatment tissue health was obtained by combining the periodontal care with the T-Scan guided occlusal adjustments.

Figure 10c. T-Scan 8 analysis at re-evaluation, 1-year post treatment. There was significantly more occlusal balance, with low-force occlusal contacts distributed on all teeth.The COF position was centered, as well.

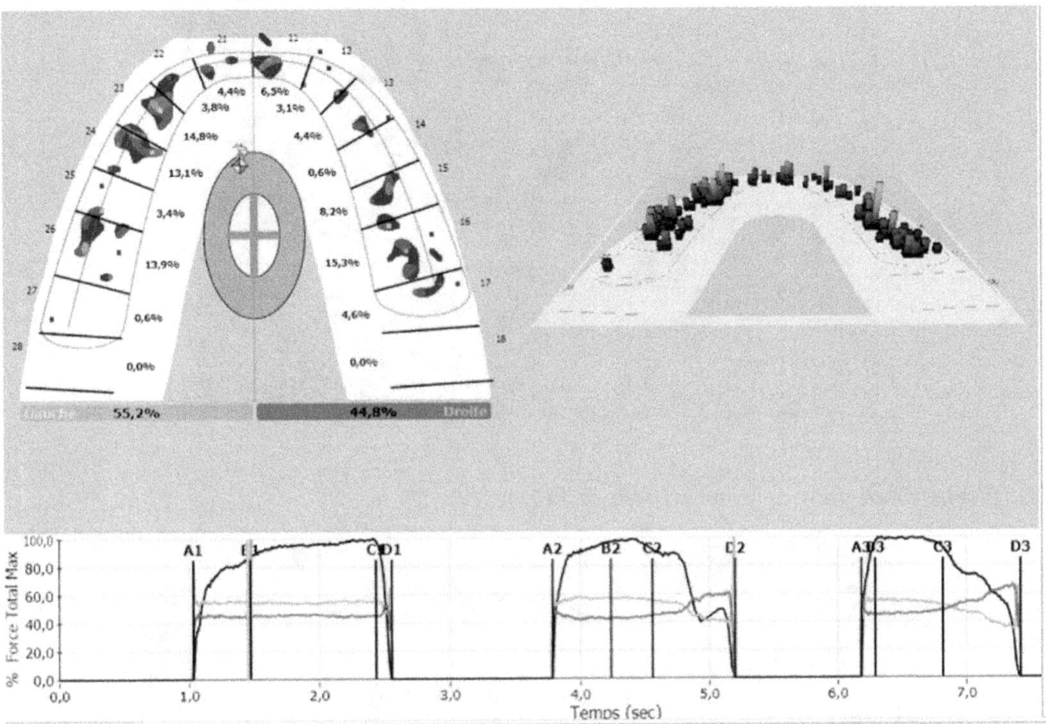

Figure 11a. Retracted frontal view in maximal intercuspation. The patient presented with periodontal pockets of > 4mm. Note the anterior spaces (known as pathologic tooth migration) resultant from alveolar bone loss.

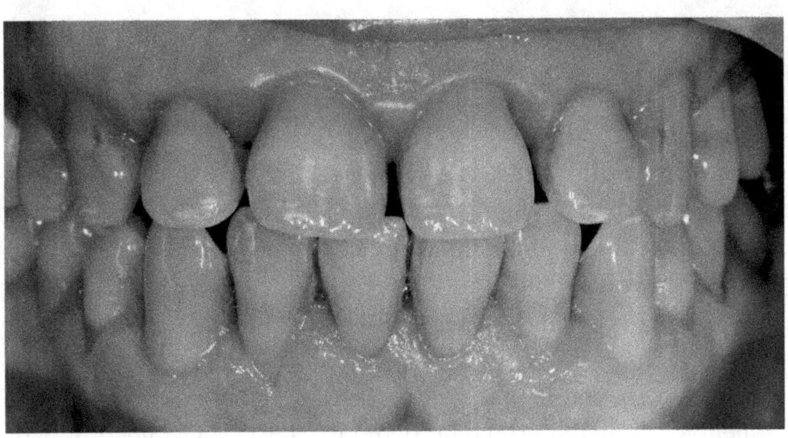

Figure 11b. Left-sided view of same patient in Figure 11a, where more pocketing, bleeding, and suppuration, was detected

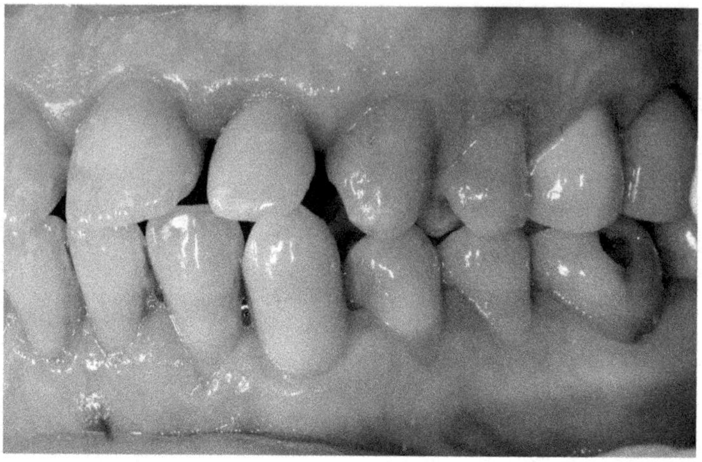

Figure 11c. Right-sided view of same patient in Figure 11a

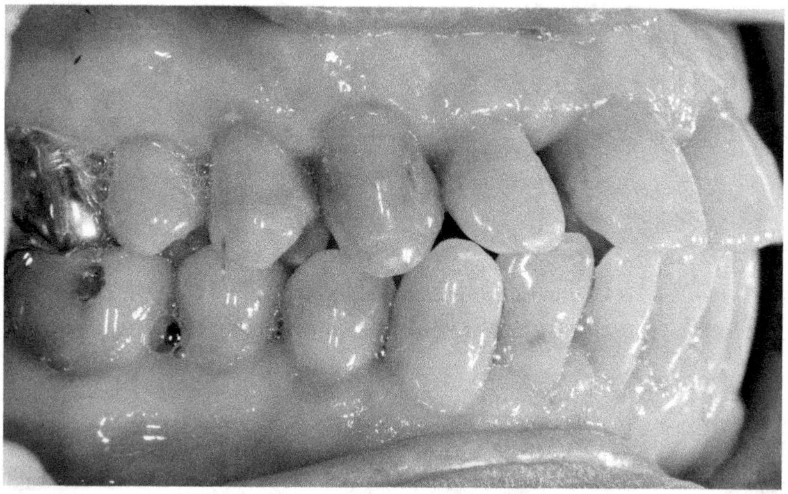

The control of balanced occlusal forces may have contributed to the improved tissue health, by redistributing the occlusal force overload away from the left side teeth, thereby minimizing the excess occlusal force as a periodontal risk factor. This is in accordance with Takeuchi's conclusions that the presence of one or more teeth with a high clinical attachment loss (CAL) and low occlusal force, might be possible risk factors for periodontal progression in the maintenance phase of periodontal therapy (Takeuchi et. al., 2010).

The hypothesis of Takeuchi suggests that the presence of an active periodontal lesion with demonstrable clinical attachment loss, can reduce the individual's "level of biting ability" (the individual's occlusal force capability, their occlusal pressure generating capability, and their amount of occlusal contact area. It has also been suggested that reduced "biting ability" can be a risk factor for the progression of periodontal disease during the maintenance phase.

Figure 11d. Pretreatment maxillary lingual occlusal view, showing widened sulci, with subgingival brown calculus, and significant tissue inflammation with edema present

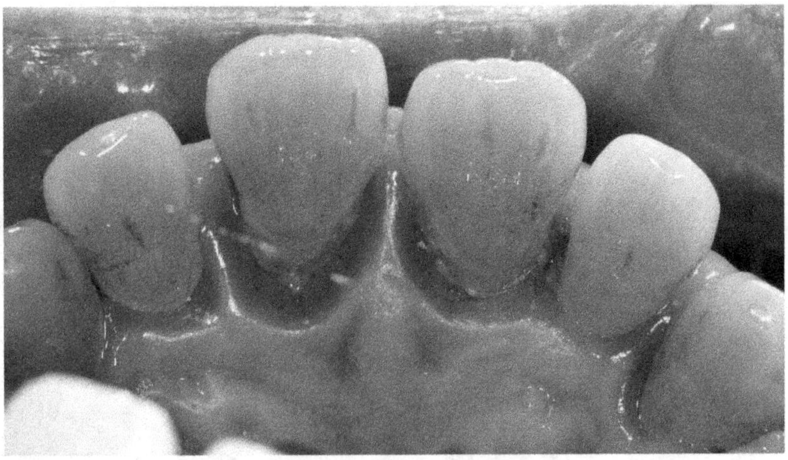

A 3-year long cohort study was performed on 223 previously treated periodontally diseased subjects using pressure-sensitive sheets that changed color to quantify static occlusal force (no timing measurement capability) (Dental Prescale, Type-R 50H; Fuji Film, Tokyo, Japan), where the occluded-through sheets were subsequently analyzed using an image scanner that measured each subject's occlusal contact area and occlusal pressure (Occluzer, FPD-707; Fuji Film, Tokyo, Japan) (Miyaura, et. al, 1999). The subjects, who all were in the maintenance phase of periodontal care but had been previously diagnosed with chronic periodontitis, received comprehensive periodontal care that included oral hygiene instruction, supra and subgingival plaque and tarter debridement, and the scaling and root planing of all pockets. The occlusal force value (N) per subject was determined from the scanned Prescale sheets, which was then compared to known human occlusal force norms for qualifying a subject's biting ability (>500 N for male subjects and >370 N for female subjects, was considered to be strong biting ability).

The authors found that the subject group that demonstrated high occlusal force capability had a better prognosis that periodontitis would not progress during maintenance (they were less likely to have periodontal disease progress or worsen), than did the group that demonstrated low occlusal force (Takeuchi et. al, 2010). This study's result also confirmed the findings of a previous cross-sectional study, in which periodontal destruction was significantly associated with the decreased biting ability of individual subjects (Takeuchi & Yamamoto, 2008).

In this presented case of chronic periodontitis (Figure 11a - l), the progression of chronic periodontitis was likely related to the significantly less occlusal force present both anteriorly, and on the right arch-half, that was in the presence of high clinical attachment loss. The patient's "biting ability" would be compromised by the poor occlusal force distribution because the left side teeth occluded firmly (generating increased occlusal force), while the right side teeth were much weaker force generators. This force imbalance meant the mandible was held up by the left teeth from fully engaging the maxilla into a solidly intercuspated position, which would likely lessen the patient's masticatory system from optimally chewing food and swallowing. This illustrated low occlusal force periodontal condition, is a very different physiologic state compared to when chronically applied excessive occlusal force causes direct occlusal trauma, and induces localized bone remodeling in response to the chronically applied

Figure 11e. Initial periodontal pocket probing described within a detailed periodontal chart. The charting noted more right-sided pockets, bleeding, and suppuration.

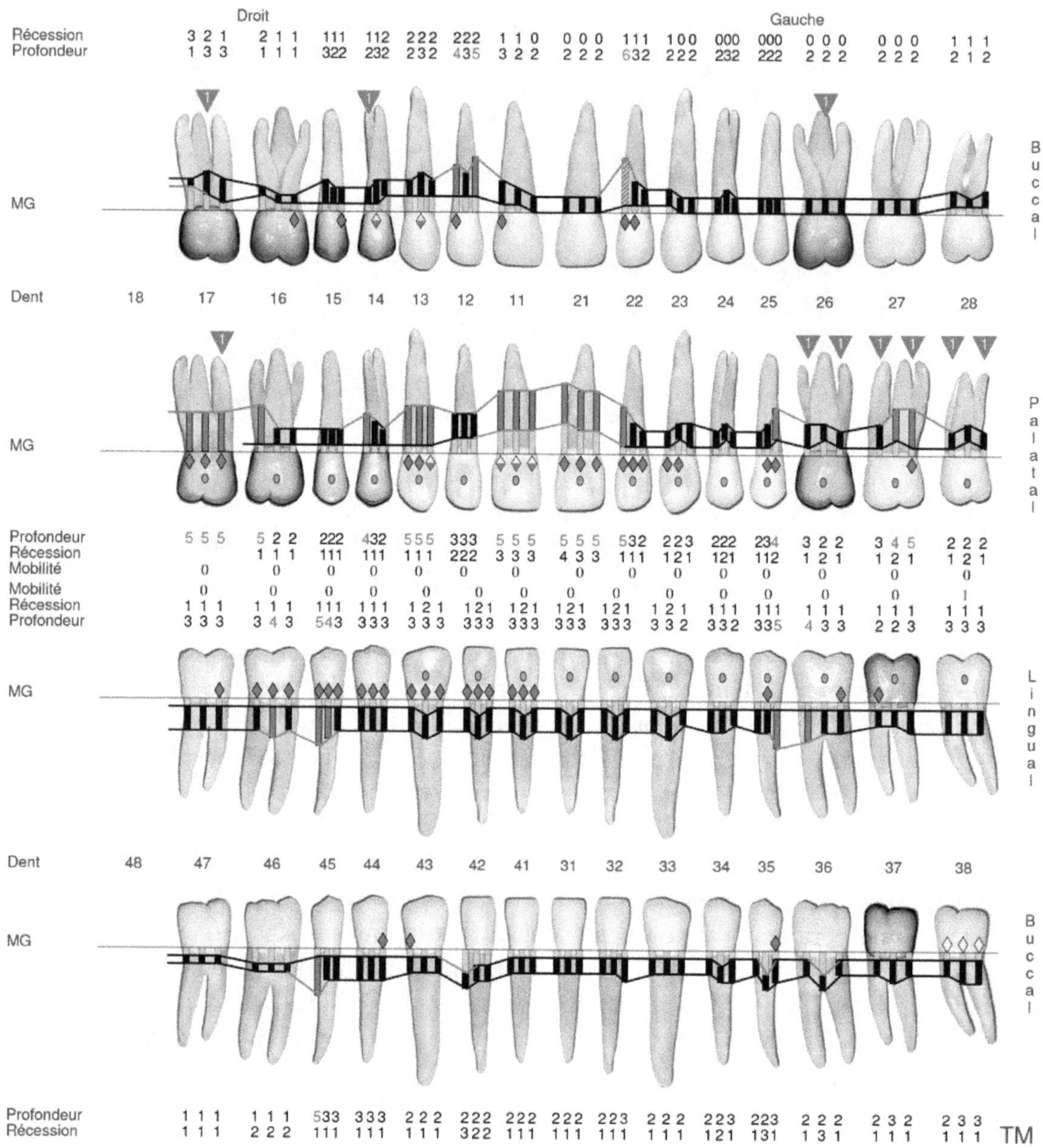

excessive occlusal force. Both of these clinical scenarios (unilateral reduced occlusal force, or contrarily localized occlusal force excess), can be diagnosed using the T-Scan system, such that both conditions should be treated accordingly during periodontal therapy.

The treatment of occlusion usually involves either a reversible approach consisting of some type of splint, or the more definitive selective reshaping of the occlusal surfaces. Orthodontic therapy is also an effective method of changing occlusal relationships and minimizing occlusal forces between opposing teeth. Appliance therapy has the advantage of being fully reversible. Selective reshaping involves

Figure 11f. Baseline T-Scan data showing an imbalance in the Center of Force, and lack of anterior tooth contact. There was twice as much occlusal force concentrated on the left arch-half compared to the right arch-half (69.4% left – 30.6% right).

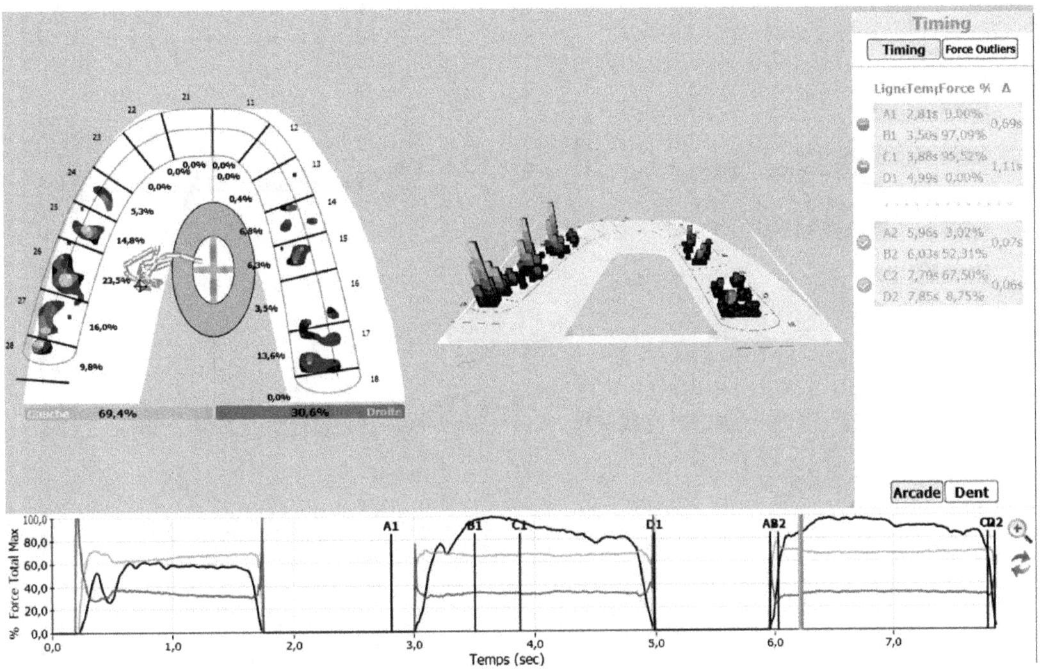

Figure 11g. T-Scan analysis showing the improved position of the Center of Force and the near-equalized overall bilateral occlusal force distribution improved from 69.4% left – 30.6% right (Figure 11f), to 56.6% left – 43.4% right.

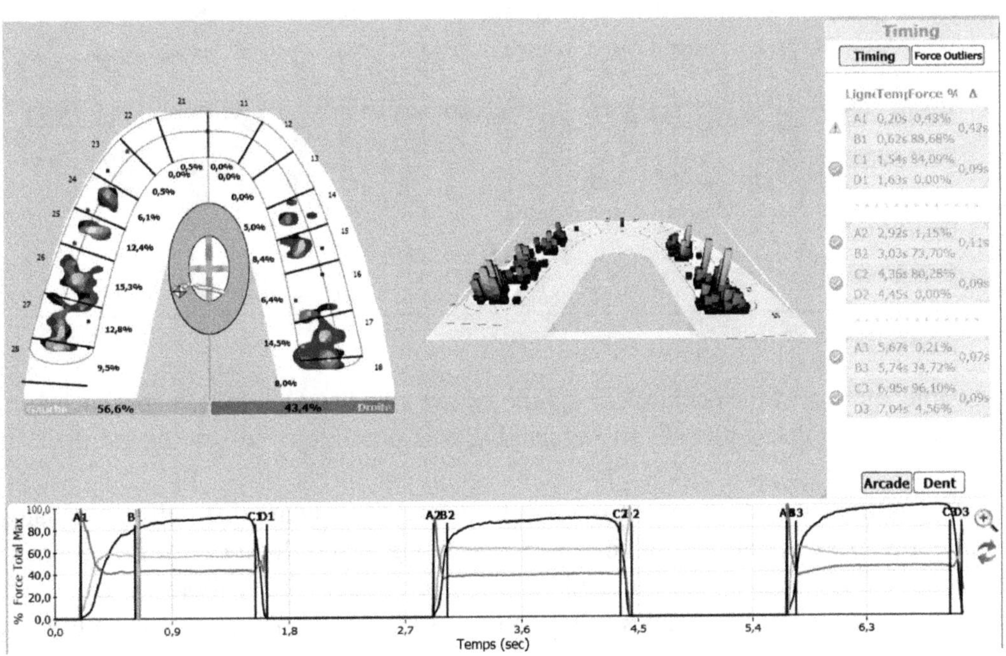

Figure 11h. Periodontal charting from control visit at one year shows reduced pocketing, suppuration and bleeding

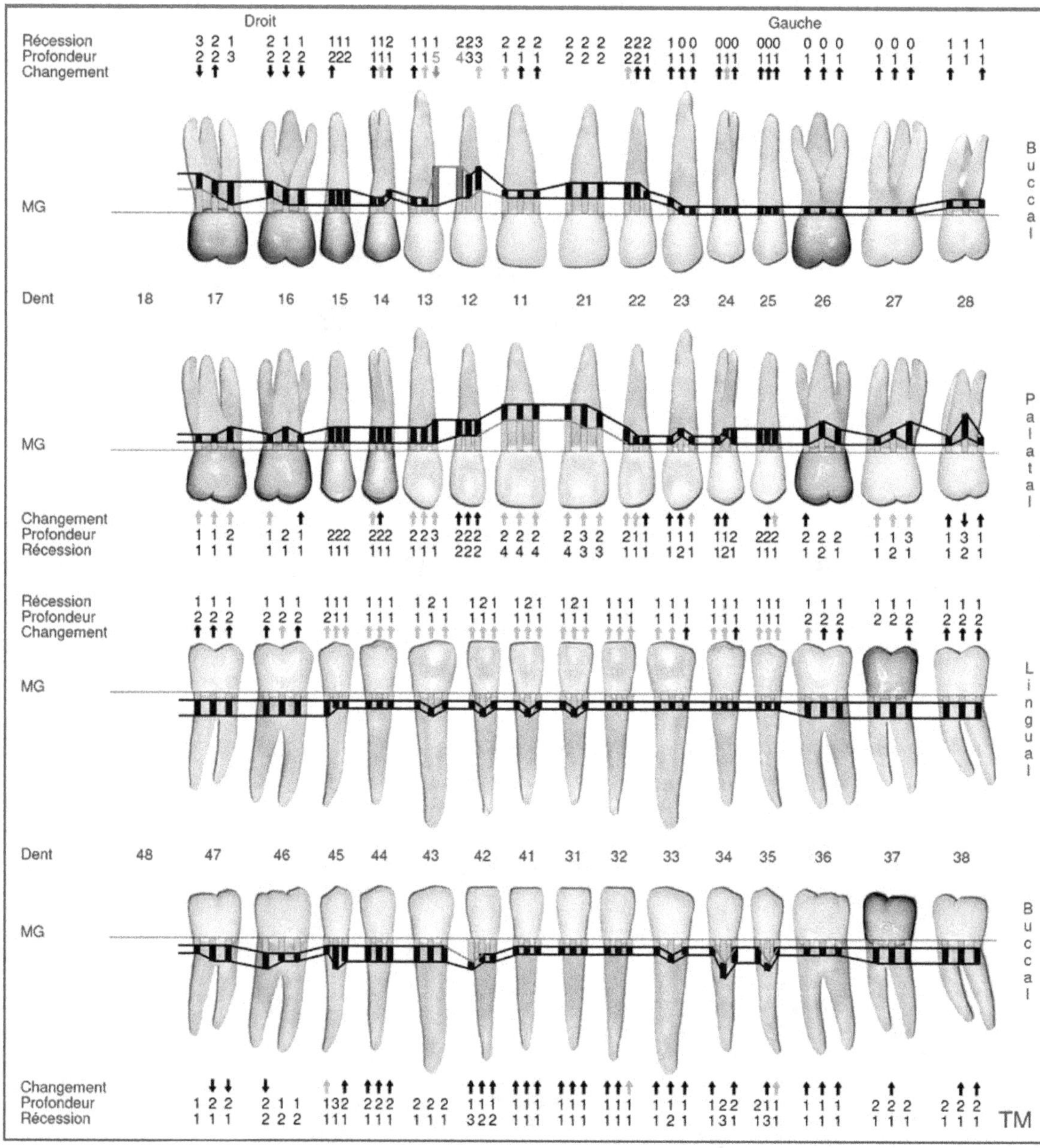

the non-reversible altering of the occlusal morphology, but an advantage of this approach compared to orthodontic treatment, is that with selective reshaping it is possible to lessen the overload applied to fragile teeth.

Measurement of the outcomes from unmeasured occlusal therapy are difficult to evaluate. In cases where the patient is experiencing discomfort from occlusal contact, the relief of heavy occlusal pressure by selective adjustment may elicit immediate relief of the patient's symptoms. However, in most periodontally diseased cases, the changes in outcome from occlusal treatment can only be measured

Figure 11i. The anterior maxillary occlusal lingual view, post treatment. Note the improved tissue color and the lack of edema present with no subgingival tarter causing tissue breakdown.

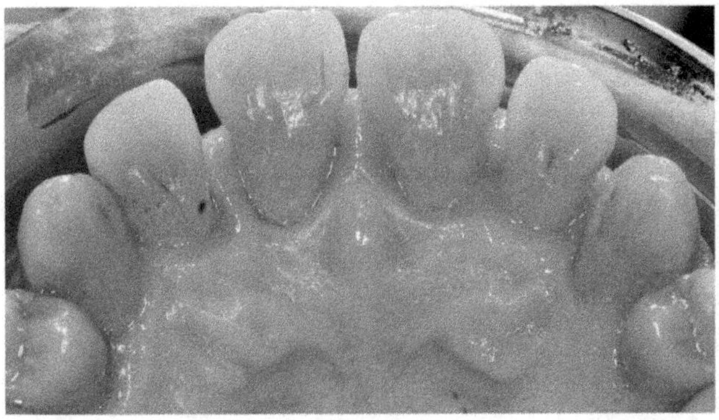

Figure 11j. The right-sided view of same patient in Figure 11c, 1- year post treatment

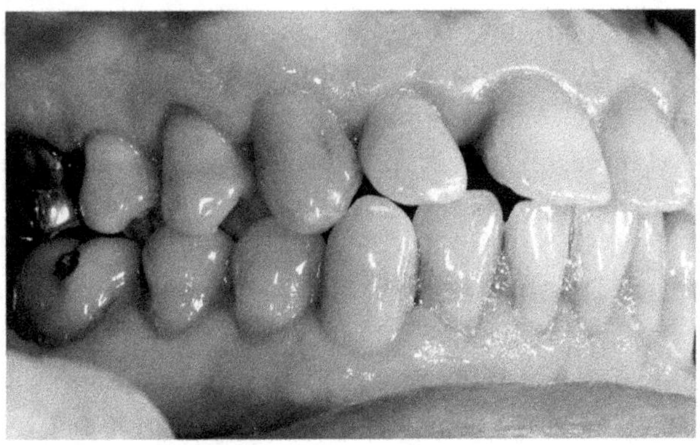

Figure 11k. The left-sided view of same patient in Figure 11b, 1- year post treatment. No pocketing, bleeding, and or suppuration was detected.

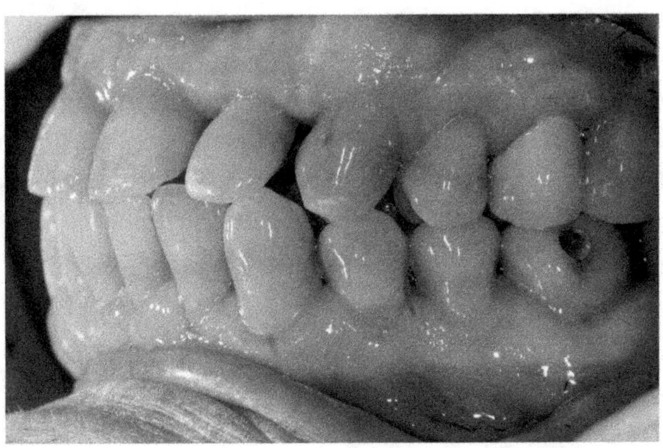

Figure 11l. The retracted frontal view in maximal intercuspation 1-year post treatment. Improved tissue health is readily visible.

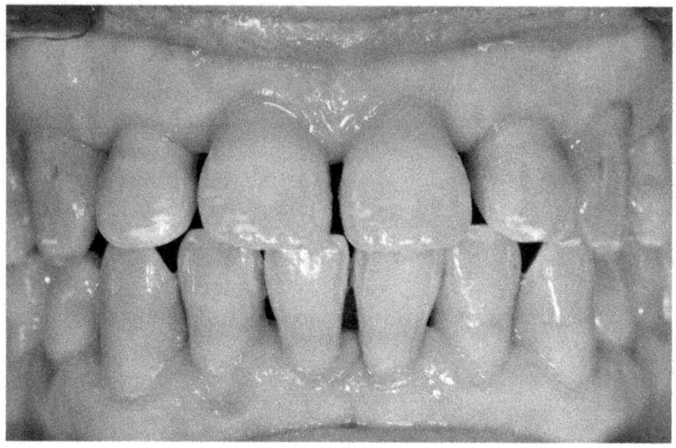

in terms of decreased mobility and long-term favorable results obtained from the rendered periodontal therapy. It is important to understand that because periodontal disease results from a combination of risk factors and contributing causes, long-term favorable outcomes are probably due to the elimination of all the risk factors. The treatment of periodontal disease then attempts to control the risk factors for the disease, including occlusal force, and smoking habits, as well as the debridement of deeper pockets which harbor reservoirs of plaque and bacteria.

Occlusion during the Maintenance Phase of Periodontal Therapy

The objective of periodontal maintenance therapy is to control the progression of periodontal disease, and to prevent its recurrence. Some studies have shown a correlation between changes in periodontal parameters and the occlusal contacts (Takeuchi et. al., 2010), such that control of the occlusal factors could be linked to good post-treatment healing. Despite the small number of publications relating to this topic, it is recommended that clinicians should continue to check the stability of the occlusal contacts over time. In this respect, the T-Scan system is a great asset, because it makes it possible to compare different recordings of the same patient made over passing time. It provides a veritable dynamic memory for the practitioner, while creating an occlusal history of the patient's disease state.

The post-treatment occlusal status can be used as a reference for assessing improvements obtained from treatment, and for future comparisons made during the maintenance phase. During therapy as well as during maintenance, any tooth loss will modify the occlusal force distribution, such that T-Scan data can provide a reliable method for periodontists to analyze the occlusal consequences of such changes in a patient's long-term periodontal status. Changes that result in a deleterious occlusal force distribution can be readily corrected when guided by recently recorded T-Scan data.

SOLUTIONS AND RECOMMENDATIONS

The successful treatment of periodontal disease requires the control of all contributory risk factors. The treatment of occlusal discrepancies and occlusal trauma should be viewed in the context of attempting to control one of the risk factors contributing to periodontal disease progression. If occlusal discrepancies exist in the presence of active periodontal disease, the occlusal factors should be controlled by minimizing the occlusal forces and their impact on compromised teeth. Computer-guided occlusal treatment should be rendered within the periodontal treatment plan, to lessen occlusal overload to any periodontally compromised teeth. This will assist in improving periodontal treatment outcomes, providing for lessened tooth mobility, and reducing the formation of abfractive root defects that compromise tissue attachment levels.

Therefore, it is this author's recommendation that the field of Periodontics, and specifically Periodontists themselves, at this time in the digital era of Dental Medicine, seriously consider employing computer-guided, T-Scan based force control, as part of managing occlusal force-related periodontal risk factors. It is this author's additional recommendation that occlusal treatment should be performed where indicated, as a routine part of periodontal therapy even in the absence of significant tooth mobility.

FUTURE RESEARCH DIRECTIONS

In the long term, it would be interesting to study the integration of computerized occlusal analysis into the everyday practice of Periodontology. Measured control of the occlusal factors would undoubtedly facilitate the identification of positive and negative responders to treatment among patients undergoing active periodontal disease treatment. The challenge will be to find a way to perform a Randomized Controlled Trail on the relationship between occlusion and periodontal disease. The T-Scan system could help to identify more occlusal parameters that could help clinicians stabilize periodontally compromised patients over the long-term.

A study could be designed and performed to compare periodontal treatment rendered with and without T-Scan-guided occlusal force control using 2 groups; one with T-Scan occlusal corrections as part of treatment, and one without, where all other risk factors are matched, and all subjects are preliminarily assessed with the T-Scan.

It would be also very interesting to analyze how occlusal forces contribute to favorable healing after periodontal surgery. Indeed, two groups of patients which both need periodontal surgery could be followed in the days after surgery, to correlate a possible influence of occlusal forces on the mucosal healing time, as well as on the quality of the healing across equal time frames.

The T-Scan system could be also very helpful in analyzing healing after implant treatment. One challenge of implant treatment is to restore the patient with a functioning prosthesis, as soon as is feasible, post implantation. Immediate loading is a non-predictable technique because of the difficulties of controlling occlusal contact forces after implant placement. Two groups of patients could be analyzed in a clinical study; one with the T-Scan system controlling the immediately loaded occlusion, and one group solely treated with articulating paper. The results of this type of study could help clinicians to determine a method that predictably increased successful outcomes when immediately loading implant restorations.

Some authors describe employing progressive loading on implants (Misch et. al., 2004). But, the lack of an appropriate technology to prove the degree of loading during the progressive load period, and the true impact of occlusion or the absence of occlusion, on the stability of recently installed implants, has proved difficult to assess in a study environment. A double blind randomized controlled study with two implant prosthesis groups could be designed, where one group undergoes T-Scan guided occlusal force control following initial implant placement and loading, while the other group has no T-Scan guided occlusal control after implant placement. The findings of this type of study could demonstrate if a relationship exists between applied occlusal forces and the degree of peri-implant bone density obtainable around progressively loaded implant prostheses.

CONCLUSION

The correlation between periodontal status and occlusal force remains a matter of debate. Occlusal force, which is a mechanical stress applied to the supportive tissues, has always been considered to not initiate, nor accelerate, periodontal attachment loss resultant from inflammatory periodontal disease. However, the absence of a validated device or quantifying method for analyzing the occlusion, has contributed to the confusion and questions that exist in the scientific community about the relationship between periodontal disease and occlusion.

The T-Scan system is an occlusal measurement technology that is definitively more reproducible than are articulating paper markings, providing the Periodontist with an objective analysis of the relative occlusal forces of many tooth contacts, thereby making it possible to demonstrate periodontal disease progression that has been influenced occlusally. Moreover, T-Scan data can guide the diagnosis and treatment of periodontal disease, and be included as a monitoring device during periodontal maintenance.

REFERENCES

Bernhardt, O., Gesch, D., Look, J. O., Hodges, J. S., Schwahn, C., Mack, F., & Kocher, T. (2006). The influence of dynamic occlusal interferences on probing depth and attachment level: Results of the Study of Health in Pomerania (SHIP). *Journal of Periodontology*, *77*(3), 506–516. doi:10.1902/jop.2006.050167 PMID:16512766

Branschofsky, M., Beikler, T., Schafer, R., Flemming, T. F., & Lang, H. (2011). Secondary trauma from occlusion and periodontitis. *Quintessence International*, *42*(6), 515–522. PMID:21519589

Burgett, F. G., Ramfjord, S. P., Nissle, R. R., Morrison, E. C., Charbeneau, T. D., & Caffesse, R. G. (1992). A randomized trial of occlusal adjustment in the treatment of periodontitis patients. *Journal of Clinical Periodontology*, *19*(6), 381–387. doi:10.1111/j.1600-051X.1992.tb00666.x PMID:1634627

Bush, F. M. (1984). Occlusal therapy in the management of chronic orofacial pain. *Anesthesia Progress*, *31*(1), 10–16. PMID:6375467

Carranza, F. A. Jr. (1987). *Glickman's Periodontology*. Philadelphia, PA: WB Saunders, Co.

Celenza, F. V. (1984). The theory and clinical management of centric positions: II. Centric relation and centric relation occlusion. *The International Journal of Periodontics & Restorative Dentistry*, *4*(6), 62–86. PMID:6597180

Ericsson, I., & Lindhe, J. (1977). Lack of effect of trauma from occlusion on the recurrence of experimental periodontitis. *Journal of Clinical Periodontology*, *4*(2), 115–127. doi:10.1111/j.1600-051X.1977.tb01891.x PMID:266504

Ericsson, I., & Lindhe, J. (1982). Effect of longstanding jiggling on experimental marginal periodontitis in the beagle dog. *Journal of Clinical Periodontology*, *9*(6), 497–503. doi:10.1111/j.1600-051X.1982.tb02111.x PMID:6960025

Fleszar, T. J., Knowles, J. W., Morrison, E. C., Burgett, F. G., Nissle, R. R., & Ramfjord, S. P. (1980). Tooth mobility and periodontal therapy. *Journal of Clinical Periodontology*, *7*(6), 495–505. doi:10.1111/j.1600-051X.1980.tb02156.x PMID:6938529

Foz, A. M., Artese, H. P., Horliana, A. C., Pannuti, C. M., & Romito, G. A. (2012). Occlusal adjustment associated with periodontal therapy--a systematic review. *Journal of Dentistry*, *40*(12), 1025–1035. doi:10.1016/j.jdent.2012.09.002 PMID:22982113

Gher, M. E. (1996). Non-surgical pocket therapy: dental occlusion. *Annals of Periodontology, 1*(1), 567-580. doi: 10.1902/annals.1996.1.1.567

Glickman, I. (1967). Occlusion and the periodontium. *Journal of Dental Research*, *46*(1), 53–59. doi:10.1177/00220345670460014101 PMID:5227129

Green, M. S., & Levine, D. F. (1996). Occlusion and the periodontium: A review and rationale for treatment. *Journal of the California Dental Association*, *24*(10), 19–27. PMID:9120603

Hallmon, W. W. (1999). Occlusal trauma: effect and impact on the periodontium. *Annals of Periodontology, 4*(1), 102-108. doi: 10.1902/annals.1999.4.1.102

Harrel, S. K., & Nunn, M. E. (2001). The effect of occlusal discrepancies on periodontitis II. Relationship of occlusal treatment to the progression of periodontal disease. *Journal of Periodontology*, *72*(4), 495–505. doi:10.1902/jop.2001.72.4.495 PMID:11338302

Harrel, S. K., & Nunn, M. E. (2009). The association of occlusal contacts with the presence of increased periodontal probing depth. *Journal of Clinical Periodontology*, *36*(1), 1035–1042. doi:10.1111/j.1600-051X.2009.01486.x PMID:19930093

Kaku, M., Uoshima, K., Yamashita, Y., & Miura, H. (2005). Investigation of periodontal ligament reaction upon excessive occlusal load-osteopontin induction among periodontal ligament cells. *Journal of Periodontal Research*, *40*(1), 59–66. doi:10.1111/j.1600-0765.2004.00773.x PMID:15613081

Kantor, M., Polson, A. M., & Zander, H. A. (1976). Alveolar bone regeneration after removal of inflammatory and traumatic factors. *Journal of Periodontology*, *47*(12), 687–695. doi:10.1902/jop.1976.47.12.687 PMID:825630

Kardesler, L., Buduneli, N., Cetinkalp, S., & Kinane, D. F. (2010). Adipokines and inflammatory mediators after initial periodontal treatment in patients with type 2 diabetes and chronic periodontitis. *Journal of Periodontology*, *81*(1), 24–33. doi:10.1902/jop.2009.090267 PMID:20059414

Karolyi, M. (1901). Beobachtungen über pyorrhea alveolaris. *Öst. Ung. Vierteeljschr Zahnheilk*, *17*, 279.

Karpinia, K., Magnusson, I., Gibbs, C., & Yang, M. C. (2004). Accuracy of probing attachment levels using a CEJ probe versus traditional probes. *Journal of Clinical Periodontology*, *31*(3), 173–176. doi:10.1111/j.0303-6979.2004.00464.x PMID:15016020

Keown, A. J., Bush, M. B., Ford, C., Lee, J. J., Constantino, P. J., & Lawn, B. R. (2012). Fracture susceptibility of worn teeth. *Journal of the Mechanical Behavior of Biomedical Materials*, *5*(1), 47–256. doi:10.1016/j.jmbbm.2011.08.028 PMID:22100100

Keown, A. J., Lee, J. J., & Bush, M. B. (2012). Fracture behavior of human molars. *Journal of Materials Science. Materials in Medicine*, *23*(12), 2847–2856. doi:10.1007/s10856-012-4756-6 PMID:22956116

Lang, N. P., & Tonetti, M. S. (1996). Periodontal diagnosis in treated periodontitis. Why, when and how to use clinical parameters. *Journal of Clinical Periodontology*, *233*(Pt. 2), 240–250. doi:10.1111/j.1600-051X.1996.tb02083.x PMID:8707984

Lee, J. J., Kwon, J. Y., Chai, H., Lucas, P. W., Thompson, V. P., & Lawn, B. R. (2009). Fracture modes in human teeth. *Journal of Dental Research*, *88*(3), 224–228. doi:10.1177/0022034508330055 PMID:19329454

Lindhe, J., & Ericsson, I. (1976). The influence of trauma from occlusion on reduced but healthy periodontal tissues in dogs. *Journal of Clinical Periodontology*, *3*(2), 110–122. doi:10.1111/j.1600-051X.1976.tb01857.x PMID:1064595

Lindhe, J., & Ericsson, I. (1982). The effect of elimination of jiggling forces on periodontally exposed teeth in the dog. *Journal of Periodontology*, *53*(9), 562–567. doi:10.1902/jop.1982.53.9.562 PMID:6957593

Lindhe, J., Karring, T., & Lang, N. (2008). *Clinical Periodontology and Implant Dentistry* (5th ed.). Oxford, UK: Blackwell Publishing.

Lindhe, J., & Svanberg, G. (1974). Influence of trauma from occlusion on progression of experimental periodontitis in the beagle dog. *Journal of Clinical Periodontology*, *1*(1), 3–14. doi:10.1111/j.1600-051X.1974.tb01234.x PMID:4532114

Misch, C. E., Wang, H. L., Misch, C. M., Sharawy, M., Lemons, J., & Judy, K. W. (2004). Rationale for the application of immediate load in implant dentistry: Part I. *Implant Dentistry*, *13*(3), 207–217. doi:10.1097/01.id.0000140461.25451.31 PMID:15359155

Miyaura, K., Matsuka, Y., Morita, M., Yamashita, A., & Watanabe, T. (1999). Comparison of biting forces in different age and sex groups: A study of biting efficiency with mobile and non-mobile teeth. *Journal of Oral Rehabilitation*, *26*(3), 223–227. doi:10.1046/j.1365-2842.1999.00364.x PMID:10194731

Nunn, M. E., & Harrel, S. K.Relationship of Initial Occlusal Discrepancies to Initial Clinical Parameters. (2001). The effect of occlusal discrepancies on periodontitis. I. Relationship of initial occlusal discrepancies to initial clinical parameters. *Journal of Periodontology*, *72*(4), 485–494. doi:10.1902/jop.2001.72.4.485 PMID:11338301

Orban, B., & Weinmann, J. P. (1933). Signs of traumatic occlusion in average human jaws. *Journal of Dental Research*, *13*, 216.

Oringer, R. J., Fiorellini, J. P., Koch, G. G., Sharp, T. J., Nevins, M. L., Davis, G. H., & Howell, T. H. (1997). Comparison of manual and automated probing in an untreated periodontitis population. *Journal of Periodontology*, *68*(12), 1156–1162. doi:10.1902/jop.1997.68.12.1156 PMID:9444589

Parameter on occlusal traumatism in patients with chronic periodontitis. American Academy of Periodontology. (2000). *Journal ofPeriodontology*, *71*(5 Suppl.), 873-875. doi: 10.1902/jop.2000.71.5-S.873

Polson, A. M. (1974). Trauma and progression of marginal periodontitis in squirrel monkeys. II. Co-destructive factors of periodontitis and mechanically-produced injury. *Journal of Periodontal Research*, *9*(2), 108–113. doi:10.1111/j.1600-0765.1974.tb00661.x PMID:4277746

Polson, A. M., Kennedy, J. E., & Zander, H. A. (1972). Effect of traumatic injury on the progression of marginal periodontitis. *Journal of Periodontal Research*, *10*, 17. PMID:4272216

Polson, A. M., Kennedy, J. E., & Zander, H. A. (1974). Trauma and progression of marginal periodontitis in squirrel monkeys. I. Co-destructive factors of periodontitis and thermally-produced injury. *Journal of Periodontal Research*, *9*(2), 100–107. doi:10.1111/j.1600-0765.1974.tb00660.x PMID:4277745

Polson, A. M., Meitner, S. W., & Zander, H. A. (1976). Trauma and progression of marginal periodontitis in squirrel monkeys IV. Reversibility of bone loss due to trauma alone and trauma superimposed upon periodontitis. *Journal of Periodontal Research*, *11*(5), 290–298. doi:10.1111/j.1600-0765.1976.tb00083.x PMID:133236

Quirynen, M., Bollen, C. M., Vandekerckhove, B. N., Dekeyser, C., Papaioannou, W., & Eyssen, H. (1995). Full- vs. partial-mouth disinfection in the treatment of periodontal infections: Short-term clinical and microbiological observations. *Journal of Dental Research*, *74*(8), 1459–1467. doi:10.1177/00220345950740080501 PMID:7560400

Rees, J. S. (2001). An investigation into the importance of the periodontal ligament and alveolar bone as supporting structures in finite element studies. *Journal of Oral Rehabilitation*, *28*(5), 425–432. doi:10.1046/j.1365-2842.2001.00686.x PMID:11380782

Rosling, B., Nyman, S., Lindhe, J., & Jern, B. (1976). The healing potential of the periodontal tissues following different techniques of periodontal surgery in plaque-free dentitions. A 2-year clinical study. *Journal of Clinical Periodontology*, *3*(4), 233–250. doi:10.1111/j.1600-051X.1976.tb00042.x PMID:1069012

Sanz, M. (2005). Occlusion in a periodontal context. *The International Journal of Prosthodontics*, *18*(4), 309–310. PMID:16052783

Stillman, P. (1917). The management of pyorrhea. *Dental Cosmos*, *59*, 405–414.

Stones, H. H. (1938). An Experimental Investigation into the Association of Traumatic Occlusion with Parodontal Disease: (Section of Odontology). *Proceedings of the Royal Society of Medicine*, *31*(5), 479–495. PMID:19991440

Takeuchi, N., Ekuni, D., Yamamoto, T., & Morita, M. (2010). Relationship between the prognosis of periodontitis and occlusal force during the maintenance phase – a cohort study. *Journal of Periodontal Research*, *45*(5), 612–617. doi:10.1111/j.1600-0765.2010.01273.x PMID:20546114

Takeuchi, N., & Yamamoto, T. (2008). Correlation between periodontal status and biting force in patients with chronic periodontitis during the maintenance phase of therapy. *Journal of Clinical Periodontology*, *35*(3), 215–220. doi:10.1111/j.1600-051X.2007.01186.x PMID:18190555

Waerhaug, J. (1979). The angular bone defect and its relationship to trauma from occlusion and downgrowth of subgingival plaque. *Journal of Clinical Periodontology*, *6*(2), 61–82. doi:10.1111/j.1600-051X.1979.tb02185.x PMID:287677

Weinmann, J. (1941). Progress of gingival inflammation into the supporting structures of the teeth. *The Journal of Periodontology*, *12*, 71–82.

Yoshinaga, Y., Ukai, T., Abe, Y., & Hara, Y. (2007). Expression of receptor activator of nuclear factor kappa B ligand relates to inflammatory bone resorption, with or without occlusal trauma, in rats. *Journal of Periodontal Research*, *42*(5), 402–409. doi:10.1111/j.1600-0765.2007.00960.x PMID:17760817

ADDITIONAL READING

Dawson, P. E. (2006). *Functional Occlusion: From TMJ to Smile Design* (pp. 1–648). Maryland Heights, MO: Elsevier Health Sciences.

Goudot, P., Lacoste, J. P., & Fumat, C. (2013). *Guide Pratique d'Implantologie* (pp. 1–248). Paris, France: Elsevier Health Sciences.

Lindhe, J., Lang, N. P., & Karring, T. (2009). *Clinical Periodontology and Implant Dentistry*. Oxford, UK: Wiley.

Misch, C. E. (2008). *Contemporary Implant Dentistry* (pp. 1–1102). Maryland Heights, MO: Mosby Elsevier.

Newman, M. G., Takei, H. H., Klokkevold, P. R., & Carranza, F. A. (2011). *Carranza's Clinical Periodontology* (pp. 1–872). Maryland Heights, MO: Elsevier Health Science Division.

Okeson, J. P. (2007). *Management of Temporomandibular Disorders and Occlusion* (pp. 1–640). St. Louis, MO: Elsevier Health Sciences Division.

KEY TERMS AND DEFINITIONS

Full Mouth Disinfection: An intense course of treatment for periodontitis, typically involving scaling and root planning in combination with adjunctive use of local antimicrobials, such as chlorhexidine, applied to the diseased tissues by various intraoral methods. The aim of this therapy is complete debridement of all periodontal pocket areas within a very short time frame (in 24 hours), to minimize the chance of re-infection from pathogens that reside in other oral niches like the tongue, tonsils, and non-treated periodontal pockets.

Jiggling: When an applied constraint to a tooth alternates in two opposite directions (i.e. only buccal-lingual or only mesial-distal), where the tooth no longer is able to move in any given direction. Jiggling is different from the movement resultant from the continuous unidirectional force applied by an orthodontic device. Functional (non-constrained) mobility is therefore stronger, and more uncontrolled compared to the mobility induced by orthodontic treatment, which is somewhat controlled.

Occlusal Trauma: Occlusal trauma describes changes in the periodontal state due to the applied force of the masticatory muscles.

Periodontal Attachment Loss: A reduction in the connective tissue attachment to both the root of the tooth and to the alveolar bone. It is usually caused by persistent inflammation of the gingival and periodontal tissues, and can be worsened by occlusal trauma.

Periodontal Disease: An inflammatory disease process affecting the soft and hard structures that support the teeth, often caused by local pathogens combined with other contributory risk factors.

Periodontal Maintenance Therapy: Following active periodontal therapy, maintenance is necessary to preserve the results obtained during the active therapy, and to prevent further periodontal disease breakdown. Maintenance is an extension of active periodontal therapy, requiring the combined efforts of both the Periodontist and the patient.

Primary Occlusal Trauma: Occlusal trauma observed on teeth without reduced periodontal bone height.

Secondary Occlusal Trauma: Occlusal trauma observed on teeth with reduced periodontal bone height.

This work was previously published in the Handbook of Research on Computerized Occlusal Analysis Technology Applications in Dental Medicine edited by Robert B. Kerstein, DMD, pages 791-828, copyright year 2015 by Medical Information Science Reference (an imprint of IGI Global).

Chapter 3
Force Finishing in Dental Medicine:
A Simplified Approach to Occlusal Harmony

Sushil Koirala
Thammasat University, Thailand & Vedic Institute of Smile Aesthetics (VISA), Nepal

ABSTRACT

This chapter introduces the Force Finishing concept that is based upon the T-Scan technology. During case finishing, the aesthetic components are clinically visible and guided by the subjective analyses of the patient and the clinician. Alternatively, the case occlusal force components are invisible and do not become apparent until their adverse effects become chronic. When the force components are not properly addressed, clinicians may encounter Occlusal Force Disorder (OFD) symptomatology. Often, clinicians focus on the aesthetic finishing while placing a low priority on the occlusal Force Finishing by relying on subjective articulating paper mark interpretation and the patient's subjective "feel" with which to guide occlusal adjustments. Because articulating paper is a poor indicator of occlusal force and timing, the T-Scan technology can greatly improve the occlusal case finishing. This chapter details how to integrate the Force Finishing concept into conventional case finishing to simplify achieving occlusal force harmony in every case.

INTRODUCTION

It is now more than 100 years that both dentists and researchers have debated how to identify and define concepts of Dental Occlusion that could be practically applied in both diagnostic and therapeutic situations. Occlusion has been, and still to some extent, is a controversial discipline, as there are numerous questions related to occlusal characteristics which have not yet been answered with scientific certainty. There are many diverse and polarized opinions regarding this subject that are seldom based on current scientific evidence, such as the etiology of Bruxism, the role of occlusion in Temporomandibular Disorders (TMD), Orthodontic treatment and its effects on TMD pain, and determining a correct mandibular position as a reference point for treatment.

DOI: 10.4018/978-1-5225-1903-4.ch003

Clinicians around the world routinely perform various diagnostic and therapeutic procedures that involve Dental Occlusion (fillings, crowns, bridges, removable prosthesis, implant supported restorations, full mouth reconstruction, and orthodontics). However, there is a lack of scientific studies verifying the success of the different advocated concepts of occlusion used restoratively and during occlusal therapy. Nor are the methods to validate or the variable of an individual clinician's knowledge, clinical skills, and comfort zone with successfully treating occlusal problems. Generally, during the undergraduate education, dental students are not fully trained in Dental Occlusion. When these new graduates enter into clinical practice and begin accepting complex clinical cases to treat, many become confused with the differing theoretical recommendations and varied concepts about Dental Occlusion that are taught within academic and clinical Dental Medicine.

This chapter first discusses the many mandibular positional theories and the controversies surrounding each one, based upon their available clinical evidence. Next, the occlusal and other intraoral forces (applied stresses) are briefly discussed, that act on the Stomatognathic system during function and parafunction. Lastly, the chapter introduces the *Force Finishing* concept and its protocol to diagnose, prevent, and manage the occlusal force disorders in clinical practice.

Occlusion in Dental Medicine is a Mixture of Science and Art

The study of occlusion in Dental Medicine has two components; the science and the art. The science component of occlusion addresses how teeth fit together, and how the forces generated within the masticatory system affect the teeth and supportive structures. However, the subjective response of the patient to their occlusal "feel", and its customized management by clinicians is more of an art than a science.

Human beings are blessed with excellent adaptive capacity, hence, it is not surprising to observe that many patients adopt various occlusal schemes delivered by differing clinicians, that are based upon the clinician's knowledge, occlusal skill, and comfort rendering the occlusal treatment. Hence, in the clinical practice of occlusion, a clinician must follow some scientific basis, and use his or her artistic skills to respect the patient's ability to physiologically adapt.

A review of the literature regarding the history of Dental Occlusion suggests that occlusion can be divided into three physiologic stages (Dawson, 1989; Moffett, Johnson, & McCabe et al.,1964; Okeson, 1993; Ramfjord & Ash, 1983):

- **Normal Occlusion:** Commonly known as " physiologic " occlusion, which suggests that treatment is not required.
- **Pathologic Occlusion:** Also known as "non-physiologic", which suggests that treatment may be required.
- **Therapeutic Occlusion:** Often referred as to as an "ideal" or treatment occlusion.

Additionally, there are three treatment categories routinely employed in occlusal treatment:

- **Occlusal Maintenance:** In this category, a limited number of restorations are introduced to a physiologically acceptable original occlusal scheme.
- **Occlusal Modification:** In this category, only minor to moderate changes or improvement are made to the original occlusal scheme (minor occlusion adjustment, tooth movement, or opposing

tooth restoration, or replacement), that is either physiologically acceptable, or non-physiologic and unacceptable.

- **Occlusal Re-Establishment:** In this category, major changes are required to improve a non-physiologic, unacceptable occlusal scheme. There is often a need to establish a new intercuspal position and/or establish a new occlusal vertical dimension.

Clinically, the maintenance and modification categories are considered easier to accomplish when compared to the re-establishment category, because the maintenance and modification categories are founded on both the existing intercuspal position and the pre treatment vertical dimension of occlusion. However, when an occlusal scheme requires re-establishment of a new intercuspal position and/or vertical dimension, a new reference position is required, because the original intercuspal position is no longer available for clinician to use as the reference point. This is one of the major clinical areas in Dental Medicine where many clinicians may become confused as to how to design a new occlusal scheme.

Mandibular Position Theories

Confusion generally arises resultant from the various differing theories available, regarding the selection of a reference position for the newly-determined, proper mandibular relation. These theories, known as *Mandibular Position Theories*, differ in where the mandibular position should be located during the diagnosis and treatment, with regards to the position of the mandibular condyle within the glenoid fossa of the Temporomandibular joints. The selected condyler position directly affects the occlusion because the condyles and the teeth each occupy opposite ends of the solid mandible.

The differing mandibularposition theories are:

- **Intercuspal Position (A Tooth Contact Dedicated Position; ICP):** This tooth contact guided mandibular position is the most reproducible reference position.

This tooth contact position is where the mandibular closing muscles contract with maximum contractile activity (Miller, 1966). In a physiologically accepted mandibular position, ICP is the most used reference position in a day- to-day restorative dental practice. The sensory input received from the periodontal ligament sensory mechanoreceptors and from existing muscle memory, allows the mandible to open and close rapidly and repeatedly, and intercuspate all occluding teeth in the same mandibular position.

A small percentage of the subjects (10% to 14%) demonstrate an identical ICP in the Centric Relation (CR) position, where CR = ICP naturally) (Beyron, 1969; Rieder, 1978). However, a much large percentage of individuals demonstrate an ICP - CR difference of approximately 0.1 to 1.5 mm (between the retruded centric position (RCP) and ICP). This 1.5 mm positional displacement is known as a Centric Slide, which occurs in all three planes. In one study, the ICP-CR slide was measured to be 0.1 to 1.5 mm vertically, 0.1 to 1.0 mm horizontally, and less that 1 mm transversely (Rieder, 1978).

Alternative Mandibular Position Theories to ICP

Clinicians may encounter an unacceptable ICP during patient evaluations, such that three alternative concepts that can be used to relate the mandible to the cranium on a relatively repeatable basis. These three theories are:

- **Centric Relation:** Based upon a Temporomandibular joint-ligamentous position.
- **Neuromuscular:** Based upon a muscle-dedicated position.
- **Anterior Protrusion:** Based upon a radiographic determination of the condyle located on the articular eminence.

Additional clinical literature describes using various other muscles to establish the mandibular relationship. These techniques rely on the tongue, the closest speaking space (Pound, 1976), the rest position (Thompson, 1964), or patient voluntarily repeated mandibular closure. However, these methods have not been deemed reliable or easily standardized.

- **Centric Relation Theory (TM Joint-Ligamentous Dedicated Position):** This concept was first described in 1935 (Schuyler, 1935). It should be noted that the definition of Centric Relation has changed within the literature, due to improvements in mandibular manipulation techniques and new knowledge regarding the anatomic and physiologic position of the condyle.
  Earlier definitions describe Centric Relation (CR) as the most superior retruded position of the condyles. (Boucher, 1963; Posselt, 1952; Boucher, 1970). Since this position is determined mainly by the ligaments of the TMJ, it was described as ligamentous position. It became popular among Prosthodontists because CR was a reproducible mandibular position that could facilitate the construction of complete dentures (Boucher, 1970). It has been suggested that the condyles should be in their most superior *posterior* position against the eminentia, irrespective of vertical dimension or tooth position (Dawson, 1989). However, with more recent understanding of the biomechanics and function of the TMJ, the most superior retruded position has been questioned, such that presently, the most superior *anterior* position (Dawson's position) of the condyle has been deemed the most orthopedically stable position of the condyle in the fossa. The 7th edition of the Glossary of Prosthodontic Term defines Centric Relation as the maxillomandibular relationship in which the condyles articulate with the thinnest avascular portion of their respective disks, with the complex in the anterior-superior position against the slopes of the articular eminencies (Van Blarcom, 1999). It should be noted that when posterior force is applied to the mandible, it is resisted in the Temporomandibular joint by the inner fibers of the Temporomandibular ligament. If this ligament is tight, there may be very little difference between the most superior retruded position, the most superior position (Dawson's position), and the most anterior-superior position (Okeson, 2013). But, if the ligament is loose or elongated, an anterioposterior range of movement can occur while the condyle remains in its most superior position (Okeson, 2013).
  Locating the Centric Relation position can, at times be clinically difficult to achieve. To reproduce the Centric Relation position predictably, there are two accepted clinical techniques routinely employed to locate CR:
- **Bimanual Manipulation:** This is one of the most reproducible manipulation techniques available (Dawson, 1989). In this technique, the patient is reclined and with their chin directed upward. The clinician places four fingers along the lower border of the mandible, with the small finger placed behind the mandibular angle, making sure the fingers are positioned on bone and not on the soft tissue of the neck. Both thumbs should meet over the mandibular symphysis near the chin. Then the clinician applies a downward force with the thumbs to the chin, while an upward force is applied to the angle of mandible by the fingers, so that the condyles are seated in the glenoid fossae antero-superiorly.

- **Functional Manipulation:** This technique uses the patient's muscles to seat the condyles. This is achieved by placing an occlusal stop in the anterior section of the mouth, and asking the patient to attempt to close their posterior teeth. This can be accomplished using a Lucia jig (Lucia, 1960), a leaf gauge(Downs, 1988; Long, 1973; McHorris, 1985), or an anterior deprogrammer (Solow, 2013). The concept behind this technique is that when only the anterior teeth occlude (disengaging the posterior teeth), the directional force provided by the elevator muscles (the temporalis, masseter, and medial pterygoid) will seat the condyle with the articular disc interposed, in a antero-superior position within the glenoid fossae (the CR position).
  For a detailed description of Centric Relation concepts, and how to assess the Centric Relation Prematurity with the T-Scan, refer to Chapter 14.
- **Neuromuscular Theory; A Muscle Dedicated Position Known as Myocentric:** In the neuromuscular concept (Jankelson, 1969), the advocated, most optimal condylar position is located through the use of trans-cutaneous electrical nerve stimulation (TENS) that causes an electrically-induced relaxation of elevator muscles. The elevator muscles are electrically pulsed, or simulated at regular intervals, in an attempt to produce muscle relaxation reducing their electromyographic (EMG) activity to the lowest level possible. This electrically-reduced new relaxed muscle length and mandibular position, is then considered to be the neuromuscular position of choice.
  This TENS determined rest position represents the point at which the forces of gravity are pulling the mandible down to equal the elasticity of the elevator muscles and ligaments that support the mandible (viscoelastic tone). It should be noted that, the mandibular position of the lowest EMG activity does not always create a reasonable rest position from which the mandible should function, as it may be found at 8 to 9 mm from the intercuspal position. The postural rest position is located 2 to 4 mm below intercuspal position (Rugh & Drago, 1981; Manns, Zuazola, & Sirhan, 1990). Studies have shown that the intercuspal position (ICP) resulting from this technique is always anterior to the original ICP (Bessette & Quinlivan, 1973; Remien & Ash, 1974).
  Clinicians should recognize thatwhen using the neuromuscular technique three clinical situations may arise:
- The new mandibular position is always found to be downward and forward to the seated condylar position.
- The new mandibular position is almost always found to be at an increased vertical dimension.
- Patent's head position can change the acquired maxilla-mandibular relationship.
- The neuromuscular position must be maintained with at least an orthotic device, or when required, through significant prosthodontic reconstruction that must re-occlude all 28 teeth.
  For a detailed description of Neuromuscular concepts and methods, utilizing TENS with the T-Scan, refer to Chapter 17.
- **The Anterior Protrusive Position Theory, known as the Gelb 4/7 position:** In this approach theocclusion is determined by how the muscles brace the components of the Temporomandibular joint against the articular eminence.
  The Gelb 4/7 mandibular position (Gelb & Gelb, 1991) can be determined by radiological assessment using appliances to open the occlusion and reposition the mandible, forward and downward of the true center of the glenoid fossa. This Gelb radiological assessment of the TM Joints is not always appropriate to determine the condylar position, because no soft tissue can be imaged (without an MRI). Additionally, various topographic surveys of non-symptomatic subjects have shown there exists great variation in condylar position (Blaschke & Blaschke, 1981; Pullinger, Hollender, &

Solberg,1985). A variety of articular disc thicknesses and shapes allows for physiologic condylar seating of the condyle/disc/fossa assembly, which prevents the use of a standardized measurement to determine a true condyle position.

When choosing the concept of locating a proper reference mandibular position for any proposed occlusal treatment, the clinician must recognize that any protruded mandibular position requires extensive orthodontics, orthognathic surgery, or restoration, to establish an evenly distributed posterior tooth occlusion. Further, building an occlusion in a protruded position exposes the patient to the risk that posterior tooth contact can result in the development of an interference to the natural arc of mandibular closure. This occurs when the mandible does not stay in its established protruded position, because the condyle is not physiologically positioned within the glenoid fossae.

Laterotrusive Concepts of Occlusion

Based upon on the laterotrusive movements made from Centric Occlusion, various concepts of functional occlusion have been recognized and advocated as physiologic:

- Balanced occlusion (McLean, 1938; Woda, Vigneron, & Kay, 1979);
- Canine-protected occlusion (D'Amico, 1958; Gysi,1915; Kaplan,1963; Stuart & Stallard,1963; Reynolds,1971; McAdam,1976; Lucia,1983; Schwartz,1986);
- Group function occlusion (MacMillan, 1930; Schuyler,1961; Alexander, 1963 Mann & Pankey; 1963; Beyron,1964);
- Mixed canine-protected and group function (Rinchuse & Sassouni, 1982);
- Flat plane (attrition) occlusion (Begg, 1954; DeShields, 1978);.
- Measured immediate (time-based) anterior guidance control over the duration of the posterior disclusion (Kerstein, 1993).

However, among these lateroturs ive movement-based occlusion concepts, balanced and flat plane occlusion are presently advocated for use with denture patients, specifically for force-related reasons, and are no longer advocated for use with natural tooth occlusion. In the natural dentition, group function is quite common. However group function should not be considered as a part of a therapeutic occlusion, because group function occlusion allows for greater occlusal force application to the teeth, because molar and premolar lateral excursive contacts result in higher levels of muscle contractions, than when a canine protected occlusion is established (Kerstein & Radke, 2012). Hence, of all the available concepts to apply to a lateroturs ive movement occlusal scheme, the canine protected occlusion is optimal, because of its protective and low-muscle activating nature regarding its affect on the masticatory system.

For descriptions of many key occlusal concepts, refer to the Force Finishing facts within this chapter, as well as Chapter 7, which describes the concepts regarding measured, immediate (time-based) anterior guidance.

Commonly Agreed Upon Occlusal Concepts Shared by the Differing Mandibular Position Theories

Despite their theoretical mandibular position differences, all of the mandibular positional theories agree on the following four concepts, which are related to occlusal contacts and occlusal force (Dawson, 2007; Glickman, 1979; McNeil, 1997; Okeson, 2003):

- **How Teeth Should Meet During Mandibular Closure:** All teeth should occlude simultaneously and bilaterally during any mandibular closure movement.
- **How the Occlusal Load Should Be Distributed Within the Dental Arch:** An equal percentage of occlusal force should be shared between the right and left arch- halves.
- **How the Occlusal Load Should Be Distributed on Teeth:** An equal percentage of occlusal force should be distributed on each tooth's cross-arch counterpart tooth.
- **The Time Duration of Lateral Excursive Interfering contacts:** The anterior teeth should immediately disclude the posterior teeth during excursive movements.

Whatever the mandibular position theory (reference position) is adopted in clinical practice, the clinician must always understand that during any act of occlusal functioning (both in function or para-function), various forces (stresses) are generated within the masticatory system. An ongoing physiologic balance is required between the applied occlusal stresses and the adaptive capacity of the supporting tissues (the teeth, the periodontium, the masticatory muscles, the mandibular bone, the Temporomandibular joints, and the associated supporting structures), to maintain the long-them health,function and aesthetics of Stomatognathic system.

Hence, when selecting a mandibular position for treatment, the clinician must consider the clinical effects the selected mandibular position will have on the final occlusion, and the extent of treatment required to achieve the treatment goals. It is always advisable to choose the most conservative occlusal treatment approach. This lessens for the patient, both the biological and financial cost of the treatment.

Occlusal Forces are the Keys to Occlusal Harmony

A patient's psychology, health, function and aesthetics, are the four fundamental components of any preventative, therapeutic, and cosmetic dental treatment, that is designed to achieve healthy, harmonious, and beautiful smiles. The clinical sequence of how these core components are practically involved within a restorative treatment plan, have been arranged in the Smile Design Wheel (Figure 1) (Koirala, 2009), which can guide clinicians to preserve tooth structure, prolong tooth longevity, reduce treatment cost, lessen the number of restoration replacement cycles in a lifetime, increase patient confidence and trust in the clinician, while enhancing the image of the profession during dental treatment. The wheel specially focuses on function as one of the critical factors for long-term clinical success, because function is directly related to the occlusion, which generates various forces and stresses that occur within the masticatory system of a patient.

The establishment of the patient's oral health, proper function, and smile aesthetics is directly related with the overall harmony of his/her teeth, muscles, TM joints, and airway (known as the TMJA system). Any occlusal modification and/or rehabilitative procedures contemplated, should always consider isolating and treating the underlying functional and para-functional forces, for long-term clinical case success.

Figure 1. The Smile Design Wheel. It includes the components of psychology, health, function, and aesthetics, all of which should be considered during any comprehensive dental treatment. Reprinted from Koirala, S. (2009). Smile Design Wheel: A practice approach to smile design. Cosmetic Dentistry Science and Beauty, 3, 24-28. © [2006] [Courtesy of Nepal Dental Association]. Used with permission.

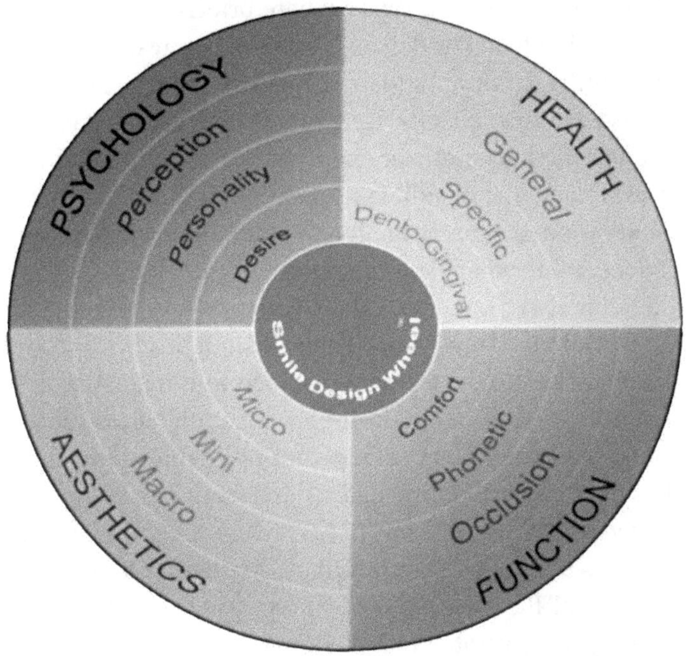

When such forces are not properly analyzed, and not properly lessened through the finishing treatment procedures, clinicians may encounter various clinical complications:

- Damaged restorations (veneers, onlays, crowns, and bridges),
- Fractured teeth,
- Tooth mobility,
- Abnormal tooth wear and tooth sensitivity,
- Pain in the teeth, muscles, and Temporomandibular joints,
- Other signs and symptoms of occlusal force disorders (OFD).

Mastication and Tooth Contacts Forces

The Stomatognathic system is a complex unit designed to carry out three major functions:

- Mastication,
- Swallowing,
- Speech.

These functions are basic to life, but are also secondary functions that aid in respiration, and the expression of human emotion.

Muscles contraction is the means by which mandibular motion and craniomandibular forces are generated, which is intimately involved with the functioning of the dentition. The geometry of the craniofacial skeleton with muscles attached, are all related to the tooth compressions that occur when the mandible is in motion, which generates occlusal forces between the mandible and the cranium. Hence, mastication, and the resultant forces will be discussed here briefly:

Mastication is the act of chewing food (Anderson, 1988) and represents the initial stages of digestion. It is a complex function that utilizes not only the masticatory muscles, the teeth, and the periodontal supportive structures, but also the lips, cheeks, tongue, and the salivary glands. Mastication is made up of rhythmic, and well-controlled separations and closures of the maxillary and mandibular teeth. Each opening and closing movement the mandible makes represents a chewing stroke, such that similar chewing strokes are repeated over and over, as the food is broken down. Studies show that during act of mastication, tooth contact does occur, where few contacts occur when the food is initially introduced into the mouth, but then as the bolus is broken down, the frequency of tooth contacts increases (Anderson & Picton, 1957; Ahlgren, 1966). In the final stage of mastication just prior to swallowing, tooth contact occurs during every stroke but forces to the teeth are deemed minimal (Adams & Zander, 1964).

The amount of the force placed on the teeth during mastication varies greatly from individual to individual. It is generally found that males can occlude with more force than can females. In one study it was reported that a female's maximal occluding load ranged from 79 - 99 lbs. (35.8 - 44.9 kg.), whereas a male's occluding load varied from 118 - 142 lbs. (53.6 - 64.6 kg.) (Brekhus, 1941). The greatest maximal occlusal force reported was 975 lb. (443 kg.) (Gibbs, Mahan, & Mauderli, 1986). It has also been noted that the maximal amount of the force applied to a molar is usually several times higher than is applied to an incisor. One studydemonstrated that the range of maximal force applied to the first molar was 91- 198 lbs. (41.3 - 89.8 kg.), whereas the maximal force applied to the central incisors was 29 - 51 lbs. (13.2 - 23.1 kg.) (Howell & Manly, 1948). The maximal occluding force appears to increase with age through adolescence (Garner & Kotwal, 1973; Worner & Anderson, 1944). Moreover, it has been demonstrated that with practice and exercise, an individual can increase their maximal occluding force over time (Brekhus, 1941; Worner, 1939; Worner & Anderson, 1944; Kiliardus, Tzakis, & Carlsson, 1995; Waugh, 1939).

Facial skeletal relationships may also play role in increased occlusal strength. The type of foods and their consistency also affect the applied force that occurs during chewing. One study reported that chewing carrots produced approximately 30 lbs. (14 kg.) of force on the teeth, whereas chewing meat produced only 16 lbs. (7 kg.) (Anderson, 1981). It has also been demonstrated that tooth pain (Goldreich, Gazit, Lieberman, & Rugh, 1994), or muscle pain (Bakke & Michler, 1991) reduced the amount of generated force during chewing. When foods are tougher, chewing occurs predominantly in the first molar and premolar region (Brudevold, 1951; Lundgren & Laurell, 1986; Michael, Javid, Colaizzi, & Gibbs, 1990), but during any normal chewing cycle, the greatest amount of force is applied to the first molar region (Howell & Brudevold, 1950). It has been estimated that during each chewing stroke, an average of 58.7 lbs. of force is applied to the teeth for 115 milliseconds (Gibbs, Mahan, Lundeen, Brehnan, & Walsh, 1981). This yields an applied load of 6.75 lb./sec./chew (pounds per second per chew) (Lundeen & Gibbs, 1982). If a human makes 1800 chews during an average day, it equals 12,150 lb./sec./per day of occlusal force that is applied during chewing functional activity. However, the occluding force of patients who wear complete dentures is ¼ that of a patient who chews with natural teeth (Michael, Javid, Colaizzi, & Gibbs, 1990).

Swallowing and Tooth Contacts Forces

The act of swallowing requires a series of coordinated muscular contractions that move a bolus of food from the oral cavity, through the esophagus, to the stomach. It consists of voluntary, involuntary, and reflex muscular activities. The teeth are brought up into their maximum intercuspal position (ICP) during swallowing, which properly stabilizes the mandible by fixing its position against the maxilla, so that contraction of the suprahyoid and infrahyoid muscles can control the hyoid bone during swallowing.

There are two type of swallowing:

- Somatic (adult); and
- Visceral (infantile).

In somatic swallowing, the teeth are used to stabilize the mandible, but during infantile swallowing, the mandible is braced when the tongue is placed forward and between the dental arches or gum pads (Cleall, 1965). This type of swallowing remains with the child until the posterior teeth erupt.

The effects of the applied force during swallowing in asymptomatic adults depends on the mid-swallow tooth contact durations, and their frequency. The average tooth contact during swallowing lasts about 683 milliseconds (Suit, Gibbs, & Benz, 1975). It is interesting to note that the tooth contact duration present in a single swallow, is three times longer than is present in a single chewing stroke. Also, the force applied to the teeth during swallowing is approximately 66.5lbs., which is 7.8 lb.greater than the force applied during mastication (Suit, et al., 1975).

A few studies have demonstrated that the swallowing cycle occurs 590 times during a 24-hour period (Schneyer, Pigman, Hanahan, & Gilmore, 1956; Flanagan, 1963):

- 146 swallowing cycles during eating,
- 349 swallowing cycles between meals while awake,
- 50 swallowing cycles during sleep.

The lower levels of salivary flow present during sleep result in less human need to swallow.

Speech and Tooth Contacts Forces

Speech is the third major function of the masticatory system. Speech occurs when a volume of air is forced by the diaphragm, out from the lungs through the larynx and the oral cavity. Controlled contraction and relaxation of the vocal cords and the bands of the larynx create sounds with the desired pitch (Jenkins, 1974). By varying the relationships of the lips and tongue to the palate and teeth, a human can produce a variety of sounds (Jenkins, 1974). However, tooth contacts do not routinely occur during speech, such that no tooth contact force is generated during any action of speech.

Parafunctional Habits and Forces

Mastication, swallowing and speaking are considered the vital functions of masticatory system. The rest of the activities are considered "non-functional" or parafunctional. Parafunctions are popularly thought of as self-destructive oral habits, because they are perceived to result from a type of patient self-aggression towards the patients' own body. The following are the so-called parafunctional habits:

- Long durations of teeth clenching,
- Nighttime teeth grinding as is seen in Bruxism,
- Sustained contractions of the muscles of mastication (without dental contact), chewing on the lips, cheeks, or tongue,
- Tongue thrust,
- Nail chewing, cuticle chewing,
- Chewing different objects,
- Patient self-altering of their mandibular posture.

All these parafunctional habits produce some type of force within the masticatory system. Their deleterious effects depend upon the magnitude, direction, duration, and the frequency the force is applied to the system.

Influence of Parafunctional Bruxing and Clenching on Occlusal Forces

Among the commonly observed oral parafunctional habits, Bruxism and clenching produce heavy occlusal forces within the masticatory system. These activities can occur subconsciously, such that the patient is often is unaware they are actively parafunctioning.

To understand the influence of parafunctional activities in development of occlusal forces disorders (OFD), it is important to compare normal functional activity with the parafunctional activities of Bruxism and Clenching.

- **Intensity of Dental Contacts:** The higher the intensity of the dental contacts, the greater is the force that affects the masticatory system.

During normal mastication, a human routinely generates 20.7- 26.6 kg. of force, while in swallowing a human ranges from 25.0 - 30.2 kg. (Gibbs, Mahan, & Lundeen, 1981). However, during parafunction (during sleep associated bruxism), a human can generate an average of 42.3 kg., ranging between 15.6 kg. - 81.2 kg. (Nishigawa, Bando, & Nakano, 2001), which is almost double those of normal mastication and swallowing.

- **Frequency of Dental Contacts:** The frequency of occlusal contacts is one of the major factors guiding occlusal force generation, because without tooth contact significantly less force is generated.

In normal function, occlusal contact occurs for 17.5 minutes during a 24-hour period (Graf, 1969; Glickman, 1972). However during parafunction, the frequency of contact increases, such that occlusal contact occurs for 30 -170 minutes in 8 hours of sleep (Brewer & Hudson, 1961), and 38.7 - 162 minutes per full night of sleep (Trenouth, 1976).

- **Duration of Bruxism Events:** It has been shown that bruxism events in chronic bruxism patients were of longer durations (27 seconds/ hour), than were those of non-bruxing patients (7.4 seconds/ hour) (Baba, Clark, Watanabe, & Ohiyama, 2003)
- **Direction of Occlusal Forces:** Forces that are developed horizontally and laterally over the teeth during excursive movements, increase the probability of damage to the supporting structures, when compared to more vertically aligned forces.

In normal mastication and swallowing function, there exists a predominance of vertical mandibular movements, despite the rotary path the mandible takes during chewing. Vertical occlusal forces are better supported by the tooth-periodontium complex than are lateral stresses. It is important to note that during parafunctional activity, mainly eccentric mandibular movements occur.

- **Mandibular Position :** Most functional activities are carried out in the intercuspal position so that occlusal stability is enhanced, because the distribution of the functional forces is spread over several teeth. This minimizes the potential harm to any individual tooth (Okeson, 2003).

In contrast, parafunctional activities are mainly carried out with the mandible in eccentric positions, where there are only few dental contacts in play, and the condyles are displaced from a stable Centric Relation (Schulte, 1983). When powerful parafunctional forces are loaded over a few teeth, with the mandible in an unstable condylar position, a high probability of sustaining pathologic effects on the teeth, the muscles, and the TM joints, is created.

- **Reduced Influence of Protective Reflexes:** The neuromuscular reflexes present during functional activities protect the Stomatognathic structures against potential harmful forces. However, during parafunctional activities, the protective neuromuscular reflexes appears to be reduced.

Bruxism appears to cause an increase in the excitation thresholds of some receptors, which adapt, and have less physiologic control over the inhibition of mandibular muscle activity (Miralles, Carvajal, Manns, & Rossi, 1980; Muhlbrat, Jenz, & Luks, 1976). This allows for the development of greater occlusal forces during parafunctional activity, thereby increasing the probability of damaging Stomatognathic system structures. Hence, the degree of force and the duration of tooth contact engagements during parafunctional activity, pose a much more serious consequence to the masticatory system than do those resulting from normal functional activity.

Lastly, habits that introduce extraoral forces are also important causes of functional force disturbances present within the masticatory system. Behaviors such as holding a telephone between the chin and shoulders, resting the mandible in the hands while sitting at a table, or playing certain musical instruments, also apply force to the Stomatognathic structures (Howard, 1991; Bryant, 1989). Any force applied to the mandible, either intraorally or extraorally, must be identified as a potential contributing factor to observed functional disturbances present in the masticatory system (Chun & Koskinen-Moffett, 1990).

The Definition, Classification, Etiology, and the Signs and Symptoms of Occlusal Force Disorders (OFD)

Occlusal stability exists when the various components of the masticatory system operate in an integrated and harmonized manner. The physiological tolerance level (the resistive and adaptive capacities) of the patient plays a vital role in maintaining occlusal force harmony. If the occlusal forces exceed the physiologic tolerance limitations of the patient, the system can breakdown, which usually begins with the "weakest link" within the individual's Stomatognathic apparatus. Hence, Occlusal Force Disorders (OFD) can be defined as:

- The disorders of teeth, muscles, Temporomandibular joints, and airway, resultant from excess occlusal force which is greater than the individual's adaptive capacity.

Etiology of OFD

When a person uses their Stomatognathic system both functionally and parafunctionally, forces are constantly generated within the masticatory system, which are then disseminated through a series of complex physiological and biological process that take place within the body. With physiologic loading, there is a balance between the synthesis and breakdown within the tissues (both catabolic and anabolic activity). When occlusal loading exceeds these physiologic limits, protective and compensatory mechanisms are recruited to prevent or limit damage, or support the repair of the damage. For example, when some of the molar teeth are missing for a long period of time without being replaced, the neighboring teeth commence migrating to super erupt or tilt. This diminishes the size of the edentulous space so that other teeth absorb the altered occlusal force pattern, attempting to compensate for the tooth position changes so as to balance the total masticatory load (Seligman & Pulinger,1991; Tallents, Macher, Kyranides, Katzberg, & Moss, 2002; Kahn, Tallents, Katzberg, Moss, & Murphy, 1999; Kahn, Tallents,, Katzberg, Moss, & Murphy, 1998; Roberts, Tallents, & Katzberg, 1987; Ishimaru, Handa, Kurita, & Goss, 1994; Kawata, Niida, & Kawasoko, 1994; Kawata, Niida, & Kawasoko, 1997).

Tissues that undergo decreased loading show decreases in anabolic activity, such that insufficient cellular matrix is produced. In contract, tissue overloading initially induces an adaptive responses like hypertrophy and hyperplasia, both which that persist until the adaptive capacity is exceeded, which leads to cell damage and possibly cell necrosis (apoptosis). Therefore, when the capacity of the Stomatognathic system's complex load-absorbing system is exceeded or reduced, the fibrocartilage, the synovial membrane, the subchondral bone, the capsular ligaments, and the masticatory muscle tissues, may all become damaged (Stegenga, 2001; De Bont, Dijkgraaf, & Stegenga, 1997). Therefore, OFD results from ongoing disharmony of the functional forces within the masticatory system.

There are four major factors that directly or indirectly affect the force components of the masticatory system:

- **Morphological Factors:** The morphological components of the Stomatognathic system are established by the type and patterns of growth and development, which are generally guided by genetic and environmental factors.

The morphological factors that are related to force outcome, can be further divided into:

- **Dental Type:** Intercuspal position contacts (ICP), the angle of the tooth contacts, the type of tooth contacts present in an excursive movement, and the anterior-posterior contact location.
- **Articulation Type:** The condylar position.
- **Cranio-Facial Type:** Dolichofacial, Mesofacial, or Brachyfacial, which describe genetically differing skeletal Vertical Dimension of Occlusion conditons, directly affect the generation of force magnitude.
- **Pathophysiologic Factors:** Tooth decay and periodontal disease affects the occlusal force balance due to the loss of tooth and periodontal supporting tissues. Force disharmony can also be created by trauma (micro and macro), or upper airway obstruction, which leads to the formation of anterior open occlusion, oral breathing, and snoring and obstructive sleep apnea. Sleep breathing disorders can promote parafunctional habits like clenching and grinding, which produce high occlusal force within the masticatory system.
- **Parafunctional Habit and Psychosocial Factors:** The etiology of parafunctional habits is still not fully understood, but may have a partial etiology resultant from long Disclusion Time (Kerstein, 1995). Most clinicians and authors consider that parafunctional habits are closely related to various psychosocial factors like depression, anxiety, stress, emotional sensitivity, hyperactivity, and personality type. Parafunctional habits like clenching and bruxing of teeth can be a fundamental cause of OFD, because these activities generate high occlusal forces within the masticatory system.

For comprehensive management of any occlusal force disorder, a detailed clinical history, clinical examination, and suitable diagnostic tests are required to recognize the "weakest link" (the teeth-periodontium, muscles, Temporomandibular Joints, or airway complex) within the patient's Stomatognathic system. Once the weakest link is identified, then a treatment plan must include a suitable minimally invasive approach to optimize the occlusal force distribution, thereby limiting and preventing the occlusal force disorders sequelae (Figure 2a - i).

To guide clinicians in making a proper diagnosis of OFD, the sign and symptoms of OFD can be classified into 4 clinical categories:

Type I Occlusal Force Disorder: Teeth and Periodontal Complex

- **Teeth:** Excessive tooth wear (attrition), abfraction formation, tooth fracture, enamel cracking, tooth mobility, frequent restoration failure, implant prosthesis screw loosening, dentinal hypersensitivity, pulpitis, pulpal necrosis, pulpal atrophy, pulpal dystrophic calcification, and tooth pain upon occluding.
- **Periodontium:** Tooth hypermobility, gingival recession, thickening of the lamina dura, tooth migration.
- **Alveolar Bone:** Angular bone loss, the presence of Tori and Exostoses, and dehiscence.

Figure 2a. Example of occlusal force disorders: Multiple abfraction. Note there are abfractions present on the mandibular anterior teeth due to significant friction present during the protrusive movement.

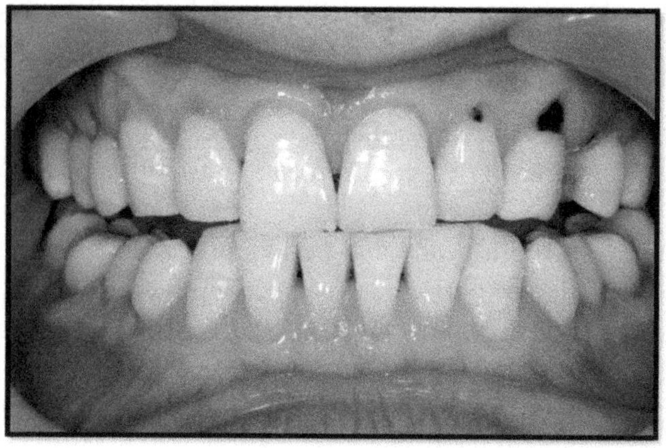

Figure 2b. Example of occlusal force disorders: Tongue indentation of a patient who is a heavy clencher

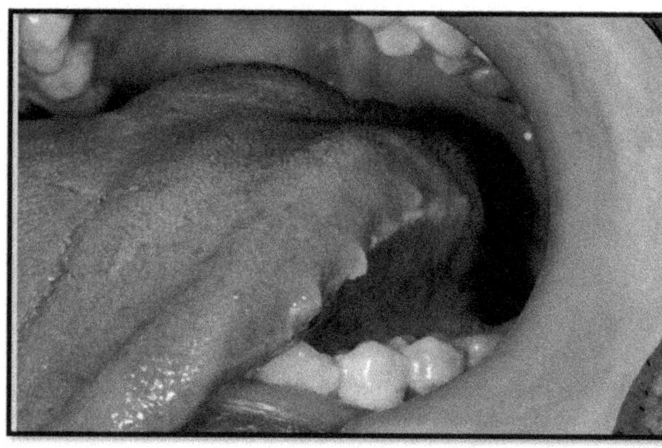

Figure 2c. Example of occlusal force disorders: Cheek marks (Linea Alba) resultant from heavy teeth clenching

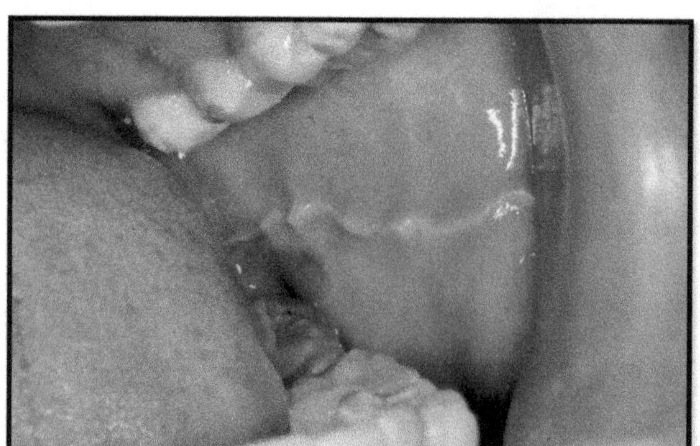

Figure 2d. Example of occlusal force disorders: Cracked enamel due to excessive occlusal load

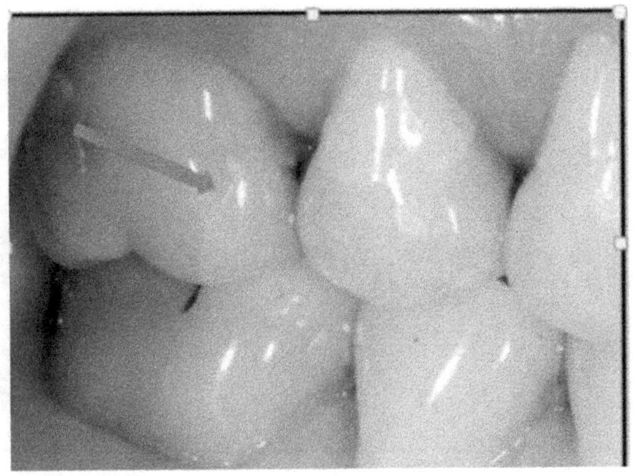

Figure 2e. Example of occlusal force disorders: Fracture of the ceramic layer of a PFM crown, due to a high concentration of occlusal force present on that restoration

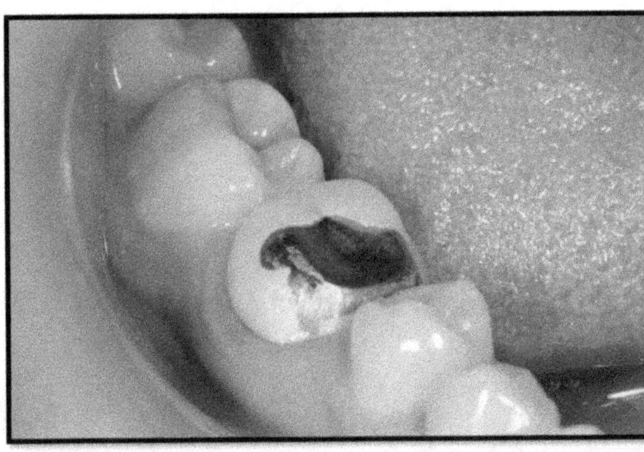

Figure 2f. Example of occlusal force disorders: Exostoses formed from heavy occlusal forces

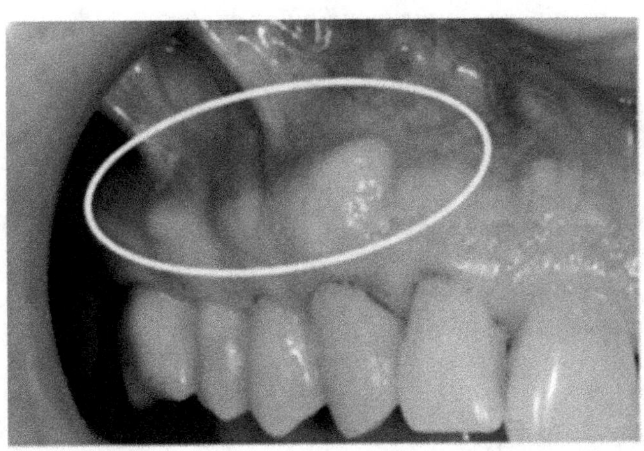

Figure 2g. Example of occlusal force disorders: Severe attrition due to heavy bruxism

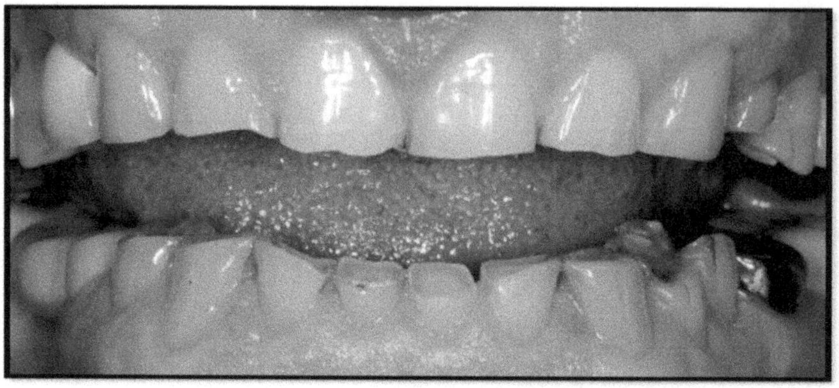

Figure 2h. Occlusal force disorder signs: Panoramic radiograph of a heavy bruxer. Note the flat cusps and minimal enamel present on the posterior teeth, both visible in the radiograph.

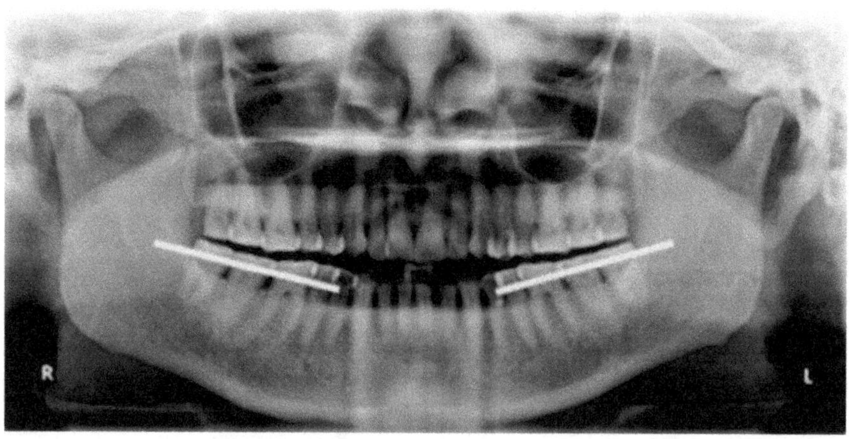

Figure 2i. Occlusal force disorder signs: Panoramic radiograph of a person with hypertrophic masseter muscles. Note the bilateral prominence of the mandibular angles.

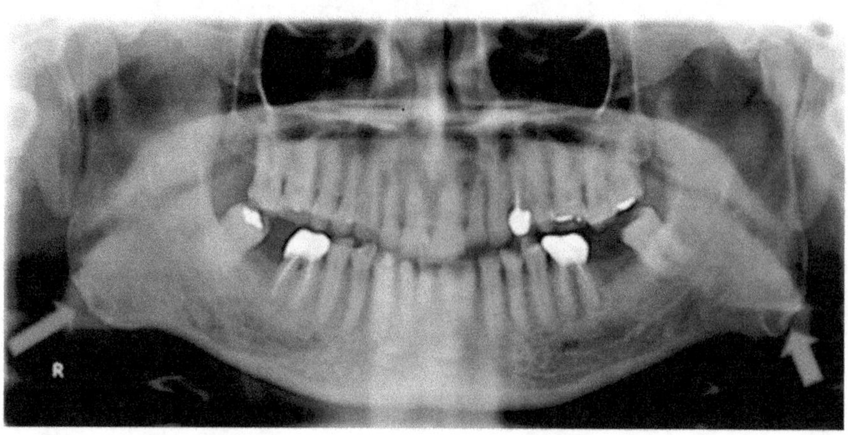

Type II Occlusal Force Disorder: Muscle Complex

- **Masticatory Muscles:** Tender to palpation, masticatory muscle hypertrophy, muscle incoordination, muscle fatigue, muscle hyperactivity, pain, discomfort, and reduced range of mandibular motion, deviated range of motion, temporal headache, and earache.
- **Lips, Cheek, Tongue:** Cheek marks (Linea alba), traumatic ulcers, tongue indentation.

Type III Occlusal Force Disorders: Mandible and Temporomandibular Joint Complex

- **Mandible and TM Joints:** Movement deviation, internal disk derangement, clicking sounds, structural deformation, maxillomandibular TM joint asymmetry, TM joint discomfort and pain. TM Joint degenerative changes, and locking and dislocation.

Type IV Occlusal Force Disorder: Airway Complex

Obstruction of oral respiration distracts the throat muscles from the forces exerted by the tongue, cheeks, and lips upon the maxillary arch.

- **Maxillary Airway:** The main characteristics of a compromised airway complex (upper airway obstruction and breathing mode) are the presence of hypertrophied tonsils or adenoids, mouth breathing, anterior open occlusion, crossbite, excessive anterior facial height, incompetent lip posture, excessive appearance of maxillary anterior teeth, narrow external nares, and a "V-shaped" maxillary arch.

These characteristics generally are related to occlusal force imbalances present within the Stomatognathic system, which over the long-term, promote the development of any of the above noted occlusal force disorders.

Various studies and experiments have shown the interrelationship between airway, mode of breathing, malocclusion, and the craniofacial growth pattern. These studies advocate that there exists a "form follows function" relationship. Dysfunction of the human airway and breathing can cause malocclusion and skeletal deformation, which can result in an increase in total anterior face height, which mostly contributes to more vertical development of the lower anterior face (Linder-Aronson, 1970; Hannukseal, 1981; Bresolin, Shapiro, Dhapito, Chapko, & Dessel, 1983 ; Trask, Shipiro, & Shapiro; 1987; Hannukseal, 1981; Sassuni, Shnorhokain, Beery, Zullo, & Friday, 1982; Woodside, Linder-Aronson, 1979). Concomitantly, an increase in mandibular plane, the gonial angle, and the tipping of the palate can also be found. In these instances, facial prognathism has been reported to be decreased (Linder- Aronson, 1970; Hannukseal, 1981; Sassuni, et al., 1982; Bresolin, et al., 1983; Trask, et al., 1987; Bresolin, et al., 1983; Linder- Aronson, 1970; Hannukseal, 1981; Subtelny,1980; Tarvonen, & Kosko, 1987; Freng, 1979)

Within the literature, several mechanisms have been suggested that act on the development of the maxilla and other skeletal structures, during impaired nasal breathing, which are atrophy of nasal cavity resultant from inactivity, and an upward direction of the airstream affecting the formation of the palate (Michel, Lippen, Wangen & Zungendruk, 1908),while raising negative pressure in the nasal cavity (Kantorowicz, 1916; Wustrow, 1915). The contemporary belief is that alterations in postural muscle activity influence the position of the teeth and the growth behavior of some of the craniofacial structures (Linder-Aronson, 1970; Linder-Aronson, 1974; Harvold, Tormer, Vangervik, & Chierici, 1981). An alternative hypothesis has suggested that soft tissue stretching mechanisms elicit a morphogenetic response that leads to the same structural results (Solow & Kreiberg, 1977).

General practitioners are in a unique position to screen patients for the recognizable signs and symptoms of airway complex problems, including snoring and obstructive sleep apnea. Early diagnosis and intervention are essential to prevent future airway disease complexities, while limiting potential extensive and invasive treatment methods. However, a clinician must always be careful when designing a treatment plan and selecting therapeutic treatment methods, because individual variation in response to treatment should be expected due to the alteration in airway patency and breathing mode. As a result, there are considerable controversies that still exist within the literature regarding the "form-function relationship" (Whitaker, 1911; Emslie, Massler, & Zwemer, 1952; Kingsley, 1888; McKenzie, 1909; James & Hastings, 1932; Gwynne- Evans & Ballard, 1957).

It should be noted that, the signs and symptoms of the differing occlusal force disorder types are not mutually exclusive. There are interrelationship between the signs and symptoms of each of the OFD categories, because various imbalanced Stomatognathic forces are the causative factors for OFD, whereby many or all of the above-listed signs and symptoms of OFD may occur simultaneously. As such, the treatment planning of OFD requires the taking a detailed oral patient history, performing a thorough clinical examination, and having the patient undergo suitable diagnostic testing, to verify the specific clinical signs and symptoms of an OFD that are present.

MAIN FOCUS OF CHAPTER

Force Finishing in Dental Medicine: A Simplified Approach to Occlusal Force Harmony

Achieving occlusal harmony in Dental Medicine necessitates the balancing of the occlusal force components with the resistive and adaptive capacity of the patient's TMJA Complex. Regardless of the occlusal concept a clinician adopts, if the occlusal forces at the completion of treatment are not harmonized, they may negatively affect the success of the treatment result, thereby compromising long-term health, function, and craniofacial aesthetics.

The concept of Force Finishing was introduced by this author in 2011, during the 2nd biennial scientific conference, "*Minimally Invasive Cosmetic Dentistry with Computerized Occlusion* ", presented at the South Asian Academy of Aesthetic Dentistry (SAAAD), in Bangalore, India. The goal for presenting the Force Finishing concept was to simplify the clinical approach of obtaining occlusal harmony in cosmetic dental cases (Figure 3).

It is interesting to note that cosmetic dentists spend significant clinical time and effort on the aesthetic end-results, because the aesthetic components are visible to both the clinician and the patient, where the outcome can immediately be appreciated. However, the force components are invisible, and their negative effects are not easily appreciated clinically, until the effects become chronic. Another reason that role of force components in case finishing has been undermined, is because clinicians rely solely on articulating paper marks when performing occlusal adjustments, believing (incorrectly) that the occlusal forces are visible to them, within the shapes and color-depth of the markings. Hence, the concept

Figure 3. The occlusal force harmony cycle. This schematic diagram shows the flow of occlusal force harmony and disharmony, occlusal force disorders, and the role of Force Finishing in re-establishing occlusal force harmony.

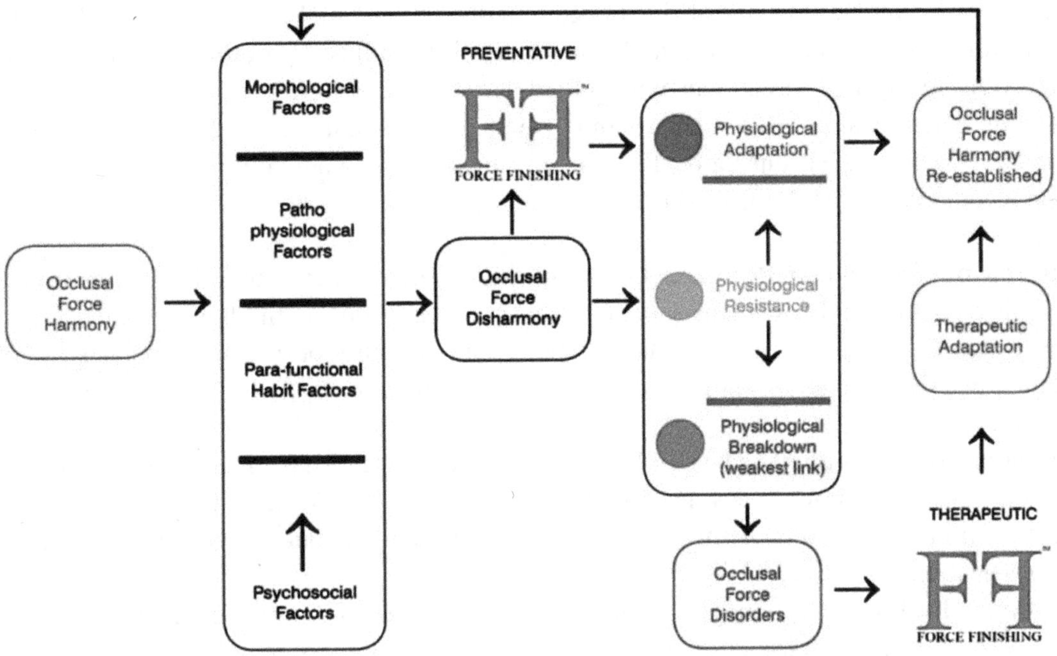

of Force Finishing was first introduced to cosmetic dentists, to help them better understand the role that masticatory forces have on the long-term clinical success of installed cosmetic dental restorations.

Morphological, pathophysiological, parafunctional habits and psychosocial issues, are the four major contributing factors that directly or indirectly affect the force components of the masticatory system. If the occlusal forces generated during either function and/or para-function becomes imbalanced, occlusal force disharmony will likely occur. The early detection and timely application of the preventative force finishing protocol can help support the masticatory system to achieve physiological adaptation (the green light within the schematic diagram), so that no signs and symptoms of an occlusal force disorder are visible and experienced by the patient. However, if the occlusal force imbalances are ignored and not resolved quickly, there will likely be two resultant possibilities:

- **Physiological Resistance (Yellow Light within the Schematic Diagram):** Here the system may moves towards gaining physiologic adaptation (the green light within the schematic diagram). This will occur if the patient's self-adaptation capacity is strong enough.
- **Physiological Breakdown (Red Light within the Schematic Diagram):** This will occur at the weakest link of TMJA complex, where the signs and symptoms of an occlusal force disorder become apparent. Once OFD signs and symptoms are detected, a suitable therapeutic treatment is necessary, which can include therapeutic force finishing procedures to support the masticatory system with balanced occlusal forces. This will aid in a faster therapeutic adaptation leading to the re-establishment of occlusal force harmony within Stomatognathic system.

Force Finishing should not be confused with conventional Occlusal Equilibration (Dawson, 2008), or unmeasured occlusal adjustment procedures (Koirala, 2011; Kerstein, 2010; Kerstein, 1993). Force Finishing is based upon normal human masticatory physiology and the occlusal force facts and figures that were derived from various scientific studies (cited in the below Force Finishing Clinical Facts). Force Finishing plays a major role in establishing structural stability, by optimizing the occlusal force distribution during any dental treatment, whether it is a restorative case, in periodontal therapy, in prosthodontic reconstruction, after orthodontic tooth movement, or when using therapeutic oral appliances.

There are five basic areas during occlusal scheme preparation where clinicians can control the occlusal force components (McNeil, 1997):

- **Intercuspal Position (ICP) Contacts:** The restorative dentists can control which teeth come into complete contact, and how many tooth contacts are present during the ICP closure.
- **Excursive Contacts:** By altering the number type, and duration of tooth contacts in eccentric excursions, the restorative dentist can change the muscular contraction levels and the distribution of forces.
- **Angle of Tooth Contacts:** The depth of the overbite, or steepness of the anterior guidance will have an impact on how forces are distributed (Katona, 1989; Weinberg & Kruger, 1995). The angle of impact will not only affect the distribution of the force, but also the ability of the muscles of mastication to contract.
- **Condylar Position:** The condylar position chosen, will have a dramatic impact on the clinician's ability to control which teeth contact each other, and when they contact.
- **Vertical Dimension of Occlusion (VDO):** The Vertical Dimension of Occlusion can be opened or closed when restoring at least one arch. Decreasing the vertical dimension can increase the occlusal forces, but only to the point of maxillomandibular over closure, which then weakens patient contraction strength capability.

Force Finishing Types

Based upon the patient's psychological make-up, their health, their functional and aesthetic requirements, and the degree of individual patient sensitivity towards their occlusal forces and occlusal contact non-simultaneity, Force Finishing can be divided into two clinical types:

- **Preventive Force Finishing (PFF):** The basic aim of preventive Force Finishing is to protect and maintain a patient's physiologically accepted, original occlusal scheme, while preventing existing restorations from failure by optimizing the occlusal force components of the Stomatognathic system.
- **Therapeutic Force Finishing (TFF):** TFF aims to customize the occlusal force components to treat the specific signs and symptoms of occlusal force disorders. Based on the patient's health and functional requirements, a direct method of TFF can be used to optimize the occlusal force components in the management of sore and hypersensitive teeth, and pain related to masticatory muscle hyperactivity. However, an indirect approach using TFF is also suitable when optimizing the occlusal force components by increasing balance, or reducing an imbalance, and by employing therapeutic oral splints in the management of Temporomandibular disorders (TMD), and snoring.

Force Finishing Core Principles

Force Finishing principles should be viewed broadly, keeping minimally invasive comprehensive treatment approaches, in mind. There are three core principles of Force Finishing that a clinician should follow, while completing occlusal treatment to achieve harmonized occlusal forces for long-term clinical success:

- Recognize the "weakest link" in a patient's Stomatognathic system, based on existing OFD signs and symptoms.
- Decide to maintain, modify, or re-establish the existing occlusion as per the patient's need and demand.
- Optimize the occlusal force components (tooth contact location, tooth contact area, tooth contact relative forces, tooth contact sequence, occlusal force distribution, Occlusion and Disclusion Times), to enhance the patient's physiologic resistive and adaptive capacity of their masticatory system.

Force Finishing Clinical Facts

These Force Finishing clinical facts are based upon this author's review of a variety of clinical publications. They are systematically organized to aid clinicians in understanding and recognizing the role the occlusal forces play in the management of a functioning occlusion.

- Unilateral tooth contacts increase force in the opposite Temporomandibular joint.
- Bilateral even tooth contacts in ICP provides more stability to the teeth, muscles and Temporomandibular joints.
- When the number of occluding teeth increases, the total percentage of force to each tooth decreases.
- The amount of the force that can be generated between teeth depends on the distance the teeth are from the Temporomandibular joint, combined with applied muscular force vectors (known as the Fulcrum Principle). Greater force can be applied to the posterior teeth than to the anterior teeth. (Howell & Manly, 1948; Manns, Miralles, Valdivia, & Bull, 1982).
- Vertical forces created by tooth contacts are well accepted by the periodontal ligament (PDL), but horizontal forces cannot be effectively dissipated (Glickman, 1963). These forces may create pathologic bone responses, or elicit neuromuscular reflex activity in an attempt to avoid, or guard against the incline plane contacts (Guichet, 1977). Hence, directing the occlusal force through the long axis of the tooth (axial loading) should be a goal of posterior tooth Force Finishing. Axial loading can be accomplished by creating cusp tip-to flat surface contacts, or by creating reciprocal incline contacts (also known as tripodization).
- Posterior teeth function effectively when accepting axial forces (axial loading) applied during intercuspated self-closure. They accept these forces well due to their position within the arch, because the applied occlusal force can be directed through their long axes, and then dissipated effectively (Okeson, 2003).
- The anterior teeth are not positioned well within the arches to accept heavy axial force. They are normally positioned at a labial angle to the direction of closure, so loading them axially is nearly impossible (Kraua, Jordon, & Abrahams, 1973).

- Anterior teeth, unlike posterior teeth, are in proper position to accept the horizontal forces of eccentric mandibular movements (Lee, 1982; Standlee, 1979; Korioth & Hannam, 1990).
- The anterior teeth should immediately disclude the posterior teeth in excursive movements (Dawson, 2007; Glickman, 1979; Okeson, 2003), resulting in friction-free excursive movements that limit wear on teeth and activate low levels of excursive muscle function (Kerstein, 2010; Kerstein & Radke 2012)
- Canines are considered to be best suited to accept the horizontal forces that occur during eccentric movements (Guichet, 1977; Standlee. 1979), because they have the longest and largest roots, and therefore the best crown/root ratio (Kraua, Jordon, & Abrahams, 1973; Lucia, 1961). Canines are surrounded by dense compact bone, which tolerates occlusal forces better than does the medullary bone found around posterior teeth. In addition, the canines provide mostly sensory input such that fewer muscles are active when canines contact during eccentric movements, than when posterior teeth contact (Ash & Nelson, 2003; Williamson & Lundquist, 1983; Kerstein & Radke, 2012).
- Lower levels of muscular activity will decrease forces applied to the dental structures and the TM joint structures, thereby minimizing pathosis. It is therefore suggested that during Force Finishing of the left and/or right laterotrusive excursion movements, "canine guidance" be the preferred excursive control, so as to best dissipate any damaging horizontal forces. When canine guidance is not possible to achieve during case finishing, the most favorable alternative is a group function that involves the canines and the 1st premolar only. Disclusion Time research has revealed that working side molar excursive contacts make the most muscle activity (Kerstein & Radke, 2012). A 1st premolar guidance surface will successfully limit molar contribution to prolonged disclusion, when required.
- Any laterotrusive contacts more posterior than the first premolar are not desirable. Molar teeth demonstrate increased amounts of muscle force than do the premolar and anterior teeth, due to their lying closer to the Temporomandibular joint fulcrum.

Force Finishing Instrumentation and Materials

The Force Finishing protocol has three fundamental steps; Force Finishing, Aesthetic Finishing, and the Finishing Evaluation. Each step requires specific instruments and materials.

For Force Finishing: To determine tooth contact locations and the size of contacts, thin (less than 20 micron thick) articulating paper (blue and red color), used in Miller articulating paper forceps is required (Figure 4).

To record digitally the occlusal contact locations and areas, the relative occlusal force distribution, the Occlusion and Disclusion Times, and the tooth contact sequence, the T-Scan 8 Computerized Occlusal Analysis technology (T-Scan 8, Tekscan, Inc. S. Boston, MA, USA) and its High Definition (HD) recording sensor are mandatory. At present, this is the only device available in the global market that can record and display for the clinician, 256 relative occlusal force levels and 0.003 second-long contact timing sequences (Figure 5).

Items like Dura green stones, diamond points, and Dura white stones are necessary to selectively contour the overly pressurized occlusal contact points during Force Finishing (Figure 6a).

For Aesthetic Finishing: This is carried out after Force Finishing procedures are completed to achieve smooth and glossy surfaces. Enamel and restorative surfaces which were adjusted for force finishing must

Figure 4. Blue and red thin articulating paper held in Miller articulating paper forceps

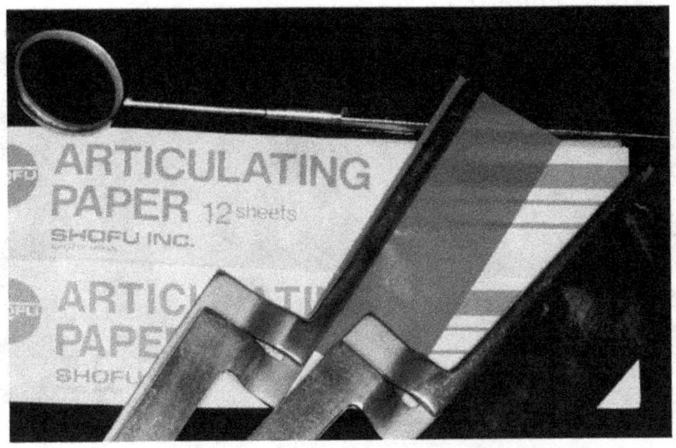

Figure 5. T-Scan 8 digital occlusal force scanning technology

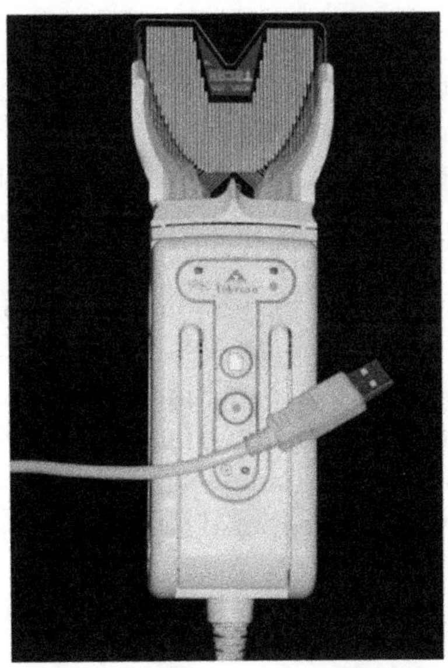

Figure 6a. The Force Finishing Kit contains contouring items, organized with coarse and fine diamond points, Dura green stones and Dura white stones (Shofu, Inc., Kyoto, Japan)

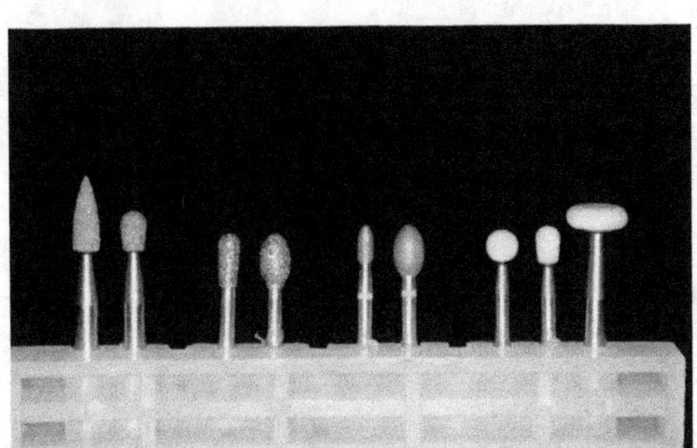

Figure 6b. The Force Finishing Kit contains finishing items, organized with diamond impregnated fine silicone points (Shofu, Inc., Kyoto, Japan)

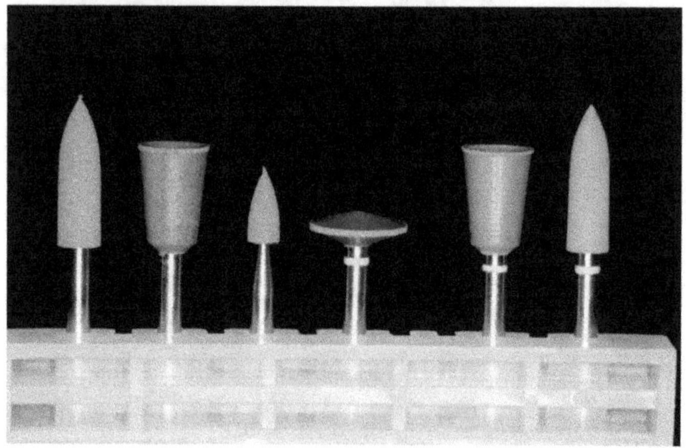

be polished meticulously, to ensure the surfaces are very smooth and highly polished. For this 2nd level of polishing, initially fine diamond impregnated points are followed by super silicone points (Figure 6b).

Finally, the surfaces are repolished with diamond paste and a Robinson bristle brush. This will help to achieve a super-high polished surface finish, with an enamel-like luster of all contoured teeth and restorations (Figure 6c).

For the Finishing Evaluation: Items like magnifying dental loupes (MiCD Loupes, Shofu, Inc., Kyoto, Japan) (Figure 7a), a digital dental camera (Eye Special II, Shofu, Inc., Kyoto, Japan) (Figure 7b) and the T-Scan 8 system are employed as the guiding tools to evaluate the Force Finishing quality.

The aesthetic outcome of any dental procedure is visible to the both patient and the clinician. However, because the force components are not visible to the naked eye, it is necessary to use a suitable digital occlusal technology in conjunction with conventional articulating paper markings. Articulating papers

Figure 6c. The Force Finishing Kit contains polishing items organized with super fine diamond impregnated silicone points, diamond paste, a polishing buff, and a Robinson brush (Shofu, Inc., Kyoto, Japan)

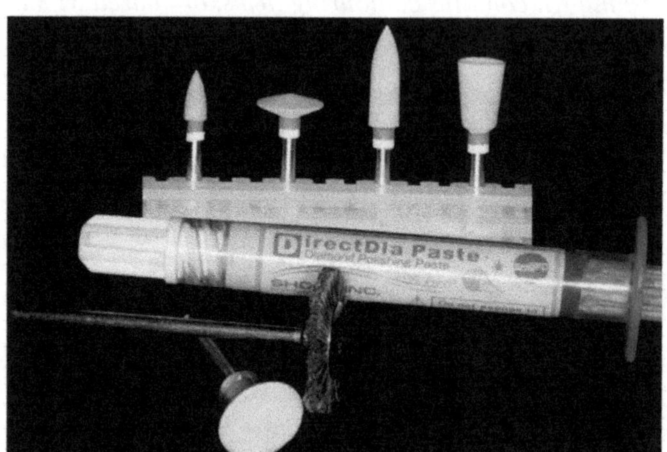

Figure 7a. MICD Dental Loupe (Shofu, Inc., Kyoto, Japan)

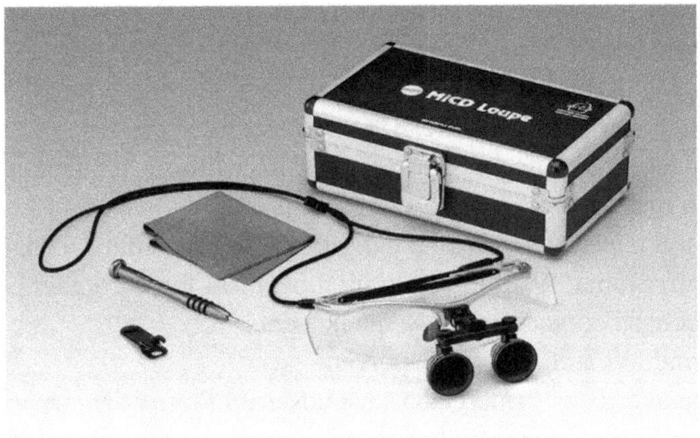

Figure 7b. Eye Special C-II digital dental camera (Shofu, Inc., Kyoto, Japan)

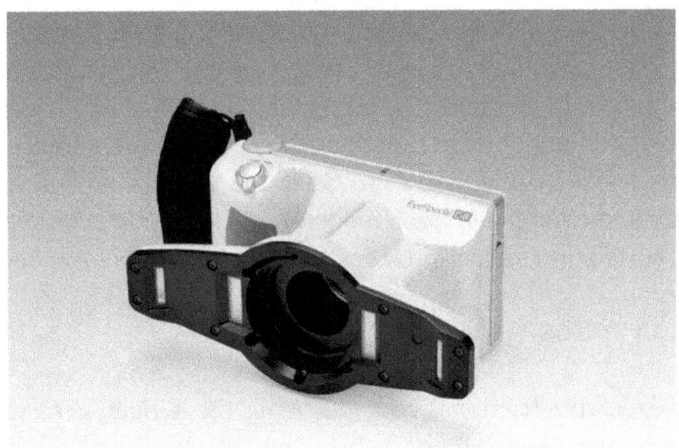

is required to mark and locate the problematic tooth contacts that are isolated by the T-Scan system as truly being problematic. After the completion of the Force Finishing process, all adjusted teeth and restorative surfaces must be polished smooth, using the previously described aesthetic finishing protocol.

Preventative Force Finishing (PFF) Clinical Protocol

The Preventative Force Finishing (PFF) protocol is employed to protect and maintain a patient's physiologically accepted original occlusal scheme, to preserve existing dental restorations and prostheses, as well as any newly installed restorations, from undergoing failure due to occlusal force disharmony.

Step I: Force Finishing During Centric Closure Movements

1. Bring all the teeth into occlusal contact by selectively adding (bonding), or subtracting (adjusting) opposing teeth or restorations, using bonding materials, the Force Finishing kit described above, and thin articulating paper with the T-Scan, as necessary.
2. Measure tooth contact relative forces and tooth contact timing sequences using the digital force scans obtained with the T-Scan.
3. Correlate the intraoral paper marks with the digital force and timing scan, by playing the recorded force movie frame-by-frame, to adjust early high occlusal force contact points one-by-one,based upon the T-Scan occlusal contact timing sequence data.
4. Equalize the right and left arch half force percentages.
5. Distribute nearly equal force percentage on each posterior tooth counterpart (i.e. the left first molar region should be nearly equal to the right first molar region's force percentage), again one-by-one.
6. Keep light tooth contacts (less force percentage) in the anterior region, but there should be definitive anterior contact where possible, or there will be increased potential for prolonged lateral and protrusive excursive frictional contacts, to occur.
7. Check the location of Center of Force (COF) and correct it, so it travels down the middle of the 2-Dimensional ForceView window. This correction centers the distribution of all the individual contact forces within the middle of all contacting teeth.
8. In case of implant restorations, selectively adjust the natural tooth contact timing and the implant supported prosthesis contact timing, so as to delay the implant prosthesis from making contact until the teeth nearby to the implants, reach moderate occlusal contact force. This ensures the teeth make solid contact before the implant prosthesis makes initial occlusal contact.

During Excursive and Protrusive Movements

1. Evaluate opposing excursive frictional contacts using the T-Scan 8 to record the right and left excursive movements, and the protrusive movement. Playback and determine where prolonged excursive frictional contacts are present. Then use different colored articulating paper than was used when centric occlusion was evaluated, to mark the located areas of opposing surface prolonged excursive contacts.
2. Remove all prolonged frictional contacts on the restorations and/or teeth, so that the Disclusion time is reduced to $\leq$ 0.5 seconds per excursion, and the excursive movement becomes smooth and fast for the patient to accomplish (Kerstein & Wright, 1991; Kerstein, 1993).
3. Achieve canine protected guidance whenever possible with conservative minor selective coronoplasty, or by bonding composite to the lingual surface of the maxillary canines.

Step II: Aesthetic Finishing

Aesthetic Touch Up

1. Achieve natural surface details with necessary minor surface adjustments by placing texture, grooves, pits and other special surface effects into the restorations.

Polishing Sequence

1. **Pre-Polishing:** Remove any remaining surface scratches that result from the aesthetic touch up process.
2. **Polishing:** Establish a blemish free and smooth surface with no visible scratches present on the restoration.
3. **Super Polishing:** Polish the restoration to an enamel-like luster.

Step III: Finishing Evaluation

1. Evaluate the aesthetics, the health of the teeth and the gingiva, and the overall patient comfort status.
2. Confirm the Force Finishing end results by re-evaluating the occlusion with T-Scan digital occlusal force and timing analyses. Improve where required.
3. Document the final case finishing result with the digital force scan and digital photography.

Therapeutic Force Finishing (TFF) Clinical Protocol

When the occlusal force components need to be customized to treat specific signs and symptoms of occlusal force disorders, therapeutic Force Finishing can be performed on both teeth and restorations, or upon employed therapeutic oral appliances, or installed dental prostheses. In any therapeutic Force Finishing case, the patients' occlusal force disorder signs and symptoms, the number of tooth contacts, the periodontal health, the crown to root ratio, the tooth angulations, the tooth positions, the facial type and the vertical dimension of occlusion, must all be analyzed in detail, to ascertain the "weakest link" within the patient's masticatory system. Then, direct Force Finishing is performed on the teeth or on the restorations, to customize the occlusal force balance, improve the Occlusion timing and the Disclusion timing, and to remove any frictional contacts, all of which will support the healing and adaptation process of the patient's masticatory system. Alternatively when indicted, indirect Force Finishing can be done to customize the occlusal force components (to increase balance, or reduce an imbalance), using therapeutic oral splints or prostheses that do not involve altering the natural teeth, or changing any existing restorations.

The clinician must keep the following points in mind when performing Therapeutic Force Finishing:

1. The force percentage must be distributed as per the periodontal health, root and occlusal surface area available, and the available numbers of load bearing teeth
2. Reduce the occlusal load percentage on weak teeth that present with compromised periodontal bone support, are mobile, and/or present as painful or hypersensitive teeth, so as to support the natural healing process
3. Remove excursive frictional forces on painful, mobile, and hypertensive teeth
4. In cases of masticatory muscle pain symptoms, reduce the Disclusion Time, and balance the occlusal forces by using conservative tooth contouring methods (combining bonding and coronoplasty). However, if conservative methods are not possible to safely accomplish the needed occlusal changes, use a therapeutic oral appliance and reduce on its occlusal table the Disclusion Time, while also balancing the closure occlusal forces.

5. Once the signs and symptoms of OFD have subsided from treatment, then preventative Force Finishing can be performed, to aid in maintaining long-term functional occlusal health.

Force Finishing Clinical Case Presentation

Force Finishing can be applied in every field of Dental Medicine where occlusion is involved. The Orthodontist is one whose work always involves occlusion, as is the clinician who regularly fabricates full mouth reconstruction, performs smile makeovers, places multiple restorations at one time, fabricates implant supported prostheses, and treats Temporomandibular disorders with occlusal adjustment. Clinicians who perform these procedures would obtain significant benefits from employing Force Finishing with the T-Scan technology in clinical practice.

As mentioned earlier, Force Finishing has two components; Preventative (PFF) and Therapeutic (TFF). Presented below are three clinical cases of Force Finishing, that illustrate both PFF and TFF, to aid the reader in understanding the simplicity of, and the clinical benefits of using Force Finishing in daily clinical practice.

Case I: Preventative Force Finishing (PFF) in Full Mouth Reconstruction of a Severely Worn Smile

A 55 year-old male reported with complaints of having a severely worn smile resultant from his longstanding chronic habit of nighttime bruxing. Through the years, the patient tried to maintain and protect his teeth by having multiple crowns and bridges placed. However, due to his chronic habit of bruxism, all of his natural teeth and his porcelain fused to metal crown and bridges, were being worn away (Figure 8a - e).

After a thorough clinical case analysis, an occlusal analysis with the T-Scan was performed. The detected occlusal force pattern was very imbalanced, as the molars were taking most of the occlusal load. Hence, the Center of Force icon was shifted far to the posterior, indicating poor anteroposterior occlusal force balance, with slightly more force on right half of the arch (Figure 9).

The excursive scan data of the right and left lateral excursive movements, showed the presence of working side group function. There was no canine guidance acting to minimize the muscular forces created from the existing posterior excursive frictional contacts (Figures 10a - d).

A micro - invasive, full mouth reconstruction using indirect composite restorations that would be installed with Force Finishing, was proposed to the patient. The fundamental aim of the treatment was to establish occlusal harmony (Force Balance), improve the anterior guidance function, and restore the lost aesthetics, without sacrificing any tooth structure to maintain the vitality of all worn teeth. In this case, Ceramage indirect composite restorations were used (Ceramage, Shofu, Inc., Kyoto, Japan) (Figure 11a - c), to completely restore the worn teeth with overlays, without requiring any invasive tooth preparation, other than to micro-etch the tooth structure required for restorative material chemical bonding (Figures12a - d).

Once these laboratory-fabricated indirect composite overlays were seated and bonded to place, the case was completed using the Force Finishing protocol that was previously described under Preventative Force Finishing.

Post insertion and after Force Finishing, the occlusal forces in maximum intercuspation were balanced, demonstrating proper force distribution on each tooth, and in both arch-halves (45.4% to 54.6%) (Figure 13). Note that the Center of Force icon, which was previously positioned in the posterior right

Figure 8a. Severely worn smile shown from the frontal view. Note that because of the high masticatory forces, both the maxillary and mandibular teeth show visible attrition. © [2013] [Courtesy of Vedic Institute of Smile Aesthetics]. Used with permission.

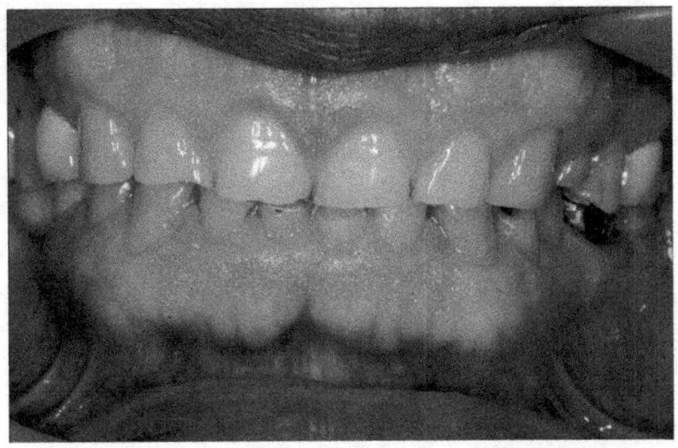

Figure 8b. Severely worn smile shown from the maxillary occlusal view. Note that the ceramic crowns show visible attrition and dentine is exposed from the attrition combined with secondary erosion. © [2013] [Courtesy of Vedic Institute of Smile Aesthetics]. Used with permission.

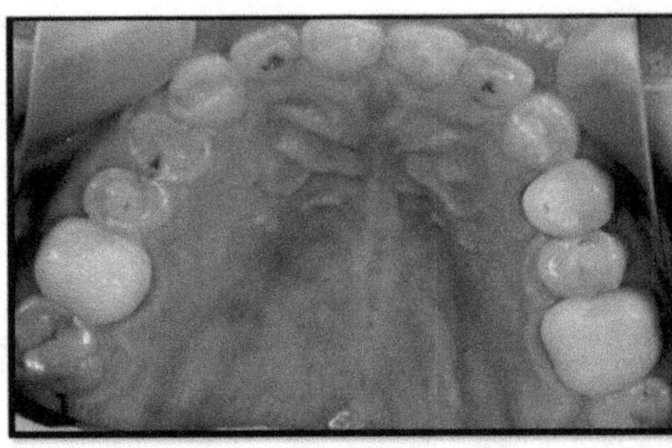

Figure 8c. Severely worn smile shown from the mandibular occlusal view. Along with the worn ceramic and metal crowns, the mandibular anterior teeth were severely worm with visibly exposed dentin. © [2013] [Courtesy of Vedic Institute of Smile Aesthetics]. Used with permission.

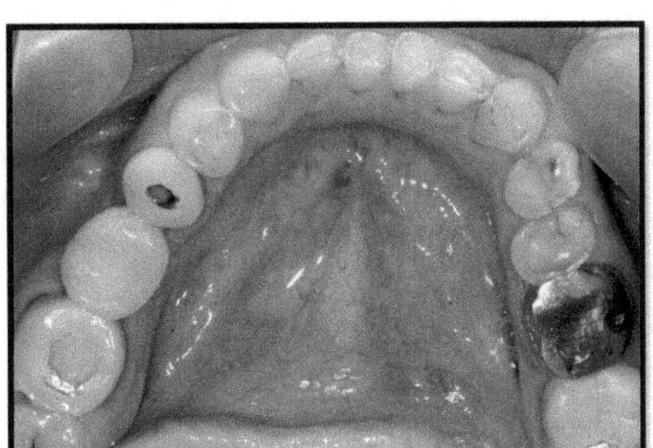

Figure 8d. Severely worn smile from the left lateral view showing attrition of the canine and premolar cusps. © [2013] [Courtesy of Vedic Institute of Smile Aesthetics]. Used with permission.

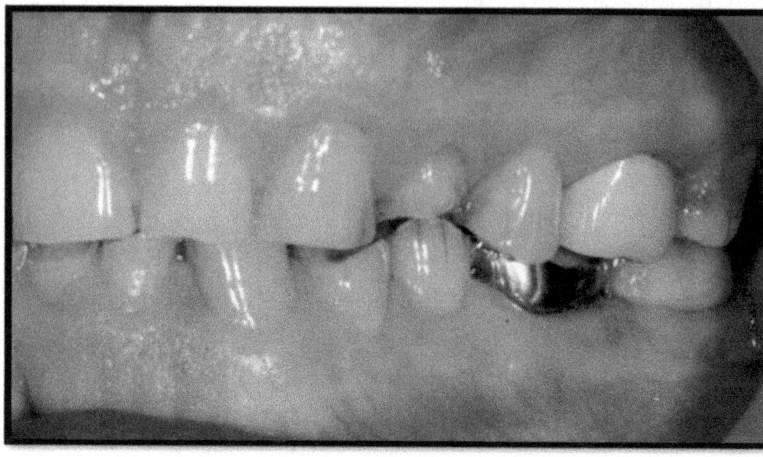

Figure 8e. Severely worn smile from the right lateral view showing attrition of the canine and the and right lateral incisors.

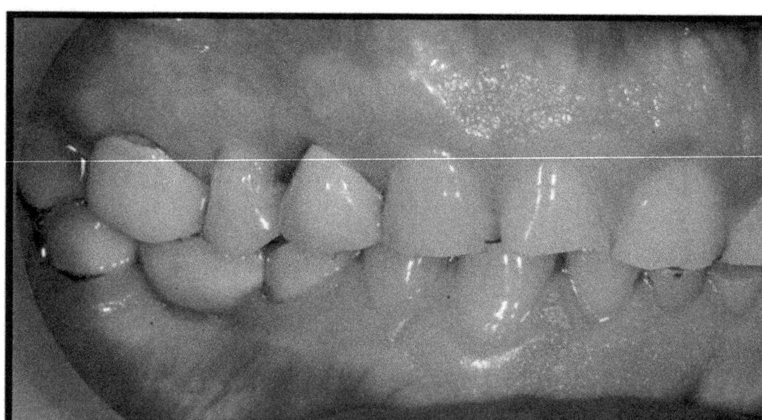

(Figure 9), was now located in the middle of the arch, indicating that the occlusal force distribution showed improved balance (Figure 13).

Since the main cause of the tooth wear in this case was bruxism, a canine-protected occlusal scheme with proper canine guidance was created, to separate the posterior teeth during the right and left excursive movements. Note in the force scan data (Figures 14a- d), that 100% canine guidance was created during both excursive movements. This will prevent any frictional forces from occurring during the restored excursive function. This type of case requires long-term follow-up force measurements recorded over time, to monitor any occlusal force distribution changes from worn materials or slight maxillomandibular relationship changes

After 12 months, this case was clinically re-evaluated, where it was observed that intact occlusal surfaces were still present, with the case demonstrating no visible signs of fracture and/or restorative

Figure 9. Force scan showing maximum intercuspation. The right and left arch halves are almost balanced, however the molars are receiving most of the occlusal load. The Center of Force icon is far to the right posterior, with no occlusal contacts visible on the majority of the anterior teeth.

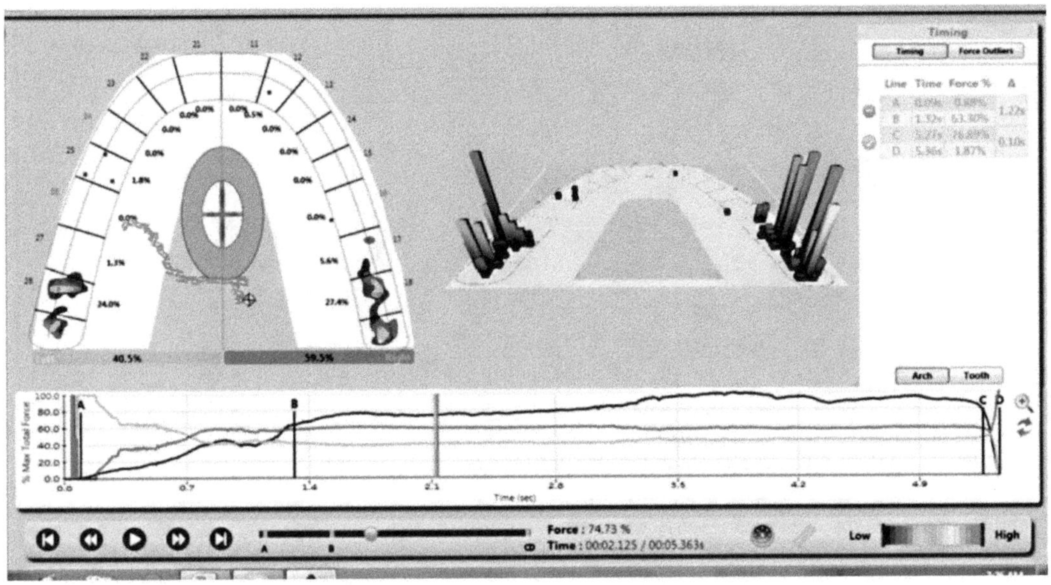

Figure 10a. Force scan view of the right lateral excursive movement, 0.14 seconds after line C, which is where the excursion commenced. There is lack of canine guidance, as all right posterior teeth are in contact in the excursion. No guiding contacts are present on the anterior teeth to lift apart he posteriors. *© [2013] [Courtesy of Vedic Institute of Smile Aesthetics]. Used with permission.*

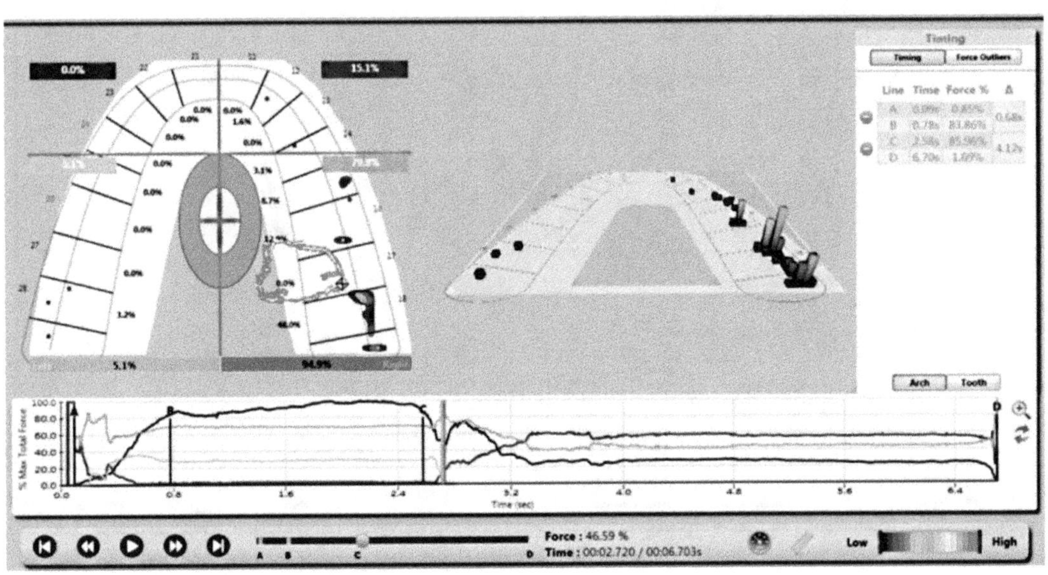

Figure 10b. Force scan view of the right lateral excursive movement. Again there is a lack of canine guidance as the right 2nd molar is still in contact after 1.46 seconds into the right excursive movement. © [2013] [Courtesy of Vedic Institute of Smile Aesthetics]. Used with permission.

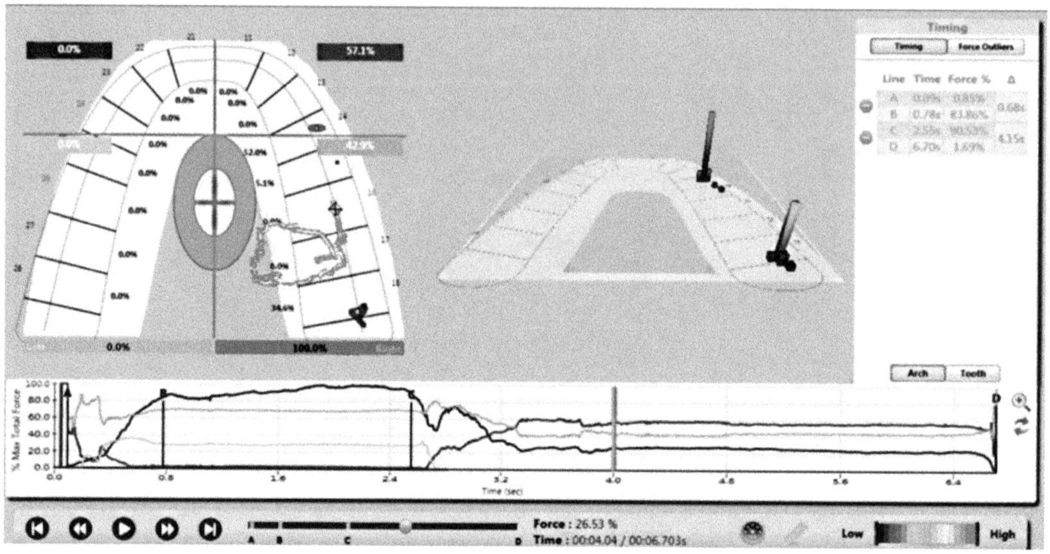

Figure 10c. Force scan view of the left lateral excursive movement 0.321 seconds after line C where the excursion was commenced. There is a lack of canine guidance, as all the left working side posterior teeth are in contact within a group function. There is a balancing side right second molar contact present, as well. © [2013] [Courtesy of Vedic Institute of Smile Aesthetics]. Used with permission.

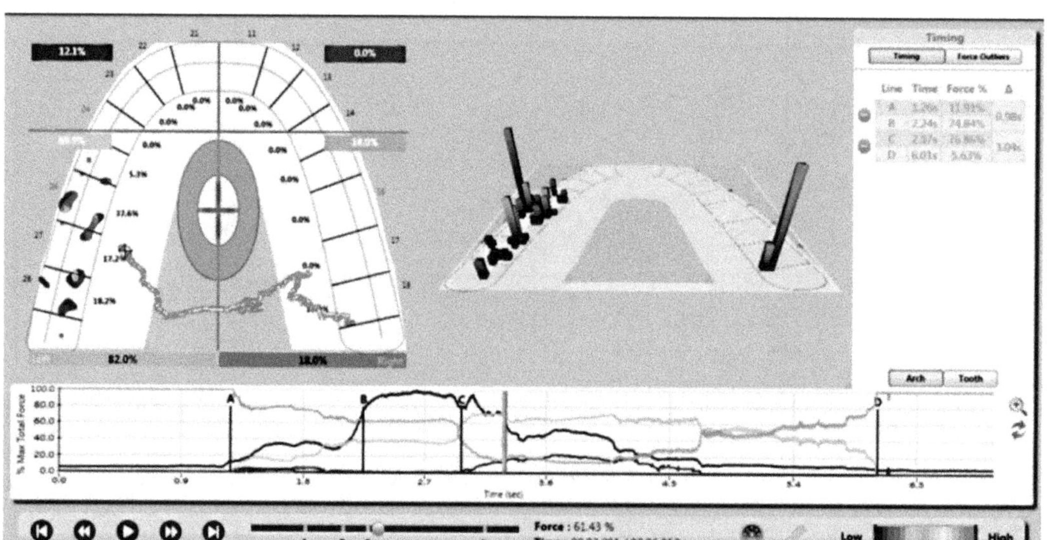

failure (Figures 15a- f). Only the surface gloss of the restorations was dulled, which is a normal occurrence when employing composite restorative materials. During a follow-up visit, super polishing was performed again, using the polishing Force Finishing kit.

Figure 10d. Force scan view later within the left lateral excursive movement, 1.214 seconds after excursive commencement. There remains in contact the left working side posterior group function and a forceful balancing contact on the right second molar. © [2013] [Courtesy of Vedic Institute of Smile Aesthetics]. Used with permission.

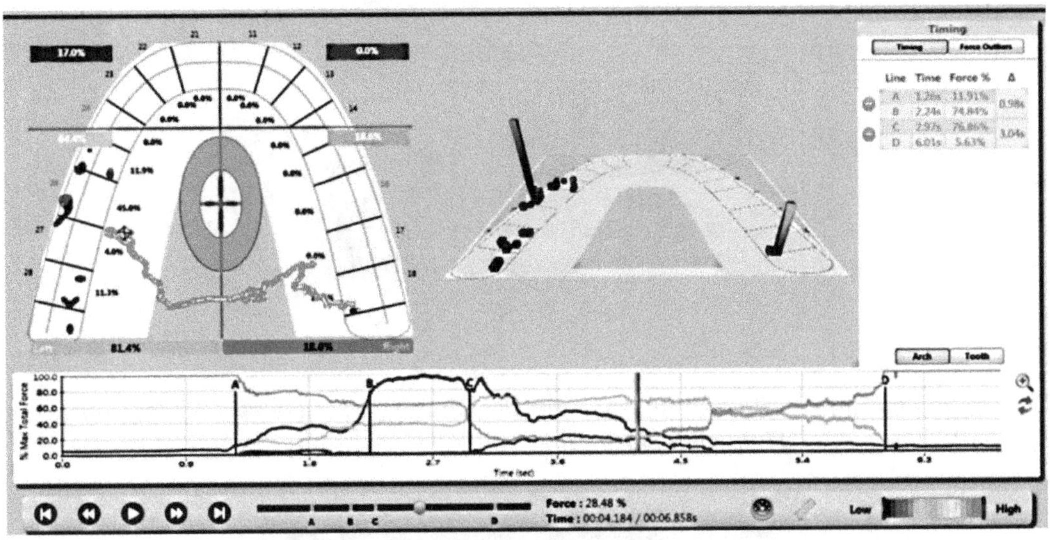

Figure 11a. Ceramage indirect composite system (Shofu, Inc., Kyoto, Japan). © [2013] [Courtesy of Vedic Institute of Smile Aesthetics]. Used with permission.

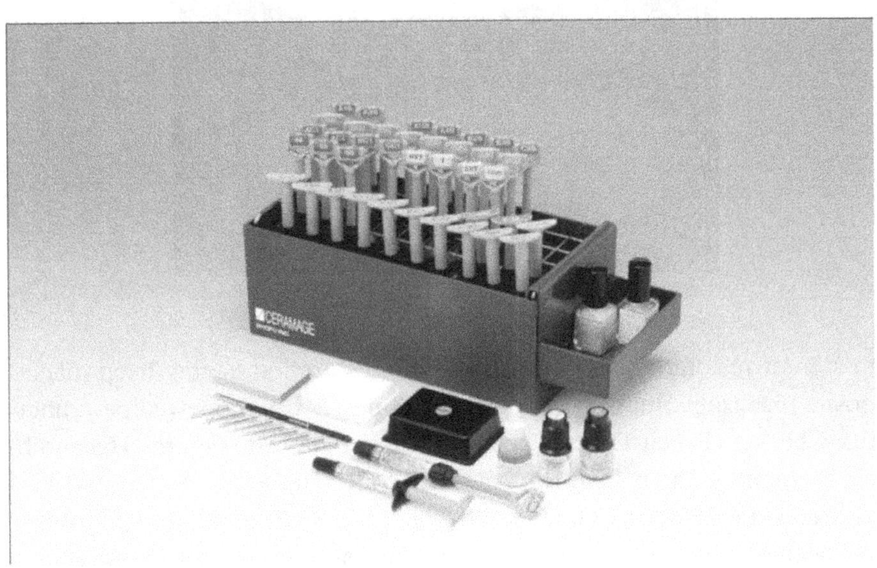

12 month post insertion, the force scan data illustrated that the occlusal force balance had slightly changed to a 41.9% left - 58.1% right distribution. The Center of Force icon was still located near the center of the arch. However, the mandibular path of closure had changed somewhat, compared to immediate post insert.

Figure 11b. Ceramage indirect composite light curing system (Shofu, Inc., Kyoto, Japan). © [2013] [Courtesy of Vedic Institute of Smile Aesthetics]. Used with permission.

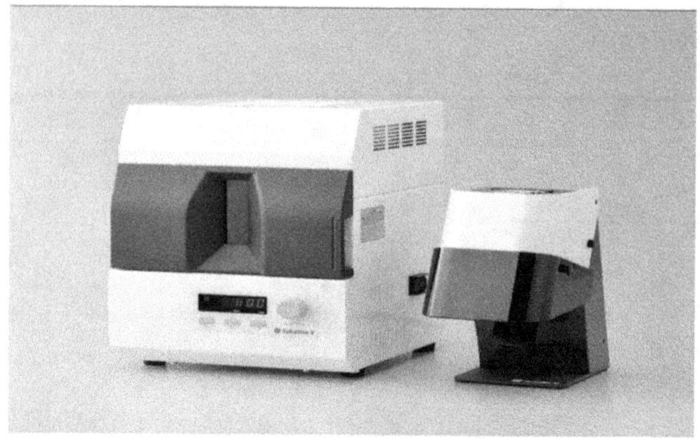

Figure 11c. Upper anterior overlays fabricated using the Ceramage system. © [2013] [Courtesy of Vedic Institute of Smile Aesthetics]. Used with permission.

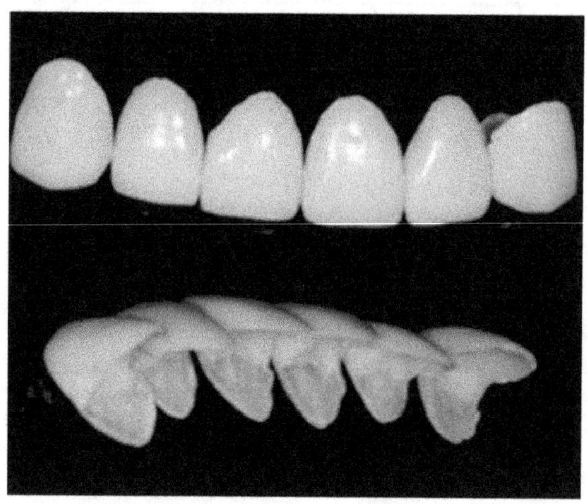

There was no sign of restorative fracture despite the restoration having been made by softer (than porcelain) composite materials. But the patient had begun to exhibit renewed parafunction, which was revealed in a Brux-Checker (Scheu-Dental, Germany) overnight test (Figures 16a and b).

However after 26 months, the patient re-visited for follow up and reported that his parafunctional habit was slowly increasing, despite the quality of the existing occlusal scheme (Figures 17 - 20b). Brux-Checker was used again for one night, which showed that intense nighttime parafunction had returned (Figure 21).

Since the full mouth reconstruction had been completed with a non-invasive, adhesive technique using indirect composite restorative material which was softer than porcelain, the restorations were kind to the enamel, the masticatory muscles, and the Temporomandibular Joints, despite that the patient demonstrated parafunctional habits, one year post treatment. Of note was that after 22 months the occlusal cusps of the soft composite restorations were found to be somewhat worn, but not fractured.

Figure 12a. Maxillary arch occlusal view after complete restoration with indirect composite Ceramage overlays. The occlusion was force finished using articulating paper and the T-Scan 8. © [2013] [Courtesy of Vedic Institute of Smile Aesthetics]. Used with permission.

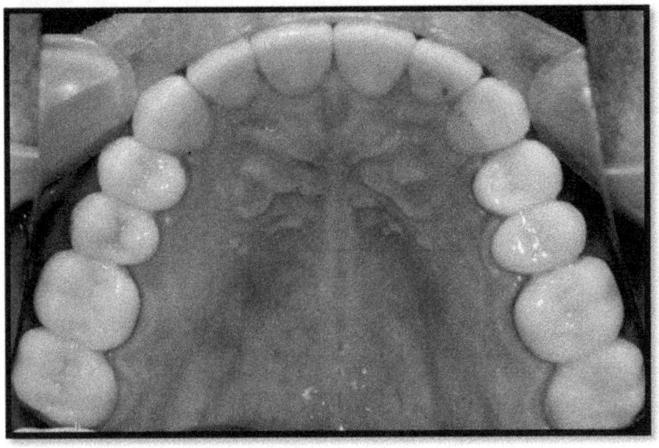

Figure 12b. Mandibular arch occlusal view after complete restoration with indirect composite Ceramage overlays. The occlusion was force finished using articulating paper and the T-Scan 8. © [2013] [Courtesy of Vedic Institute of Smile Aesthetics]. Used with permission.

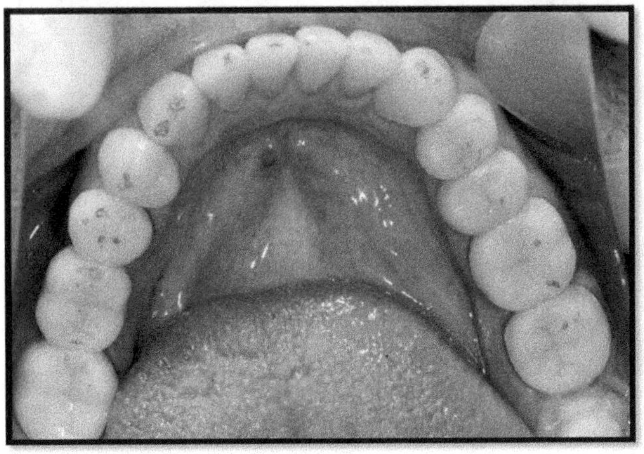

Had the full mouth reconstruction been completed using harder restorative materials like porcelain, metal, or zirconia, the effect of the parafunctional occlusal forces would have been visible within the masticatory muscles or the TM joints function. The beauty of using composite restorative materials in this type of severely worn dentition, is that the clinician can readily reconfigure the occlusion either by selective adjustment, or by bonding any worn areas back into full function. These corrective procedures can then be followed-up with appropriate Force Finishing assessments. Because the patient had persistent bruxism, he was advised to wear a night guard to protect the restorations until the re-restorative occlusal balancing, was accomplished.

Figure 12c. Right lateral view after complete restoration with Ceramage indirect composite overlays. © [2013] [Courtesy of Vedic Institute of Smile Aesthetics]. Used with permission.

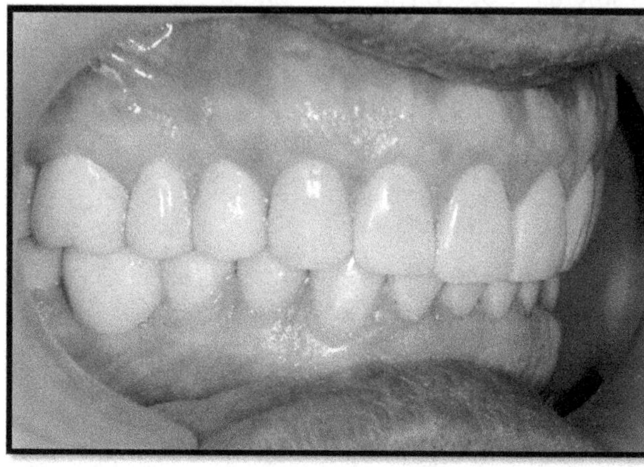

Figure 12d. Left lateral view after complete restoration with Ceramage indirect composite overlays. © [2013] [Courtesy of Vedic Institute of Smile Aesthetics]. Used with permission.

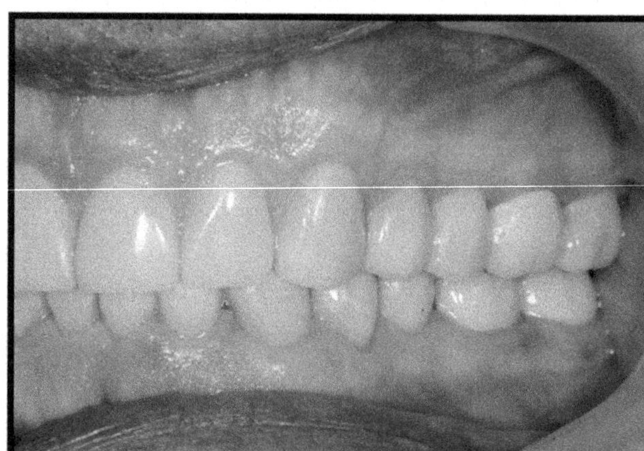

Case II: Preventative Force Finishing in Complete Dentures - The Conventional Approach vs. the Digital Approach

A 76 year-old Sherpa from Tibet presented with the desire to have a new maxillary complete denture fabricated. The rendered treatment consisted of a new maxillary complete denture and a new mandibular cast partial denture (Figure 24).

At delivery, the case was initially finished conventionally using only articulating paper combined with patient oral "feel" feedback. After, the case was re-evaluated using digital occlusal force scanning with the T-Scan 8 system. When articulating paper markings were used alone, although the forces in right and left arch halves were properly balanced, there was excess force accumulation located in the canine and premolar regions (Figure 25). It should be noted that a high concentration of occlusal force located solely on one tooth or restoration, might lead to the development of an occlusal force disorder. Hence,

Figure 13. Note the changes to the occlusal force pattern after proper Force Finishing. The force percentage between the right and left arch halves was 49.8% left - 50.2% right, in maximum intercuspation. The Center of Force icon is near the middle of the arch, and the force on each tooth is properly distributed. The COF path of closure begins near tooth #11 and #21 then centers slightly towards left side. © [2013] [Courtesy of Vedic Institute of Smile Aesthetics]. Used with permission.

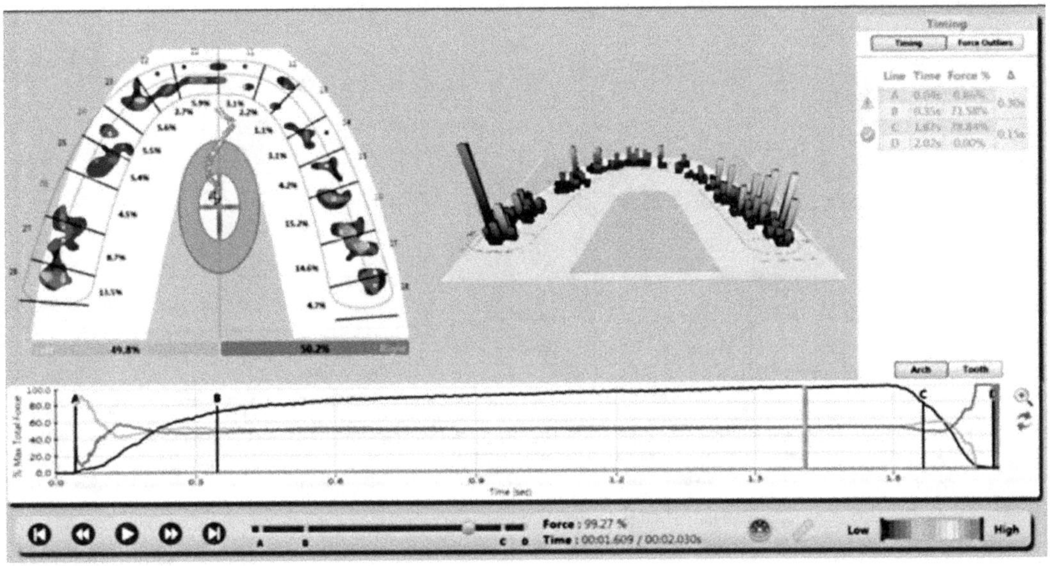

Figure 14a. Force Scan data of the right lateral excursive movement showing the right canine accepting 55% of the excursive forces 0.118 seconds after excursive commencement (past line C). © [2013] [Courtesy of Vedic Institute of Smile Aesthetics]. Used with permission.

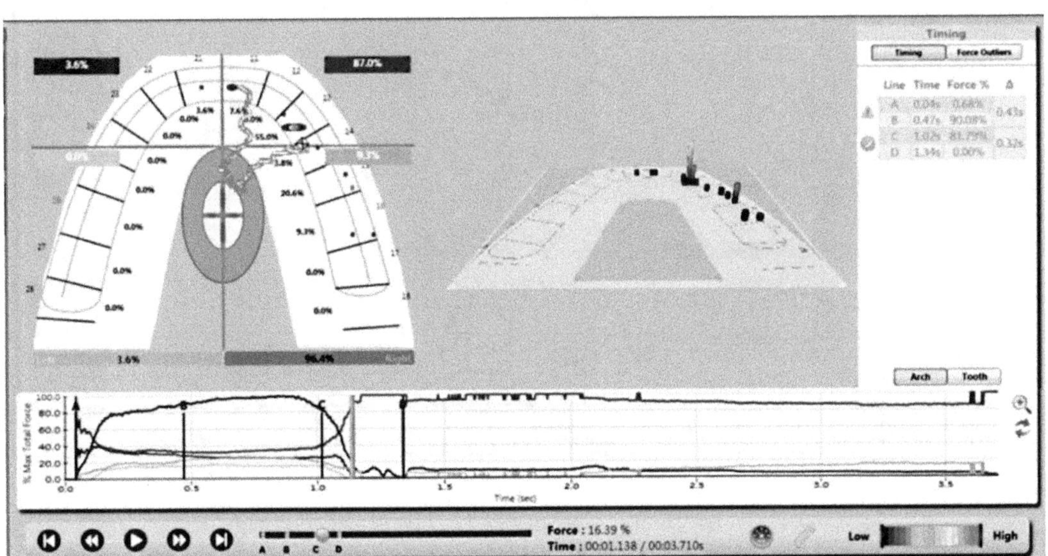

Figure 14b. Force Scan data of the right lateral excursive movement showing the right canine accepting 100% of the excursive forces 0.241 seconds after excursive commencement (past line C). © [2013] [Courtesy of Vedic Institute of Smile Aesthetics]. Used with permission.

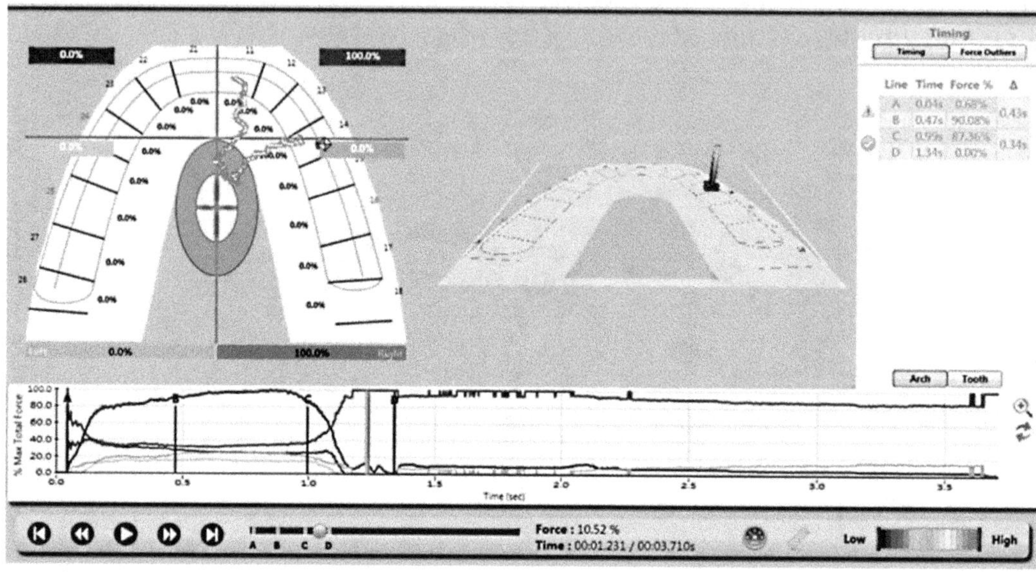

Figure 14c. Force Scan data of the left lateral excursive movement 0.914 seconds after excursive commencement. © [2013] [Courtesy of Vedic Institute of Smile Aesthetics]. Used with permission.

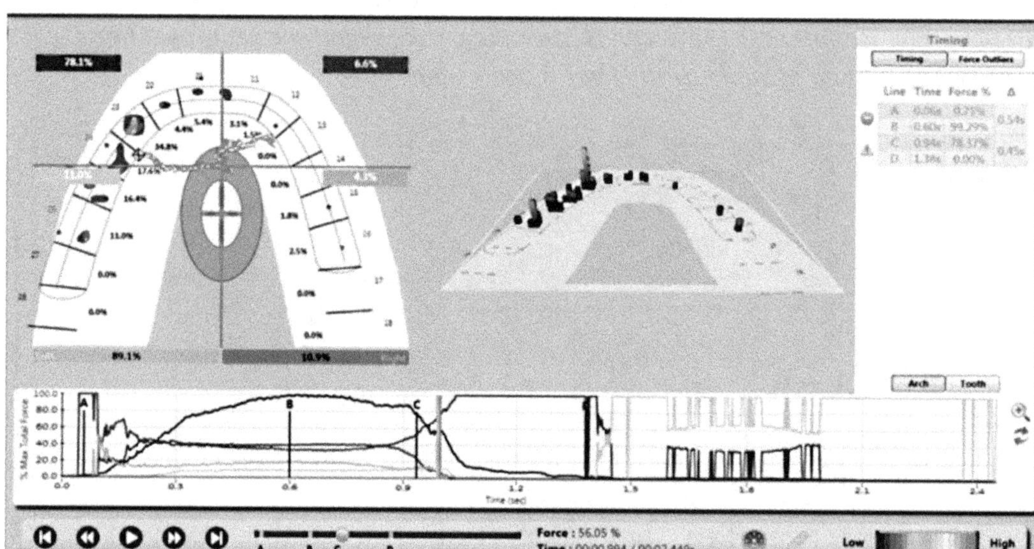

Figure 14d. Force Scan data of the left lateral excursive movement showing the left canine accepting 100% of the excursive forces 0.276 seconds from excursive commencement. © [2013] [Courtesy of Vedic Institute of Smile Aesthetics]. Used with permission.

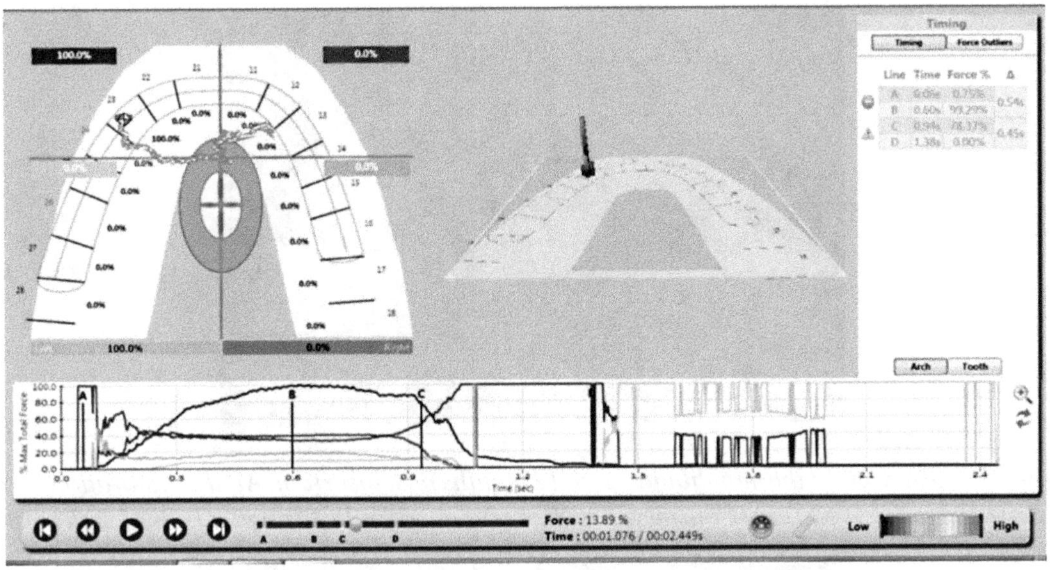

Figure 15a. Frontal view of the restorations 12 months, post insertion. The restorations are intact with no sign of fractures or porcelain chipping. However, after one year, the restorations have lost their aesthetic gloss, requiring re-polishing. © [2013] [Courtesy of Vedic Institute of Smile Aesthetics]. Used with permission.

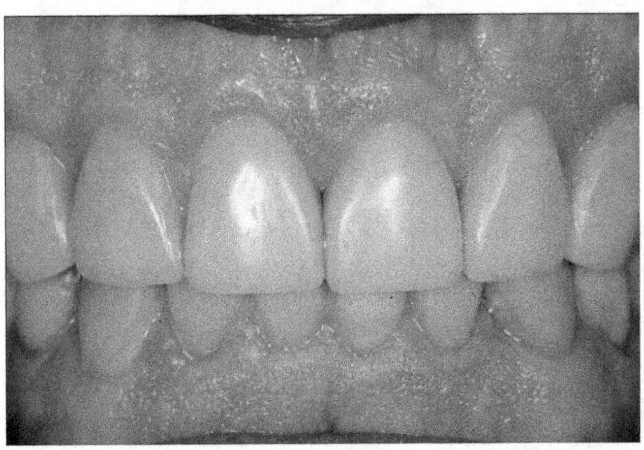

the case was re-balanced employing Force Finishing with the T-Scan as the guiding tool (Figure 26), to reduce the high forces in the premolar area. Additionally, the total force was balanced both tooth-wise, and arch-half-wise, the Center of Force icon was relocated into the middle of the distribution of teeth, and the path of closure was redirected onto the arch half midline, indicating that all teeth contacted simultaneously.

Figure 15b. Occlusal view of the maxillary arch 12 months post insertion. The patient is not wearing a night guard, but the restorations are intact with no sign of fracture. © [2013] [Courtesy of Vedic Institute of Smile Aesthetics]. Used with permission.

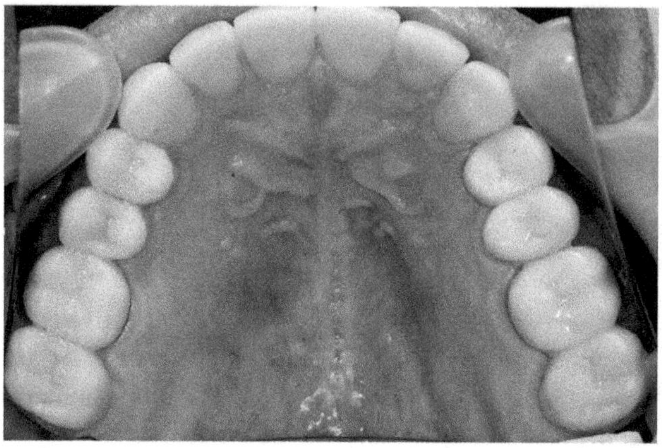

Figure 15c. Occlusal view of the mandibular arch 12 months post insertion. All the restorations are intact with no sign of fracture. © [2013] [Courtesy of Vedic Institute of Smile Aesthetics]. Used with permission.

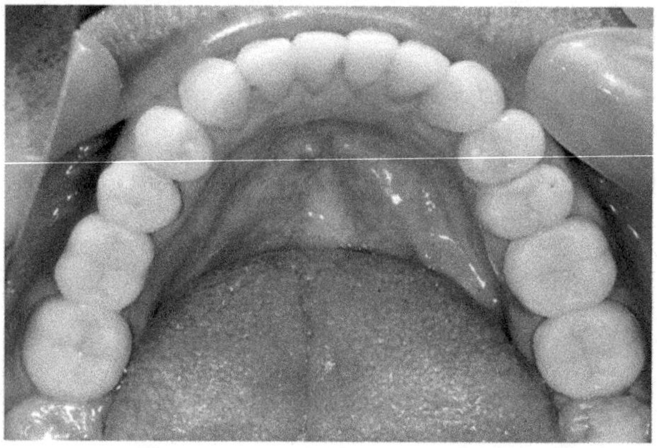

Figure 15d. The right lateral view 12 months post insertion. All of the buccal cusps of the restorations are still intact. © [2013] [Courtesy of Vedic Institute of Smile Aesthetics]. Used with permission.

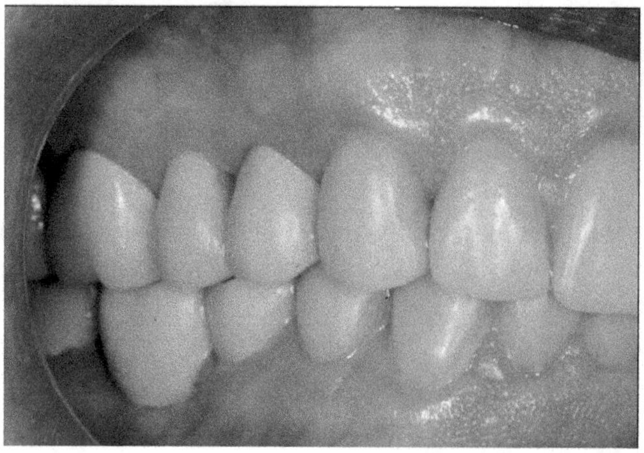

Figure 15e. The left lateral view 12 months post insertion. All the buccal cusps of the restorations are still intact

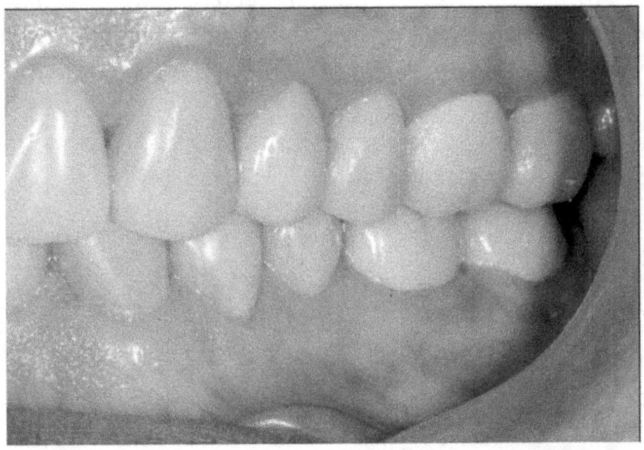

Figure 15f. The restoration after cosmetic touch up polishing

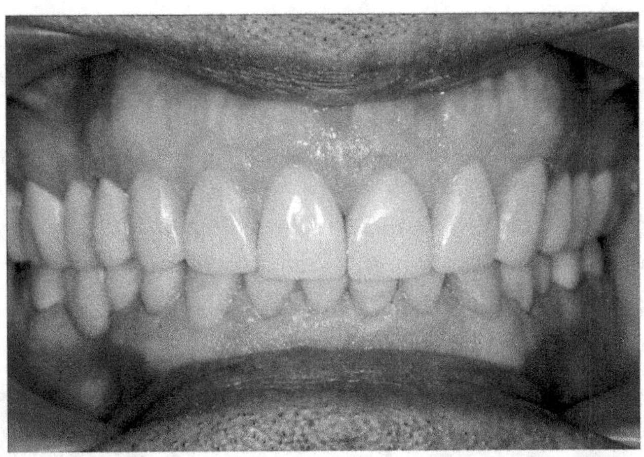

Case III: Therapeutic Force Finishing (TFF) in TMD Management

Occlusal force disharmony is considered a fundamental factor in the etiology of Temporomandibular Disorders (TMD) (Glaros, Glass, & McLaughlin, 1994; Arbree, Campbell, Renner, & Goldstein, 1995; Dawson, 1999). Therefore, a major aim of any TMD management should be to balance any detected occlusal force imbalance, either by selectively increasing the load in a patient with a healthy TMJA complex, or by decreasing the load in a compromised one. To accomplish these load changes to the TMJA complex, four major categories of TMJA Harmony oral appliances have been described (Koirala, 2013):

- **Type I:** Protective Appliances that protect the teeth and the supportive arches.
- **Type II:** Growth Appliances that guide the growth of the dental and skeletal patterns.

Figure 16a. 12-month post insertion, the force scan data illustrated occlusal force balance had changed to become 41.9% left - 58.1% right. The Center of Force icon was still located near the center of the arch. However, the mandibular path of closure had changed compared to immediate post insertion. The COF trajectory after 12 months indicates the right side forces rise in time much earlier than the left side forces. © [2013] [Courtesy of Vedic Institute of Smile Aesthetics]. Used with permission.

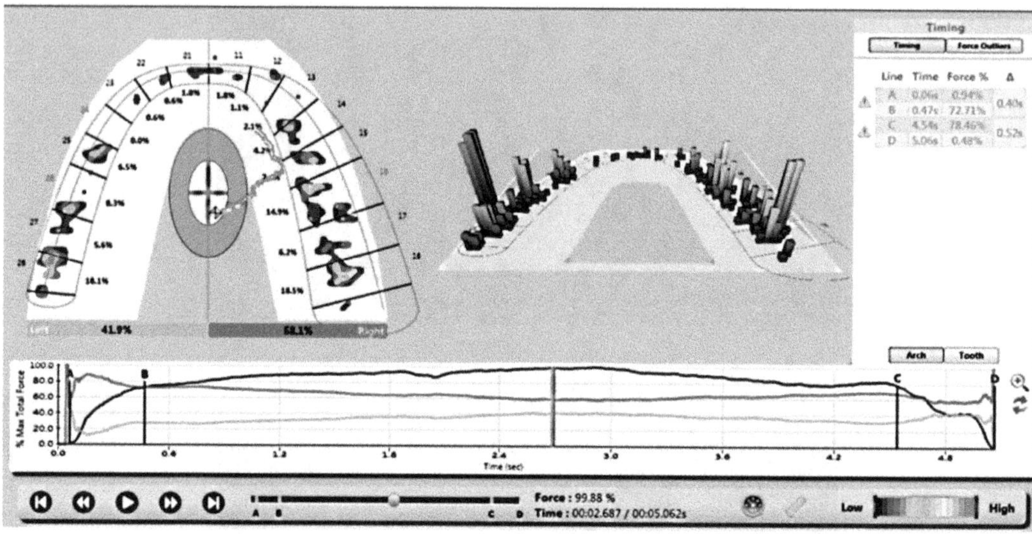

Figure 16b. The patient used a Brux-Checker, which showed he had begun to exhibit some renewed teeth clenching (similar contact marks are visible bilaterally). Since the occlusal forces remained balanced and the load was properly distributed resultant from the insertion Force Finishing, clinically there were no restorative factures detected. © [2013] [Courtesy of Vedic Institute of Smile Aesthetics]. Used with permission.

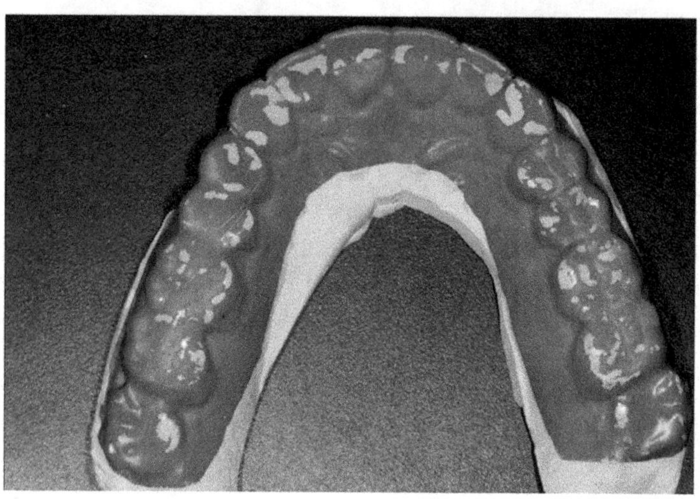

Figure 17. Maxillary occlusal view follow-up photograph, 26 months post insertion. Note all restorations are intact. © [2013] [Courtesy of Vedic Institute of Smile Aesthetics]. Used with permission.

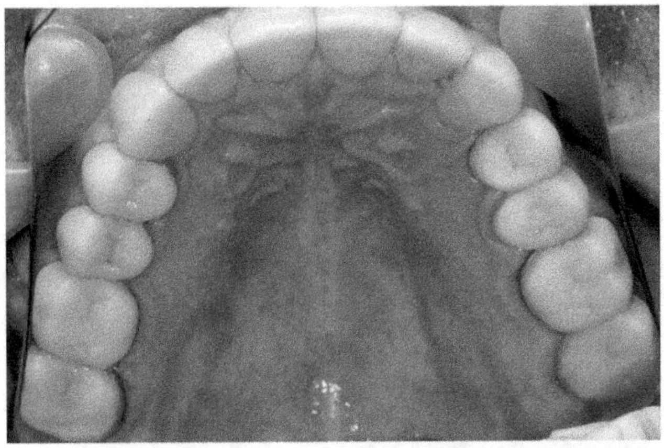

Figure 18. Mandibular occlusal view follow-up photograph 26 months post insertion. There are no restorative fractures visible. © [2013] [Courtesy of Vedic Institute of Smile Aesthetics]. Used with permission.

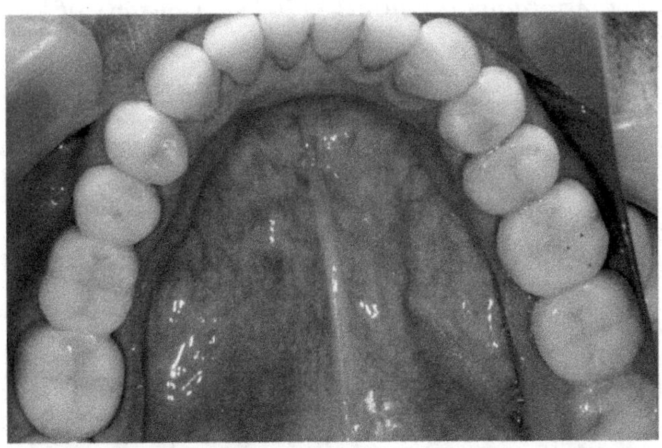

Figure 19. Frontal view photograph with all restorations intact, 26 months post insertion. © [2013] [Courtesy of Vedic Institute of Smile Aesthetics]. Used with permission.

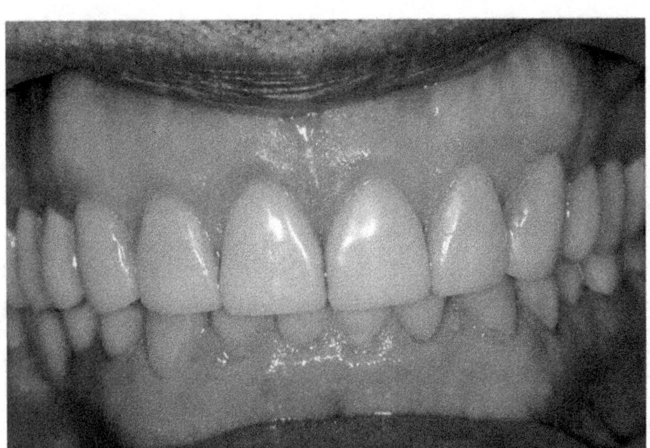

Figure 20a. The left lateral view, 26 months post insertion. All the buccal cusps of the restorations are still intact, with no sign of restoration fracture. © [2013] [Courtesy of Vedic Institute of Smile Aesthetics]. Used with permission.

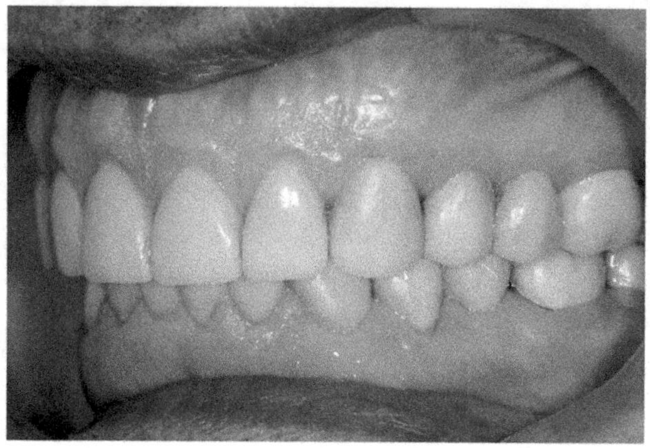

Figure 20b. The right lateral view, 26 months post insertion. All of the buccal cusps of the restorations are still intact with no sign of restoration fracture. © [2013] [Courtesy of Vedic Institute of Smile Aesthetics]. Used with permission.

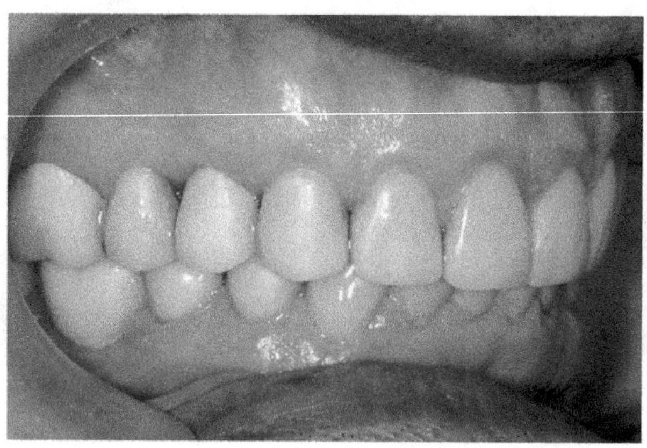

- **Type III:** TMD Appliances that support masticatory muscles and Temporomandibular joint health:
  - Muscle Type.
  - TM Joint Type.
- **Type IV:** Sleep Appliances that reduce airway obstruction.

To ensure these oral appliances will induce changes in the occlusal loading that occur in both function and parafunction, it is always advisable to use the Force Finishing process during the appliance delivery.

In general, clinicians employ two different Type III - TMD appliances:

- **Muscle Type:** Stabilization Appliance.
- **TM Joint Type:** Re-positioning Appliance.

Figure 21. Nighttime bruxism detected on the Brux-Checker, 26 month post insertion. Note that the teeth contact marks are more visible on the left side of the Brux-Checker, which corresponded with the T-Scan detected force imbalance, shown in Figure 22 (Figures 22 - 23b). © [2013] [Courtesy of Vedic Institute of Smile Aesthetics]. Used with permission.

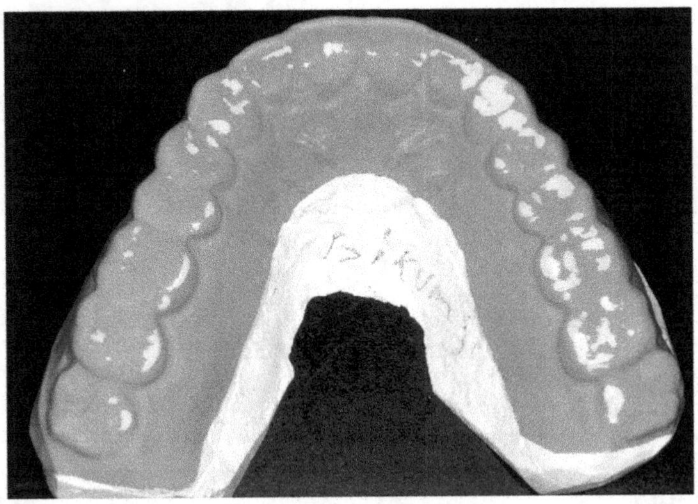

Figure 22. Force Scan data 26 months post restoration. The force balance had changed drastically with 18.3% of the occlusal force on left side, and 81.7% on the right side. The Center of Force icon was located in the right posterior area. This force imbalance resulted from the re-occurrence of the patient's bruxism habit. Note the grinding marks present on the Brux-Checker in Figure 21. © [2013] [Courtesy of Vedic Institute of Smile Aesthetics]. Used with permission.

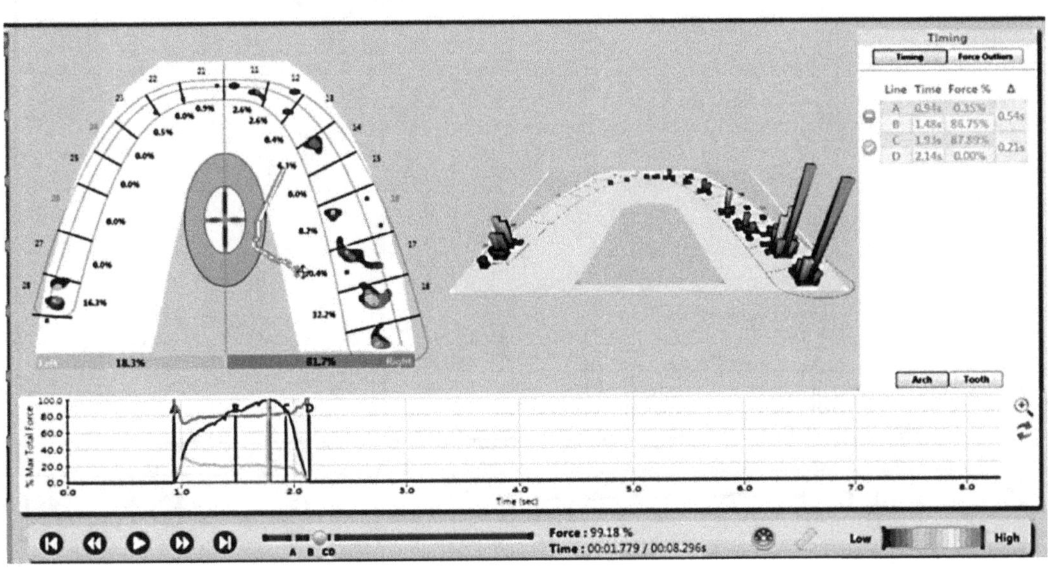

Figure 23a. Force Scan data of the right lateral excursive movement, 0.128 seconds after excursive commencement (line C), 26 months post insertion. © [2013] [Courtesy of Vedic Institute of Smile Aesthetics]. Used with permission.

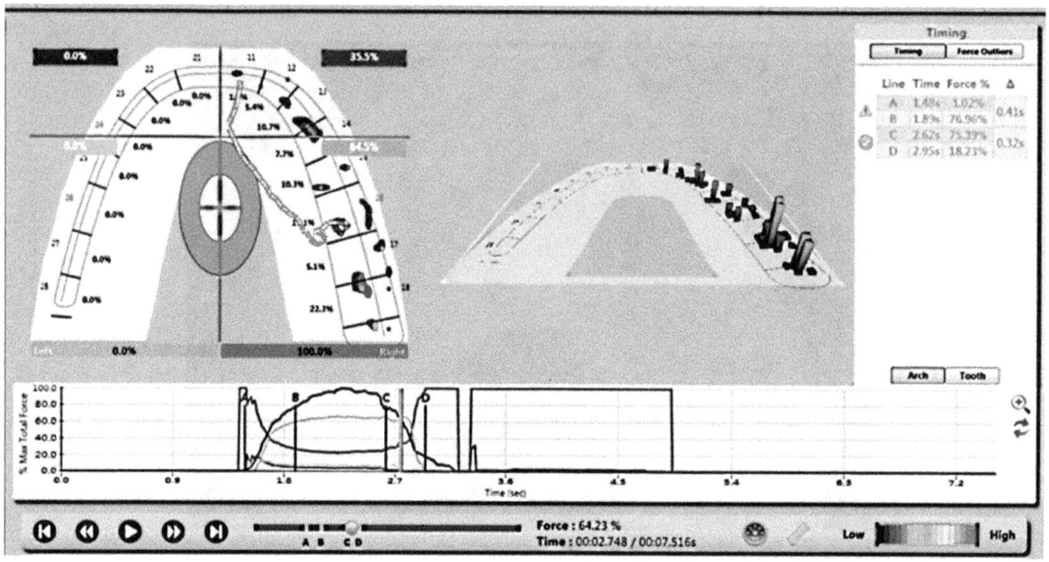

Figure 23b. Force Scan data of the right lateral excursive movement 0.378 seconds after excursive commencement (line C), 26 months post insertion. © [2013] [Courtesy of Vedic Institute of Smile Aesthetics]. Used with permission.

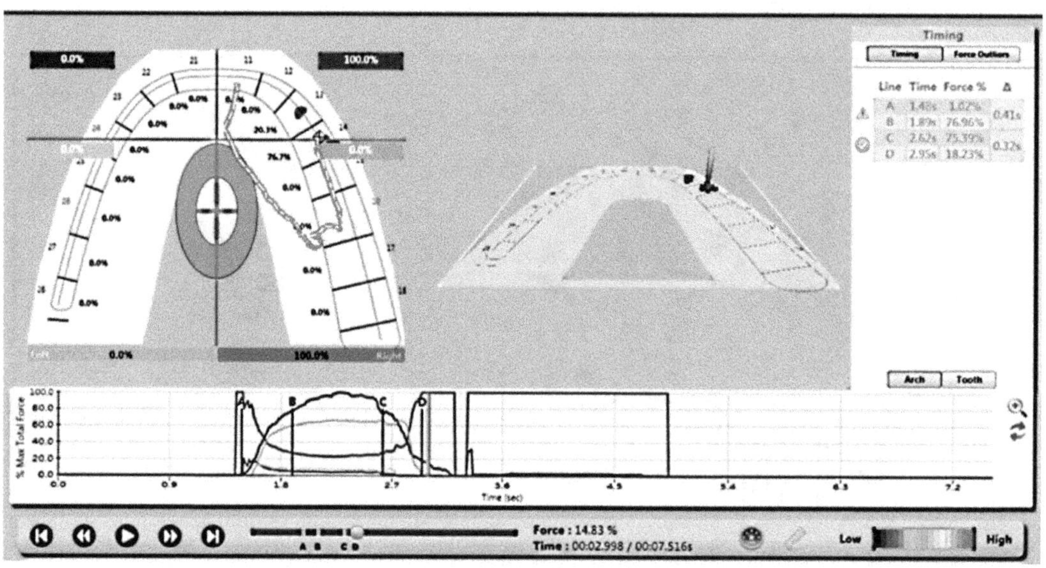

Figure 23c. Force Scan data of the left lateral excursive movement 0.446 seconds after excursive commencement (line C), 26 months post insertion. © [2013] [Courtesy of Vedic Institute of Smile Aesthetics]. Used with permission.

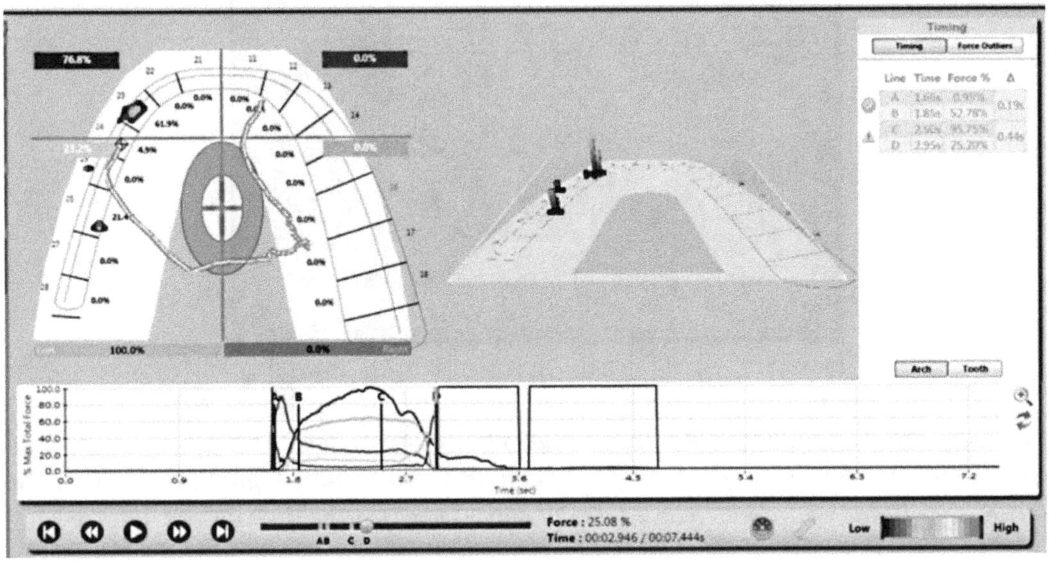

Figure 23d. Force Scan data of the left lateral excursive movement 0.576 seconds after excursive commencement (line C), 26 months post insertion. © [2013] [Courtesy of Vedic Institute of Smile Aesthetics]. Used with permission.

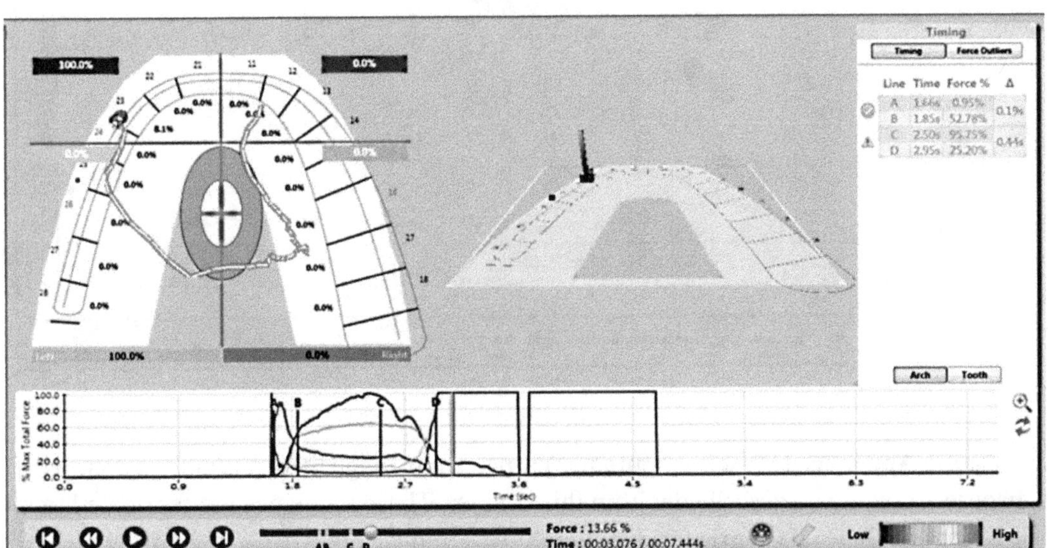

Figure 24. Delivery of a maxillary complete denture against a mandibular cast partial denture.

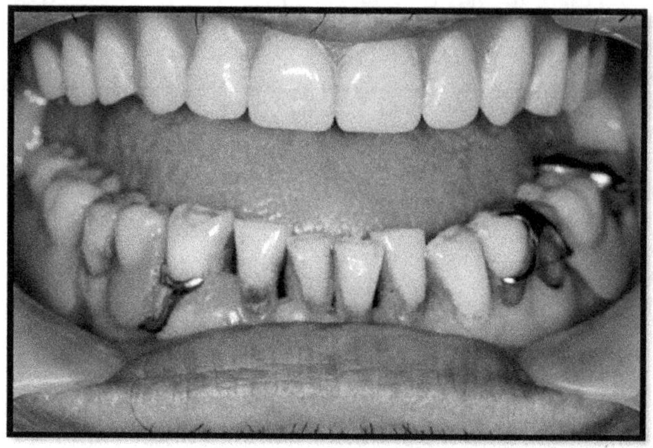

Figure 25. Using articulating paper marks and subjective patient "feel", the forces were balanced bilaterally, but excess force was accumulated in the canine and premolar region (25%). Note the Center of Force trajectory began near tooth #25, and then moved towards the arch center.

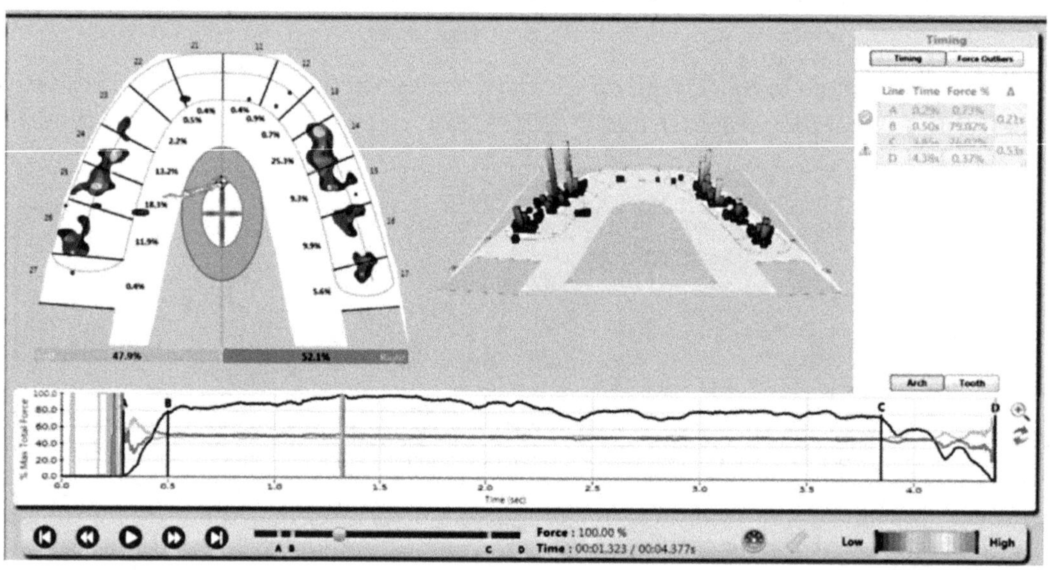

A Stabilization Appliance (Muscles Appliance) is used to manage the signs and symptoms of muscle complex disorders previously described within this chapter. These appliance are fabricated to minimize the Centric Relation (CR) and Centric Occlusion (CO) discrepancy (CR-CO), to harmonize the occlusal forces during normal function, and to create canine guidance to reduce the excursion frictional forces during function and parafunction (Chu, 1996; Segu, Sandrini, Lanfranchi, & Collesano, 1999; Pettengill, Growney, Jr., Schoff, & Kenworthy, 1998; Wassell, Adams, & Kelly, 2006).

Alternatively, a TM joint Repositioning Appliance is used to manage the signs and symptoms of Temporomandibular Joint complex disorders. This appliance is considered to be a healing and support

Figure 26. After digital Force Finishing using the T-Scan 8, the high forces in the premolar area were reduced, the overall force distribution was balanced, the Center of Force icon was located in the middle of the contacting teeth, and the trajectory path indicated all teeth contacted simultaneity.

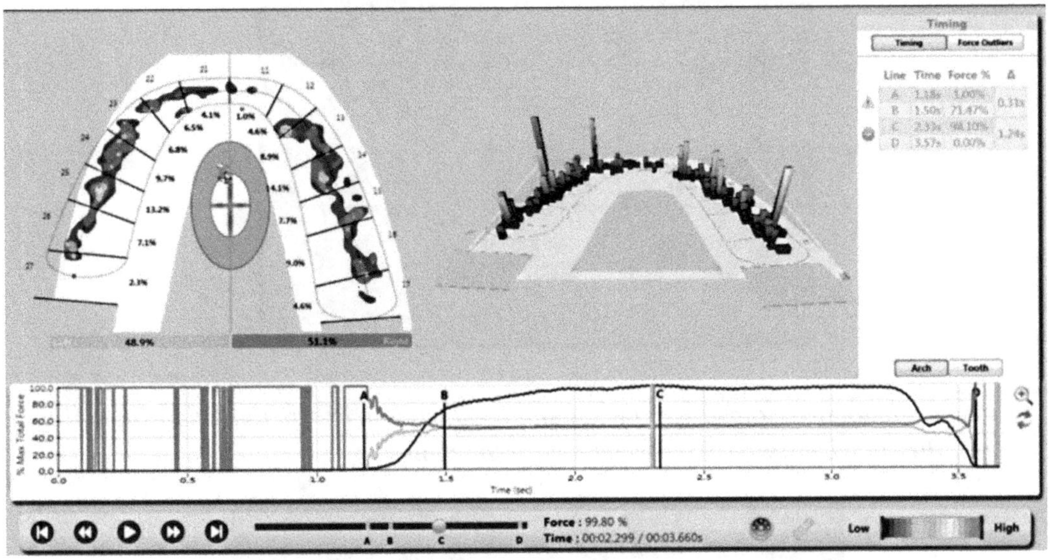

appliance, where the position of the condyle within the TM joints is changed to attempt to re-capture the disk, enhance the healing process of the retrodiscal tissues, and to induce positive osseous changes (remodeling) within the condylar bone (Farrar, 1972; Williamson, 2005; Williamson & Rosenzweig, 1998; Niemann, 1999; Gelb & Gelb, 1991).

Canine guidance is often not created with this appliance, because as its' name suggests, the aim of this appliance is to modify the mandible's condylar position, by incorporating a special acrylic ramp that guides the path of mandibular closure towards the desired position. However, occlusal force harmony is maintained in the new mandibular position by establishing on the appliance at insertion, a Force Finished and optimized occlusal force distribution.

The goal of employing either of these appliances is to harmonize the masticatory forces, by modifying the patient's tooth contact characteristics (contact location, contact time-sequencing, the Occlusion and Disclusion timing, and the contact forces), in the clinician's chosen Temporomandibular joint position. The precision of the occlusal force harmony installed upon the appliance, plays a vital role in achieving predictable physical improvements. Hence, it is always wise to use the Force Finishing protocol when delivering these devices to achieve early therapeutic recovery.

A 29-year-old female presented for a post orthodontic cosmetic touch up, with complaints of post-orthodontic facial and mandibular muscle pain, with headache. The patient was aware of her parafunctional habit, as she heavily bruxed on her orthodontic retainer every night, perforating it in a few sites. The patient was given a Brux-Checker to wear, just before going to bed for one night, to observe evidence of her bruxing habit (Figures 27a - d).

A thorough clinical examination revealed that the patient presented with a 2.5 mm CR - CO discrepancy (Figures 28 and 29). When the patient was recorded with the T-Scan system, the posterior molars exhibited forceful lateral excursive contacts that demonstrated long Disclusion Time bilaterally (Figures 30a and 30b).

Figure 27a. Before orthodontic treatment. Note the deep bite and the Class II Division II maxillomandibular relation. Picture courtesy by Dr. Situlal Pradhan (Orthodontist).

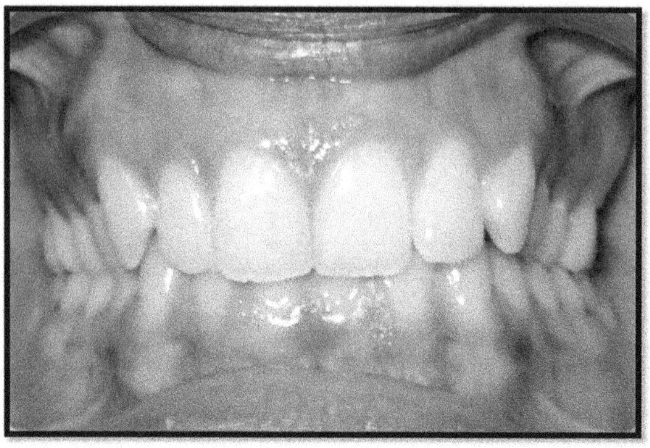

Figure 27b. Post orthodontic treatment that was completed without extraction, and with molar distalization (Dr. Situlal Pradhan), followed by cosmetic case finishing.

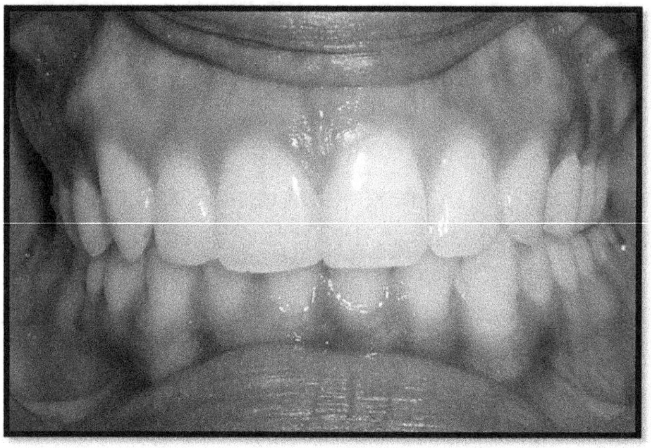

Figure 27c. A 2 mm thick, post orthodontic vacuum retainer. The patient bruxed during sleep causing perforations of the retainer at the molar and canine regions.

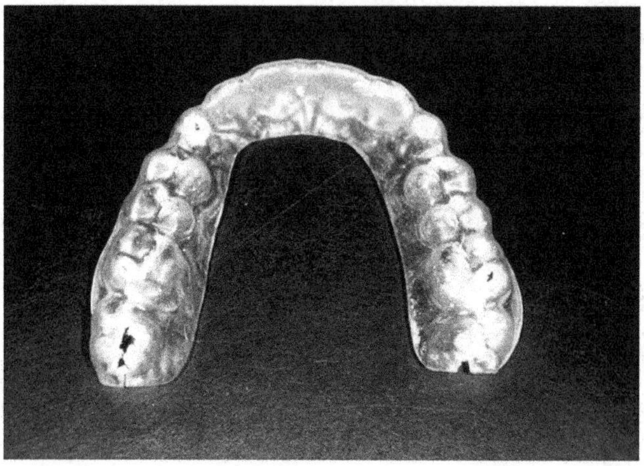

Figure 27d. To reconfirm the patient's Bruxism habit, a color-coded, ultra-thin Brux-Checker (0.1 mm thick) was worn just before going to bed. Note the signs of bruxing are visible (the white marks), which occurred on the same teeth that previously perforated the orthodontic retainer.

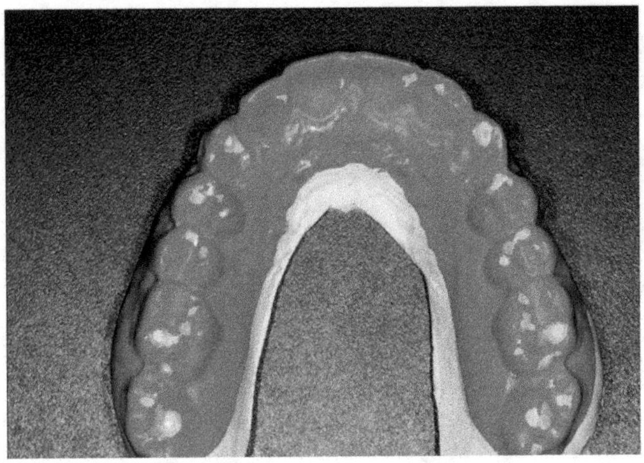

Figure 28. Force scan data of a manipulated Centric Relation closure, where the CR - CO discrepancy was almost 2.5 mm. Note the occlusal balance is uneven in CR (44.9% right - 55.1% left). with the Center of Force icon located slightly to the right posterior of centered. The right arch half had more total tooth contacts than the left, with the most individual tooth force concentrated on the right second molar (24.7%).

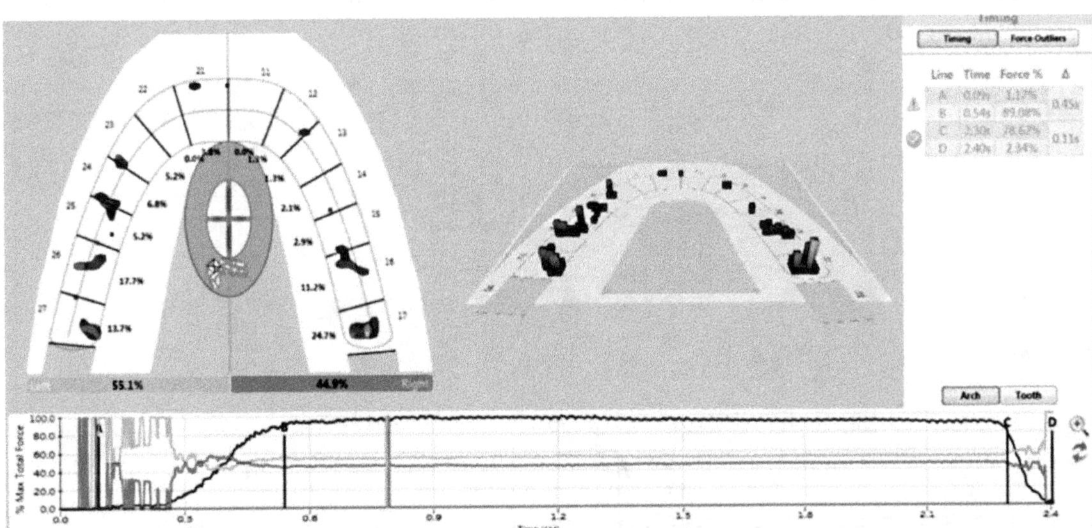

Since the patient herself was a dentist, and aware of her problems, she elected to not undergo an occlusal equilibration (Dawson, 2008), or Immediate Complete Anterior Guidance Development (ICAGD) (Kerstein, 1992), due to her (emotional) resistance to having her natural teeth reshaped with coronoplasty procedures. Instead, the patient was treated using a Stabilization Appliance that incorporated cuspid guid-

Figure 29. Force scan data of Maximum Intercuspation (MIP). The occlusal force balance was nearly equal (49.9% right- 50.1% left side). The Center of Force trajectory hugged the right midline, and finished near the middle of the aches when all teeth finally were in contact.

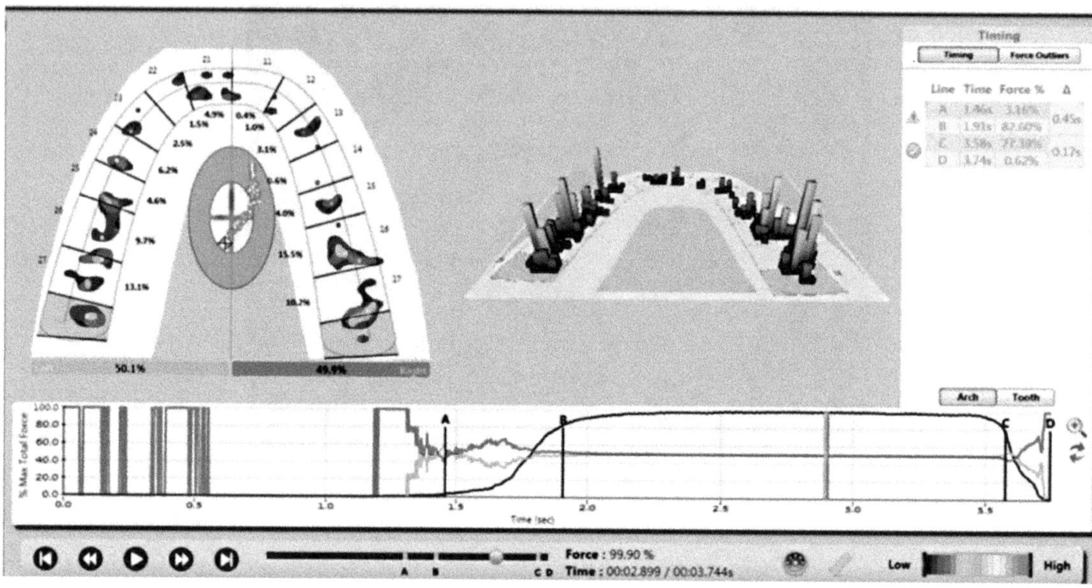

Figure 30a. The Force scan data of the right lateral excursive movement 0.137seconds after excursive commencement (line C).

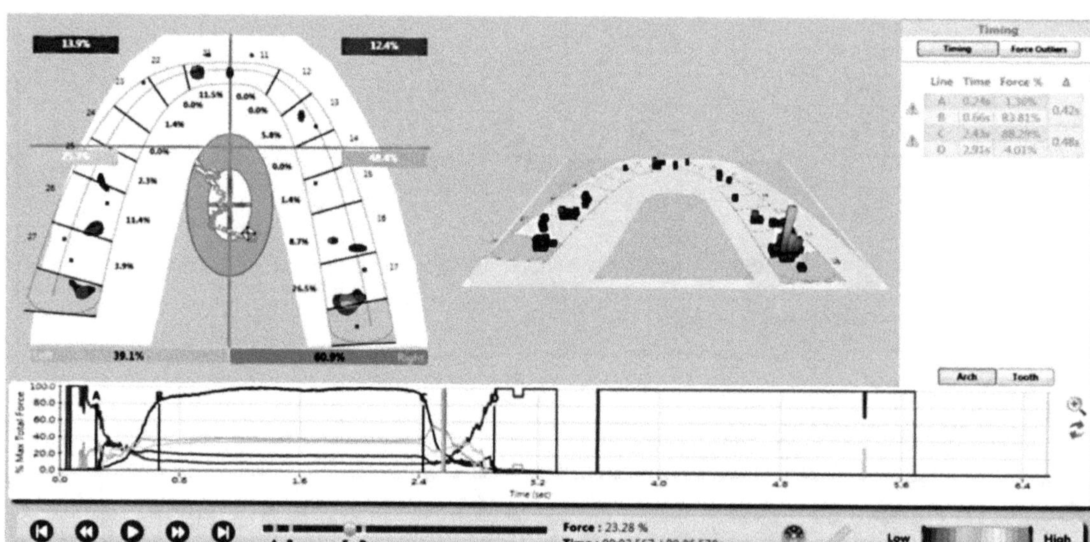

Figure 30b. Force scan of right lateral excursive movement 0.705 seconds after excursive commencement (line C), with the right canine accepting 100% of the excursive forces.

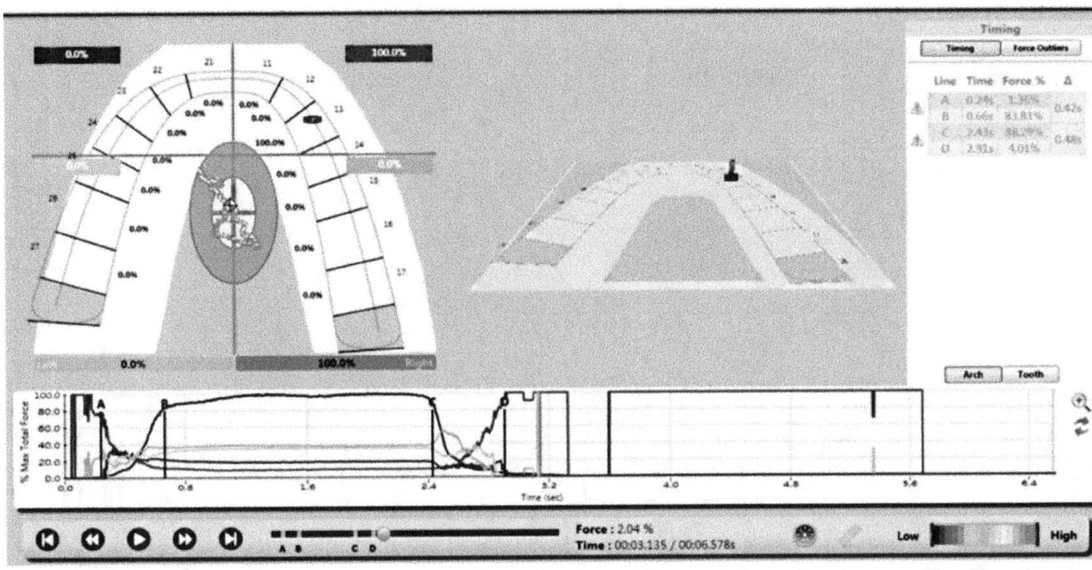

Figure 30c. Force scan of left lateral excursive movement 0.151 seconds after excursive commencement (line C), showing posterior contacts are present within the early excursion.

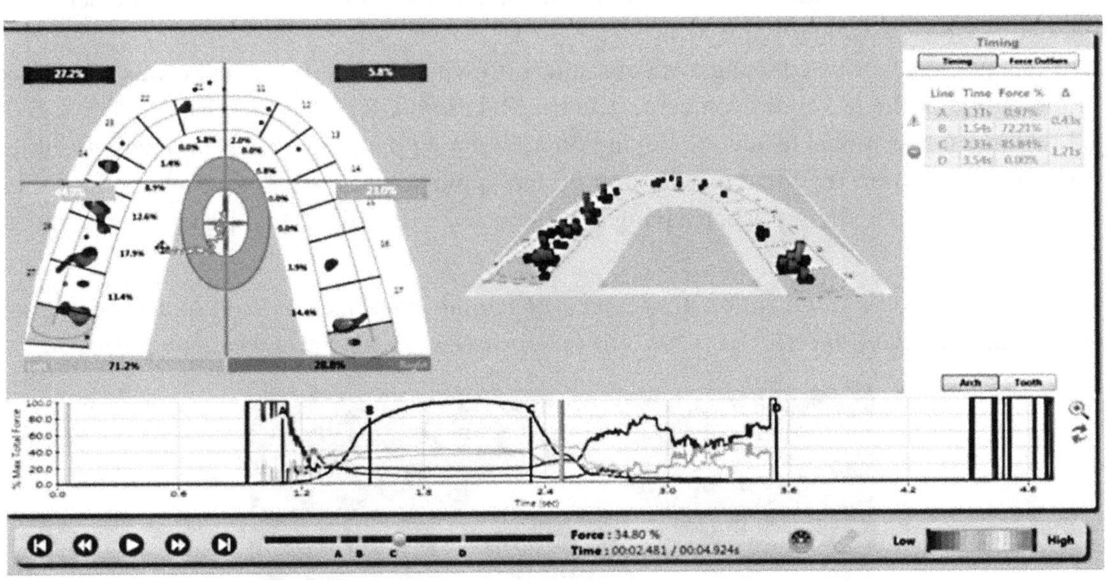

Figure 30d. Force scan of left lateral excursive movement 0.617 seconds after excursive commencement (line C), showing posterior contacts are still involved in the excursion, despite the left anterior guiding contacts.

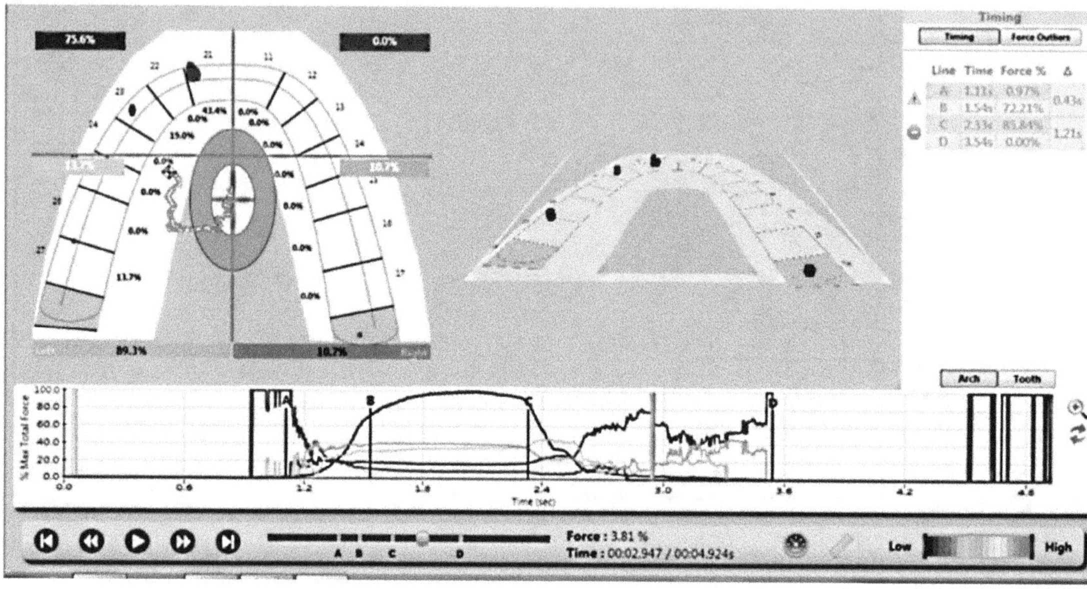

ance, to both balance her occlusion and lessen the molar excursive movement friction present, thereby reducing her Disclusion Time (Figure 31a).

The appliance was fabricated using a vacuum plate, to which cold-cured acrylic was added occlusally that broughtg all the teeth into contact in Centric Relation (CR) (Figure 31b). The occlusion was adjusted with the conventional technique relying on articulating paper markings and patient subjective "feel" (Figure 31c). After, the force distribution on the appliance was reassessed using the T-Scan 8, which showed that despite the appliance having been adjusted with articulating paper and patient "feel",

Figure 31a. TMJA Type III Stabilization Appliance with canine guidance. This appliance treats masticatory muscle pain and discomfort. It also helps to protect at-risk tooth structure during bruxism.

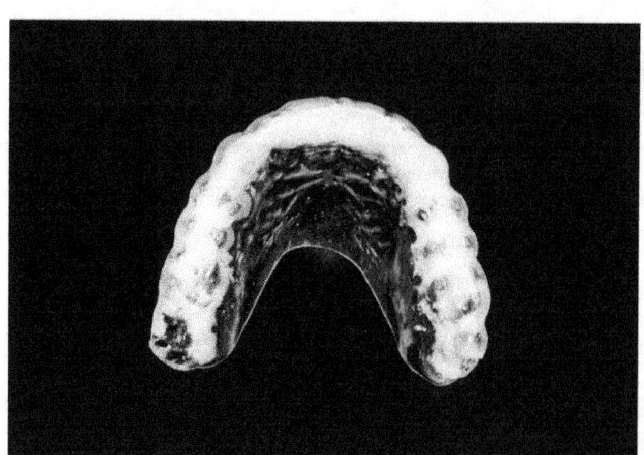

the occlusal forces were not distributed properly. There was more total force present on the right side (56.8% right - 43.2% left), and the Center of Force Trajectory moved from anterior to posterior staying mostly right of the midline (Figure31d).

Then the appliance was then finished using the Therapeutic Force Finishing protocol (Figure 31d), whereby the occlusal forces were measurably balanced, bilaterally. The Center of Force Trajectory lied on the midline and was very short in length, indicating that the simultaneous MIP contacts demonstrated improved overall force balance.

Then, a small amount of acrylic was added intraorally to create canine guidance and excursive movement control (Figures 32a and 32b), which was then recorded for the presence of short Disclusion Time. There was no prolonged posterior excursive interferences present resultant from the bilaterally smooth, canine guidance contacts.

At two weeks post splint insert, the patient reported that her pain was subsiding, as long as she wore the appliance. Since the patient presented with a CR-CO discrepancy, it was decided to change the vacuum retainer to a wrap-around retainer, which would better allow the recent orthodontically moved teeth to settle, naturally (Figure 33). Follow-up force scans of both CR and CO were performed after 5 months of settling (Figures 34a and 34b), and then again at 6 months (Figure 35a and 35b). This case demonstrates the value of Force Finishing in orthodontic case finishing.

It was interesting to note that the muscle pain had subsided within two weeks of wearing the appliance. However, after six months' time, Brux-Checker revealed that the patient still bruxed heavily at night (Figure 36), but the patient reported she did not experience any significant pain or discomfort. This case illustrates that TMD is a complex issue, where the clinician needs to account for all factors that cause occlusal force disharmony, and then adopt the most minimally invasive treatment approach to treat each patient's specific TM disorder.

Figure 31b. Frontal view of the patient wearing the Stabilization Appliance

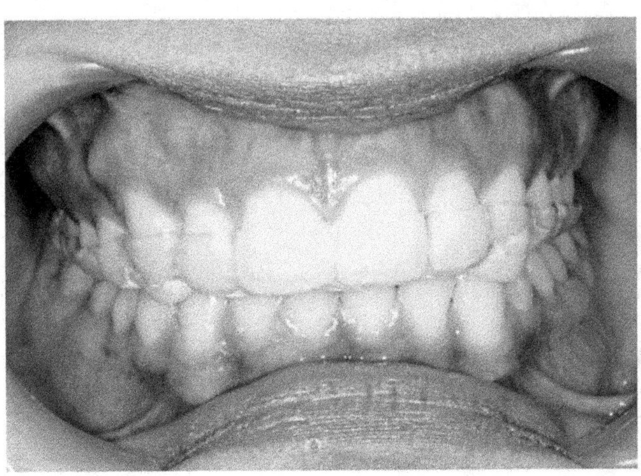

Figure 31c. Force scanning with the appliance in Centric Relation (CR). The occlusion was adjusted with articulating paper markings and patient subjective "feel" only. The forces were poorly distributed properly, with more total force on the right side (56.8% right- 43.2% left). The Center of Force Trajectory moved anteroposteriorly right of the midline.

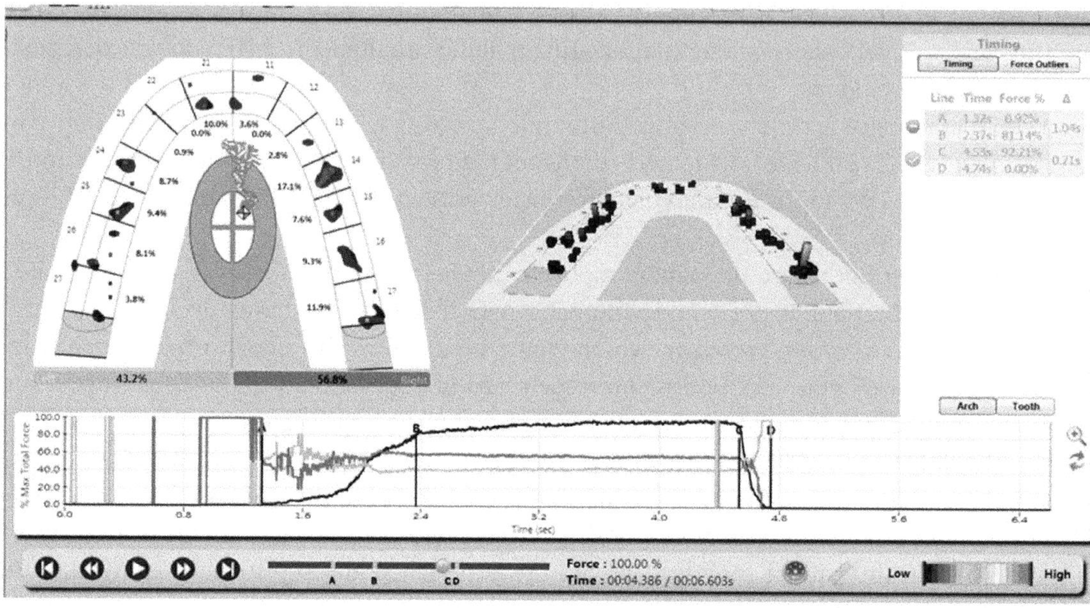

Figure 31d. The Forced Finished appliance in CR. Note the Center of Force Trajectory is very tight to the midline and short in length, indicating that simultaneous contacts have improved occlusal force balance

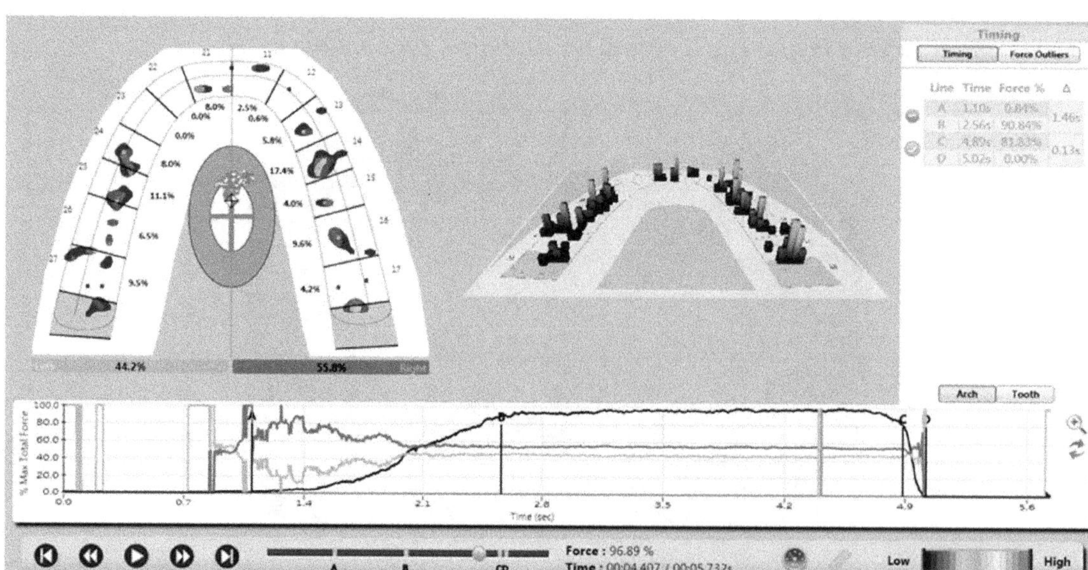

Figure 32a. Left lateral view showing canine guidance developed on the appliance to reduce the Disclusion Time

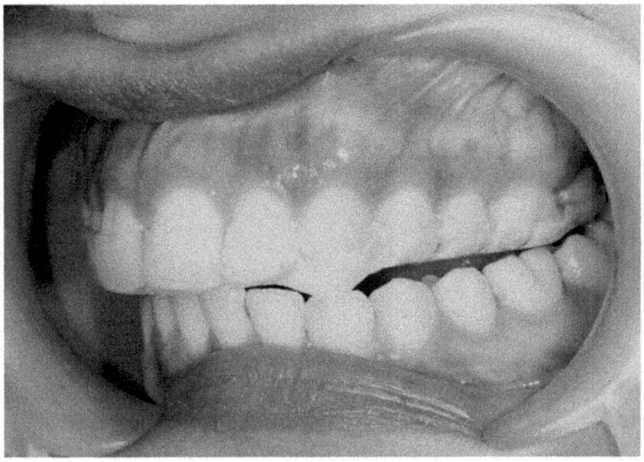

Figure 32b. Right lateral view showing canine guidance developed on the appliance to reduce the Disclusion Time

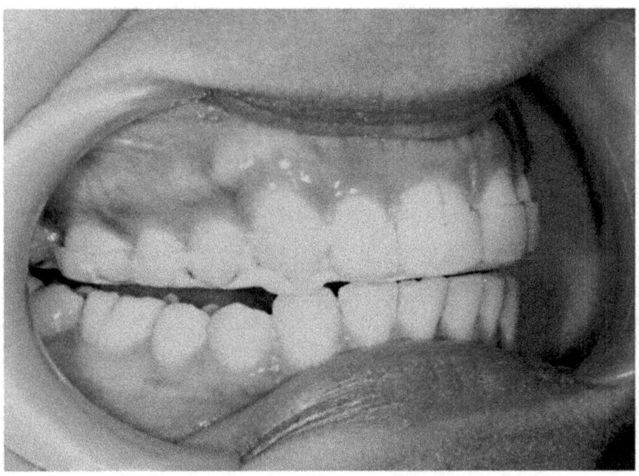

Solutions and Recommendations

There exists a trend in Dental Medicine, to move towards the digital approach because it is based on objective occlusal data. Diagnostic monitoring where clinicians employ digital technologies that provide objective data and measured physical information, which accurately and non-subjectively, describes a patient's conditional state, are being employed on wide scale basis in many Dental Medicine disciplines. The traditional subjective and analog approach of diagnosing occlusal problems and formulating a treatment plan, is slowly being replaced by the inclusion of computer-based devices within the diagnostic process. Moreover, during occlusal and reconstructive treatment procedures, it would benefit Dental Medicine greatly if clinicians were routinely and predictably, achieving high quality and precise treatment occlusal case end-results. This is only possible if measurement participates in the evaluation of a

Figure 32c. The left lateral excursive recording of the appliance. The Disclusion Time equaled 0.29 seconds (≤ 0.5 is physiologic).

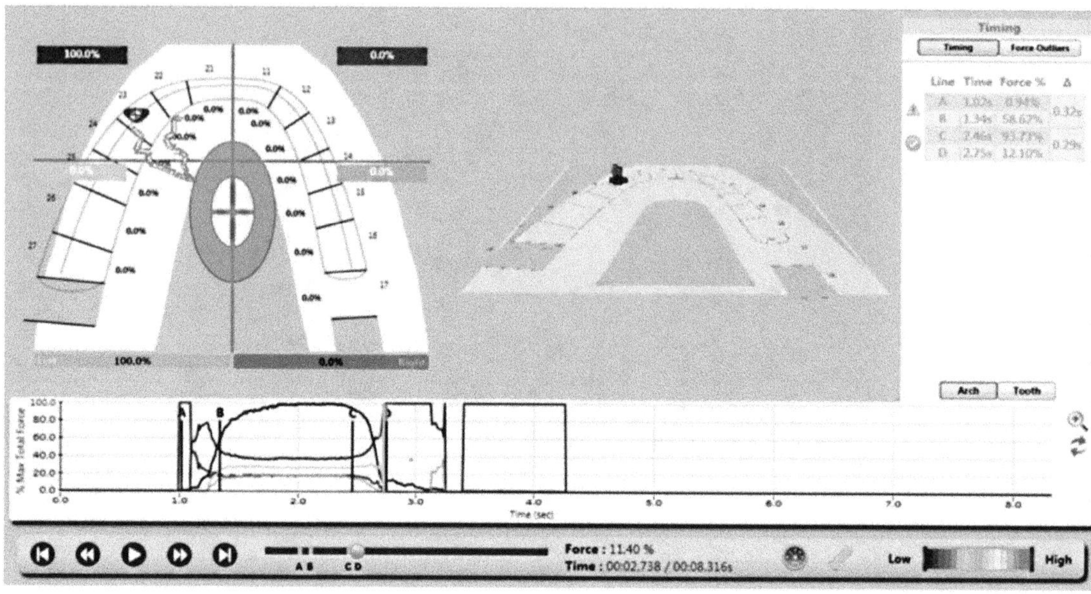

Figure 32d. Right lateral excursive recording of the appliance. The Disclusion Time equaled 0.24 seconds (≤ 0.5 is physiologic)

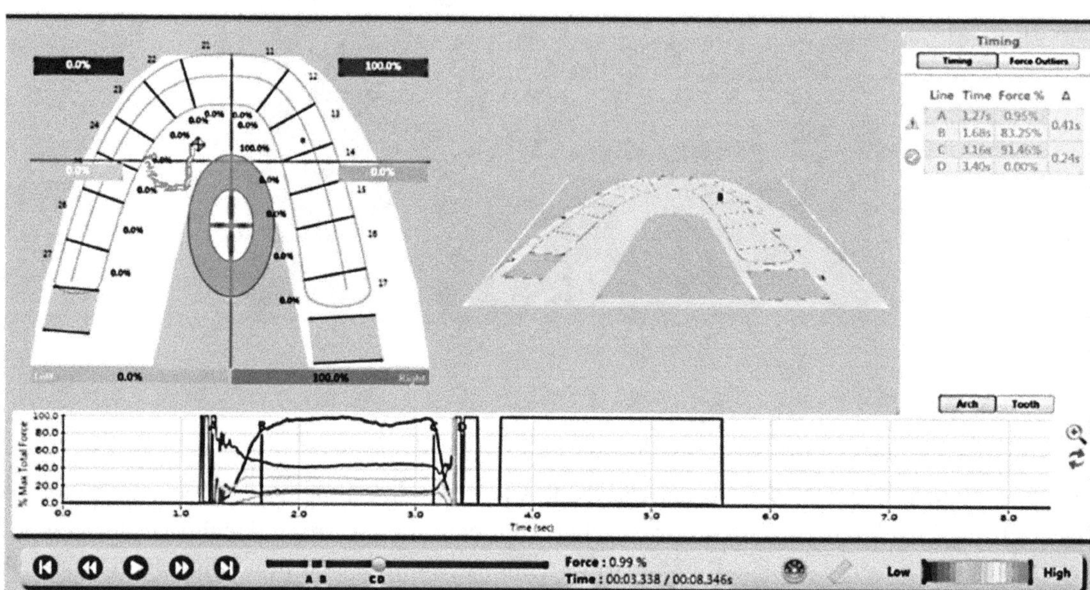

Figure 33. After appliance therapy, a wrap-around retainer was instituted to enhance post orthodontic natural tooth settling

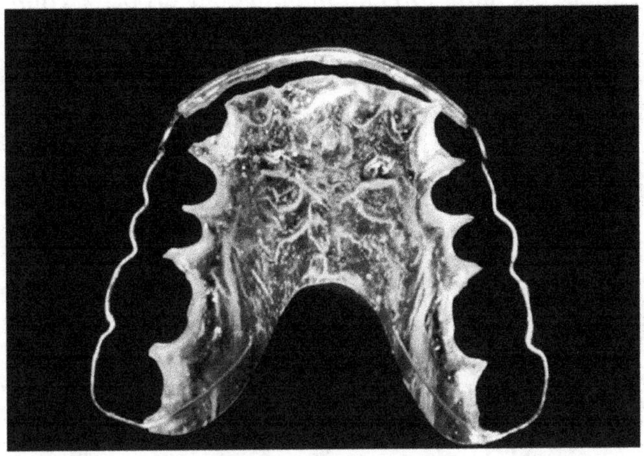

Figure 34a. CO force scan after 5 months of tooth settling where the posterior teeth are taking more load than in Figure 31c. There was improved, shared arch-half force balance.

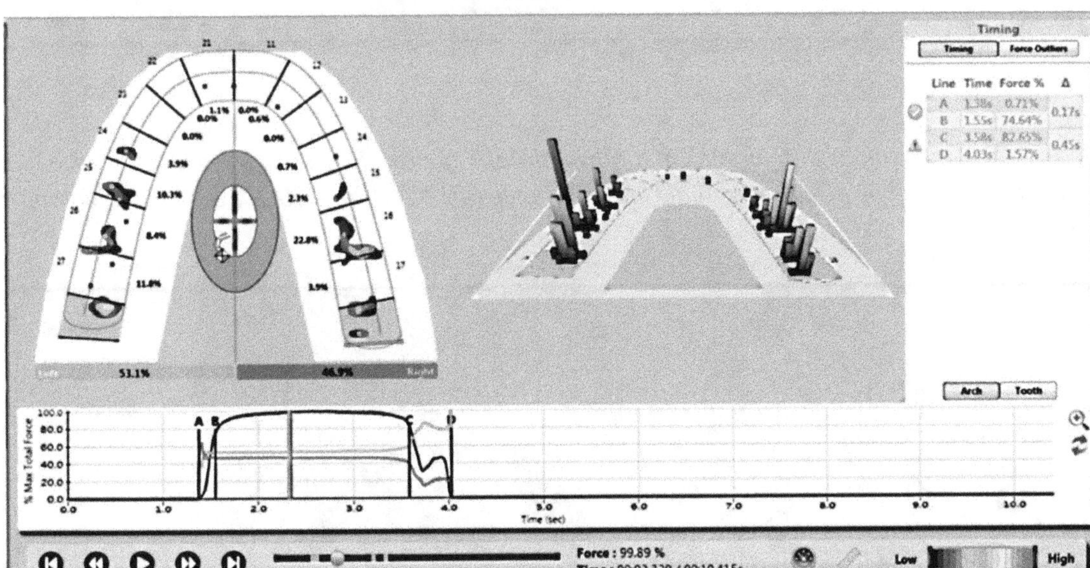

patient's Stomatognathic system, rather than allowing clinicians to continue to use the *hit or miss*, subjective methods involving stone casts, wax wafers, silicone imprints, and dental articulating papers. Dental Medicine should call on clinicians to incorporate digital diagnostic case recording and case monitoring devices in clinical practice, to open the doors into daily clinical, and practice-based research studies.

Within both the PFF and TFF Force Finishing protocols, a clinician records all the required digital occlusal data, before, during, and after case finishing. The T-Scan's objective occlusal data becomes a reliable source and reference for occlusal force disease (OFD) screening, when diagnosing occlusal problems, preventing the destructive effects of occlusal disease from continuing, during treatment planning to

Figure 34b. Centric Relation (CR) force scan after 5 months of settling, when the posterior teeth demonstrate increased loads. This change was similar that seen in Centric Occlusion (Figure 34a). However in CR, the right side of the arch was more forceful than the left s (60.1% right - 39.9% left).

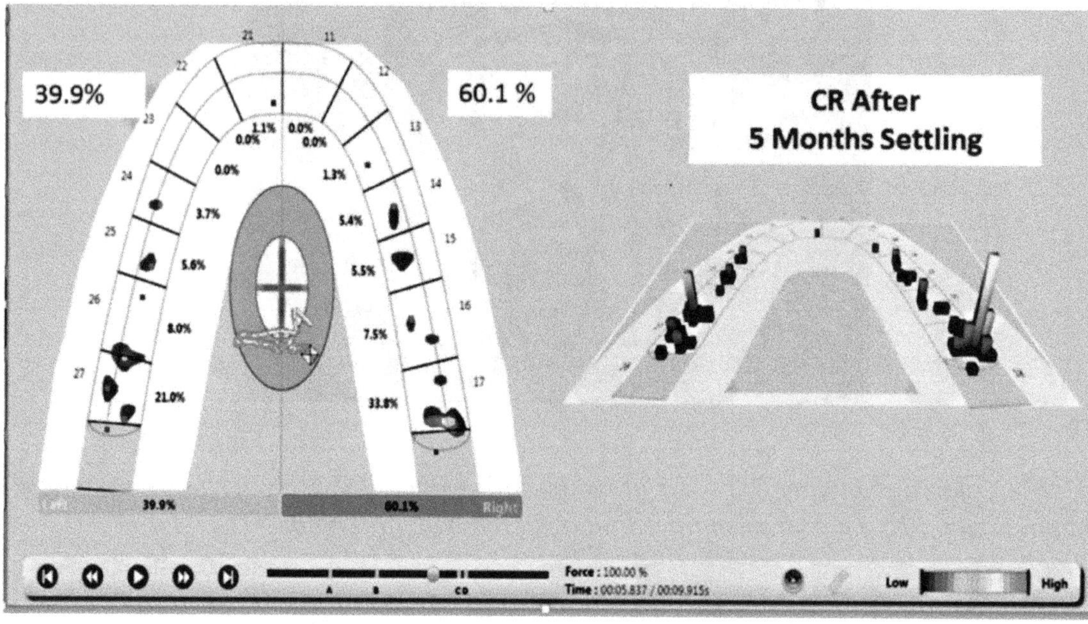

Figure 35a. CO force scan after 6 months of tooth settling. The posterior teeth show better force balance and demonstrate equally shared arch - half force balance (49.9% Right- 50.1% left),when compared to Figure 34a.

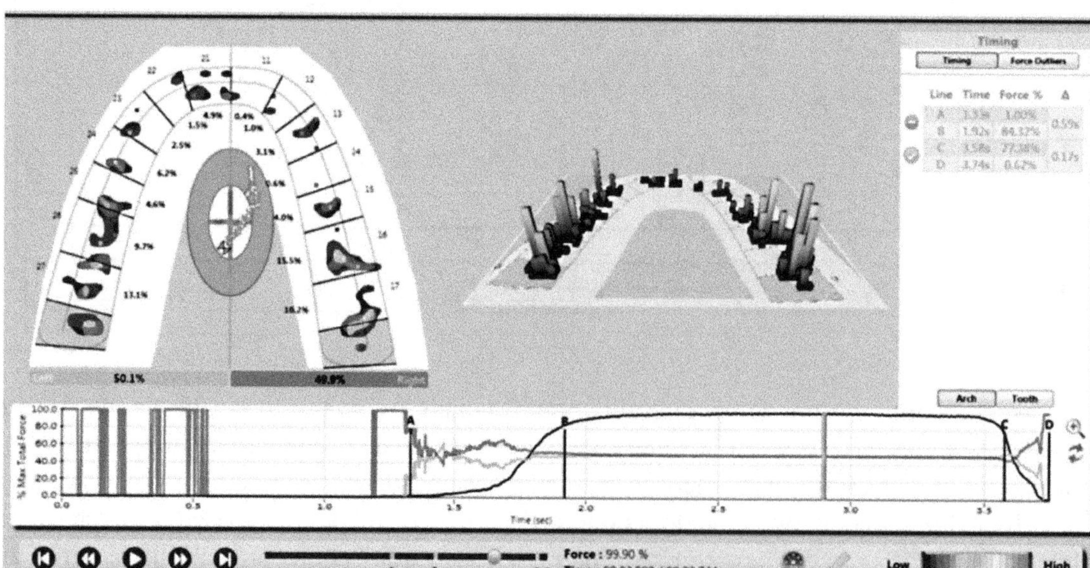

Figure 35b. Centric Relation (CR) after 6 month of tooth settling. The Center of Force trajectory in CR is not yet consistent. Hence, the case is planned for T-Scan guided occlusal adjustments one year after tooth settling, with follow up occlusal force scanning, as needed.

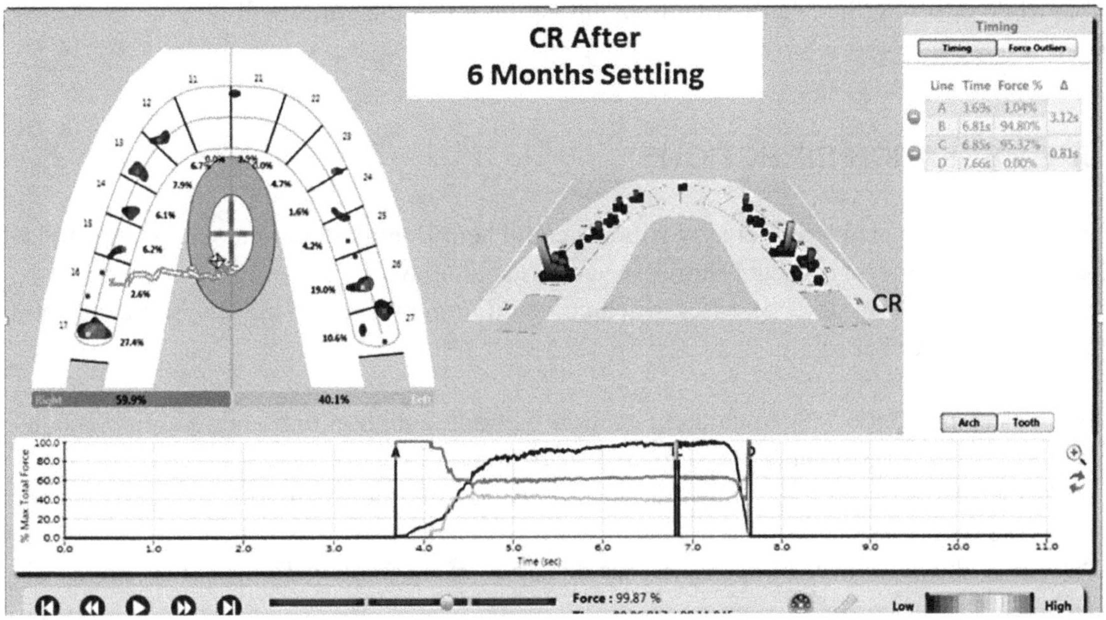

Figure 36. To reconfirm the patient's Bruxism habit, a color-coded, ultra-thin Brux-Checker (0.1 mm thick) was used again after six months time. The signs of bruxing (the white marks) are still visible, as they were in Figure 27d.

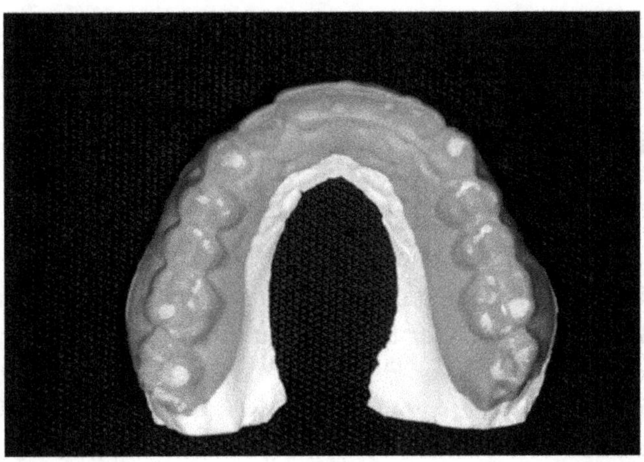

lessen the potential progressive effects of occlusal disease, and to monitor the treatment end-result over the long-term to reduce the possibility of occlusal disease reoccurrence. This author strongly recommends that clinicians utilize Preventative Force Finishing (PFF) in occlusally force sensitive cases, such as during full mouth reconstruction, implant prosthodontic reconstruction, smile makeovers, orthodontic case-finishing, and during cases involving complex multiple restorations.

Lastly, it is this author's hope that the T-Scan technology and the Force Finishing approach will be adopted by educators and clinicians, so that they will better objectively manage occlusal forces. This will help prevent and drastically reduce unwanted, premature case failures resultant from occlusal force overload, while ensuring the health, function, and aesthetics of the smile will be preserved for longer periods of time.

FUTURE RESEARCH DIRECTIONS

A simple occlusal data analysis of elderly patients could help Dental Medicine obtain new clinical evidence evaluating long-term clinical restorative success and failure.

Specifically, long-term practice-based research could employ the T-Scan 8 system and the Force Finishing concept together to:

- Stud post-orthodontic T-Scan guided retention vs. traditional non-digital retention procedures for differences in the resultant occlusal force distribution.
- Study the role occlusal forces play in crestal bone loss in both periodontal disease and peri-implant disease.
- Determine the prevalence of occlusal force disharmony observed in Temporomandibular disorder patients.
- Determine the occlusal force quality present in an asymptomatic population.

CONCLUSION

This chapter explained the Force Finishing concept, and its clinical role in comprehensive Dental Medicine. Force Finishing aids the clinician in achieving case-after case, high quality and precise treatment end-results, when installing prosthetic dentistry, adhesive dentistry, orthotic devices, and implant prostheses, and after orthodontics during the settling period following bracket and wire removal.

In the performance of clinical dental procedures, ranging from single restorations to complex case management like during full mouth reconstruction involving dental implants, often the occlusal force components of the final case are neglected and misunderstood. As such, the physical strength of the restorative materials is still an important topic. In restorative dentistry, clinicians are tempted to choose restorative materials that are much stronger than the natural teeth, hoping the selected material will overcome any potential restoration fracture. This "hope" is deeply rooted in that the majority of clinicians around the world that do not objectively Force Finish their clinical cases and completely depend on articulating paper mark Subjective Interpretation combined with patient proprioceptive feedback. Restorative clinicians must understand that overcoming the restoration fracture through material choice ignores the underling force factors, thereby shifting the effects of occlusal force overload from the restoration, to other areas like the periodontium, the masticatory muscles, and the Temporomandibular joints. Interestingly, in the field of Orthodontics, where clinician routinely change the patient's occlusion during their treatment procedures, there is no priority given to Force Finishing, yet orthodontic cases frequently encounter treatment relapse, which is a direct response to masticatory force disharmony.

In order to achieve the maximum therapeutic effects from any dental treatment, it is necessary for clinicians to understand the force components involved in a patient's masticatory system. With the advancement in the science and technology ofadhesive restorative materials, and the availability of the T-Scan Occlusal Analysis system, that can measure relative occlusal forces precisely in real-time, a modern clinician can predictably treat simple to complex cases in conservative ways, so that the biologic cost of the treatment can be drastically reduced, while the quality of the occlusal care rendered, is greatly raised.

REFERENCES

Adams, S. H., & Zander, H. A. (1964). Functional tooth contacts in lateral and centric occlusion. *The Journal of the American Dental Association*, *69*, 465–743. PMID:14198784

Ahlgren, J. (1966). Mechanism of mastication. *Acta Odontologica Scandinavica*, *24*(Suppl. 44), 100–109.

Alexander, P. C. (1963). Analysis of the cuspid protected occlusion. *The Journal of Prosthetic Dentistry*, *66*(2), 309–317. doi:10.1016/0022-3913(63)90176-8

Anderson, D. J. (1981). Measurement of stress in mastication. *Journal of Dental Research*, *35*(5), 671–674. doi:10.1177/00220345560350050301 PMID:13367283

Anderson, D. J., & Picton, D. C. A. (1957). Tooth contact during chewing. *Journal of Dental Research*, *36*(1), 21–26. doi:10.1177/00220345570360011301 PMID:13398499

Anderson, D. M. (1988). *Dorland's Illustrated Medical Dictionary* (28th ed.). Philadelphia, PA: W.B. Saunders.

Ash, M. M., & Nelson, S. J. (2003). *Wheeler's dental anatomy, physiology, and occlusion* (8th ed.). St. Louis, MO: CV Mosby.

Baba, K., Clark, G. T., Watanabe, T., & Ohiyama, T. (2003). Bruxism forces detection by a piezoelectric film-based recording device in sleeping humans. *Journal of Orofacial Pain*, *17*, 58–64. PMID:12756932

Bakke, M., & Michler, L. (1991). Temporalis and masseter muscle activity in patients with anterior open bite and craniomandibular disorders. *Scandinavian Journal of Dental Research*, *99*(3), 219–228. PMID:1871532

Begg, P. R. (1954). Stone Age man's dentition. *American Journal of Orthodontics*, *40*(4), 298–312. doi:10.1016/0002-9416(54)90092-5

Bessette, R. W., & Quinlivan, J. T. (1973). Electromyographic evaluation for the Myo-monitor. *The Journal of Prosthetic Dentistry*, *30*(1), 91–24. doi:10.1016/0022-3913(73)90073-5 PMID:4513524

Beyron, H. (1969). Optimal occlusion. In *Symposium on Occlusion: Dental Clinics of North America*, (vol. 13, pp. 537-554). Academic Press.

Blaschke, D. D., & Blaschke, T. J. (1981). Normal TMJ bone relationships in centric occlusion. *Journal of Dental Research*, *60*, 98–104. doi:10.1177/00220345810600021901 PMID:6936462

Boucher, C. O. (1963). *Current Clinical Dental Terminology*. St. Louis, MO: C.V. Mosby.

Boucher, C. O. (1970). *Swenson's Complete Dentures* (6th ed.). St. Louis, MO: C.V. Mosby.

Brekhus, P. H., Armstrong, W. D., & Simon, W. J. (1941). Stimulation of the muscles of mastication. *Journal of Dental Research*, *20*(2), 87–92. doi:10.1177/00220345410200020801

Bresolin, D., Shapiro, P. A., Dhapito, E. E., Chapko, M. K., & Dessel, S. (1983). Mouth breathing in allergic children: Its relationship to dentofacial development. *American Journal of Orthodontics*, *83*(4), 334–340. doi:10.1016/0002-9416(83)90229-4 PMID:6573147

Brewer, A. A., & Hudson, P. C. (1961). Application of miniature electronic devices for the study of tooth contact in complete dentures. *The Journal of Prosthetic Dentistry*, *11*(1), 62–68. doi:10.1016/0022-3913(61)90111-1

Brudevold, F. (1951). A basic study of the chewing forces of a denture wearer. *The Journal of the American Dental Association*, *43*, 45–51. PMID:14841027

Bryant, G. W. (1989). Myofascial pain dysfunction and viola playing. *British Dental Journal*, *166*(9), 335–336. doi:10.1038/sj.bdj.4806830 PMID:2713183

Byron, H. (1964). Occlusal relations and mastication in Australian Aborigines. *Acta Odontologica Scandinavica*, *22*(6), 597–678. doi:10.3109/00016356409058580 PMID:14280848

Chun, D. S., & Koskinen-Moffett, L. (1990). Distress, mandibular habits, and connective tissue laxity as predisposing factors to TMJ sounds in adolescents. *Journal of Craniomandibular Disorders*, *4*(30), 165–176. PMID:2098392

Cleall, J. F. (1965). Study of form and function. *American Journal of Orthodontics*, *51*(8), 566–594. doi:10.1016/0002-9416(65)90028-X PMID:14331958

D'Amico, A. (1958). The canine teeth - normal functional relations of the natural teeth of man. *Journal of the Californian Dental Association*, *26*, 6–23.

Dawson, P. E. (1989). *The evaluation, diagnosis, and treatment of occlusal problems* (2nd ed.). St. Louis, MO: C.V. Mosby.

Dawson, P. E. (2007). *Functional occlusion: from TMJ to smile design* (Vol. 1). St. Louis, MO: C.V. Mosby.

De, B. (1997). Epidemiology and natural progression of articular Temporomandibular disorders. *Oral Surgery, Oral Medicine, Oral Pathology, Oral Radiology, and Endodontics*, *83*(1), 72–76. doi:10.1016/S1079-2104(97)90094-9 PMID:9007927

DeShields, R. W. (1978). Gnathological considerations of a controversial nature. *Dental Survey*, *54*, 12–18. PMID:284997

Downs, D. H. (1988). An investigation into condylar position with leaf gauge and bimanual manipulation. *The Journal of Gnathology*, *7*, 75–81.

Emslie, R. D., Massler, M., & Zwemer, J. D. (1952). Mouth breathing: Etiology and effects. *The Journal of the American Dental Association*, *44*, 506–521. PMID:14917514

Flangan, J.B. (1963). The 24 hour pattern of swallowing in man. *Journal of Dental Research, 43*(165), 1072.

Freng, A. (1979). Restricted nasal respiration, influence on facial growth. *International Journal of Pediatric Otolaryngology, 1*(3), 249–254. doi:10.1016/0165-5876(79)90019-3 PMID:552382

Garner, L. D., & Kotwal, N. S. (1973). Correlation study of incisive biting forces with age, sex and anterior occlusion. *Journal of Dental Research, 52*(4), 698–702. doi:10.1177/00220345730520041001 PMID:4515849

Gelb, M. L., & Gelb, H. (1991). Mandibular orthopedic repositioning therapy. *Cranio Clinics International, 1*(2), 81–98. PMID:1811812

Gibbs, C. H., Mahan, P. E., Lundeen, H. C., Brehnan, K., Walsh, E. K., & Holbrook, W. B. (1981). Occlusal forces during chewing and swallowing as measured by sound transmission. *The Journal of Prosthetic Dentistry, 46*(4), 443–449. doi:10.1016/0022-3913(81)90455-8 PMID:6946215

Gibbs, C. H., Mahan, P. E., Mauderli, A., Lundeen, H. C., & Walsh, E. K. (1986). Limits of human bite strength. *The Journal of Prosthetic Dentistry, 56*(2), 226–229. doi:10.1016/0022-3913(86)90480-4 PMID:3463748

Glickman, I. (1963). Inflammation and trauma from occlusion. *The Journal of Periodontology, 34*(5), 15–39.

Glickman, I. (1972). *Clinical Periodontology* (4th ed.). Philadelphia, PA: W.B. Saunders and Co.

Glickman, I. (1979). *Clinical Periodontology* (5th ed.). Philadelphia, PA: W.B. Saunders and Co.

Goldreich, H., Gazit, E., Lieberman, M. A., & Rugh, J. D. (1994). The effect of pain from orthodontic arch wire adjustment on masseter muscle electromyographic activity. *American Journal of Orthodontics and Dentofacial Orthopedics, 106*(40), 365–370. doi:10.1016/S0889-5406(94)70057-5 PMID:7942651

Graf, H. (1969). Bruxism. *Dental Clinics of North America, 13*, 659–665. PMID:5256151

Guichet, N. E. (2010). Occlusion: A teaching manual, Anaheim, California, 1977, The Denar Corporation. guided occlusal adjustments. *Compendium of Continuing Education, 31*(7), 530–543.

Gwynne-Evans, E., & Ballard, C.F. (1957). Discussion on the mouth breather. *Proceedings of the Royal Society of Medicine, 51*, 279-285.

Gysi, A. (1915). Masticating efficiency in natural and artificial teeth. *Dental Digest, 21*, 74–78.

Hannukseal, A. (1981). The effect of moderate and severe atrophy on the facial skeletal. *European Journal of Orthodontics, 3*(3), 187–193. doi:10.1093/ejo/3.3.187 PMID:6943033

Harvold, E. P., Tormer, B. S., Vangervik, K., & Chierici, G. (1981). Primate experiments on oral respiration. *American Journal of Orthodontics, 79*(4), 359–372. doi:10.1016/0002-9416(81)90379-1 PMID:6939331

Howard, J. A. (1989). Temporomandibular joint disorders, facial pain and dental problems of performing artists. *Journal of Craniomandibular Disorders: Facial & Oral Pain, 3*, 71–74. PMID:2606999

Howell, A. H., & Brudevold, F. (1950). Vertical forces used during chewing of food. *Journal of Dental Research*, *29*(2), 133–136. doi:10.1177/00220345500290020401 PMID:15415485

Howell, A. H., & Manly, R. S. (1948). An electrical strain gauge for measuring oral forces. *Journal of Dental Research*, *27*(6), 705–712. doi:10.1177/00220345480270060701

Ishimaru, J., Handa, Y., Kurita, K., & Goss, A. N. (1994). The effects of occlusal loss on normal and pathological temporomandibular joints: An animal study. *Journal of Cranio-Maxillo-Facial Surgery*, *2*(2), 95–102. doi:10.1016/S1010-5182(05)80018-6 PMID:8021325

James, W. W., & Hastings, S. (1932). Discussion on mouth breathing and nasal obstruction. *Proceedings of the Royal Society of Medicine*, *25*, 1343. PMID:19988850

Jankelson, B. (1969). Electronic control of muscle contraction: A new clinical era in occlusion and prosthodontics. *Scientific and Educational Bulletin*, *2*, 29–31. PMID:4949886

Jenkins, G. N. (1974). *The physiology and biochemistry of the mouth* (4th ed.). Oxford, UK: Blackwell Scientific Publications.

Kahn, J., Tallents, R. H., Katzberg, R. W., Moss, M. E., & Murphy, W. C. (1998). Association between Dental Occlusion variables and intraarticular temporomandibular joint disorders: Horizontal and vertical overlap. *The Journal of Prosthetic Dentistry*, *79*(6), 658–662. doi:10.1016/S0022-3913(98)70072-1 PMID:9627894

Kahn, J., Tallents, R. H., Katzberg, R. W., Moss, M. E., & Murphy, W. C. (1999). Prevalence of dental occlusal variables and intra articular temporomandibular disorders: Molar relationship, lateral guidance, nonworking side contacts. *The Journal of Prosthetic Dentistry*, *82*(4), 410–415. doi:10.1016/S0022-3913(99)70027-2 PMID:10512959

Kantorowicz, A. (1916). Uber den Mechanismus der Kiefe deformierung beibe hinderter Atmnug. *Deutsch Mschr Zahnheilk*, *34*, 225.

Kaplan, R. L. (1963). Concepts of occlusion: Gnathology as a basis for a concept of occlusion. *Dental Clinics of North America*, *7*, 577–590.

Katona, T. R. (1989). The effect of cusp and mandibular morphology on the forces on the teeth and the temporomandibular joint. *Journal of Oral Rehabilitation*, *16*(2), 211–219. doi:10.1111/j.1365-2842.1989.tb01335.x PMID:2715869

Kawata, T., Niida, S., & Kawasoko, S. (1997). Morphology of the mandibular condyle in "toothless" osteopetrotic (op/ op) mice. *Journal of Craniofacial Genetics and Developmental Biology*, *17*, 198–203. PMID:9493078

Kerstein, R. B. (1993). A comparison of traditional occlusal equilibration and immediate complete anterior guidance development. *The Journal of Cranio-Mandibular Practice*, *11*, 126–140. PMID:8495505

Kerstein, R. B. (2010). Reducing chronic masseter and temporalis muscular hyperactivity with computer-guided occlusal adjustments. *Compendium of Continuing Education*, *31*(7), 530–543. PMID:20879206

Kerstein, R. B., & Radke, J. (2012). Masseter and temporalis excursive hyperactivity decreased by measured anterior guidance development. *The Journal of Cranio-Mandibular Practice*, *30*(4), 243–254. PMID:23156965

Kerstein, R. B., & Radke, J. (2013). Clinician accuracy when subjectively interpreting articulating paper markings. *The Journal of Craniomandibular & Sleep Practice*, *32*(1), 13–23. PMID:24660642

Kerstein, R. B., & Wright, N. (1991). An electromyographic and computer analysis of patients suffering from chronic myofascial pain dysfunction syndrome, pre and post - treatment with immediate complete anterior guidance development. *The Journal of Prosthetic Dentistry*, *66*(5), 677–686. doi:10.1016/0022-3913(91)90453-4 PMID:1805009

Kiliardus, S., Tzakis, M. G., & Carlsson, G. E. (1995). Effects of fatigue and chewing training on maximal bite force endurance. *American Journal of Orthodontics and Dentofacial Orthopedics*, *107*(4), 372–379. doi:10.1016/S0889-5406(95)70089-7 PMID:7709901

Kingsley, N.W. (1888). *A treatise on oral deformities as a branch of mechanical surgery*. New York, NY: D. Appleton, Co.

Koirala, S. (2009). Smile Design Wheel: A practice approach to smile design. *Cosmetic Dentistry Science and Beauty*, *3*, 24–28.

Koirala, S. (2011). MiCD -Customized case finishing concept & clinical protocol. *MiCD Clinical Journal*, *1*(1), 32–42.

Koirala, S. (2013). TMJA Harmony Appliances in Dental Medicine. *TMJA Harmony Workshop Manual*, *1*, 1–65.

Korioth, T. W. P., & Hannam, A. G. (1990). Effect of bilateral asymmetric tooth clenching on load distribution at the mandibular condyle. *The Journal of Prosthetic Dentistry*, *64*(1), 62–78. doi:10.1016/0022-3913(90)90154-5 PMID:2384899

Kraua, B. S., Jordon, R. E., & Abrahams, L. (1973). *Dental anatomy and occlusion*. Baltimore, MD: Waverly Press.

Lee, R. L. (1982). *Anterior guidance advances in occlusion*. Boston, MA: John Wright, PSG.

Linder-Aronson, S. (1970). Adenoids: Their effect on mode of breathing and nasal airflow and their relationship to characteristics of the facial skeleton and the dentition. *Acta Oto-Laryngologica*, *265*(Supplement), 1–132.

Linder-Aronson, S. (1974). Effects of adenoidectomy on dentition and nasopharynx. *American Journal of Orthodontics*, *65*(1), 1–15. doi:10.1016/0002-9416(74)90153-5 PMID:4525094

Long, J. H. (1973). Locating Centric Relation with a leaf gauge. *The Journal of Prosthetic Dentistry*, *29*(6), 608–610. doi:10.1016/0022-3913(73)90267-9 PMID:4513791

Lucia, V. O. (1960). Centric relation: Theory and practice. *The Journal of Prosthetic Dentistry*, *10*(5), 849–856. doi:10.1016/0022-3913(60)90118-9

Lucia, V. O. (1961). *Modern gnathology concepts*. St. Louis, MO: C.V. Mosby.

Lucia, V. O. (1983). *Modern gnathological concepts up-dated.* Chicago: Quintessence.

Lundeen, H. C., & Gibbs, C. H. (1982). Advances. In *Occlusion* (pp. 89–107). Boston, MA: John Wright, PSC.

Lundgren, D., & Laurell, L. (1986). Occlusal force pattern during chewing and biting in dentitions restored with fixed bridges of cross- arch extension. *Journal of Oral Rehabilitation, 13*(1), 57–71. doi:10.1111/j.1365-2842.1986.tb01556.x PMID:3511198

MacMillan, H. W. (1930). Unilateral vs bilateral balanced occlusion. *The Journal of the American Dental Association, 17*, 1207–1220.

Mann, A. W., & Pankey, L. D. (1954). Concepts of occlusion. The PankeyMann philosophy of occlusal rehabilitation. *The Journal of Prosthetic Dentistry, 4*, 440–245.

Manns, A., Miralles, R., Valdivia, J., & Bull, R. (1989). Influence of variation in anteroposterior occlusal contacts on electromyographic activity. *The Journal of Prosthetic Dentistry, 61*(5), 617–623. doi:10.1016/0022-3913(89)90288-6 PMID:2746532

Manns, A., Zuazola, R. V., & Sirhan, R. M. (1990). Relationship between the tonic elevator mandibular activity and the vertical dimension during the stages of vigilance and hypnosis. *The Journal of Cranio-Mandibular Practice, 8*(2), 163–170. PMID:2073696

McAdam, D. B. (1976). Tooth loading and cuspal guidance in canine and group -function occlusions. *The Journal of Prosthetic Dentistry, 35*(3), 2832–2890. doi:10.1016/0022-3913(76)90252-3 PMID:1062598

McHorris, W. H. (1985). Occlusal adjustment via selective cutting of natural teeth, part 1. *The International Journal of Periodontics & Restorative Dentistry, 5*, 8–25.

McKenzie, D. (1909). Adenoids, deformities of the palate, and artificial infants feedings. An analysis of 222 cases. *British Dental Journal, 30*, 159.

McLean, D. W. (1938). Physiologic vs. pathologic occlusion. *The Journal of the American Dental Association, 25*, 1583–1594.

McNeil, C. (1997). *Science and Practice of Occlusion.* Carol Stream, IL: Quintessence Publishing.

Michael, C. G., Javid, N. S., Colaizzi, F. A., & Gibbs, C. H. (1990). Biting strength and chewing forces in complete denture wearers. *Journal of Prosthetic Dental Medicine, 63*(5), 549–553. doi:10.1016/0022-3913(90)90074-M PMID:2338667

Michel, A., Lippen, K., & Wangen, V. (1908). Zungendruk. Dtsch. Mschr. *Zahnheilk, 26*, 527.

Miralles, R., Carvajal, E., Manns, A., & Rossi, E. E. (1980). Studio comparative de umbralespresorreceptivos en dientes con normofuncion vs. hiperfuncion o trauma occlusal. *Revista Dental de Chile*, 3–7.

Muhlbrat, L., Jenz, K. P., & Luks, D. (1976). Die Beruhrungschwellebeigesunden und erkranktenParodontien. *Deutsch Zahnarztz, 31*, 306–312.

Nishigawa, K., Bando, E., & Nakano, M. (2001). Quantitative study of bite force during sleep-associated bruxism. *Journal of Oral Rehabilitation, 28*(5), 485–491. doi:10.1046/j.1365-2842.2001.00692.x PMID:11380790

Okeson, J. P. (2003). *Management of temporomandibular disorders and occlusion* (5th ed.). St. Louis, MO: C.V. Mosby and Co.

Okeson, J. P. (2013). *Management of Temporomandibular Disorders and Occlusion* (7th ed.). St. Louis, MO: C.V. Mosby Elsevier, Inc.

Posselt, U. (1952). Studies in the mobility of the human mandible. *Acta Odontologica Scandinavica, 10*(Suppl), 19.

Pound, E. (1976). Controlling anomalies of vertical dimension and speech. *The Journal of Prosthetic Dentistry, 36*(2), 124–135. doi:10.1016/0022-3913(76)90134-7 PMID:789862

Pullinger, A. G., Hollender, L., Solberg, W. K., & Petersson, A. (1985). A tomographic study of mandibular condyle position in an asymptomatic population. *The Journal of Prosthetic Dentistry, 53*(5), 706–713. doi:10.1016/0022-3913(85)90029-0 PMID:3858537

Remien, J. C. II, & Ash, M. M. Jr. (1974). Myo – monitor centric: An evaluation. *The Journal of Prosthetic Dentistry, 31*(2), 137–145. doi:10.1016/0022-3913(74)90048-1 PMID:4520661

Reynolds, J. M. (1971). The organization of occlusion for natural teeth. *The Journal of Prosthetic Dentistry, 26*(1), 56–67. doi:10.1016/0022-3913(71)90029-1 PMID:5281471

Rieder, C. E. (1978). The prevalence and magnitude of mandibular displacement in a survey population. *The Journal of Prosthetic Dentistry, 39*(3), 324–329. doi:10.1016/S0022-3913(78)80105-X PMID:273095

Rinchuse, D. J., & Sassouni, V. (1982). An evaluation of eccentric occlusal contacts in orthodontically treated subjects. *American Journal of Orthodontics, 82*(3), 251–256. doi:10.1016/0002-9416(82)90146-4 PMID:6961798

Roberts, C. A., Tallents, R. H., Katzberg, R. W., Sanchez-Woodworth, R. E., Espeland, M. A., & Handelman, S. L. (1987). Comparison on internal derangements of the TMJ with occlusal findings. *Oral Surgery, Oral Medicine, and Oral Pathology, 63*(6), 645–650. doi:10.1016/0030-4220(87)90361-6 PMID:3473388

Rugh, J. D., & Drago, C. J. (1981). Vertical dimension: A study of clinical rest position and mandibular muscle activity. *The Journal of Prosthetic Dentistry, 45*(6), 670–675. doi:10.1016/0022-3913(81)90426-1 PMID:6941018

Sassuni, V., Shnorhokain, H., Beery, Q., Zullo, T., & Friday, G.A. (1982). Influence of perennial allergic rhinitis (PAR) on facial type L. *Journal of Allergy and Clinical Immunology, 69*(149), 29-64.

Sataloff, R., Brandfonbrener, A., & Lederman, T. (1991). *Editor's Textbook of Performing Arts Medicine*. New York, NY: Raven Press.

Schneyer, L. H., Pigman, W., Hanahan, L., & Gilmore, R. W. (1956). Rate of flow of human parotid, sublingual, and submaxillary secretions, during sleep. *Journal of Dental Research, 35*(1), 109–144. doi:10.1177/00220345560350010301 PMID:13286394

Schulte, W. (1983). *Die exzentrische okklusion*. Berlin, Germany: Quintessenz Verlag.

Schuyler, C. H. (1935). Fundamental principles in the correction of occlusal disharmony, natural and artificial. *The Journal of the American Dental Association, 22*, 1193–1202.

Schuyler, C. H. (1961). Factors contributing to traumatic occlusion. *The Journal of Prosthetic Dentistry, 11*(4), 708–716. doi:10.1016/0022-3913(61)90179-2

Schwartz, H. (1986). Occlusal variations for reconstructing the natural dentition. *The Journal of Prosthetic Dentistry, 55*(1), 101–105. doi:10.1016/0022-3913(86)90084-3 PMID:3511222

Seligman, D. A., & Pulinger, A. G. (1991). The role of functional relationships in temporomandibular disorders. *Journal of Craniomandibular Disorders, 5*, 265–279. PMID:1814969

Shipiro, G. C., & Shapiro, P. A. (1987). The effects of perennial allergic rhinitis on dental and skeletal development: A comparison of sibling pairs. *American Journal of Orthodontics and Dentofacial Orthopedics, 92*(4), 286–293. doi:10.1016/0889-5406(87)90328-3 PMID:3477946

Solow, B., & Kreiberg, S. (1977). Soft-tissue stretching: A possible control factor in craniaofacial morphogenesis. *Scandinavian Journal of Dental Research, 85*, 505–507. PMID:271349

Standlee, J. P., Caputo, A. A., & Ralph, J. P. (1979). Stress transfer to the mandible during anterior guidance and group function in centric movements. *The Journal of Prosthetic Dentistry, 34*(1), 35–45. doi:10.1016/0022-3913(79)90353-6 PMID:281524

Stegenga, B. (2001). Osteoarthritis of the temporomandibular joint organ and its relationship to disc displacement. *Journal of Orofacial Pain, 15*, 193–205. PMID:11575190

Stuart, C. H., & Stallard, C. E. (1982). Concepts of occlusion -what kind of occlusion should recusped teeth be subject to? *American Journal of Orthodontics, 82*, 251–256. PMID:6961798

Subtelny, J. D. (1980). Oral rcspiration: Facial maldevelopment and corrective dentofacial orthopedics. *The Angle Orthodontist, 50*, 147–164. PMID:6996532

Suit, S. R., Gibbs, C. H., & Benz, S. T. (1976). Study of gliding tooth contacts during mastication. *Journal of Periodontology, 47*(6), 331–334. doi:10.1902/jop.1976.47.6.331 PMID:1064720

Tallents, R. H., Macher, D. J., Kyranides, S., Katzberg, R. W., & Moss, M. E. (2002). Prevalence of missing posterior teeth and intra articular temporomandibular disorders. *The Journal of Prosthetic Dentistry, 87*(1), 45–50. doi:10.1067/mpr.2002.121487 PMID:11807483

Tarvonen, P. L., & Kosko, K. (1987). Craniofacial skeleton of seven year old children with enlarged adenoids. *American Journal of Orthodontics and Dentofacial Orthopedics, 91*(4), 300–304. doi:10.1016/0889-5406(87)90170-3 PMID:3471072

Thompson, J. R. (1964). The rest position of the mandible and its significance to dental science. *The Journal of the American Dental Association, 33*, 151–180. PMID:21010948

Trask, G. M., Shipiro, G. C., & Shapiro, P. A. (1987). The effects of perennial allergic rhinitis on dental and skeletal development: A comparison of sibling pairs. *American Journal of Orthodontics and Dentofacial Orthopedics, 92*(4), 286–293. doi:10.1016/0889-5406(87)90328-3 PMID:3477946

Trenouth, M. J. (1979). The relationship between bruxism an temporomandibular joint dysfunction as shown by computer analysis of nocturnal tooth contact patterns. *Journal of Oral Rehabilitation, 6*(1), 81–87. doi:10.1111/j.1365-2842.1979.tb00408.x PMID:282418

Van Blarcom, C. W. (1999). *The Glossary of Prosthodontic Terms* (7th ed.). St. Louis, MO: C.V. Mosby.

Waugh, L. M. (1939). Dental observation among Eskimos. *Journal of Dental Research, 16*, 355–356.

Weinberg, L. A., & Kruger, B. (1995). A comparison of implant / prosthesis loading with four clinical variables. *The International Journal of Prosthodontics, 50*, 421–433. PMID:8595100

Whitaker, R. H. R. (1911). The relationship of nasal obstruction to contracted arches and dental irregularities. *Dentist's Record, 31*, 425.

Williamson, E. H., & Lundquist, D. O. (1983). Anterior guidance: Its effect on the elecromyographic activity of temporal and masseter muscles. *The Journal of Prosthetic Dentistry, 49*(6), 816–823. doi:10.1016/0022-3913(83)90356-6 PMID:6576136

Woda, A., Vigneron, P., & Kay, D. (1979). Non-functional and functional occlusal contacts: A review of the literature. *The Journal of Prosthetic Dentistry, 42*(3), 335–341. doi:10.1016/0022-3913(79)90226-9 PMID:383965

Woodside, D. G., & Linder-Aronson, S. (1979). The channelization of upper and lower anterior face heights compared to population standards in mates between ages six to twenty years. *European Journal of Orthodontics, 1*(1), 24–40. doi:10.1093/ejo/1.1.25

Worner, H. K. (1939). Ganthodynamics: The measurement of biting forces with a new design of ganthodynamometer. *Australian Dental Journal, 43*, 381–386.

Worner, H. K., & Anderson, M. N. (1944). Biting force measurements in children. *Australian Dental Journal, 48*, 1–5.

Wustrow, E. (1915). ZurKritik der Ursachen der kieferanomalien. *Deutsch Mschr Zahnheilk, 34*.

ADDITIONAL READING

Ash, M. M., & Ramfjord, S. P. (1995). *Occlusion*. Philadelphia, PA: W.B. Saunders Co.

Baad-Hansen, L., Jadidi, F., Castrillon, E., Thomsen, P. B., & Svensson, P. (2007). Effect of a nociceptive trigeminal inhibitory splint on electromyographic activity in jaw closing muscles during sleep. *Journal of Oral Rehabilitation, 34*(2), 105–111. doi:10.1111/j.1365-2842.2006.01717.x PMID:17244232

Carey, J. P., Craig, M., Kerstein, R. B., & Radke, J. (2007). Determining a relationship between applied occlusal load and articulation paper mark area. *The Open Dental Journal, 1*(1), 1–7. doi:10.2174/1874210600701010001 PMID:19088874

Ciavarella, D., Mastrovincenzo, M., Sabatucci, A., Parziale, V., Granatelli, F., Violante, F., & Chimenti, C. (2010). Clinical and computerized evaluation in study of temporomandibular joint intracapsular disease. *Minerva Stomatologica, 59*(3), 89–101. PMID:20357736

Coleman, T. A., Grippo, J. O., & Kinderknecht, K. E. (2003). Cervical1 Dentin Hypersensitivity. Part III: Resolution following occlusal equilibration. *Quintessence International, 34*, 427–434. PMID:12859087

Garrido Garcia, V. C., Garcia Cartagena, A., & Gonzalez Sequeros, O. (1997). Evaluation of occlusal contacts in maximum intercuspation using the T-Scan system. *Journal of Oral Rehabilitation*, *24*(12), 899–903. doi:10.1046/j.1365-2842.1997.00586.x PMID:9467991

Grippo, J. O., Simring, M., & Coleman, T. A. (2012). Abfraction, Abrasion, Biocorrosion, and the Enigma of Noncarious Cervical Lesions: A 20-Year Perspective. *Journal of Esthetic and Restorative Dentistry*, *24*(1), 10–23. doi:10.1111/j.1708-8240.2011.00487.x PMID:22296690

Harper, K. A., & Setchell, D. J. (2002). The use of shimstock to assess occlusal contacts: A laboratory study. *The International Journal of Prosthodontics*, *15*, 347–352. PMID:12170848

Harrel, S. K., Nunn, M. E., & Hallmon, W. W. (2006). Is there an association between occlusion and periodontal destruction?: Yes- occlusal forces can contribute to periodontal destruction. *The Journal of the American Dental Association*, *137*(10), 1381–1389. doi:10.14219/jada.archive.2006.0049 PMID:17012716

Kamyszek, G., Ketcham, R., Garcia, R. Jr, & Radke, J. (2001). Electromyographic evidence of reduced muscle activity when ULF-TENS is applied to the Vth and VIIth cranial nerves. *The Journal of Cranio-Mandibular Practice*, *19*(3), 162–168. PMID:11482827

Kerstein, R. B. (2011). Health and harmonized function with computer guided force management. *Cosmetic Dentistry*, *5*(2), 6–12.

Kerstein, R. B. (2011). The new rules of occlusion to apply during MICD Cosmetic Reconstruction. *MICD Journal*, *1*(1), 6–16.

Kerstein, R. B., Lowe, M., Harty, M., & Radke, J. (2006). A Force reproduction analysis of two recording sensors of a computerized occlusal analysis system. *The Journal of Cranio-Mandibular Practice*, *24*(1), 15–24. PMID:16541841

Khan, A., & Hargreaves, K. M. (2010). *Animal models of orofacial pain. Analgesia* (pp. 93–104). New York, NY: Humana Press.

Koos, B., Godt, A., Schille, C., & Goz, G. (2010). Precision of an instrumentation-based method of analyzing occlusion and its resulting distribution of forces in the dental arch. *Journal of Orofacial Orthopedics*, *71*(6), 403–410. doi:10.1007/s00056-010-1023-7 PMID:21082303

Koos, B., Holler, J., Schille, C., & Godt, A. (2012). Time-dependent analysis and representation of force distribution and occlusion contact in the masticatory cycle. *Journal of Orofacial Orthopedics*, *73*(3), 204–214. doi:10.1007/s00056-012-0075-2 PMID:22580427

Mahan, P. E., Wilkinson, T. M., Gibbs, C. H., Mauderli, A., & Brannon, L. S. (1983). Superior and inferior bellies of the lateral pterygoid muscle EMG activity at basic jaw positions. *The Journal of Prosthetic Dentistry*, *50*(5), 710–718. doi:10.1016/0022-3913(83)90214-7 PMID:6580440

Qadeer, S., Kerstein, R. B., Yung-Kim, R. J., Huh, J. B., & Shin, S. W. (2012). Relationship between articulation paper mark size and percentage of force measured with computerized occlusal analysis. *Journal of Advanced Prosthodontics*, *4*(1), 7–12. doi:10.4047/jap.2012.4.1.7 PMID:22439094

Raphael, K. G., & Ciccone, D. S. (2008). *Psychological aspects of chronic orofacial pain. Orofacial pain and headache* (pp. 57–74). Edinburgh, Scotland: Elsevier. doi:10.1016/B978-0-7234-3412-2.10004-5

Saad, M. N., Weiner, G., Ehrenberg, D., & Weiner, S. (2008). Effects of load and indicator type upon occlusal contact markings. *Journal of Biomedical Materials Research. Part B*, *85*(1), 18–22.

Sierpińska, T., Gołebiewska, M., & Długosz, J. W. (2006). The relationship between masticatory efficiency and the state of dentition at patients with non-rehabilitated partial loss of teeth. *Advances in Medical Sciences*, *51*(Suppl. 1), 196–199. PMID:17458090

Sierpinska, T., Golebiewska, M., & Lapuc, M. (2008). The effect of mastication on occlusal parameters in healthy volunteers. *Advances in Medical Sciences*, *53*(2), 316–320. doi:10.2478/v10039-008-0049-1 PMID:19095582

Stern, K., & Kordaß, B. (2010). Comparison of the Greifswald Digital Analyzing System with the T-Scan III with respect to clinical reproducibility for displaying occlusal contacts. *Journal of Craniomandibular Function*, *2*, 107–119.

Tarantola, G., Becker, I. M., Gremiilion, H., & Pink, F. (1998). The Effectiveness of Equilibration in the Improvement of Signs and Symptoms in the Stomatognathic System. *International Journal of Periodontal and Restorative Dentistry*, *18*(6), 595–603. PMID:10321174

KEY TERMS AND DEFINITIONS

Force Finishing: A clinical concept and technique employed to optimize the occlusal force components of the masticatory system, using objective T-Scan based occlusal force and timing measurements. The goals are to obtain ideal occlusal force and timing occlusal clinical parameters, so that long-term health, function, and craniofacial aesthetics are maintained.

Occlusal Force Disorders: The disorders of teeth, muscles, Temporomandibular joints, and airway, resultant from the presence of excess occlusal force that is greater than the individual's resistive and adaptive capacity.

Occlusal Harmony: The Physiologic and functional balance of the occlusion.

Occlusion: The physiologic action that generates occlusal forces within the Stomatognathic system.

Preventative Force Finishing: A procedure to optimize the occlusal force components of the masticatory system, to protect and maintain a physiologic, accepted original occlusal scheme, while preventing existing restorations from future failure.

Therapeutic Force Finishing: A procedure to customize the occlusal force components in the treatment of the specific signs and symptoms of occlusal force disorder conditions.

TMJA Harmony: The physiologic and functional harmony of the entire Stomatognathic system; the teeth, muscles, Temporomandibular joints, and airway.

This work was previously published in the Handbook of Research on Computerized Occlusal Analysis Technology Applications in Dental Medicine edited by Robert B. Kerstein, DMD, pages 905-973, copyright year 2015 by Medical Information Science Reference (an imprint of IGI Global).

Chapter 4
Dental Tissue Engineering Research and Translational Approaches towards Clinical Application

Athina Bakopoulou
Aristotle University of Thessaloniki, Greece

Werner Geurtsen
Medical University of Hannover, Germany

Gabriele Leyhausen
Medical University of Hannover, Germany

Petros Koidis
Aristotle University of Thessaloniki, Greece

ABSTRACT

Stem cell-based dental tissue regeneration is a new and exciting field that has the potential to transform the way that we practice dentistry. It is, however, imperative its clinical application is supported by solid basic and translational research. In this way, the full extent of the potential risks involved in the use of these technologies will be understood, and the means to prevent them will be discovered. Therefore, the aim of this chapter is to analyze the state-of-the-science with regard to dental pulp stem cell research in dental tissue engineering, the new developments in biomimetic scaffold materials customized for dental tissue applications, and to give a prospectus with respect to translational approaches of these research findings towards clinical application.

INTRODUCTION

Dental diseases, such as caries, periodontitis, tooth loss, and orofacial/dental trauma are major public health problems worldwide, with a profound effect on an individual's quality of life (Petersen, et al., 2005). The experience of pain, problems with eating, chewing, smiling, and communication due to missing, discoloured, or damaged teeth have a major impact on people's daily lives and well-being. It is estimated that teeth congenital abnormalities account for 20% of all inherited disorders (Line, et al., 2003; Kousssoulakou, et al., 2009), whereas, dental pathology occupies a leading position in the list of human diseases. In addition, dental infectious diseases, such as periodontitis, have an associated risk of

DOI: 10.4018/978-1-5225-1903-4.ch004

systemic complications (e.g. diabetes, cardiovascular diseases, etc.) and therefore an impact on general health. All these factors have led to increased demand for effective management of dental diseases and replacement of missing tooth structures/teeth. Current strategies of replacement are based on non-biological artificial substitutes, such as dental fillings, fixed and removable partial dentures supported by teeth and/or implants, complete dentures, etc. All these substitutes have several disadvantages, including uncomfortable sensation, insufficient biocompatibility, damage to the surrounding tissues and unpredictable long-term therapeutic efficacy (Dodson, 2006; Jung, et al., 2008). The need for alternative therapies is evident in reports by the United States Department of Health and Human Services (USDHHS, 2000) and WHO Global Oral Health Data Bank, which reveal startling statistics about the high incidence of tooth loss and edentulism.

Recent progress in dental tissue engineering methodologies have provided the opportunity for novel and innovative alternative therapies based on regeneration strategies of the lost dental, periodontal and bone tissues in the craniofacial area (Sartaj & Sharp, 2006). These regenerative approaches are mainly based on the use of stem cells in combination with biomimetic scaffolds and relevant growth and differentiation factors, which make the classical tissue engineering triad (Vats, et al., 2005). It is envisioned that these novel regenerative therapies will be based on the use of bioengineering methods to regenerate the lost dental or surrounding bone tissues from easily harvested, donor-derived autologous tissues (Zivkovik, et al., 2010). It is also expected that these strategies will significantly reduce the cost of dental care. According to the 2006 National Health Expenditure Accounts, the annual US expenditures on dental services totaled 91.5 billion dollars (NHEA, 2006). It is estimated that 90% of adults have caries lesions and that 40% of the Western population is missing one or more teeth (Hacking, et al., 2009; Garcia-Godoy & Murray, 2006). Tissue engineering strategies for tooth replacement could potentially account for 90 million instances of caries, 45 million fractured or avulsed teeth, and 21 million procedures for endodontic surgery each year only in the USA (Garcia-Godoy & Murray, 2006).

However, before moving from reparative treatment to regenerative therapy in dentistry several scientific challenges must be addressed. First, a profound understanding of the developmental and functional characteristics of the dental organ must be acquired, including the complex cell interactions leading to dental tissue development, but also the regenerative processes that take place as a response to external stimuli. But even if this knowledge is acquired, the major challenge will then be the translational pathway from the basic scientific data through the in vitro studies, animal studies and clinical studies to commercialization and finally availability to the patient, who will be the final recipient of this knowledge and technology. Several questions will have then to be answered. For example, how several risks will be outweighed, including the possibility of transformation of the stem cells after implantation, the risk of unwanted contamination with pathogens during these procedures or the possible immugenicity of these cells on the recipient (Casagrande, et al., 2011). Another critical issue is how to deliver the right signals at the right place and time, which prerequisites a profound understanding of the molecular signals orchestrating cell function during odontogenesis. Moreover, what is the role of the cells going to be: replacement of the endogenous cell population or a biological "factory" by secreting matrix, growth factors, etc.?

One of the most important and decisive evolutions towards the development of novel therapeutic strategies for the regeneration of lost or damaged oral tissues was the discovery and characterization of stem cells of dental origin. Molecular biology studies focused on these cells have certainly significantly improved our understanding of tooth development. In addition, this knowledge has been applied in translational studies that aim at the use of these stem cells in clinical settings where the regeneration of dental and craniofacial tissues is indicated. Dental tissue-derived stem cells have been shown to be capable of regenerating dentin-pulp complexes in animal studies (Codeiro, et al., 2008; Demarco, et al., 2010). In addition, other studies have expanded the potential of these cells in the treatment of diseases, such as muscular dystrophies, critical size bone defects, spinal cord injury, etc. (Kerkis, et al., 2008; Seo, et al., 2008; Nosrat, et al., 2001).

Studies focused on the cellular and molecular mechanisms of odontogenesis have also provided very important information on the signaling pathways and morphogenetic factors regulating dentinogenesis. Growth factors, such as Bone Morphogenetic Proteins (BMPs), Platelet-Derived Growth Factor (PDGF), Vascular Endothelial Growth Factor (VEGF), as well as other morphogenetic molecules, such as Bone Sialoprotein (BSP), Dentin Matrix Protein (DMP-1), etc. have been characterized for their important role during odontogenic/regenerative processes and can therefore be beneficially used during dental tissue engineering applications (Goldberg, et al., 2009).

Finally, significant progress has been also accomplished on the development of novel biodegradable and biocompatible scaffolds. Mimicking natural extracellular matrix, scaffolds provide the 3D environment that allows for the adhesion, proliferation, migration, and finally differentiation of the seeded stem cells until they begin to secrete and shape their own microenvironment. A wide range of biomaterials have been proposed for this purpose, including porous ceramics, natural ECM-derived scaffolds (e.g. collagen), polymeric hydrogels, nanofibers, and microparticles (Galler, et al., 2011). The future development of biomimetic scaffolds customized for dental tissue regeneration will provide the tools to create customized microenvironments with defined properties for dental tissue engineering applications.

There is no doubt that stem cell-based dental tissue regeneration is a new and exciting field that has the potential to transform the way that we practice dentistry. It is, however, imperative its clinical application to be supported by solid basic and translational research. In this way, the full extent of the potential risks involved in the use of these technologies will be understood and the means to prevent them will be discovered. In this chapter, the *"state of the science"* of dental tissue engineering research will be analyzed and a prospectus of the translational possibilities of its findings towards clinical application will be given.

STEM CELL RESEARCH IN DENTAL TISSUE ENGINEERING: STATE OF THE SCIENCE

Tooth Structure and Development: A Basis for Dental Tissue Regeneration

Tissue regeneration in postnatal life recapitulates events that occur in the normal course of embryonic development and morphogenesis. Both processes are equally regulated through the interaction of highly conserved families of proteins and gene products. Therefore, an in depth understanding of the cellular and molecular interactions occurring during tooth morphogenesis is a basic prerequisite before proceeding to dental tissue regeneration strategies. The aim of regenerative dentistry is to re-create stepwise *in vitro* all the processes that occur during the development of the tooth organ and to safely transfer them into the clinical application (Saber, 2009).

The tooth organ is comprised of 4 major tissues: enamel, dentin, cementum and dental pulp. Its main body is consisted of dentin, a calcified tissue, mainly composed of collagen (90%) and non-collagenous proteins, such as Dentine Sialophosphoprotein (DSPP) and Dentine Matrix Protein (DMP-1). The deposition of hydroxyapatite minerals on this matrix gives rise to the mature calcified dentin (Bluteau, et al., 2008). Dentine surrounds the pulp, which is rich in fibroblast- like cells, blood vessels and nerves. The upper part of the dentine is covered by a layer of enamel, the hardest tissue of the human body, which is collagen-free. Its main proteins are amelogenin (90%), ameloblastin, enamelin, amelotin, tuftelin, and odontogenic ameloblast associated proteins (ODAM) (Sire, et al., 2007). The tooth root firmly supports the tooth within an alveolar socket by means of the periodontium. Cementum, periodontal ligament, and alveolar bone are the periodontal tissues that support teeth into the oral cavity (Koussoulakou, et al., 2009).

For permanent teeth, the template for these tissues is established during fetal development around the 20th week. Tooth development is the cumulative result of complex reciprocial interactions between different tissues, namely, the ectodermal-derived oral epithelium and neural crest–derived ectomesenchyme (Sharpe, 2001; Tucker & Sharpe, 1999). These interactions progressively transform the tooth primordia into complex mineralized structures of various cell types and progresses through 4 widely recognized stages of tooth development (Mitsiadis, et al., 2010): the bud, cap, bell, and crown stages. The first event in tooth development is the thickening of the oral epithelium and its proliferation into the underlying mesenchyme in the form of the cellular cord called dental lamina. The oral epithelium possesses the inductive capability for odontogenesis, which leads to the conditioning of the underlying mesenchyme. At the bud stage, the dental mesenchyme acquires odontogenic potential. At the cap stage epithelial components undergo specific folding, which is accompanied by the formation of the enamel knot under the influence of BMP-4. The enamel knot represents the signaling center that determines tooth morphogenesis, apoptosis, and definite tooth morphology and is formed by subsets of cells that express BMPs, FGFs, Wnt factors, and Shh, which are the main highly conserved gene families regulating odontogenesis (Imai, et al., 1998; Mitsiadis, et al., 2010). By the late cap stage, enamel knots disappear by apoptosis (Vaahtokari, et al., 1996). At the cap stage mesenchyme undergoes cytodifferentiation into two distinct types of cells: dental papilla cells and dental follicle cells (Koussoulakou, et al., 2009). At the bell stage, the tooth germ consists of the enamel organ (epithelial component) and dental mesenchyme consisting of the dental papilla and the dental follicle. Four cell layers form the epithelial component during late odontogenesis: the inner dental epithelium (future ameloblasts), stratum intermedium, stellate reticulum, and outer dental epithelium. The dental mesenchyme is also composed of different cell types, such as odontoblasts, sub-odontoblastic layer cells, dental papilla cells and dental follicle cells. Ameloblasts and odontoblasts are highly differentiated cells that synthesize and secrete the organic components of the enamel and dentin respectively (Bluteau, et al., 2008; Mitsiadis, et al., 2010). How this terminal differentiation is achieved is not yet understood. It has been proposed that Notch Signaling pathway, an evolutionarily conserved intercellular signaling mechanism that is mainly mediated through the Jag2 receptor and regulated through FGF and BMP signals, plays a pivotal role in ameloblast lineage commitment from the earliest stages of odontogenesis and is therefore indispensable for normal tooth development (Mitsiadis, et al., 2010).

After the crown formation, the apical mesenchyme of the dental papilla continues to proliferate to form the developing periodontium. Cells from the dental follicle give rise to cementoblasts (forming the cementum that covers the dentin of the root), fibroblasts (generating the periodontal ligament), and osteoblasts (elaborating the alveolar bone). At the same time, cells of the cervical loop proliferate and form the bilayer Hertwig's epithelial root sheath and produce the basement membrane that contains chemotactic proteins that would induce cementoblast differentiation (Slavkin, et al., 1989). One of these proteins is the Cementum Attachment Protein (CAP) whose role is in recruiting putative cementoblast precursors from the dental ectomesenchyme (Zeichner-David, et al., 2003). Transcription factors as-

Figure 1. Cell cultures of DPSC, SCAP, and SHED cells

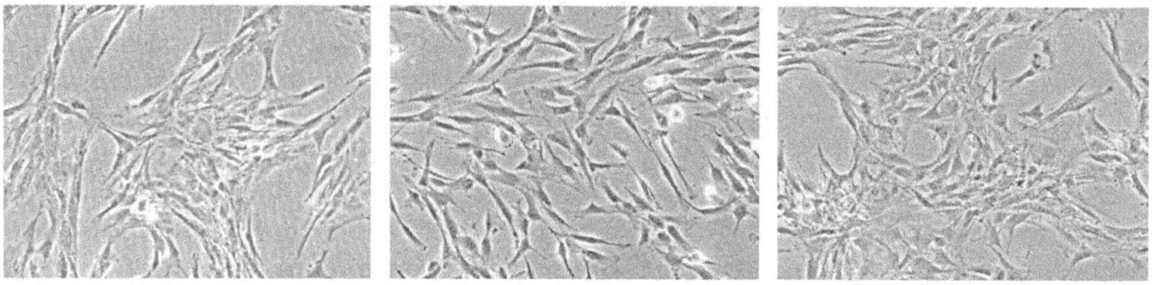

sociated with root development include two members of the homeobox family of transcription factors: Dlx2 and Dlx3 (Lezot, et al., 2000).

All the above complex signaling interactions overall determine the formation, position, and overall shape of tooth development (Tucker & Sharpe, 1999; Thesleff, et al., 2001; Honda, et al., 2008; Kapadia, et al., 2007; Salazar-Ciudad, 2008) (Figure 1). They are mediated by signaling molecules mostly belonging to four conservative gene families (Bluteau, et al., 2008):

1. Tumor Growth Factor Beta (TGF-β) superfamily, with members, such as BMP-2 and BMP- 4, which are key signaling molecules in regulating epithelial-mesenchymal interactions during odontogenesis (Kratochwil, et al., 1996; Nadiri, et al., 2004; Vainio, et al., 1993).
2. Molecules of the Fibroblast Growth Factor (FGF) family, such as FGF-3, -4, -8, and -10, which are involved in cell proliferation and regulation of the expression of specific target genes in teeth (Bei & Maas, 1998; Kettunen, et al., 1998).
3. Wingless integrated (Wnt), such as Wnt- 3, -7b, -10a, and -10b, which have essential roles as regulators of cell proliferation, migration and differentiation during tooth initiation and morphogenesis (Dassule & McMahon, 1998).
4. Other diffusible factors such as Sonic Hedgehog (SHH), which also contribute to both initiation and subsequent dental morphogenesis (Khan, et al., 2007). These genes encode transcription factors that regulate the synthesis of various signaling factors (Thesleff, et al., 2001).

All the above signaling factors mediate inductive interactions between the odontogenic tissue layers and affect cell multiplication, cell death, and cytodifferentiation (Matalova, et al., 2004).

Cell Sources for Dental Tissue Engineering

As tooth formation results from epithelial-mesenchymal interactions, two different populations of multipotent stem cells have to be considered: Epithelial Stem Cells (EpSC), which will give rise to enamel tissue and Mesenchymal Stem Cells (MSC) that will form the dentin-pulp complex and periodontium (cementum, periodontal ligament, and alveolar bone).

A stem cell is defined as a cell that can continuously produce unaltered daughters and furthermore, has the ability to generate cells with different and more restricted properties. Stem cells can divide either symmetrically (allowing the increase of stem cell number) or asymmetrically. Asymmetric divisions keep the number of stem cells unaltered and are responsible for the generation of cells with different properties. These cells can either multiply (progenitors or transit amplifying cells) or be committed to terminal differentiation. Progenitors and transit amplifying cells have a limited lifespan and therefore can only reconstitute a tissue for a short period of time when transplanted (Bluteau, et al., 2008).

Until now, several potential stem cell sources, with an ability of self-renewal and multi-lineage differentiation have been proposed as suitable precursors for dental tissue regeneration. There are two main types of stem cells: Embryonic Stem Cells (ESC), which are derived from blastocysts and Adult Stem Cells (ASC), which are derived from adult tissues. Both ESC cells and ASC cells have been shown to be capable of differentiating toward dental cells (Zhang, et al., 2006; Yen & Sharpe, 2008). In the clinical setting, the use of ESC is, however, subjected to ethical concerns. For this reason, most recent studies have focused on the localization of sites in adult tissues, where specific populations of ASC reside. ASC are quiescent, slow-cycling, undifferentiated cells, which are surrounded by neighboring cells and extracellular matrix. This microenvironment is specific for each stem cell compartment but is likely to be influenced by common factors, such as vasculature or loading pressure. The specialized microenvironment, housing ASC and transient amplifying cells or progenitors, forms a "niche." Understanding these microenvironments and their regulation is the key for the successful reproduction of such niches and for the *ex vivo* engineering of an organ with ensured functional homeostasis (Mitsiadis, et al., 2011). The basic problem when using ASC as stem cell source are the difficulties encountered during their *in vitro* expansion. It is questioned whether epigenetic (e.g. homing receptor/ligand expression, cytokine/growth factor production, lineage commitment/differentiation, programmed senescence, etc.) and genetic alterations (e.g. transformation, fusion, gene transfer, etc.) occurring during expansion culture may affect their therapeutic potential in a positive or negative way (Javazon, 2004). For example, the changes shown might be beneficial for site-specific utilization but detrimental for systemic administration. Because the capacity to expand stem cells in culture is an indispensable step for regenerative medicine, a considerable effort has been made to evaluate the consequences of the cultivation on stem cell behavior.

Finally, another proposed alternative cell source may be the so called "inducible pluripotent stem cells (iPS) (Takahashi, et al., 2006). iPS cells are reprogrammed cells derived from adult tissue, usually by the addition of several promoters (Chang & Cotsarelis, 2007; Pera & Hasegawa, 2008). iPS cells represent a novel renewable source of tissue precursors, with pluripotent properties, but lacking the ethical limitations of ESC. Current research focuses on improving induction strategies and on demonstrating the proof-of-principle that iPS cells can be differentiated into a variety of cell types. Although the prospect of using patient-specific iPS cells has much appeal from an ethical and immunologic perspective, the limitations of the technology from the standpoint of reprogramming efficiency and therapeutic safety necessitate much more in-depth research before the initiation of human clinical trials (Robbins, et al., 2010).

Epithelial Stem Cells (EpSC)

Finding a suitable epithelial stem cell source is one of the most challenging goals of dental tissue engineering strategies. The major problem is that dental epithelial cells, such as ameloblasts, are eliminated soon after tooth eruption and therefore, are no more present in human adult teeth (Bluteau, et al., 2008). In several studies, EpSC have been isolated from newborn or juvenile animals, usually from third molar teeth. In these studies, epithelia were removed and cells dissociated enzymatically. Precursors were then amplified and associated with MSC (originated from the same tooth) *in vitro* in contact with biomaterials, such as collagen sponges or synthetic polymers (Honda, et al., 2005, 2007a; Young, et al., 2002). However, this approach requires the isolation of EpSC from tooth germs of young children and is therefore unrealistic for clinical application. In other studies the rodent incisor has been used as a model of studying dental EpSC, since, in contrast to human incisors, there is an EpSC niche located at the apical part of these teeth that allows continuous growth and enamel production throughout life (Harada, et al., 1999; Kawano, et al., 2004; Mitsiadis, et al., 2007). Although this model can give important information on the mechanisms of mesenchymal-epithelial interactions in tooth formation, it is also unrealistic for clinical application, since it would require a xenogenic introduction of rodent cells in the human environment. For all these reasons, seeking for other sources, such as non-dental EpSC (Ohazama, et al., 2004b) that will be genetically engineered to acquire odontogenic potential is one of the main goals of current dental tissue engineering strategic.

Mesenchymal Stem Cells (MSC)

Mesenchymal Stem Cells (MSC), with a capacity of self renewal and multi-lineage differentiation, have attracted worldwide attention during the past few years as attractive progenitor cell sources for tissue engineering and regeneration. However, the basic question of how to define an MSC remains a point of discussion and controversy. Given the lack of universally accepted criteria for defining an MSC, the Mesenchymal and Tissue stem cell Committee of the International Society for Cellular Therapy (ISCT) proposed a set of standards to define human MSC for both laboratory-based scientific investigations and pre-clinical studies (Dominici, et al., 2006; Karp, et al., 2009). As part of the minimal criteria, human MSC must adhere to tissue culture plastic. Be positive for CD105, CD73, and CD90, and negative for CD45, CD34, CD14, or CD11b, CD79a, or CD19, and HLA-DR and must be able to differentiate into osteoblasts, adipocytes, and chondroblasts under standard *in vitro* differentiating conditions. Given the heterogeneity of typical MSC culture procedures and a lack of enforcement of the above mentioned characterization criteria, definitive conclusions based on the literature are often difficult to surmise (Karp, et al., 2009).

The potential use of different types of MSC for tooth regeneration and repair has been extensively studied in the last years. In the field of dentistry, several potential sources of MSCs have been identified as candidates for dental tissue engineering. These include MSCs from bone marrow (BMMSC) (Hu, et al., 2006a, 2006b; Yu, et al., 2007; Li, et al., 2007), adipose tissues (Wu, et al., 2008; Jing, et al., 2008), umbilical cord blood (Mareshi, et al., 2001), and dental tissues (Huang, et al., 2009), the last being the most obvious and promising candidates. The first type of dental stem cells was isolated from human pulp tissue and termed Dental Pulp Stem Cells (DPSCs) (Gronthos, et al., 2000). This was followed by the isolation of other dental MSCs types, including stem cells from human exfoliated deciduous teeth (SHED) (Miura, et al., 2003), periodontal ligament stem cells (PDLSC) (Seo, et al., 2004) and, most recently, MSCs residing in the apical papilla of developing teeth (SCAP) (Sonoyama, et al., 2008; Abe, et al., 2008). Recent studies have also identified a population of stem cells in the dental follicle, referred to as Dental Follicle Stem Cells (DFSC) (Morsczeck, et al., 2009; Yao, et al., 2008). There are concerns regarding the development and differentiation of stems cells in non-fetal environments, such as the adult mouth; however, a review of the literature suggests that adult tissues are capable of odontogenesis (Yen & Sharpe, 2008).

Dental tissue-derived MSC are characterized by their multipotentiality and ability to differentiate into several cell-restricted lineages, such as osteo/odontogenic, adipogenic, neurogenic, chondrogenic, and myogenic, when grown under defined culture conditions (Wei, et al., 2007; Zhang, et al., 2006a; Koyama, et al., 2009; d'Aquino, et al., 2007). One of the most striking features for dental tissue engineering applications is their odontogenic differentiation potential. Previous studies have shown that dental MSCs, including DPSC, SHED, and SCAP are capable to differentiate into odontoblastic lineages *in vitro*.

Several surface markers have been found to be expressed by dental MSCs, including STRO-1, CD146, CD105, CD106/VCAM, CD117 (c+kit), CD44, CD90, CD34, TGFαRII, FGFR3, Flt-1 (VEGF receptor 1), etc. (Huang, et al., 2009). In addition, other premature embryonic stem cell markers, including Oct4, Nanog, stage specific embryonic antigens (SSEA-3, SSEA-4) and tumor recognition antigens (TRA-1-60, TRA-1-81) have been also identified (Kerkis, et al., 2006).

The precise relationship among different stem cell types as candidates for dental tissue engineering still remains unclear. Below, we describe the basic characteristics of different MSC types of dental origin (Figure 1).

Adult Dental Pulp Stem Cells (DPSC)

Previous studies have shown that the mature dental pulp contains precursor cells involved in repair processes under appropriate signals (About & Mitsiadis, 2001; Tecles, et al., 2005). When the signal is mild, as for example slowly progressing dentinal caries, pulp tissue responds through reactionary dentinogenesis. During this physiological repair process, reactivated odontoblasts and/or cells located in the Hoehl's layer produce a mineralized dentin barrier, in the form of tubular orthodentin or as an osteodentin-like layer (Goldberg, 2011). However, in more severe dentinal injuries, such as pulp exposure, the subjacent odontoblastic layer may be severely affected or destroyed (de Souza Costa, et al., 2007; Murray, et al., 2002). In this case, stem/progenitor cells from the pulp core are triggered by the inflammatory signals to recruit towards the specific intrusion point at the dentin-pulp border. These cells then differentiate into secreting odontoblast- or osteoblast-like cells, producing a reparative ortho- or osteo-dentin barrier, in order to repair the damage (Goldberg, 2011). Several groups during the past few years have attempted to isolate and characterize these putative stem/progenitor cell populations residing in dental pulp stem cell niches and to analyze the molecular mechanisms of their functional role in pulp tissue repair (Schmalz & Galler, 2011; Mitsiadis, et al., 2011). Most studies clearly indicate that stem/progenitor cells isolated from the dental pulp and expanded *in vitro* are characterized by significant heterogeneity, expressed through multiple phenotypic differences, which most probably reflect distinct functional properties (Huang, et al., 2009). There is already evidence that there are significant variations in the odontogenic potential of single colony-derived populations isolated from the dental pulp, reflecting differences in their genotypic and protein expression patterns (Gronthos, et al., 2002). It has been found that two-thirds of the single-colony derived DPSC are able to form the same amount of dentin as multi-colony DPSC. This is further supported by the fact that DPSC isolated with enzyme treatment of pulp tissues form CFU-Fs with various characteristics (Gronthos, et al., 2002; Huang, et al., 2006). There are different cell densities of the colonies, suggesting that each cell clone may have a different growth rate, whereas different cell morphologies and sizes may be observed within the same colony. When seeded onto dentin, some DPSCs convert into odontoblast-like cells with a polarized cell body and a cell process extending into the existing dentinal tubules (Huang, et al., 2006).

In addition to their odontogenic potential, subpopulations of DPSC also possess an ability of *in vitro* multilineage differentiation towards adipogenic, neurogenic osteogenic, chondrogenic, and myogenic phenotypes, also supported by their gene expression patterns (Zhang, et al., 2006a, 2006b; d'Aquino, et al., 2007). In addition, transplantation of *ex vivo* expanded DPSC mixed with Hydroxyapatite/Tricalcium Phosphate (HA/TCP) leaded to the formation of ectopic pulp-dentin-like tissue complexes in immunocompromised mice (Gronthos, et al., 2000; Batouli, et al., 2003). These pools of heterogeneous DPSC form vascularized pulp-like tissue and are surrounded by a layer of odontoblast-like cells expressing Dentin Sialophosphoprotein (DSPP), which produces dentin containing dentinal tubules similar to those in natural dentin.

Stem Cells from Human Exfoliated Deciduous Teeth (SHED)

Recent findings demonstrated the isolation of mesenchymal progenitors from the pulp of human deciduous teeth (SHED) (Miura, et al., 2003). These cells exhibited a higher proliferation rate and population doublings compared to other MSC types, such as DPSC and BMMSC. They also showed high plasticity and multi-lineage differentiation potential (Huang, et al., 2009). Apart from the expression of several MSC markers (Bakopoulou, et al., 2011a), SHED also express neuronal and glial cell markers, which may be related to the neural-crest-cell origin of the dental pulp (Chai, et al., 2000). Concerning their neural potential, SHED were able to form sphere-like clusters when cultured in neurogenic medium. This is due to the highly proliferative cells, which aggregate in clusters that either adhere to the culture dish or float freely in the culture medium. These neural cells were positive for markers, including βIII-tubulin, GAD and NeuN. In addition, SHED can survive after injection into the dentate gyrus of the hippocampus of immunocompromised mice for more than 10 days and express neural markers, such as neurofilament (Huang, et al., 2009).

In vivo SHED can induce bone or dentin formation but, in contrast to DPSC, SHED failed to produce a dentin-pulp complex (Miura, et al., 2003). Another important feature of these cells after *in vivo* transplantation is their osteo-inductive capacity. All single-colony-derived SHED clones tested were capable of inducing bone formation in immunocompromised mice, while only one-fourth of the clones had the potential to generate ectopic dentin-like tissue (Miura, et al., 2003). SHED were also able to form an osteo-inductive template in immunocompomised mice that caused the recruitment of host murine ostegenic cells and finally the repair of critical sized calvarial defects (Seo, et al., 2008).

Stem Cells from the Apical Part of the Papilla (SCAP)

Stem cells with a very high proliferation and odontogenic differentiation potential have been also isolated from the apical part of the human dental papilla (SCAP), which is an easily accessible source, usually available from human immature third molars (Huang, et al., 2008). The apical papilla is the precursor tissue of the radicular pulp, and therefore, it is speculated that it gives rise to the coronal dentin by producing odontoblasts (Huang, et al., 2009). However, the apical papilla is an anatomically distinct area compared to the dental pulp and there is an apical cell-rich zone lying between these two tissues. Similar to DPSC and SHED, *ex vivo* expanded SCAP can undergo odontogenic, as well as adipogenic and neurogenic differentiation *in vitro* (Figure 2). However, recently published data by our group have shown that SCAP are more robust compared to DPSC derived from the same donor in terms of proliferation rate and odontogenic differentiation potential, which makes them very attractive candidates for dental tissue engineering applications (Bakopoulou, et al., 2011b). Finally, the capacity of SCAP to differentiate into functional dentinogenic cells has been verified by the same approaches used for other dental MSC types.

Figure 2. Multilineage differentiation of SCAP cells towards osteogenic, adipogenic, and neurogenic cell lineages

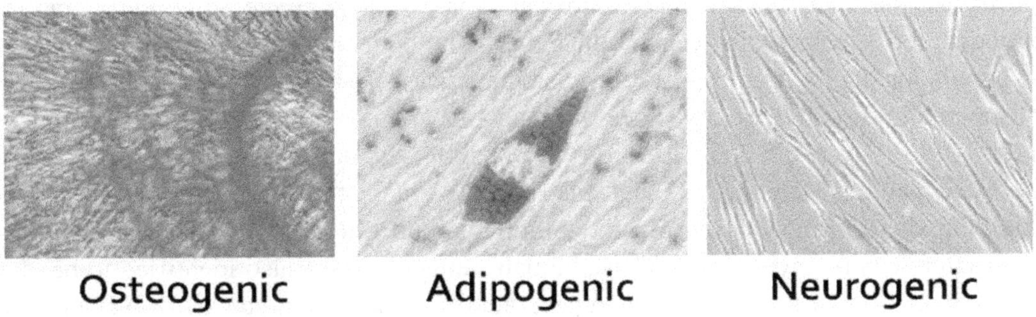

A typical dentin-pulp-like complex is generated when SCAP are transplanted into immunocompromised mice in an appropriate carrier matrix (Sonoyama, et al., 2006; Huang, et al., 2008; Abe, et al., 2008).

Dental Follicle Stem Cells (DFSC)

DFSC have been isolated from human dental follicles of impacted third molars (Honda, et al., 2010). Compared to other MSC types, DFSC form only low numbers of adherent clonogenic colonies when released from the tissue following enzymatic digestion. They also express stem cell markers, including Notch-1, STRO-1, nestin, collagen type I, Bone Sialoprotein (BSP), Osteocalcin (OCN), and Fibroblast Growth Factor Receptor (FGFR)1-IIIC (Morsczeck, et al., 2005). STRO-1 positive DFSC can differentiate into cementoblasts *in vitro* (Kemoun, et al., 2007) when stimulated with rhBMP-2 and rhBMP-7 or Enamel Matrix Derivatives (EMD) for 24 hrs. This is confirmed by the up-regulation of putative cementoblast markers, such as Cementum Attachment Protein (CAP) and Cementum Protein-23 (CP-23). In addition, other studies have shown that DFSC have the capacity for osteogenesis, adipogenesis, and neurogenesis (Jo, et al., 2007; Luan, et al., 2006; Kemoun, et al., 2007; Morsczeck, et al., 2005, 2009), whereas their capacity for chondrogenesis is still questioned (Yao, et al., 2008; Lindroos, et al., 2008). Significant differences in their multi-differentiation potential were also recorded among different clonal derived and expanded DFSC, strongly suggesting the significant heterogeneity of the cell populations derived from dental follicle biopsies.

DFSC have been also found able to form cementum *in vivo* (Handa, et al., 2002), while immortalized dental follicle cells are able to re-create a new Periodontal Ligament (PDL) after *in vivo* implantation (Yokoi, et al., 2007). Transplantation of DFSC by the same methods as described for other dental MSC generates a structure comprised of fibrous or rigid tissue. These transplants expressed human-specific transcripts for BSP, OCN and collagen type I. Gene expression was increased more than 100 times for BSP and OCN and was decreased for collagen type I transcripts after transplantation into immunocompromised mice. However, there was no dentin, cementum, or bone formation observed in the transplant *in vivo*. The authors explained that it could be due to the low number of cells in the original cultures (Morsczeck, et al., 2005, 2009).

Periodontal Ligament Stem Cells (PDLSC)

There is evidence that PDL contains progenitor cells that maintain tissue homeostasis and regeneration of periodontal tissue, including cementum and alveolar bone. Enzyme digestion treatment of PDL releases a population of clonogenic cells with characteristics of postnatal stem cells (Seo, et al., 2004). These cells maintain certain plasticity, since they can adopt adipogenic, osteogenic, and chondrogenic phenotypes *in vitro* (Gay, et al., 2007; Lindroos, et al., 2008; Xu, et al., 2009). These cells express also MSC-associated markers, including STRO-1, CD105, CD90, and other CDs, scleraxis, nestin, etc. (Seo, et al., 2004). Finally, after in vivo transplantation into immunocompromised mice a typical cementum/PDL-like structure can be regenerated. These human stem cells were also identified to be closely associated with the trabecular bone next to the regenerated PDL, suggesting their involvement in alveolar bone regeneration (Seo, et al., 2004).

Scaffold Materials used for Dental Tissue Engineering

For most regenerative strategies, a scaffold is used to provide a structure on which cells may adhere, grow, and spatially organize. Therefore, scaffolds are considered a critical component of tissue engineering. The ideal scaffold should mimic the Extra Cellular Matrix (ECM) to provide appropriate mechanical support and biochemical stimulation. It should provide chemical stability and physical properties matching the surrounding tissues with respect to cell compatibility, adhesion performance, cell proliferation, controlled degradation, and mechanical strength. Moreover, it should manipulate cell behaviors to achieve the desired functions, such as proliferation, differentiation, and matrix remodeling (Galler, et al., 2011; Casagrande, et al., 2011). In addition, regarding dentin-pulp-complex engineering, the scaffold should be able to compensate tissue-specific problems, such as possible contamination of the root canal, vascularization, and innervation of a long and narrow space and incorporation of growth and differentiation factors relevant to odontoblast differentiation and mineralized dentin formation.

Various scaffold materials have been employed recently in tooth regeneration protocols, including long-lasting porous bioceramics (e.g. hydroxyapatite, β-tricalcium phosphate, or their combination HA/TCP), naturally occurring molecules of intermediate duration (e.g. collagen and chitosan), relatively short-lasting polymers, such as Polyglycolic Acid (PGA), Polylactic Acid (PLA), Polyglycolic Acid-Poly-L-Lactic Acid (PGA-PLLA), and Polylactic Polyglycolic Acid (PLGA), and most recently synthetic hydrogel materials (e.g. polyethylene glycol/PEG and self-assembling peptides-SEP) (Galler, et al., 2011; Moioli, et al., 2007; Yuan, et al., 2011). Each material offers a unique chemistry, composition, structure, degradation profile, and possibility for modification.

The first scaffold material used after isolation and *in vitro* characterization of dental pulp stem cells from deciduous and permanent teeth was the biphasic system Hydroxyapatite/Tricalcium Phosphate (HA/TCP), that combined with the cells allowed the formation of dentin, bone, and dentin-pulp-like complexes *in vivo* (Gronthos, et al., 2000; Miura, et al., 2003). Furthermore, 3D CaP porous granules were able to support odontogenic development, as determined by the expression of dentin-associated genes, matrix synthesis, and mineralization (Nam, et al., 2011). Transplantation of a root-shaped HA/TCP block loaded with swine-SCAP and coated with Gelform containing PDLSC into the extraction socket of a minipig lower incisor showed the successful regeneration of the root/periodontal structure over which a porcelain crown could have been placed (Sonoyama, et al., 2006). Overall, ceramic scaffolds present important advantages, such as porous structure and chemical texture that promotes MSC differentiation and mineralization of the extracellular matrix (El-Ghannam, 2005), while the most important is the lack of toxic byproducts usually released by polymeric materials. Moreover, ceramic scaffolds can be used as carriers of growth factors, angiogenetic agents, drugs, and cell differentiation products formulating the proper microenvironment (Gerhardt, et al., 2010).

Synthetic polymers, as well as biologic molecules, such as type I collagen have been also widely applied in dental and bone tissue engineering, showing promising results. Scaffolds made of synthetic polymers allow for the manipulation of their physicochemical properties such as degradation rate, pore size, and mechanical resistance. They are also inexpensive and easy to prepare. The most common synthetic polymers in tissue engineering are PLLA, PGA, and the copolymer PLGA. These scaffolds are biodegradable and biocompatible and allow for cell growth and differentiation, making them highly suitable for tissue engineering applications (Young, et al., 2002; Cordeiro, et al., 2008; Sakai, et al., 2010). One of the first examples of successful replacement of scaffold by dental tissues was the use of copolymers (PGA/PLLA and PLGA) in combination with porcine third molar fully dissociated tooth buds that allowed for the engineering of complex dental structures with characteristics similar to the crowns of natural teeth (Young, et al., 2002). In addition, promising results have been achieved in studies by Nör's group (Codeiro, et al., 2008; Sakai, et al., 2010), which demonstrated the formation of a vascularized pulp-like tissue, odontoblast-like cells and newly generated dentin after seeding SHED into PLA in dentin disks (tooth slice/scaffold model). Similarly, Huang *et al.* (2010) observed soft tissue and new dentin deposition after transplantation of SCAP into PGLA in an empty root canal space, whereas El-Backly *et al.* (2008) also regenerated a dentin-pulp like tissue using a stem cell/poly (lactic-co-glycolic) acid scaffold construct in a rabbit model. Furthermore, Duailibi *et al.* (2004) observed dentin regeneration after seeding tooth bud cells onto Polyglycolic Acid (PGA) and incubating in rat jaws for 12 weeks. A main disadvantage of these already used polymer scaffolds is, however, the lack of cell-specific chemical information that is physiologically found in the normal ECM.

In contrast, collagen scaffolds offer the chemical and structural information of the ECM but are difficult to customize for specific applications. Because of their biological origin, they are also afflicted with the risk of transmitting animal-associated pathogens or provoking an immunoresponse. However, they are proposed for regeneration of the pulp and/or periodontal tissues, as they can be easily injectable in combination with stem cells and growth factors. Prescott *et al.* (2008) were able to regenerate a pulp-like tissue by using DPSCs seeded on a collagen scaffold and incorporating DMP-1 as growth factor. In addition, most recently, formation of regenerated pulp tissue with good vascularization and new dentine deposition was achieved in the pulp-chamber space, where pulp tissues were previously removed by pulpotomy and replaced with stem/progenitor cells in a collagen scaffold (Iohara, et al., 2009).

From a translational standpoint, it would be beneficial for scaffolds designed for dental pulp tissue engineering purposes to be made of injectable materials. The goal of these injectable scaffolds is to allow for stem cell transplantation throughout the full extent of the root canal and pulp chamber. An excellent example of such an approach was recently described by Galler *et al.* (2011) that generated self-assembling multidomain peptide hydrogels with the addition of a matrix metalloprotease 2 specific cleavage site and a cell adhesion motif (i.e., RGD), which enhanced cell survival and induced cell motility. These scaffolds provide a promising approach for tissue engineering, since they allow for a 'bottomup' approach of generating ECM-like materials, which offer high control at the molecular level and produce injectable materials ideally suited for small defects.

Growth Factors/Morphogenetic Factors and Dental Tissue Regeneration

Growth and morphogenetic factors are proteins that bind to specific membrane receptors and trigger signalling pathways that coordinate several cellular functions. These molecules play a critical role during tissue development, but also during tissue regeneration/repair (Casagrande, et al., 2011). Indeed, it is known that factors, such as TGF-α, BMPs, Platelet-Derived Growth Factor (PDGF), Fibroblast Growth Factor (FGF), and Vascular Endothelial Growth Factor (VEGF) are incorporated into the dentin matrix during dentinogenesis and are retained there as "fossilized" molecules, but remaining protected in an active form through interaction with other components of the dentin matrix (Smith, et al., 1998; Finkelman, et al., 1990). These molecules have been characterized for their important role during odontogenic/regenerative processes and can therefore be beneficially used during dental tissue engineering applications. Among those, BMP-2 (Saito, et al., 2004), BMP-4 (Nakashima, et al., 1994), and BMP-7 (Andelin, et al., 2003) have been shown to direct pulp progenitor/stem cell differentiation into odontoblasts resulting in dentin formation, which makes BMP family the most likely candidate for dental tissue engineering applications. Promising results were shown by autogenous transplantation of recombinant human BMP2 (rBMP2)-treated culture pellets of porcine cells into the amputated pulp of dog teeth, resulting in the formation of reparative dentin with odontoblast-like cells to be attached to the newly formed osteodentin after 4 weeks (Iohara, et al., 2004). Other studies with rBMP2 also showed promising results by stimulating adult pulp stem cell differentiation *in vitro* (Nakashima, et al., 1994; Saito, et al., 2004), while rBMP 2, -4, -7 also induced formation of reparative dentin *in vivo* (Nakashima, et al., 1994). Moreover, the application of recombinant human insulin-like growth factor-1 together with collagen has been found to induce complete dentin bridging and tubular dentin formation (Lovschall, et al., 2001).

Often as a result of their physiologic solubility, growth factors like BMPs are applied at levels in excess of their endogenous expression (McKay & Sandhu, 2002). These higher loading levels can result, however, in unwanted side-effects and limited spatial control. Microencapsulation (Carrasquillo, et al., 2003) or binding of these factors to the scaffold (Lin, et al., 2008) can relieve problems related to loss of activity of diffusion of the molecules from the scaffold. Microparticles containing growth factors or drugs are another example of the use of microscale technologies to control the activity of cells (Cheng, et al., 2006). For example, PLGA microspheres that release VEGF have been delivered into a porous scaffold to provide sustained growth factor release for up to 21 days (Ennett, et al., 2006).

Figure 3 presents the various types of stem cells, biomimetic scaffolds and relevant growth/morphogenetic factors, already applied in dental tissue engineering, which consist the "tissue engineering triad."

STEM CELL-BASED THERAPY FOR DENTAL TISSUE/ WHOLE TOOTH ENGINEERING

Enamel Regeneration

Enamel is the hardest mineralized tissue in the human body. It is comprised of nanorod-like hydroxyapatite crystals arranged into highly organized micro architectural units called enamel prisms (Bluteau, et al., 2008). The ameloblasts which are responsible for enamel development are lost after tooth eruption, making enamel a non-regenerating tissue (Zivkovic, et al., 2010). Therefore, engineering human enamel still remains a major challenge.

Figure 3. Stem cells, biomimetic scaffolds, and growth/morphogenetic factors applied in dental tissue engineering

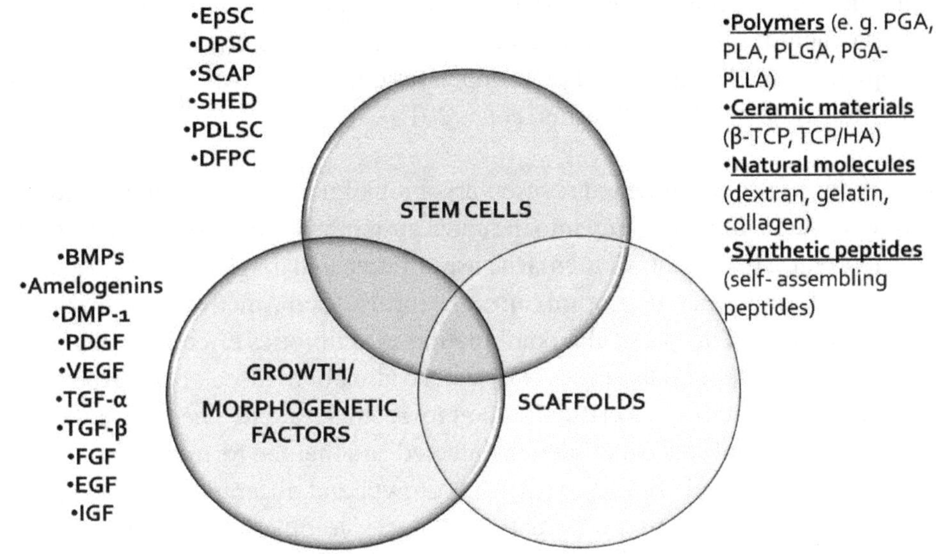

Previous attempts to engineer enamel focused exclusively on its chemical synthesis. Chen *et al.* (2005, 2006a) synthesized and modified a hydroxyapatite nanorod surface with monolayers of surfactants to create specific surface characteristics that allowed the nanorods to self-assemble into an enamel prism-like structure at a water/air interface. The size of the synthetic hydroxyapatite nanorods can be controlled and synthesized nanorods were similar in size to both human and rat enamel crystals. Wang *et al.* (2009) also achieved direct growth of human enamel-like structures on the human tooth by using fluorapatite/phosphoric acid pastes. The newly formed calcium phosphate crystals showed the ability to self-assemble into an ordered microstructure similar to those seen in human enamel.

Another strategy to regenerate human enamel relies on cell-mediated tissue engineering by combining epithelial and mesenchymal cells of various origins that possess odontogenic potential. Several attempts have been made to form teeth *in vivo* by recombining dental epithelial and mesenchymal tissues with very promising results. In these studies single cell suspensions were obtained after fully dissociating rat, pig or mice tooth germs, then seeded onto the surface of selected biomaterials (e.g. collagen-coated polyglycolic acid, calcium phosphate material, collagen sponges) and successfully re-implanted into immunocompromised animals (Duailibi, et al., 2004; Honda, et al., 2006, 2007a, 2007b; Hu, et al., 2006b; Robey, et al., 2005; Young, et al., 2002; Yu, et al., 2008; Sumita, et al., 2009; Takahashi, et al., 2010). All these reports describe the presence of both dentin and enamel after retrieval of the transplanted tissues. This indicates that the recombined cells could re-organize themselves and form individual layers and furthermore, that they can differentiate properly into odontoblasts and ameloblasts. Therefore, this approach is attractive for future application of bioengineered tooth formation in the human jaw. However, it remains an open question the selection of the most appropriate human epithelial stem cell population derived from adult human tissues that will be able to give rise to ameloblasts producing enamel. Recently, BMSC were shown to acquire ameloblast characteristics when interacting with the dental mesenchyme (Hu, et al., 2006a). However, further research is needed towards this direction, emphasizing the importance of their microenvironment.

Dentin/Pulp Complex Regeneration

Several tissue engineering approaches have been proposed in order to regenerate a functional dentin-pulp complex. These include (1) root canal revascularization via blood clotting, (2) scaffold/stem cells/growth factors implantation, (3) engineered pulp implantation, (4) three-dimensional cell printing, and (5) gene therapy (Murray, et al., 2007; Sharma, et al., 2010).

1. Several case reports have documented revascularization of necrotic root canal systems by disinfection followed by establishing bleeding into the canal system via overinstrumentation (Banchs, et al., 2004). An important aspect of these cases is the use of intracanal irrigants (NaOCl and chlorhexdine) with placement of antibiotics (e.g. a mixture of ciprofloxacin, metronidazole, and minocycline paste) for several weeks. This particular combination of antibiotics effectively disinfects root canal systems (Sato, et al., 1996) and increases revascularization of avulsed and necrotic teeth (Ritter, et al., 2004), suggesting that this is a critical step in revascularization. The revascularization method assumes that the root canal space has been disinfected and that the formation of a blood clot yields a matrix (e.g. fibrin), which is rich in constituent growth and differentiation factors and that traps cells capable of initiating new tissue formation. A bacteria impermeable seal of the access opening provided by an adequate thickness restorative material is mandatory to prevent any bacterial infiltration and destruction of the neo tissue (Sharma, et al., 2010). The advantages of this approach is the simplicity and low cost, without the need for expensive biotechnology. Furthermore, the pulp regeneration from a patient's own blood cells avoids the possibility of immune rejection and pathogen transmission. However, concerns still remain on the oxygen supply for the cells in the coronal portion of the root canal system and on the functionality of the regenerated pulp tissue. It is still questionable whether the neo tissue contains functional odontoblasts that get attached in the canal walls and whether the newly deposited hard tissue has the histologic picture of cementum, bone, dentin, or osteodentin (Sharma, et al., 2010).
2. Another pulp regeneration approach relies on the classical tissue engineering triad (stem cells/scaffolds/growth factors constructs). With the advances of tissue engineering techniques, it is now possible to seed stem cells onto a three-dimensional conductive scaffold matrix, rich in bioactive signaling molecules and grown in an appropriate culture medium. This artificial pulp construct generated in the laboratory can be then transplanted into the pulp cavity. Several potential postnatal stem cell sources have been proposed for this purpose, including, skin, buccal mucosa, fat and bone marrow (Murray, et al., 2007), with stem cells from dental origin (DPSC, SHED, etc) being the most obvious and promising candidates. Gebhardt *et al.* (2009) showed that pulp constructs could be created using polymer and collagen scaffolds seeded with DPSC. Both these scaffolds showed better cell survival compared to calcium phosphate scaffolds. Gotlieb *et al.* (2008) also concluded that pulp tissue constructs made with polylactic acid polymer and collagen seeded with SHED could be implanted into cleaned and shaped root canals. The implantation of DPSC seeded on a collagen scaffold and combined with Dentin Matrix Protein 1 (DMP1) in the site of injury, can induce an organized matrix formation similar to that of pulpal tissue, which might lead to hard tissue formation (Prescott, et al., 2008). However, in certain studies, collagen scaffolds impregnated with pulp cells have shown to undergo significant contraction both *in vivo* and *in vitro,* which could affect pulp tissue regeneration (Huang, et al., 2008; Chan, et al., 2005). PLG matrices seeded with DPSC have shown good cellular adhesion with no observable contraction, suggesting their use as

a suitable carrier (Huang, et al., 2008). Zhang *et al.* (2006b), observed successful dental pulp stem cell growth on spongeous collagen, porous ceramic and fibrous titanium mesh scaffolds that were implanted into nude mice. In a recent study, pulp like tissue was shown to regenerate in emptied root canal space, with odontoblast like cells producing dentin like tissue on existing dentinal walls, when SCAP and DPSC seeded onto poly lactide/glycolide scaffolds were inserted into tooth fragments and transplanted into immunocompromised mice (Huang, et al., 2009). It was also reported that Treated Dentin Matrix (TDM) can serve as both scaffold and inductive microenvironment, and DFPC is a suitable cell type for complete and prefabricated shaped dentin regeneration (Guo, et al., 2009). Further research needs to be conducted to identify an optimum matrix deemed suitable for carrying pulp stem cells/growth factors into the pulp space and maintaining their survival.

3. Another pulp regeneration approach includes the implantation of engineered 3D tissue construct into a pulp cavity. This is an attractive approach but requires construction of precise 3D models for each individual pulp cavity. Moreover, an effective delivery system that will allow introduction of these constructs into narrow canal spaces has to be developed. Injecting a soft scaffold matrix impregnated with pulp stem cells and growth factors into areas with accessibility constraints like the root canal system can overcome difficulties associated with implanting a rigid matrix. Scaffold materials that can be injected include synthetic hydrogels, such as poly-ethylene-glycol polymers (Trojani, et al., 2005). Modifying hydrogel polymers with peptides like arginine, glycine, or aspartic acid have helped in improving cell adhesion and matrix synthesis rendering them suitable for this specific use (Galler, et al., 2011). These injectable materials can be also loaded with angiogenic factors, such as VEGF, in order to induce angiogenesis of the newly formed pulp tissue. Despite these advances, hydrogels are still at an early stage of research and this type of delivery system, although promising, has yet to be proven to be functional *in vivo*.

   Another approach for delivering engineered tissue into the pulp cavity includes the *in vitro* development of cell sheets. The cultured pulp tissue is grown in sheets *in vitro* on biodegradable polymer nanofibers or on sheets of extracellular matrix proteins, such as collagen I or fibronectin (Huang, et al., 2006). The advantage of having the cells aggregated together is that it localizes the postnatal stem cells in the root canal system. The disadvantage of this technique is, however, that implantation of sheets of cells may be technically difficult.

4. Several other approaches have been proposed for the regeneration of the dentin-pulp complex, among those the three-dimensional cell printing. In this method, an ink-jet-like device is used to dispense layers of cells suspended in a hydrogel to recreate the structure of the tooth pulp tissue. The three-dimensional cell printing technique can be used to precisely position cells and this method has the potential to create tissue constructs that mimic the natural tooth pulp tissue structure (Barron, et al., 2005).

5. Finally, gene therapy has been also proposed for dental pulp tissue engineering. This method is based on the introduction of genes into target cells with the aim of altering their phenotype or protein expression profiles. Transfection is the use of chemical (calcium phosphate, lipids, polymers, and proteins) or physical (electropolation, microinjection, naked DNA) methods for introducing DNA into recipient cells, where as transduction is the use of viral vectors for introducing DNA (Edwards, et al., 2006). One use of gene delivery in endodontics would be to deliver mineralizing genes into pulp tissue to promote tissue mineralization. Successful bone induction has been reported after application of the BMP family members BMP-2,-4,-7 and -9 by gene therapy using viral vectors (Alden, et al., 2002). Transplantation of cultured dermal fibroblasts expressing virally mediated

BMP has induced reparative dentin formation in exposed pulps with reversible pulpitis (Rutherford, et al., 2001). Mineralized tissue has shown to effectively form after BMP2 transfected DPSC seeded onto ceramic scaffolds were implanted into nude mice (Yang, et al., 2009). However, potentially serious health hazards exist with the use of gene therapy; these arise from the use of the vector (gene transfer) system, rather than the genes expressed. Prolonged expression by integration of the gene/viral vector into the target cell genome may also result in tumor formation (Edwards, et al., 2006). Therefore, extended research is needed before clinical application.

Periodontal Ligament Regeneration

The periodontium is comprised of tissues (cementum, periodontal ligament, alveolar bone, and gingiva) that surround, support, and anchor the tooth. Loss of this tissue is broadly referred to as periodontal disease. Currently, the methods to reconstitute lost periodontal structures have relied on conventional mechanical techniques (root debridement) and anti-infective modalities to prevent its further regression, followed by a range of regenerative procedures. These mainly include Guided Tissue Regeneration (GTR), which uses biomaterials (barrier membranes) to prevent ingrowth of epithelial cells while providing a protected niche for repair by periodontal cells. GTR has been used alone or in combination with bone replacement grafts (autografts, demineralized freeze-dried bone allografts, bovine-derived xenografts) and/or exogenous growth factors, such as BMP-2 and-7, PDGF, IGF-1 and FGF-2, which have been shown promising for periodontal repair (Taba, et al., 2005; Hacking, et al., 2009; Chen, et al., 2010).

However, current clinical approaches and emerging paradigms have been shown to have variable rather than restricted regenerative outcomes or need to be further developed for clinical use respectively. For a variety of reasons (such as oral hygiene, defect size, infection, and many others), injured or diseased periodontium may not be capable of repairing itself in many, if not all, cases, by means of wound healing and tissue re-growth (Polimeni, et al., 2006). The poor innate ability of damaged periodontal tissues to regenerate and the limited extent of possible tissue regeneration in periodontal defects demonstrate the need for developing clinically effective procedures to regenerate enough healthy periodontal tissues to restore the periodontium's original architecture and function (Villar, et al., 2010; Reynolds, et al., 2010; Trombelli, et al., 2005; Chen, et al., 2010).

Recent approaches using tissue-engineering technology have utilized scaffold materials in combination with stem cells of dental origin for periodontal tissue regeneration. Different types of scaffolds/stem cells combinations have been proposed, including collagen sponges seeded with periodontal ligament cells (Nakahara, et al., 2004) or Hydroxyapatite/Tricalcium Phosphate (HA/TCP) scaffolds seeded with Periodontal-Ligament (PDL) Derived Stem Cells (PDLSC) (Liu, et al., 2008).

Most recently, therapeutics based on endogenous regenerative technology have been proposed as a very promising approach towards periodontal tissue regeneration (Chen, et al., 2010). This approach aims to stimulate latent self-repair mechanisms of the patient and harness the host's innate capacity for regeneration. This is basically accomplished by localized delivery of growth factors loaded in appropriate scaffolds (e.g. fibrin or hydrogel injectable scaffolds), sometimes also in association with commercialized products (e.g. bone grafts, morphogenetic factors) to create a material niche in an injured site that stimulates the recruitment of progenitor/stem cells from neighboring tissues (cell homing) for *in situ* periodontal regeneration. After reaching the injured site these host stem cells can then differentiate into PDL-forming cells, mineral-forming cementoblasts and/or bone-forming osteoblasts (Chen, et al., 2010; Zaky, et al., 2009). A variety of signaling molecules have been proposed for this purpose, specifically

BMP-2 and-7, PDGF, TGF-β, VEGF, EGF, FGF) and IGF-1 among others (Lee, et al., 2010; Chen, et al., 2009; Werner, et al., 2003). Enamel Matrix Proteins (EMP), produced by Hertwig's epithelial sheath, have been also proposed for this purpose, as they play an important role in cementogenesis and in the development of the periodontal attachment apparatus. There is some evidence that these proteins also play a role in regeneration of periodontal tissues after periodontal therapy. *In vitro* studies have shown that EMP added to cultures of periodontal fibroblasts result in enhanced proliferation, protein, and collagen production and promote mineralization. It is believed that EMP act as a matrix enhancement factor, creating a positive environment for cell proliferation, differentiation, and matrix synthesis. In addition, a variety of scaffold materials have been proposed for the delivery of bioactive factors, including polymers, such as PGA, PLA, and their PLGA copolymer (Higuschi, et al., 1999; Takahashi, et al., 2005; Herberg, et al., 2008), Beta-Tricalcium Phosphate (β-TCP) (Sarment, et al., 2006), and natural polymers such as dextran (Chen, et al., 2006b), gelatin (Saito, et al., 2009), and collagen (Hosokawa, et al., 2000; King, et al., 2001), or combinations of the above.

The main advantage of this emerging approach (cell homing) is the avoidance of isolation, *ex vivo* culture and subsequently re-implantation of autologous stem cells. This makes this approach closer to being ready for clinical use compared to cell transplantation or gene therapy. Problems that remain to be solved are the identification of the most appropriate growth factor combinations, their optimal dosages, and the best approaches for their delivery to develop clinically meaningful therapies (Lee, et al., 2010). Currently available growth factor delivery vehicles have several drawbacks including loss of bioactivity, limited control over dose administration, non-targeted delivery, and/or lack of availability (Chen, et al., 2010). Thus, further investigation is needed to facilitate the clinical translation of the current drug carriers and delivery systems. Finally, another scientific challenge will be to mimic the natural healing process of the periodontium and the complex orchestration of structural and molecular signals presented by its natural ECM.

Whole Tooth Tissue Engineering

The replacement of lost teeth by whole tooth regeneration is one of the main goals of dental tissue engineering technology. Current efforts to reproduce a viable tooth can be broadly categorized as those based on tissue engineering techniques (scaffold-based) (Thesleff & Tummers, 2003; Duailibi, et al., 2004, 2006; Modino & Sharpe, 2005; Young, et al., 2005; Yen & Sharpe, 2008) or on developmental biology (organogenesis- or germ-tissue-based) (Yelick & Vacanti, 2006; Sharpe & Young, 2005; Sartaj & Sharpe, 2006; Nakao, et al., 2007). The first (tissue engineering) approach commonly utilizes a cell seeded scaffold to guide and support tooth formation, while the second (developmental or "organotype") approach facilitates development of a tooth from a collection of cells resembling the tooth germ (Hacking, et al., 2009).

Both techniques have been described in previous parts of this chapter, showing very promising results, although there are still several limitations. The basic problem of the scaffold approach is that it fails to reproduce the appropriate size of the tooth. This size limitation may be a consequence of the animal model or directly related to mass transfer. Animal studies using scaffold-based approaches often rely on *in vivo* maturation of a small scaffold in the renal capsule or omentum, followed by implantation into the jaw to support and develop a tooth-like structure (Young, et al., 2005; Ohazama, et al., 2004a). *In vitro* approaches generally rely on perfusion or flow-based bioreactors that facilitate a deeper exchange of molecules within the scaffold (Timmins, et al., 2007; Jaasma, et al., 2008). On the other hand, techniques based on recombination of different cell types (germ-tissue-based or scaffold-free) usually lead to teeth with normally shaped and sized crowns. In the field of dentistry, the first bioengineered tooth germ, which developed and erupted in the oral cavity as functional organ replacement therapy using this approach was recently reported by Ikeda *et al.* (2009). These results are very promising for application of bioengineered organ replacement in clinical therapy in the not so distant future.

CONCLUSION AND FUTURE PERSPECTIVES

Stem cell-based dental tissue regeneration is a novel and promising field that will change several aspects of way that we practice dentistry today (Sloan, et al., 2009). Although regeneration of whole tooth organs still remains a highly challenging goal, regeneration of the dental pulp and periodontal tissues (regenerative endodontics and periodontics) are already significantly benefiting from this innovative technology. It is also expected that a variety of bioengineered products (e.g. stem cells, material niches, tissue constructs, or engineered tissues) will be available for clinical therapies in the near future. However, a large amount of this knowledge has yet to be translated from basic science to therapeutically useful techniques applied to patients. Critical challenges still need to be resolved to achieve *de novo* tissue regeneration and morphogenesis of complex morphologies in dental and periodontal tissues. These include the problem of acquisition and *ex vivo* expansion of sufficient number of stem cells without losing their "stemness" and their engraftment at the recipient site without concerns about the short- and long-term adverse effects, such as effects of graft vs. host disease, chromosomal instability, or tumorigenicity (Bhatt, et al., 2009). Other scientific concerns are related to the present lack of tissue engineering techniques mimicking the process of tooth morphogenesis and most importantly the discovery of the most suitable substitute of the embryonic oral epithelium, which has a unique set of signals for odontogenesis. The last point is also restricted by the ethical issues on the use of human embryos (Nakahara, et al., 2007).

Future progress will depend on deep understanding of the biology of the cells used to regenerate tissues and the signaling molecules and growth factors orchestrating their function. Furthermore, the development of new biomimetic scaffold materials, customized for dental tissue regeneration will provide the necessary microenvironment for targeted applications (e.g. bone regeneration, pulp regeneration, etc). It is, therefore, clear that dental tissue regeneration needs a multidisciplinary approach derived from the cooperation of clinicians and researchers from diverse fields (e.g., biologists, biomaterial scientist, dental clinicians).

However, in order to achieve widespread clinical use, a regenerative technology must not only be scientifically sound but also cost effective, safe and clinically expedient. Although many scientific and technological components of the bioengineering paradigm are already available or emerging fast, they are most of the times uncoupled from the real economic constraints or the clinical expediency. These barriers to progress are further compounded by the significant cost-implications of current tissue engineering processes and the lack of European/International rules regarding the regulatory procedures for tissue engineering products and processes.

In conclusion, the introduction of dental stem cell–based therapy will revolutionize the way we practice dentistry, bringing a whole new concept for the treatment of tooth loss, caries, and periodontitis, as well as a variety of different conditions in the craniofacial region. However, scientific effort should focus on the potential to translate research findings into clinically applicable treatment modalities.

REFERENCES

Abe, S., Yamaguchi, S., Watanabe, A., Hamada, K., & Amagasa, T. (2008). Hard tissue regeneration capacity of apical pulp derived cells (APDCs) from human tooth with immature apex. *Biochemical and Biophysical Research Communications*, *371*, 90–93. doi:10.1016/j.bbrc.2008.04.016 PMID:18407827

About, I., & Mitsiadis, T. A. (2001). Molecular aspects of tooth pathogenesis and repair: In vivo and in vitro models. *Advances in Dental Research*, *15*, 59–62. doi:10.1177/08959374010150011501 PMID:12640742

Alden, T., Varady, P., Kallmes, D., Jane, J. A., & Helm, G. A. (2002). Bone morphogenetic protein gene therapy. *Spine*, *27*, 87–93. doi:10.1097/00007632-200208151-00016 PMID:12205425

Bakopoulou, A., Leyhausen, G., Volk, J., Tsiftsoglou, A., Garefis, P., Koidis, P., & Geurtsen, W. (2011a). Assessment of the impact of two different isolation methods on the osteo/odontogenic differentiation potential of human dental stem cells derived from deciduous teeth. *Calcified Tissue International*, *88*, 130–141. doi:10.1007/s00223-010-9438-0 PMID:21153807

Bakopoulou, A., Leyhausen, G., Volk, J., Tsiftsoglou, A., Garefis, P., Koidis, P., & Geurtsen, W. (2011b). Comparative analysis of in vitro osteo/odontogenic differentiation potential of human dental pulp stem cells (DPSCs) and stem cells from the apical papilla (SCAP). *Archives of Oral Biology*, *56*(7), 709–721. doi:10.1016/j.archoralbio.2010.12.008 PMID:21227403

Banchs, F., & Trope, M. (2004). Revascularization of immature permanent teeth with apical periodontitis: New treatment protocol? *Journal of Endodontics*, *30*, 196–200. doi:10.1097/00004770-200404000-00003 PMID:15085044

Barron, J. A., Krizman, D. B., & Ringeisen, B. R. (2005). Laser printing of single cells: Statistical analysis, cell viability, and stress. *Annals of Biomedical Engineering*, *33*, 121–130. doi:10.1007/s10439-005-8971-x PMID:15771266

Batouli, S., Miura, M., Brahim, J., Tsutsui, T. W., Fisher, L. W., & Gronthos, S. et al. (2003). Comparison of stem-cell-mediated osteogenesis and dentinogenesis. *Journal of Dental Research*, *82*(12), 976–981. doi:10.1177/154405910308201208 PMID:14630898

Bei, M., & Maas, R. (1998). FGFs and BMP4 induce both Msx1-independent and Msx1-dependent signaling pathways in early tooth development. *Development*, *125*, 4325–4333. PMID:9753686

Bernabé, E., & Marcenes, W. (2010). Periodontal disease and quality of life in British adults. *Journal of Clinical Periodontology*, *37*(11), 968–972. doi:10.1111/j.1600-051X.2010.01627.x PMID:20880054

Bhatt, A., & Le, A. D. (2009). Craniofacial tissue regeneration: Where are we? *CDA Journal California Dental Association*, *37*, 799–803. PMID:19998656

Bluteau, G., Luder, H. U., De Bari, C., & Mitsiadis, T. A. (2008). Stem cells for tooth engineering. *European Cells & Materials*, *16*, 1–9. PMID:18671204

Carrasquillo, K. G., Ricker, J. A., Rigas, I. K., Miller, J. W., Gragoudas, E. S., & Adamis, A. P. (2003). Controlled delivery of the anti-VEGF aptamer EYE001 with poly (lactic-co-glycolic) acid microspheres. *Investigative Ophthalmology & Visual Science*, *44*, 290–299. doi:10.1167/iovs.01-1156 PMID:12506087

Casagrande, L., Cordeiro, M., Nör, S. A., & Nör, J. E. (2011). Dental pulp stem cells in regenerative dentistry. *Odontology*, *99*, 1–7. doi:10.1007/s10266-010-0154-z PMID:21271319

Chai, Y., Jiang, X., Ito, Y., Bringas, P., Han, J., & Rowitch, D. H. et al. (2000). Fate of the mammalian cranial neural crest during tooth and mandibular morphogenesis. *Development*, *127*(8), 1671–1679. PMID:10725243

Chan, C., Lan, W., Chang, M., Chen, Y. J., Lan, W. C., Chang, H. H., & Jeng, J. H. (2005). Effects of TGF- betas on the growth, collagen synthesis and collagen lattice contraction of human dental pulp fibroblasts in vitro. *Archives of Oral Biology*, *50*(5), 469–479. doi:10.1016/j.archoralbio.2004.10.005 PMID:15777529

Chang, H. Y., & Cotsarelis, G. (2007). Turning skin into embryonic stem cells. *Nature Medicine*, *13*, 783–784. doi:10.1038/nm0707-783 PMID:17618266

Chen, F. M., Shelton, R. M., Jin, Y., & Chapple, I. L. (2009). Localized delivery of growth factors for periodontal tissue regeneration: Role, strategies, and perspectives. *Medicinal Research Reviews*, *29*, 472–513. doi:10.1002/med.20144 PMID:19260070

Chen, F. M., Wu, Z. F., Sun, H. H., Wu, H., Xin, S. N., & Wang, Q. T. et al. (2006b). Release of bio-active BMP from dextran-derived microspheres: A novel delivery concept. *International Journal of Pharmaceutics*, *307*, 23–32. doi:10.1016/j.ijpharm.2005.09.024 PMID:16260104

Chen, F. M., Zhang, J., Zhang, M., An, Y., Chen, F., & Wu, Z. F. (2010). A review on endogenous regenerative technology in periodontal regenerative. *Biomaterials*, *31*, 7892–7927. doi:10.1016/j.biomaterials.2010.07.019 PMID:20684986

Chen, F. M., Zhao, Y. M., Jin, Y., & Shi, S. (2011). Prospects for translational regenerative medicine. *Biotechnology Advances*, *30*(3), 658–672. doi:10.1016/j.biotechadv.2011.11.005 PMID:22138411

Chen, H., Clarkson, B. H., Sun, K., & Mansfield, J. F. (2005). Self-assembly of synthetic hydroxyapatite nanorods into an enamel prism-like structure. *Journal of Colloid and Interface Science*, *288*, 97–103. doi:10.1016/j.jcis.2005.02.064 PMID:15927567

Chen, H., Tang, Z., Liu, J., Sun, K., Chang, S. R., & Peters, M. C. (2006a). Acellular synthesis of a human enamel-like microstructure. *Advanced Materials*, *18*, 1846–1851. doi:10.1002/adma.200502401

Cheng, J., Teply, B. A., Jeong, S. Y., Yim, C. H., Ho, D., & Sherifi, I. et al. (2006). Magnetically responsive polymeric microparticles for oral delivery of protein drugs. *Pharmaceutical Research*, *23*, 557–564. doi:10.1007/s11095-005-9444-5 PMID:16388405

Cordeiro, M. M., Dong, Z., Kaneko, T., Zhang, Z., Miyazawa, M., & Shi, S. et al. (2008). Dental pulp tissue engineering with stem cells from exfoliated deciduous teeth. *Journal of Endodontics*, *34*, 962–969. doi:10.1016/j.joen.2008.04.009 PMID:18634928

d'Aquino, R., Graziano, A., Sampaolesi, M., Laino, G., Pirozzi, G., De Rosa, A., & Papaccio, G. (2007). Human postnatal dental pulp cells co-differentiate into osteoblasts and endotheliocytes: A pivotal synergy leading to adult bone tissue formation. *Cell Death and Differentiation*, *14*, 1162–1171. doi:10.1038/sj.cdd.4402121 PMID:17347663

Dassule, H. R., & McMahon, A. P. (1998). Analysis of epithelial-mesenchymal interactions in the initial morphogenesis of the mammalian tooth. *Developmental Biology*, *202*, 215–227. doi:10.1006/dbio.1998.8992 PMID:9769173

de Souza Costa, C. A., Teixeira, H. M., Lopes do Nascimento, A. B., & Hebling, J. (2007). Biocompatibility of resin-based dental materials applied as liners in deep cavities prepared in human teeth. *Journal of Biomedical Materials Research. Part B, Applied Biomaterials*, *81*(1), 175–184. doi:10.1002/jbm.b.30651 PMID:16969818

Demarco, F. F., Casagrande, L., Zhang, Z., Dong, Z., Tarquinio, S. B., & Zeitlin, B. D. et al. (2010). Effects of morphogen and scaffold porogen on the differentiation of dental pulp stem cells. *Journal of Endodontics*, *36*, 1805–1811. doi:10.1016/j.joen.2010.08.031 PMID:20951292

Dodson, T. B. (2006). Predictors of dental implant survival. *Journal of the Massachusetts Dental Society*, *54*, 34–38. PMID:16536162

Dominici, M., Le Blanc, K., Mueller, I., Slaper-Cortenbach, I., Marini, F., Krause, D., & Horwitz, E. (2006). Minimal criteria for defining multipotent mesenchymal stromal cells: The international society for cellular therapy position statement. *Cytotherapy*, *8*, 315–317. doi:10.1080/14653240600855905 PMID:16923606

Duailibi, M. T., Duailibi, S. E., Young, C. S., Bartlett, J. D., Vacanti, J. P., & Yelick, P. C. (2004). Bioengineered teeth from cultured rat tooth bud cells. *Journal of Dental Research*, *83*, 523–528. doi:10.1177/154405910408300703 PMID:15218040

Duailibi, S. E., Duailibi, M. T., Vacanti, J. P., & Yelick, P. C. (2006). Prospects for tooth regeneration. *Periodontology 2000*, *41*, 177–187. doi:10.1111/j.1600-0757.2006.00165.x PMID:16686933

Edwards, P., & Mason, J. (2006). Gene enhanced tissue engineering for dental hard tissue regeneration: (1) overview and practical considerations. *Head & Face Medicine*, *2*, 12. doi:10.1186/1746-160X-2-12 PMID:16700908

El-Backly, R. M., Massoud, A. G., El-Badry, A. M., Sherif, R. A., & Marei, M. K. (2008). Regeneration of dentine/pulp-like tissue using a dental pulp stem cell/poly(lactic-co-glycolic) acid scaffold construct in New Zealand white rabbits. *Australian Endodontic Journal*, *34*, 52–67. doi:10.1111/j.1747-4477.2008.00139.x PMID:18666990

El-Ghannam, A. (2005). Bone reconstruction: From bioceramics to tissue engineering. *Expert Review of Medical Devices*, *2*(1), 87–101. doi:10.1586/17434440.2.1.87 PMID:16293032

Ennett, A. B., Kaigler, D., & Mooney, D. J. (2006). Temporally regulated delivery of VEGF in vitro and in vivo. *Journal of Biomedical Materials Research. Part A*, *79*, 176–184. doi:10.1002/jbm.a.30771 PMID:16788907

Finkelman, R. D., Mohan, S., Jennings, J. C., Taylor, A. K., Jepsen, S., & Baylink, D. J. (1990). Quantitation of growth factors IGF-I, SGF/IGF-II, and TGF beta in human dentin. *Journal of Bone and Mineral Research*, *5*, 717–723. doi:10.1002/jbmr.5650050708 PMID:2396498

Galler, K. M., Cavender, A., Yuwono, V., Dong, H., Shi, S., & Schmalz, G. et al. (n.d). D'Souza, R. N. (2088). Self-assembling peptide amphiphile nanofibers as a scaffold for dental stem cells. *Tissue Engineering. Part A*, *14*(12), 2051–2058. doi:10.1089/ten.tea.2007.0413 PMID:18636949

Galler, K. M., D'Souza, R. N., Hartgerink, J. D., & Schmalz, G. (2011). Scaffolds for dental pulp tissue engineering. *Advances in Dental Research*, *23*, 333. doi:10.1177/0022034511405326 PMID:21677088

Garcia-Godoy, F., & Murray, P. E. (2006). Status and potential commercial impact of stem cell-based treatments on dental and craniofacial regeneration. *Stem Cells and Development*, *15*, 881–887. doi:10.1089/scd.2006.15.881 PMID:17253950

Garcia-Godoy, F., & Murray, P. E. (2012). Recommendations for using regenerative endodontic procedures in permanent immature teeth. *Dental Traumatology*, *28*(1), 33–41. doi:10.1111/j.1600-9657.2011.01044.x PMID:21794081

Gay, I., Chen, S., & Macdougall, M. (2007). Isolation and characterization of multipotent human periodontal ligament stem cells. *Orthodontics & Craniofacial Research*, *10*, 149–160. doi:10.1111/j.1601-6343.2007.00399.x PMID:17651131

Gebhardt, M., Murray, P., Namerow, K., Kuttler, S., & Garcia-Godoy, F. (2009). Cell survival within pulp and periodontal constructs. *Journal of Endodontics*, *35*(1), 63–66. doi:10.1016/j.joen.2008.09.020 PMID:19084127

Gerhardt, L. C., & Boccaccini, A. R. (2010). Bioactive glass and glass-ceramic scaffolds for bone tissue engineering. *Materials*, *3*(7), 3867–3910. doi:10.3390/ma3073867

Goldberg, M. (2011). Pulp healing and regeneration: More questions than answers. *Advances in Dental Research*, *23*, 270–274. doi:10.1177/0022034511405385 PMID:21677077

Goldberg, M., Six, N., Chaussain, C., DenBesten, P., Veis, A., & Poliard, A. (2009). Dentin extracellular matrix molecules implanted into exposed pulps generate reparative dentin: A novel strategy in regenerative dentistry. *Journal of Dental Research*, *88*, 396–399. doi:10.1177/0022034509337101 PMID:19493881

Gotlieb, E., Murray, P., Namerow, K., Kuttler, S., & Garcia-Godoy, F. (2008). An ultrastructural investigation of tissue engineered pulp constructs implanted within endodontically treated teeth. *The Journal of the American Dental Association*, *139*(4), 457–465. PMID:18385030

Gronthos, S., Brahim, J., Li, W., Fisher, L. W., Cherman, N., & Boyde, A. et al. (2002). Stem cell properties of human dental pulp stem cells. *Journal of Dental Research*, *81*, 531–535. doi:10.1177/154405910208100806 PMID:12147742

Gronthos, S., Mankani, M., Brahim, J., Robey, P. G., & Shi, S. (2000). Postnatal human dental pulp stem cells (DPSCs) in vitro and in vivo. *Proceedings of the National Academy of Sciences of the United States of America*, *97*, 13625–13630. doi:10.1073/pnas.240309797 PMID:11087820

Guo, W., He, Y., Zhang, X., Lu, W., Wang, C., & Yu, H. et al. (2009). The use of dentin matrix scaffold and dental follicle cells for dentin regeneration. *Biomaterials*, *30*(35), 6708–6723. doi:10.1016/j.biomaterials.2009.08.034 PMID:19767098

Hacking, S. A., & Khademhosseini, A. (2009). Applications of microscale technologies for regenerative dentistry. *Journal of Dental Research*, *88*(5), 409–421. doi:10.1177/0022034509334774 PMID:19493883

Handa, K., Saito, M., Yamauchi, M., Kiyono, T., Sato, S., & Teranaka, T. et al. (2002). Cementum matrix formation in vivo by cultured dental follicle cells. *Bone*, *31*, 606–611. doi:10.1016/S8756-3282(02)00868-2 PMID:12477575

Harada, H., Kettunen, P., Jung, H. S., Mustonen, T., Wang, Y. A., & Thesleff, I. (1999). Localization of putative stem cells in dental epithelium and their association with Notch and FGF signaling. *The Journal of Cell Biology*, *147*, 105–120. doi:10.1083/jcb.147.1.105 PMID:10508859

Herberg, S., Siedler, M., Pippig, S., Schuetz, A., Dony, C., Kim, C. K., & Wikesjo, U. M. (2008). Development of an injectable composite as a carrier for growth factor-enhanced periodontal regeneration. *Journal of Clinical Periodontology*, *35*, 976–984. doi:10.1111/j.1600-051X.2008.01323.x PMID:18976394

Higuchi, T., Kinoshita, A., Takahashi, K., Oda, S., & Ishikawa, I. (1999). Bone regeneration by recombinant human bone morphogenetic protein-2 in rat mandibular defects: An experimental model of defect filling. *Journal of Periodontology*, *70*, 1026–1031. doi:10.1902/jop.1999.70.9.1026 PMID:10505805

Honda, M. J., Fong, H., Iwatsuki, S., Sumita, Y., & Sarikaya, M. (2008). Tooth-forming potential in embryonic and postnatal tooth bud cells. *Medical Molecular Morphology*, *41*, 183–192. doi:10.1007/s00795-008-0416-9 PMID:19107607

Honda, M. J., Imaizumi, M., Tsuchiya, S., & Morsczeck, C. (2010). Dental follicle stem cells and tissue engineering. *Journal of Oral Science*, *52*(4), 541–552. doi:10.2334/josnusd.52.541 PMID:21206155

Honda, M. J., Ohara, T., Sumita, Y., Ogaeri, T., Kagami, H., & Ueda, M. (2006). Preliminary study of tissue-engineered odontogenesis in the canine jaw. *Journal of Oral and Maxillofacial Surgery*, *64*, 283–289. doi:10.1016/j.joms.2005.10.020 PMID:16413902

Honda, M. J., Shinohara, Y., Hata, K. I., & Ueda, M. (2007a). Subcultured odontogenic epithelial cells in combination with dental mesenchymal cells produce enamel-dentin-like complex structures. *Cell Transplantation*, *16*, 833–847. PMID:18088003

Honda, M. J., Sumita, Y., Kagami, H., & Ueda, M. (2005). Histological and immunohistochemical studies of tissue engineered odontogenesis. *Archives of Histology and Cytology*, *68*, 89–101. doi:10.1679/aohc.68.89 PMID:16079455

Honda, M. J., Tsuchiya, S., Sumita, Y., Sagara, H., & Ueda, M. (2007b). The sequential seeding of epithelial and mesenchymal cells for tissue-engineered tooth regeneration. *Biomaterials*, *28*, 680–689. doi:10.1016/j.biomaterials.2006.09.039 PMID:17045644

Hosokawa, R., Kikuzaki, K., Kimoto, T., Matsuura, T., Chiba, D., & Wadamoto, M. et al. (2000). Controlled local application of basic fibroblast growth factor (FGF-2) accelerates the healing of GBR: An experimental study in beagle dogs. *Clinical Oral Implants Research*, *11*, 345–353. doi:10.1034/j.1600-0501.2000.011004345.x PMID:11168227

Hu, B., Nadiri, A., Kuchler-Bopp, S., Perrin-Schmitt, F., Peters, H., & Lesot, H. (2006). Tissue engineering of tooth crown, root, and periodontium. *Tissue Engineering*, *12*, 2069–2075. doi:10.1089/ten.2006.12.2069 PMID:16968149

Hu, B., Unda, F., Bopp-Kuchler, S., Jimenez, L., Wang, X. J., & Haikel, Y. et al. (2006). Bone marrow cells can give rise to ameloblast-like cells. *Journal of Dental Research*, *85*, 416–421. doi:10.1177/154405910608500504 PMID:16632753

Huang, G. T. (2008). A paradigm shift in endodontic management of immature teeth: Conservation of stem cells for regeneration. *Journal of Dentistry*, *36*, 379–386. doi:10.1016/j.jdent.2008.03.002 PMID:18420332

Huang, G. T., Gronthos, S., & Shi, S. (2009). Mesenchymal stem cells derived from dental tissues vs. those from other sources: Their biology and role in regenerative medicine. *Journal of Dental Research*, *88*(9), 792–806. doi:10.1177/0022034509340867 PMID:19767575

Huang, G. T., Sonoyama, W., Chen, J., & Park, S. H. (2006). In vitro characterization of human dental pulp cells: Various isolation methods and culturing environments. *Cell and Tissue Research*, *324*(2), 225–236. doi:10.1007/s00441-005-0117-9 PMID:16440193

Huang, G. T., Sonoyama, W., Liu, Y., Liu, H., Wang, S., & Shi, S. (2008). The hidden treasure in apical papilla: The potential role in pulp/dentin regeneration and bioroot engineering. *Journal of Endodontics*, *34*, 645–651. doi:10.1016/j.joen.2008.03.001 PMID:18498881

Huang, G. T., Yamaza, T., Shea, L. D., Djouad, F., Kuhn, N. Z., Tuan, R. S., & Shi, S. (2010). Stem/progenitor cell-mediated de novo regeneration of dental pulp with newly deposited continuous layer of dentin in an in vivo model. *Tissue Engineering. Part A*, *16*(2), 605–615. doi:10.1089/ten.tea.2009.0518 PMID:19737072

Ikeda, E., Morita, R., Nakao, K., Ishida, K., Nakamura, T., & Takano-Yamamoto, T. et al. (2009). Fully functional bioengineered tooth replacement as an organ replacement therapy. *Proceedings of the National Academy of Sciences of the United States of America*, *106*, 13475–13480. doi:10.1073/pnas.0902944106 PMID:19666587

Imai, H., Osumi, N., & Eto, K. (1998). Contribution of foregut endoderm to tooth initiation of mandibular incisor in rat embryos. *European Journal of Oral Sciences*, *106*(1), 19–23. PMID:9541198

Iohara, K., Nakashima, M., Ito, M., Ishikawa, M., Nakasima, A., & Akamine, A. (2004). Dentin regeneration by dental pulp stem cell therapy with recombinant human bone morphogenetic protein 2. *Journal of Dental Research*, *83*(8), 590–595. doi:10.1177/154405910408300802 PMID:15271965

Iohara, K., Zheng, L., Ito, M., Ishizaka, R., Nakamura, H., & Into, T. et al. (2009). Regeneration of dental pulp after pulpotomy by transplantation of CD31−/CD146− side population cells from a canine tooth. *Regenerative Medicine*, *4*, 377–385. doi:10.2217/rme.09.5 PMID:19438313

Jaasma, M. J., Plunkett, N. A., & O'Brien, F. J. (2008). Design and validation of a dynamic flow perfusion bioreactor for use with compliant tissue engineering scaffolds. *Journal of Biotechnology*, *133*, 490–496. doi:10.1016/j.jbiotec.2007.11.010 PMID:18221813

Javazon, E. H., Begs, K. J., & Flake, A. W. (2004). Mesenchymal stem cells: Paradoxes of passaging. *Experimental Hematology*, *32*, 414–425. doi:10.1016/j.exphem.2004.02.004 PMID:15145209

Jing, W., Wu, L., Lin, Y., Liu, L., Tang, W., & Tian, W. (2008). Odontogenic differentiation of adipose-derived stem cells for tooth regeneration: Necessity, possibility, and strategy. *Medical Hypotheses*, *70*, 540–542. doi:10.1016/j.mehy.2007.07.010 PMID:17703893

Jo, Y. Y., Lee, H. J., Kook, S. Y., Choung, H. W., Park, J. Y., & Chung, J. H. et al. (2007). Isolation and characterization of postnatal stem cells from human dental tissues. *Tissue Engineering*, *13*, 767–773. doi:10.1089/ten.2006.0192 PMID:17432951

Jung, R. E., Pjetursson, B. E., Glauser, R., Zembic, A., Zwahlen, M., & Lang, N. P. (2008). A systematic review of the 5-year survival and complication rates of implant-supported single crowns. *Clinical Oral Implants Research*, *19*, 119–130. doi:10.1111/j.1600-0501.2007.01453.x PMID:18067597

Kapadia, H., Mues, G., & D'Souza, R. (2007). Genes affecting tooth morphogenesis. *Orthodontics & Craniofacial Research*, *10*, 237–244. doi:10.1111/j.1601-6343.2007.00407.x PMID:17973693

Karp, J. M., & Leng Teo, G. S. (2009). Mesenchymal stem cell homing: The devil is in the details. *Cell Stem Cell*, *4*(3), 206–216. doi:10.1016/j.stem.2009.02.001 PMID:19265660

Kawano, S., Saito, M., Handa, K., Morotomi, T., Toyono, T., & Seta, Y. et al. (2004). Characterization of dental epithelial progenitor cells derived from cervical-loop epithelium in a rat lower incisor. *Journal of Dental Research*, *83*, 129–133. doi:10.1177/154405910408300209 PMID:14742650

Kémoun, P., Laurencin-Dalicieux, S., Rue, J., Farges, J. C., Gennero, I., & Conte-Auriol, F. et al. (2007). Human dental follicle cells acquire cementoblast features under stimulation by BMP-2/-7 and Enamel Matrix Derivatives (EMD) in vitro. *Cell and Tissue Research*, *329*, 283–294. doi:10.1007/s00441-007-0397-3 PMID:17443352

Kerkis, I., Ambrosio, C. E., Kerkis, A., Martins, D. S., Zucconi, E., & Fonseca, S. A. et al. (2008). Early transplantation of human immature dental pulp stem cells from baby teeth to golden retriever muscular dystrophy (GRMD) dogs: Local or systemic? *Journal of Translational Medicine*, *3*, 35. doi:10.1186/1479-5876-6-35 PMID:18598348

Kettunen, P., Karavanova, I., & Thesleff, I. (1998). Responsiveness of developing dental tissues to fibroblast growth factors: Expression of splicing alternatives of FGFR1, -2, -3, and of FGFR4; and stimulation of cell proliferation by FGF-2, -4, -8, and -9. *Developmental Genetics*, *22*, 374–385. doi:10.1002/(SICI)1520-6408(1998)22:4<374::AID-DVG7>3.0.CO;2-3 PMID:9664689

Khan, M., Seppala, M., Zoupa, M., & Cobourne, M. T. (2007). Hedgehog pathway gene expression during early development of the molar tooth root in the mouse. *Gene Expression Patterns*, *7*, 239–243. doi:10.1016/j.modgep.2006.10.001 PMID:17095302

King, G. N., & Hughes, F. J. (2001). Bone morphogenetic protein-2 stimulates cell recruitment and cementogenesis during early wound healing. *Journal of Clinical Periodontology*, *28*, 465–475. doi:10.1034/j.1600-051x.2001.028005465.x PMID:11350511

Koussoulakou, D. S., Margaritis, L. H., & Koussoulakos, S. L. (2009). A curriculum vitae of teeth: Evolution, generation, regeneration. *International Journal of Biological Sciences*, *5*(3), 226–243. doi:10.7150/ijbs.5.226 PMID:19266065

Koyama, N., Okubo, Y., Nakao, K., & Bessho, K. (2009). Evaluation of pluripotency in human dental pulp cells. *Journal of Oral and Maxillofacial Surgery*, *67*, 501–506. doi:10.1016/j.joms.2008.09.011 PMID:19231772

Kratochwil, K., Dull, M., Farinas, I., Galceran, J., & Grosschedl, R. (1996). Lef1 expression is activated by BMP- 4 and regulates inductive tissue interactions in tooth and hair development. *Genes & Development*, *10*, 1382–1394. doi:10.1101/gad.10.11.1382 PMID:8647435

Lee, J., Stavropoulos, A., Susin, C., & Wikesjö, U. M. (2010). Periodontal regeneration: Focus on growth and differentiation factors. *Dental Clinics of North America*, *54*, 93–111. doi:10.1016/j.cden.2009.09.001 PMID:20103474

Lézot, F., Davideau, J. L., Thomas, B., Sharpe, P., Forest, N., & Berdal, A. (2000). Epithelial Dlx-2 homeogene expression and cementogenesis. *The Journal of Histochemistry and Cytochemistry*, *48*, 277–284. doi:10.1177/002215540004800213 PMID:10639494

Li, L., & Xie, T. (2005). Stem cell niche: Structure and function. *Annual Review of Cell and Developmental Biology*, *21*, 605–631. doi:10.1146/annurev.cellbio.21.012704.131525 PMID:16212509

Li, Z. Y., Chen, L., Liu, L., Lin, Y. F., Li, S. W., & Tian, W. D. (2007). Odontogenic potential of bone marrow mesenchymal stem cells. *Journal of Oral and Maxillofacial Surgery*, *65*, 494–500. doi:10.1016/j.joms.2006.09.018 PMID:17307598

Lin, H., Zhao, Y., Sun, W., Chen, B., Zhang, J., & Zhao, W. et al. (2008). The effect of crosslinking heparin to demineralized bone matrix on mechanical strength and specific binding to human bone morphogenetic protein-2. *Biomaterials*, *29*, 1189–1197. doi:10.1016/j.biomaterials.2007.11.032 PMID:18083224

Lindroos, B., Mäenpää, K., Ylikomi, T., Oja, H., Suuronen, R., & Miettinen, S. (2008). Characterisation of human dental stem cells and buccal mucosa fibroblasts. *Biochemical and Biophysical Research Communications*, *368*, 329–335. doi:10.1016/j.bbrc.2008.01.081 PMID:18230338

Line, S. R. P. (2003). Variation of tooth number in mammalian dentition: Connecting genetics, development, and evolution. *Evolution & Development*, *5*(3), 295–304. doi:10.1046/j.1525-142X.2003.03036.x PMID:12752768

Liu, Y., Zheng, Y., Ding, G., Fang, D., Zhang, C., & Bartold, P. M. et al. (2008). Periodontal ligament stem cell-mediated treatment for periodontitis in miniature swine. *Stem Cells (Dayton, Ohio)*, *26*(4), 1065–1073. doi:10.1634/stemcells.2007-0734 PMID:18238856

Lovschall, H., Fejerskov, O., & Flyvbjerg, A. (2001). Pulp-capping with recombinant human insulin- like growth factor I (rhIGF-I) in rat molars. *Advances in Dental Research*, *15*, 108–112. doi:10.1177/08959374010150010301 PMID:12640754

Luan, X., Ito, Y., Dangaria, S., & Diekwisch, T. G. (2006). Dental follicle progenitor cell heterogeneity in the developing mouse periodontium. *Stem Cells and Development*, *15*, 595–608. doi:10.1089/scd.2006.15.595 PMID:16978062

Mareschi, K., Biasin, E., Piacibello, W., Aglietta, M., Madon, E., & Fagioli, F. (2001). Isolation of human mesenchymal stem cells: Bone marrow versus umbilical cord blood. *Haematologica*, *86*(10), 1099–1100. PMID:11602418

Matalova, E., Tucker, A. S., & Sharpe, P. T. (2004). Death in the life of a tooth. *Journal of Dental Research*, *83*(1), 11–16. doi:10.1177/154405910408300103 PMID:14691106

McKay, B., & Sandhu, H. S. (2002). Use of recombinant human bone morphogenetic protein-2 in spinal fusion applications. *Spine*, *27*(16), 66–85. doi:10.1097/00007632-200208151-00014 PMID:12205423

Mitsiadis, T. A., Barrandon, O., Rochat, A., Barrandon, Y., & De Bari, C. (2007). Stem cell niches in mammals. *Experimental Cell Research*, *313*, 3377–3385. doi:10.1016/j.yexcr.2007.07.027 PMID:17764674

Mitsiadis, T. A., Feki, G., Papaccio, G., & Caton, J. (2011). Dental pulp stem cells niches and Notch signaling in tooth injury. *Advances in Dental Research*, *23*, 275–279. doi:10.1177/0022034511405386 PMID:21677078

Mitsiadis, T. A., Graf, D., Luder, H., Gridley, T., & Bluteau, G. (2010). BMPs and FGFs target notch signalling via jagged 2 to regulate tooth morphogenesis and cytodifferentiation. *Development*, *137*, 3025–3035. doi:10.1242/dev.049528 PMID:20685737

Miura, M., Gronthos, S., Zhao, M., Lu, B., Fisher, L. W., Robey, P. G., & Shi, S. (2003). SHED: Stem cells from human exfoliated deciduous teeth. *Proceedings of the National Academy of Sciences of the United States of America*, *100*, 5807–5812. doi:10.1073/pnas.0937635100 PMID:12716973

Modino, S. A., & Sharpe, P. T. (2005). Tissue engineering of teeth using adult stem cells. *Archives of Oral Biology*, *50*(2), 255–528. doi:10.1016/j.archoralbio.2005.01.002 PMID:15721158

Moioli, E. K., Clark, P. A., Xin, X., Lal, S., & Mao, J. (2007). Matrices and scaffolds for drug delivery in dental, oral and craniofacial tissue engineering. *Advanced Drug Delivery Reviews*, *59*, 308–324. doi:10.1016/j.addr.2007.03.019 PMID:17499385

Morsczeck, C., Götz, W., Schierholz, J., Zeilhofer, F., Kühn, U., & Möhl, C. et al. (2005). Isolation of precursor cells (PCs) from human dental follicle of wisdom teeth. *Matrix Biology*, *24*, 155–165. doi:10.1016/j.matbio.2004.12.004 PMID:15890265

Morsczeck, C., Schmalz, G., Reichert, T. E., Völlner, F., Saugspier, M., Viale-Bouroncle, S., & Driemel, O. (2009). Gene expression profiles of dental follicle cells before and after osteogenic differentiation in vitro. *Clinical Oral Investigations*, *13*(4), 383–391. doi:10.1007/s00784-009-0260-x PMID:19252934

Murray, P. E., & Garcia-Godoy, F. (2004). Stem cell responses in tooth regeneration. *Stem Cells and Development*, *13*, 255–262. doi:10.1089/154732804323099181 PMID:15186721

Murray, P. E., Garcia-Godoy, F., & Hargreaves, K. M. (2007). Regenerative endodontics: A review of current status and a call for action. *Journal of Endodontics*, *33*, 377–390. doi:10.1016/j.joen.2006.09.013 PMID:17368324

Murray, P. E., Windsor, L. J., Smyth, T. W., Hafez, A. A., & Cox, C. F. (2002). Analysis of pulpal reactions to restorative procedures, materials, pulp capping and future therapies. *Critical Reviews in Oral Biology and Medicine*, *13*, 509–520. doi:10.1177/154411130201300607 PMID:12499243

Nadiri, A., Kuchler-Bopp, S., Haikel, Y., & Lesot, H. (2004). Immunolocalization of BMP-2/-4, FGF-4, and WNT10b in the developing mouse first lower molar. *The Journal of Histochemistry and Cytochemistry*, *52*, 103–112. doi:10.1177/002215540405200110 PMID:14688221

Nakahara, T., & Ide, Y. (2007). Tooth regeneration: Implications for the use of bioengineered organs in first-wave organ replacement. *Human Cell*, *20*, 63–70. doi:10.1111/j.1749-0774.2007.00031.x PMID:17645725

Nakao, K., Morita, R., Saji, Y., Ishida, K., Tomita, Y., & Ogawa, M. et al. (2007). The development of a bioengineered organ germ method. *Nature Methods*, *4*(3), 227–230. doi:10.1038/nmeth1012 PMID:17322892

Nakashima, M. (1994). Induction of dentine in amputated pulp of dogs by recombinant human bone morphogenetic proteins-2 and -4 with collagen matrix. *Archives of Oral Biology*, *39*, 1085–1089. doi:10.1016/0003-9969(94)90062-0 PMID:7717891

Nam, S., Won, J. E., Kim, C. H., & Kim, H. W. (2011). Odontogenic differentiation of human dental pulp stem cells stimulated by the calcium phosphate porous granules. *Journal of Tissue Engineering*. Retrieved from http://www.ncbi.nlm.nih.gov/pubmed/21772958

Nosrat, I. V., Widenfalk, J., Olson, L., & Nosrat, C. A. (2001). Dental pulp cells produce neurotrophic factors, interact with trigeminal neurons in vitro, and rescue motoneurons after spinal cord injury. *Developmental Biology*, *238*, 120–132. doi:10.1006/dbio.2001.0400 PMID:11783998

Ohazama, A., Modino, S. A., Miletich, I., & Sharpe, P. T. (2004a). Stem-cell-based tissue engineering of murine teeth. *Journal of Dental Research*, *83*, 518–522. doi:10.1177/154405910408300702 PMID:15218039

Ohazama, A., & Sharpe, P. T. (2004b). TNF signalling in tooth development. *Current Opinion in Genetics & Development*, *14*, 513–519. doi:10.1016/j.gde.2004.07.008 PMID:15380242

Pera, M. F., & Hasegawa, K. (2008). Simpler and safer cell reprogramming. *Nature Biotechnology*, *26*, 59–60. doi:10.1038/nbt0108-59 PMID:18183017

Petersen, P. E., Bourgeois, D., Ogawa, H., Estupinan-Day, S., & Ndiaye, C. (2005). The global burden of oral diseases and risks to oral health. *Bulletin of the World Health Organization*, *83*(9), 661–669. PMID:16211157

Polimeni, G., Xiropaidis, A. V., & Wikesjö, U. M. (2006). Biology and principles of periodontal wound healing/regeneration. *Periodontology*, *41*, 30–47. doi:10.1111/j.1600-0757.2006.00157.x PMID:16686925

Prescott, R. S., Alsanea, R., Fayad, M. I., Johnson, B. R., Wenckus, C. S., & Hao, J. et al. (2008). In vivo generation of dental pulp-like tissue by using dental pulp stem cells, a collagen scaffold, and dentin matrix protein 1 after subcutaneous transplantation in mice. *Journal of Endodontics*, *34*, 421–426. doi:10.1016/j.joen.2008.02.005 PMID:18358888

Reich, E. (2001). Trends in caries and periodontal health epidemiology in Europe. *International Dental Journal*, *51*(6), 392–398. doi:10.1111/j.1875-595X.2001.tb00585.x PMID:11794560

Reynolds, M. A., Aichelmann-Reidy, M. E., & Branch-Mays, G. L. (2010). Regeneration of periodontal tissue: Bone replacement grafts. *Dental Clinics of North America*, *54*, 55–71. doi:10.1016/j.cden.2009.09.003 PMID:20103472

Ritter, A. L., Ritter, A. V., Murrah, V., Sigurdsson, A., & Trope, M. (2004). Pulp revascularization of replanted immature dog teeth after treatment with minocycline and doxycycline assessed by laser Doppler flowmetry, radiography, and histology. *Dental Traumatology*, *20*, 75–84. doi:10.1111/j.1600-4469.2004.00225.x PMID:15025689

Robbins, R. D., Prasain, N., Maier, B. F., Yoder, M. C., & Mirmira, R. G. (2010). Inducible pluripotent stem cells: Not quite ready for prime time? *Current Opinion in Organ Transplantation*, *15*(1), 61–67. doi:10.1097/MOT.0b013e3283337196 PMID:19855280

Robey, P. G. (2005). Post-natal stem cells for dental and craniofacial repair. *Oral Bioscience and Medicine*, *2*, 83–90.

Rutherford, R. B. (2001). BMP-7 gene transfer to inflamed ferret dental pulps. *European Journal of Oral Sciences*, *109*(6), 422–424. doi:10.1034/j.1600-0722.2001.00150.x PMID:11767280

Saber, S. E. (2009). Tissue engineering in endodontics. *Journal of Oral Science*, *51*(4), 495–507. doi:10.2334/josnusd.51.495 PMID:20032600

Saito, A., Saito, E., Handa, R., Honma, Y., & Kawanami, M. (2009). Influence of residual bone on recombinant human bone morphogenetic protein-2-induced periodontal regeneration in experimental periodontitis in dogs. *Journal of Periodontology*, *80*, 961–968. doi:10.1902/jop.2009.080568 PMID:19485827

Saito, T., Ogawa, M., Hata, Y., & Bessho, K. (2004). Acceleration effect of human recombinant bone morphogenetic protein-2 on differentiation of human pulp cells into odontoblasts. *Journal of Endodontics*, *30*(4), 205–208. doi:10.1097/00004770-200404000-00005 PMID:15085046

Sakai, V. T., Zhang, Z., Dong, Z., Neiva, K., Machado, M., & Shi, S. et al. (2010). SHED differentiate into functional odontoblasts and endothelium. *Journal of Dental Research*, *89*, 791–796. doi:10.1177/0022034510368647 PMID:20395410

Salazar-Ciudad, I. (2008). Tooth morphogenesis in vivo, in vitro, and in silico. *Current Topics in Developmental Biology*, *81*, 341–371. doi:10.1016/S0070-2153(07)81012-X PMID:18023734

Sarment, D. P., Cooke, J. W., Miller, S. E., Jin, Q., McGuire, M. K., & Kao, R. T. et al. (2006). Effect of rhPDGF-BB on bone turnover during periodontal repair. *Journal of Clinical Periodontology*, *33*, 135–140. doi:10.1111/j.1600-051X.2005.00870.x PMID:16441739

Sartaj, R., & Sharpe, P. (2006). Biological tooth replacement. *Journal of Anatomy*, *209*, 503–509. doi:10.1111/j.1469-7580.2006.00622.x PMID:17005022

Sato, I., Ando-Kurihara, N., Kota, K., Iwaku, M., & Hoshino, E. (1996). Sterilization of infected root-canal dentine by topical application of a mixture of ciprofloxacin, metronidazole and minocycline in situ. *International Endodontic Journal*, *29*, 118–124. doi:10.1111/j.1365-2591.1996.tb01172.x PMID:9206435

Schmalz, G., & Galler, K. M. (2011). Tissue injury and pulp regeneration. *Journal of Dental Research, 90*(7), 828–829. doi:10.1177/0022034511405331 PMID:21700812

Seo, B. M., Miura, M., Gronthos, S., Bartold, P. M., Batouli, S., & Brahim, J. et al. (2004). Investigation of multipotent postnatal stem cells from human periodontal ligament. *Lancet, 364*, 149–155. doi:10.1016/S0140-6736(04)16627-0 PMID:15246727

Seo, B. M., Sonoyama, W., Yamaza, T., Coppe, C., Kikuiri, T., & Akiyama, K. et al. (2008). SHED repair critical-size calvarial defects in mice. *Oral Diseases, 14*, 428–434. doi:10.1111/j.1601-0825.2007.01396.x PMID:18938268

Sharma, S., Sikri, V., Sharma, N. K., & Sharma, V. M. (2010). Regeneration of tooth pulp and dentin: Trends and advances. *Annals of Neurosciences, 17*(1), 31–43.

Sharpe, P. T. (2001). Neural crest and tooth morphogenesis. *Advances in Dental Research, 15*, 4–7. doi:10.1177/08959374010150011001 PMID:12640730

Sharpe, P. T., & Young, C. S. (2005). Test-tube teeth. *Scientific American, 293*(2), 34–41. doi:10.1038/scientificamerican0805-34 PMID:16053135

Sire, J. Y., Davit-Beal, T., Delgado, S., & Gu, X. (2007). The origin and evolution of enamel mineralization genes. *Cells, Tissues, Organs, 186*, 25–48. doi:10.1159/000102679 PMID:17627117

Slavkin, H. C., Bessem, C., Fincham, A. G., Bringas, P. J., Santos, V., Snead, M. L., & Zeichner-David, M. (1989). Human and mouse cementum proteins immunologically related to enamel proteins. *Biochimica et Biophysica Acta, 991*, 12–18. doi:10.1016/0304-4165(89)90021-4 PMID:2469482

Sloan, A. J., & Waddington, R. J. (2009). Dental pulp stem cells: What, where, how? *International Journal of Paediatric Dentistry, 19*, 61–70. doi:10.1111/j.1365-263X.2008.00964.x PMID:19120509

Smith, A. J., Matthews, J. B., & Hall, R. C. (1998). Transforming growth factor-beta1 (TGF-beta1) in dentine matrix: Ligand activation and receptor expression. *European Journal of Oral Sciences, 106*(1), 179–184. PMID:9541223

Sonoyama, W., Liu, Y., Yamaza, T., Tuan, R. S., Wang, S., Shi, S., & Huang, G. T. (2008). Characterization of the apical papilla and its residing stem cells from human immature permanent teeth: A pilot study. *Journal of Endodontics, 34*, 166–171. doi:10.1016/j.joen.2007.11.021 PMID:18215674

Sumita, Y., Tsuchiya, S., Asahina, I., Kagami, H., & Honda, M. J. (2009). The location and characteristics of two populations of dental pulp cells affect tooth development. *European Journal of Oral Sciences, 117*, 113–121. doi:10.1111/j.1600-0722.2008.00603.x PMID:19320719

Taba, M., Jin, Q., Sugai, J. V., & Giannobile, W. V. (2005). Current concepts in periodontal bioengineering. *Orthodontics & Craniofacial Research, 8*, 292–302. doi:10.1111/j.1601-6343.2005.00352.x PMID:16238610

Takahashi, C., Yoshida, H., Komine, A., Nakao, K., Tsuji, T., & Tomooka, Y. (2010). Newly established cell lines from mouse oral epithelium regenerate teeth when combined with dental mesenchyme. *In Vitro Cellular & Developmental Biology. Animal, 46*, 457–468. doi:10.1007/s11626-009-9265-7 PMID:20033791

Takahashi, D., Odajima, T., Morita, M., Kawanami, M., & Kato, H. (2005). Formation and resolution of ankylosis under application of recombinant human bone morphogenetic protein-2 (rhBMP-2) to class III furcation defects in cats. *Journal of Periodontal Research*, *40*, 299–305. doi:10.1111/j.1600-0765.2005.00794.x PMID:15966907

Takahashi, K., & Yamanaka, S. (2006). Induction of pluripotent stem cells from mouse embryonic and adult fibroblast cultures by defined factors. *Cell*, *26*(4), 663–676. doi:10.1016/j.cell.2006.07.024 PMID:16904174

Téclès, O., Laurent, P., Zygouritsas, S., Burger, A. S., Camps, J., Dejou, J., & About, I. (2005). Activation of human dental pulp progenitor/stem cells in response to odontoblast injury. *Archives of Oral Biology*, *50*(2), 103–108. doi:10.1016/j.archoralbio.2004.11.009 PMID:15721135

Thesleff, I., Keranen, S., & Jernvall, J. (2001). Enamel knots as signaling centers linking tooth morphogenesis and odontoblast differentiation. *Advances in Dental Research*, *15*, 14–18. doi:10.1177/08959374010150010401 PMID:12640732

Thesleff, I., & Tummers, M. (2003). Stem cells and tissue engineering: Prospects for regenerating tissues in dental practice. *Medical Principles and Practice*, *12*(1), 43–50. doi:10.1159/000069840 PMID:12707500

Thomson, J. A., Itskovitz-Eldor, J., Shapiro, S. S., Waknitz, M. A., Swiergiel, J. J., Marshall, V. S., & Jones, J. M. (1998). Embryonic stem cell lines derived from human blastocysts. *Science*, *282*(5391), 1145–1147. doi:10.1126/science.282.5391.1145 PMID:9804556

Timmins, N. E., Scherberich, A., Früh, J. A., Heberer, M., Martin, I., & Jakob, M. (2007). Three-dimensional cell culture and tissue engineering in a T-CUP (tissue culture under perfusion). *Tissue Engineering*, *13*, 2021–2028. doi:10.1089/ten.2006.0158 PMID:17590148

Trojani, C., Weiss, P., Michiels, J., Vinatier, C., Guicheux, J., & Daculsi, G. et al. (2005). Three dimensional culture and differentiation of human osteogenic cells in an Injectable hydroxypropyl-methylcellulose hydrogel. *Biomaterials*, *26*(27), 5509–5517. doi:10.1016/j.biomaterials.2005.02.001 PMID:15860207

Trombelli, L. (2005). Which reconstructive procedures are effective for treating the periodontal intraosseous defect? *Periodontology*, *37*, 88–105. doi:10.1111/j.1600-0757.2004.03798.x PMID:15655027

Tucker, A. S., & Sharpe, P. T. (1999). Molecular genetics of tooth morphogenesis and patterning: the right shape in the right place. *Journal of Dental Research*, *78*, 826–834. doi:10.1177/00220345990780040201 PMID:10326726

Vaahtokari, A., Aberg, T., Jernvall, J., Keränen, S., & Thesleff, I. (1996). The enamel knot as a signaling center in the developing mouse tooth. *Mechanisms of Development*, *54*, 39–43. doi:10.1016/0925-4773(95)00459-9 PMID:8808404

Vainio, S., Karavanova, I., Jowett, A., & Thesleff, I. (1993). Identification of BMP-4 as a signal mediating secondary induction between epithelial and mesenchymal tissues during early tooth development. *Cell*, *75*, 45–58. PMID:8104708

Vats, A., Bielby, R. C., Tolley, N. S., Nerem, R., & Polak, J. M. (2005). Stem cells. *Lancet*, *366*, 592–602. doi:10.1016/S0140-6736(05)66879-1 PMID:16099296

Villar, C. C., & Cochran, D. L. (2010). Regeneration of periodontal tissues: Guided tissue regeneration. *Dental Clinics of North America*, *54*, 73–92. doi:10.1016/j.cden.2009.08.011 PMID:20103473

Wang, X., Xia, C., Zhang, Z., Deng, X., Wei, S., Zheng, G., & Chen, H. (2009). Direct growth of human enamel-like calcium phosphate microstructures on human tooth. *Journal of Nanoscience and Nanotechnology*, *9*, 1361–1364. doi:10.1166/jnn.2009.C157 PMID:19441525

Wei, X., Ling, J., Wu, L., Liu, L., & Xiao, Y. (2007). Expression of mineralization markers in dental pulp cells. *Journal of Endodontics*, *33*(6), 703–708. doi:10.1016/j.joen.2007.02.009 PMID:17509410

Werner, S., & Grose, R. (2003). Regulation of wound healing by growth factors and cytokines. *Physiological Reviews*, *83*, 835–870. PMID:12843410

Wu, L., Zhu, F., Wu, Y., Lin, Y., Nie, X., & Jing, W. et al. (2008). Dentin sialophosphoprotein-promoted mineralization and expression of odontogenic genes in adipose-derived stromal cells. *Cells, Tissues, Organs*, *187*(2), 103–112. doi:10.1159/000110079 PMID:17957093

Xu, J., Wang, W., Kapila, Y., Lotz, J., & Kapila, S. (2009). Multiple differentiation capacity of STRO-1+/CD146+ PDL mesenchymal progenitor cells. *Stem Cells and Development*, *18*, 487–496. doi:10.1089/scd.2008.0113 PMID:18593336

Yang, X., van der Kraan, P., Bian, Z., Fan, M., Walboomers, X. F., & Jansen, J. A. (2009). Mineralized tissue formation by BMP2-transfected pulp stem cells. *Journal of Dental Research*, *88*(11), 1020–1025. doi:10.1177/0022034509346258 PMID:19828890

Yao, S., Pan, F., Prpic, V., & Wise, G. E. (2008). Differentiation of stem cells in the dental follicle. *Journal of Dental Research*, *87*, 767–771. doi:10.1177/154405910808700801 PMID:18650550

Yelick, P. C., & Vacanti, J. P. (2006). Bioengineered teeth from tooth bud cells. *Dental Clinics of North America*, *50*(2), 191–203. doi:10.1016/j.cden.2005.11.005 PMID:16530057

Yen, A. H., & Sharpe, P. T. (2008). Stem cells and tooth tissue engineering. *Cell and Tissue Research*, *331*, 359–372. doi:10.1007/s00441-007-0467-6 PMID:17938970

Yokoi, T., Saito, M., Kiyono, T., Iseki, S., Kosaka, K., & Nishida, E. et al. (2007). Establishment of immortalized dental follicle cells for generating periodontal ligament in vivo. *Cell and Tissue Research*, *327*, 301–311. doi:10.1007/s00441-006-0257-6 PMID:17013589

Young, C. S., Abukawa, H., Asrican, R., Ravens, M., Troulis, M. J., & Kaban, L. B. et al. (2005). Tissue-engineered hybrid tooth and bone. *Tissue Engineering*, *11*, 1599–1610. doi:10.1089/ten.2005.11.1599 PMID:16259613

Young, C. S., Terada, S., Vacanti, J. P., Honda, M., Bartlett, J. D., & Yelick, P. C. (2002). Tissue engineering of complex tooth structures on biodegradable polymer scaffolds. *Journal of Dental Research*, *81*, 695–700. doi:10.1177/154405910208101008 PMID:12351668

Yu, J., Jin, F., Deng, Z., Li, Y., Tang, L., Shi, J., & Jin, Y. (2008). Epithelial-mesenchymal cell ratios can determine the crown morphogenesis of dental pulp stem cells. *Stem Cells and Development*, *17*(3), 475–482. doi:10.1089/scd.2007.0120 PMID:18513162

Yu, J., Wang, Y., Deng, Z., Tang, L., Li, Y., Shi, J., & Yin, Y. (2007). Odontogenic capability: Bone marrow stromal stem cells versus dental pulp stem cells. *Biology of the Cell*, *99*, 465–474. doi:10.1042/BC20070013 PMID:17371295

Yuan, Z., Nie, H., Wang, S., Lee, C., Li, A., & Fu, S. Y. et al. (2011). Biomaterial selection for tooth regeneration. *Tissue Engineering. Part B, Reviews*, *17*(5), 373–388. doi:10.1089/ten.teb.2011.0041 PMID:21699433

Zaky, S. H., & Cancedda, R. (2009). Engineering craniofacial structures: Facing the challenge. *Journal of Dental Research*, *88*, 1077–1091. doi:10.1177/0022034509349926 PMID:19897785

Zeichner-David, M., Oishi, K., Su, Z., Zakartchenko, V., Chen, L. S., Arzate, H., & Bringas, P. J. (2003). Role of Hertwig's epithelial root sheath cells in tooth root development. *Developmental Dynamics*, *228*, 651–663. doi:10.1002/dvdy.10404 PMID:14648842

Zhang, W., Walboomers, X., van Kuppevelt, T., Daamen, W. F., Bian, Z., & Jansen, J. A. (2006). The performance of human dental pulp stem cells on different three dimensional scaffold materials. *Biomaterials*, *27*(33), 5658–5668. doi:10.1016/j.biomaterials.2006.07.013 PMID:16916542

Zhang, W., Walboomers, X. F., Shi, S., Fan, M., & Jansen, J. A. (2006). Multilineage differentiation potential of stem cells derived from human dental pulp after cryopreservation. *Tissue Engineering*, *12*(10), 2813–2823. doi:10.1089/ten.2006.12.2813 PMID:17518650

Zivkovic, P., Petrovic, V., Najman, S., & Stefanovic, V. (2010). Stem cell–based dental tissue engineering. *TheScientificWorldJournal*, *10*, 901–916. doi:10.1100/tsw.2010.81 PMID:20495769

KEY TERMS AND DEFINITIONS

Adult Stem Cells (ASC): Undifferentiated cells, found throughout the body after embryonic development, that multiply by cell division to replenish dying cells and regenerate damaged tissues. Also known as somatic stem cells (from Greek Σωματικός, meaning *of the body*), they can be found in juvenile, as well as adult animals and humans.

Dental Tissue Engineering: Application or use of cells, scaffolds and growth factors to restore, maintain or enhance dental tissue function.

Embryonic Stem Cells: (ECS Cells): Pluripotent stem cells derived from the inner cell mass of the blastocyst of an early-stage embryo. Human embryos reach the blastocyst stage 4–5 days post fertilization, at which time they consist of 50–150 cells. Isolating the embryoblast or Inner Cell Mass (ICM) results in destruction of the fertilized human embryo, that raises ethical issues (Thomson, et al., 1998).

Induced Pluripotent Stem (iPS) Cells: Induced pluripotent stem cells, commonly abbreviated as iPS cells are a type of pluripotent stem cell artificially derived from a non-pluripotent cell, typically an adult somatic cell, by inducing a "forced" expression of specific genes. The process of creating these cells, often referred to as "reprogramming" involves introducing a combination of three to four genes for transcription factors, delivered by retroviruses, into the somatic cell. iPS cells are similar to natural pluripotent stem cells, such as Embryonic Stem Cells (ESC), in many respects, such as the expression of certain stem cell genes and proteins, chromatin methylation patterns, doubling time, embryoid body formation, teratoma formation, viable chimera formation and potency and differentiability, but the full extent of their relation to natural pluripotent stem cells is still being assessed (Takahashi, et al., 2006).

Multipotent Stem Cells: Stem cells that can produce cells of multiple differentiated cell types, but all within a particular tissue, organ, or physiological system. For example, blood-forming (hematopoietic) stem cells are multipotent cells that can produce all cell types that are normal components of the blood. On the other hand, mesencymal stem cells are multipotent stem cells that can differentiate into a variety of cell types, including: osteoblasts (bone cells), chondrocytes (cartilage cells), adipocytes (fat cells), etc. (Karp, et al., 2009).

Stem Cell Homing: The migration of stem cells through the blood or tissue to an ultimate destination where they differentiate and replace or build tissues. Stem cell homing is triggered by interactions between the cell surface adhesion molecules (such as selectins, integrins, and ICAMs) and the cell's surrounding environment (Karp, et al., 2009).

Stem Cell Niche: The microenvironment in which stem cells are situated. During development, the niche may contain various factors and elements that alter gene expression within the stem cell, causing the cell to differentiate and proliferate into various tissues of the fetus. In developed tissue, the niche may help maintain stem cells in a quiescent state, until injury or disease signals trigger them to self-renew and differentiate to replace the damaged tissue. Niche elements may include interactions with other cells, adhesion molecules, growth factors, cytokines and parameters such as pH, ionic strength and gas composition (Li, et al., 2005).

Stem Cells: Cells that can both self-renew and differentiate into mature, specialized cells, such as blood cells, nerve cells, muscle cells, odontoblasts, etc.

Translational Medicine: Translational medicine is an evolutional concept that encompasses the rapid translation of basic research for use in clinical disease diagnosis, prevention and treatment. It follows the idea "from bench to bedside and back," and hence relies on cooperation between laboratory research and clinical care (Chen, et al., 2011).

This work was previously published in Medical Advancements in Aging and Regenerative Technologies edited by Andriani Daskalaki , pages 279-312, copyright year 2013 by Medical Information Science Reference (an imprint of IGI Global).

Chapter 5
Applications of Polymeric Micro- and Nano-Particles in Dentistry

Balasankar Meera Priyadarshini
National University of Singapore, Singapore

Nileshkumar Dubey
National University of Singapore, Singapore

ABSTRACT

The use of micro- and nanoparticles is rapidly advancing and has been most commonly used in medical and biological research that offers an encouraging scope in broad range of disciplines. Manipulation of the biomaterials to their micro- and nano-scale renders their properties and behavior different from that of the same material in the mass scale and make them more reactive than large particles. The removal of tooth structure and its restoration with synthetic material to solve the problems caused by dental caries, trauma and fracture is a practice nearly as old as dentistry. Efforts are made to create micro- and nanomaterials that can revolutionize these ancestral therapies and dental procedures. The use of these materials had shown some promising applications in caries control, endodontic therapy, regenerative dentistry, periodontology and oral biofilm management. This review aims to discuss the recent advances and future potential of polymer-based micro- and nanoparticles in dentistry.

INTRODUCTION

The prevention of tooth decay, treatment of bone loss and periodontal disease are ongoing challenges in dentistry. According to CDC, tooth decay is the most frequent childhood disease 5 times as common as asthma. LA Times came up with the fact that 42% of children are expected to have some decay by the age of 2-12 (Mascarelli, 2011). For example, in 2015-16, a UK report shows that 9.8% rise in removal of one or more teeth in children aged 10 and under (Howell, 2016). Periodontal diseases are the most

DOI: 10.4018/978-1-5225-1903-4.ch005

common infections due to the overgrowth of the dental plaque that may increase the risk of heart disease and it is estimated that 47.2% of adults aged 30 years and older has some form of periodontal disease (Dhadse, Gattani, & Mishra, 2010).

With the emergence and increase of such dental problems and continuing concerns on healthcare costs, many researchers have tried to develop new and effective treatment regimes. Such problems and needs have led to the resurgence in the use of micro- and nanomaterials in order to revolutionize the ancestral therapies and dental procedures. For example, liquids and pastes containing nano-apatite's have been used remineralization of early sub micrometer sized enamel lesions and the role of nanoparticle in the control of the oral biofilm has also been recognized (Figure 1) (Besinis, De Peralta, Tredwin, & Handy, 2015; Hannig & Hannig, 2010). Similarly, micro-/nanoparticles that can deliver antibiotics and bioactive compounds have been used to treat periodontal diseases (Yao et al., 2014).

Application of micro-/nanotechnology in dentistry aims at using these materials and theories to enhance prevention, diagnosis and treatment of injured tissues at the molecular and micro molecular levels. The high surface area to volume ratio of these materials has reportedly shown to improve the biomaterial-biological interactions (Yong, 2014). Their ability to penetrate inside locations that are inaccessible make them best suited for various site-specific delivery (Cristina Buzea & Kevin, 2007). Moreover, their stability during storage as well as in biological fluids makes them advantageous in many ways. The shape of these materials enhances their surface reactivity and renders high antibacterial action in comparison to other formulations (Khodashenas & Ghorbani). Although still evolving with their developments at infancy, these fields provide an array of possibilities that benefit the patient's health by eliminating or reducing pain associated with conventional procedures.

The use of polymeric micro-and nanoparticles has been the epicenter of extensive research in the recent years. Polymers are high performance materials predominantly used in controlled drug release due to their versatility and unique physical, chemical and structural properties that hold tremendous promise for improvements in many areas of scientific research. The use of polymers plays a major role in improving the mucoadhesive properties of nano and micro biomaterials because this improvises the interaction of polymeric particles with biological systems, especially tooth structures that are predominantly hard tissues, where it is difficult for particles to adhere. For example, both natural (e.g., chitosan and alginate) and synthetic (e.g., poly(lactic-co-glycolic acid) and poly(ε-caprolactone)) polymers have been used as carrier materials, that can be either biodegradable (e.g., poly(lactic-co-glycolic acid) or non-biodegradable (e.g., ethylcellulose) based on their ability to breakdown in a given environment.

Polymer nano and microparticles are most commonly synthesized by various methods shown in Figure 2. Other innovative procedures like dripping technique, microfluidic systems and high pressure homogenization have also been used (de Francisco, Cerquetani, & Bruschi, 2012). The dramatic impact of these materials on medicine and biology has led to applications including coatings on medical devices, wound dressing materials, antimicrobial agents, drug or gene delivery systems and bio imaging (Ambrosio & Payne, 2013; Hutter & Maysinger, 2013; Rai, Yadav, & Gade, 2009; Tsukada, Goan, & Furusawa, 2008; S. Z. Wu, Hossainy, Harish, Sanders-Millare, & Mirzaee, 2003; Zheng, Chen, Jin, Ye, & Liu, 2016). With such convincing developments in technology, micro-and nanoparticles have been anticipated to bring advances (Figure 3) and possible innovations in existing oral diagnostic and therapeutic techniques (Ozak & Ozkan, 2013). Some of the clinical aspects mentioned above (e.g., antibacterial, drug delivery) find relevance in the field of dentistry and has received significant momentum in the past few years. In this book chapter, we will mainly focus on the applications of polymer micro- and nanoparticles in dentistry.

Figure 1. (A) Diagram shows the presence of NPs (isolated particles or agglomerates) in saliva and the structure of dental tissues. The pellicle covers the superficial layer of enamel, and the oral biofilm develops on the pellicle surface. The characteristic hexagonal shape of the enamel crystallites is apparent and also the presence of the dentinal tubules in the underlying tissue of dentine. The NP–ion–protein complexes do not adhere directly to the tooth surfaces, but adhesion occurs either to the pellicle layer or the developing biofilm. (B) Schematic diagram of the oral environment, oral biofilm, and dental mineralized tissues showing the distribution of NPs and ions. Natural saliva normally contains a range of ions and proteins. In the presence of NPs, NP–ion–protein complexes are formed. Oral conditions promote particle agglomeration that results in particle sedimentation onto the dental surfaces. The pellicle has a globular structure and its proteinaceous layer facilitates the adherence of the early colonizing species necessary for the oral biofilm development. The oral biofilm and pellicle act as diffusion/permeation barriers to NPs preventing them from reaching the enamel–pellicle interface. Certain ions (F–, Cl–, SiO44–, Zn2+) are more abundant near the external surface of enamel, while others (Na+, Mg2+, CO32–) are found at higher concentrations near the dentino–enamel junction. The most commonly ions found in dentine are F–, Na+, Mg2+, and CO32–.

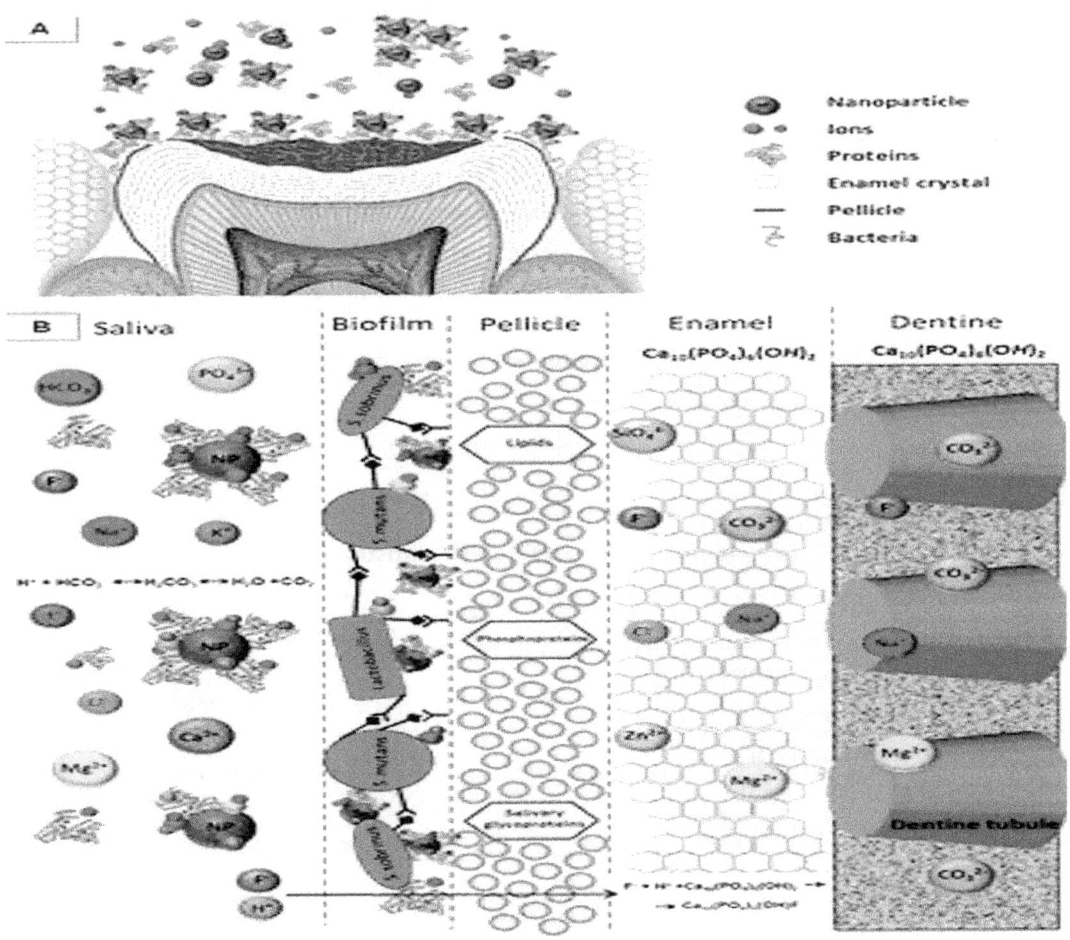

Figure 2. Various methods to synthesis micro and nanoparticles

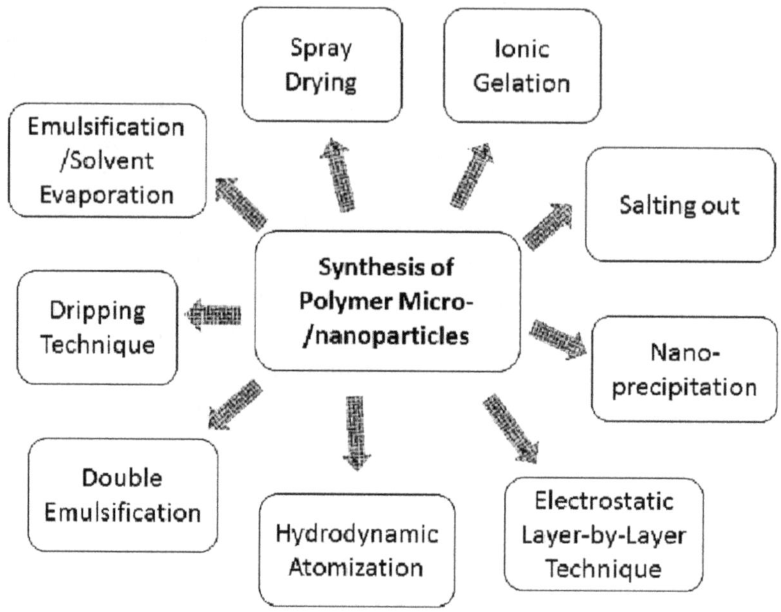

Figure 3. Different ways micro and nanoparticle can be applied to dentistry

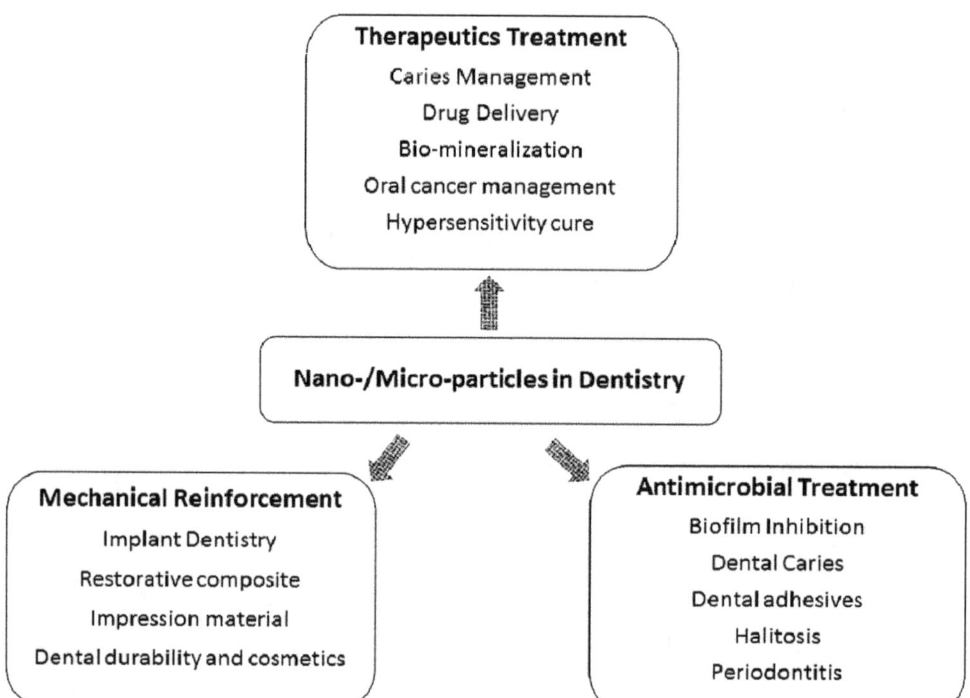

Caries Control

The microbiota present in the oral cavity is the most complex part of the human system comprising over 300 species of different bacterial, fungal and viral species (Listgarten, 1987). Most of these species associate to form biofilms that are resistant to antibiotic exposure or mechanical stress, depending on their toxicity (Avila, Ojcius, & Yilmaz, 2009). When the acid-releasing biofilms mature, they destroy the tooth structure and cause dental caries. Bacteria such as *Streptococcus mutans*, and *Lactobacillus spp* are often associated with cariogenicity (Selwitz, Ismail, & Pitts, 2007). The occurrence of caries is site-specific and the release of weak organic acids influences a drop in the pH to fall below a critical value leading to loss of calcium and phosphate (from enamel and dentin) that causes demineralization of tooth and eventual cavitation (R J Gibbons & Houte, 1975).

The process of demineralization and remineralization occurs on a daily basis and it is the balance between these two phenomena which is an important determinant of progression, arrest or reversal of the dental caries. Demineralization is reversible in its early stages and in the process of remineralization, the lost minerals can be restored to the tooth by gingival fluid or by salivary calcium and phosphate that buffers the toothbrush removal of biofilms (Melo, Guedes, Xu, & Rodrigues, 2013; Sharma, Puranik, & K.R, 2015). Various remineralization strategies have been proposed earlier focusing on restoring the mineral content of enamel and/or dentin, but the extent to which the remineralized dentin could be structurally and mechanically reconstituted remains a challenge. Although engineered nanoparticles of calcium fluoride, hydroxyapatite, bioactive glass and phosphates have frequently reported to replenish the mineral content of tooth, various studies have also utilized biodegradable polymers in order to achieve the similar effect.

The use of fluoride in inhibition of demineralization and enhancement of dental tissue remineralization has been widely acknowledged (Jorgensen, Shariati, Shields, Durr, & Proskin, 1989). Significant advancements have been made in controlling the occurrence of dental caries with the use of anti-caries fluoride such as sodium fluoride, sodium monofluorophosphate, amine fluoride and stannous fluoride (Campus, Lallai, & Carboni, 2003; Diarra, Pourroy, Boymond, & Muster, 2003; Van Rijkom, Truin, & Van't Hof, 1998; van Strijp, Buijs, & Ten Cate, 1999). The use of fluoride alone only reduces the caries progression but does not delay its development. Drawbacks such as short-term fluoride retention on the tooth surface might restrict fluoride penetration of residual plaque deposits and limits its anti-plaque activity in inaccessible areas (Watson et al., 2005). Moreover, repeated intakes of agents containing low fluoride ion concentrations might induce cytotoxicity over time. Therefore, the need for a pharmaceutical form that can improve retention and deliver sustained levels of fluoride arises (Scheifele, Studen-Pavlovich, & Markovic, 2002). The continuous release of sodium fluoride from biodegradable micron-sized polymeric carriers such as gelatin microspheres (NaF-GMS) and chitosan microparticles have shown potential anti-caries activity (Keegan et al., 2012; H. Wu et al., 2004) as indicated in Table 1. Their low molecular weight (MW) with faster rates of degradation has demonstrated efficacy against dental plaque biofilms (Chávez de Paz, Resin, Howard, Sutherland, & Wejse, 2011). Non-biodegradable polymers such as ethylcellulose have also been used to entrap various sources of fluoride such as sodium fluoride (NaF), sodium monofluorophosphate (MFP) and amino fluoride that provide a platform for inhibition of caries progression (de Francisco et al., 2012). In vivo studies on rabbit oral cavity showed that the prolonged retention at the site of dental plaque has contributed to its potential to restrain demineralization even at low concentrations (H. Wu et al., 2004). The bioadhesive property of gelatin and chitosan microparticles previously reported as a crucial factor for prolonging the retention time in mucosal tissues, might serve as an important clinical advantage (Kawaguchi, 2000; J. J. Wang et al., 2011). Farnesol-loaded nanoparticles have shown to disrupt *Streptococcus mutans* 4 fold more effectively than free Farnesol. The release of Farnesol is pH defendant as nanoparticles undergo core destabilization at acidic pH (Figure 4) (Horev et al., 2015).

With the recognition of these agents as effective antibacterial and antibiofilm agents from the province of research workers to clinicians, newer approaches with a potential to eliminate bacteria and supersede these agents were investigated. In such context, the use of light as an effective antibacterial agent came under scrutiny (Wilson, 1993). Photodynamic therapy (PDT) is a therapeutic process that combines the effect of light and photosensitive agents called photosensitizers and renders an antibacterial effect (Longo et al., 2012). Nano and micro-sized particles functionalized with various photoactive compounds have shown to combat the antimicrobial resistance and enhance antimicrobial PDT (a-PDT). Since dental caries are localized, the limitations of traditional dental treatments have prompted the use of PDT as an alternative protocol (Banfi et al., 2006).

Chitosan is a natural polymer obtained from the exoskeleton of crustaceans and often used in drug delivery. Annie Shrestha et al has shown that the dual property of photoactivable chitosan nanoparticles surface functionalized with rose-bengal (CSRBnp) has resulted in the targeted elimination of *E. faecalis* biofilms and simultaneous restoration of the structural as well as mechanical integrity of the infected root dentin matrix (Annie Shrestha, Hamblin, & Kishen, 2014). The same group of researchers has demonstrated diminished antibacterial activity of chitosan nanoparticulates (CS-NP)-modified root canal sealers in comparison to that incorporated with nanoparticles of zinc oxide (ZnO-NP). The limited release of CS-NP from the sealer and the variation in their bactericidal mechanisms could have attributed to this difference (Anil Kishen, Shi, Shrestha, & Neoh, 2008). Moreover, CS-NP require longer interaction time for complete elimination of biofilms and their penetration might be restricted by the extracellular polymeric substance surrounding the biofilm mass (Upadya, Shrestha, & Kishen, 2011). The involvement of FDA-approved synthetic polymers like poly(D,L-lactide-co-glycolide) (PLGA) in dentistry have been well recognized (Maria Justina Roxana Virlan & Bogdan, 2015). Studies have shown that the encapsulation of active compounds like photosensitizers (methylene blue) and recombinant proteins in PLGA micro and nano-sized particles have improved the anti-planktonic as well as anti-biofilm activities of these delivery carriers exhibiting enhanced bacterial uptake and phototoxicity (Klepac-Ceraj et al., 2011; Zhao et al., 2006). The potential of these nanocarriers to diffuse inside biofilms and release the drug in an active form is an important criteria allowing the encapsulation phenomena to be extended for various bacteriostatic and bactericidal agents with promising prospects in vaccine delivery (Zhao et al., 2006). Polymers modified with quaternary ammonium salts have been frequently used in dentistry along with the use of composite resins (He, Söderling, Vallittu, & Lassila, 2013; Sun et al., 2011). Quaternary ammonium-loaded polyethylenimine (QAS-PEI) nanoparticles incorporated in dental composites were effective against *S. mutans* for over a month without altering the original mechanical properties of the composite (Nurit Beyth, Yudovin-Farber, Bahir, Domb, & Weiss, 2006; N. Beyth, Yudovin-Farber, Perez-Davidi, Domb, & Weiss, 2010).

Periodontics

Periodontal diseases (PD) or Periodontitis is a collective term that refers to a combination of multiple inflammatory diseases leading to slow, irreversible damage that affect the supportive structures surrounding the teeth such as gum, alveolar bone and the periodontal ligament (Armitage, 1999; Socransky &

Figure 4. Structure and function of nanoparticles and properties of used polymers. (A) Depiction of the chemistry and self-assembly of diblock copolymers. Cationic and pH-responsive ~20 kDa diblock copolymers with equivalent first- to second-block molecular weights and PDI of 1.1 were synthesized by two-step RAFT polymerizations, as indicated, and self-assembled into micelle-based nanoparticles in aqueous solutions via sonication. (B) Structures of control polymers utilized to isolate required physico-chemical characteristics for binding to dental surfaces. (C) Proposed mode of action of pH-responsive nanoparticles for prevention and/or treatment of biofilms. RAFT is reversible addition–fragmentation chain transfer polymerization. PDI is polydispersity index; ECT is the chain transfer agent (CTA), 4-cyano-4-[(ethylsulfanylthiocarbonyl)sulfanyl]pentanoic acid; AIBN is the initiator, 2,2-azobis(isobutyronitrile); DMF is dimethylformamide; DP is degree of polymerization

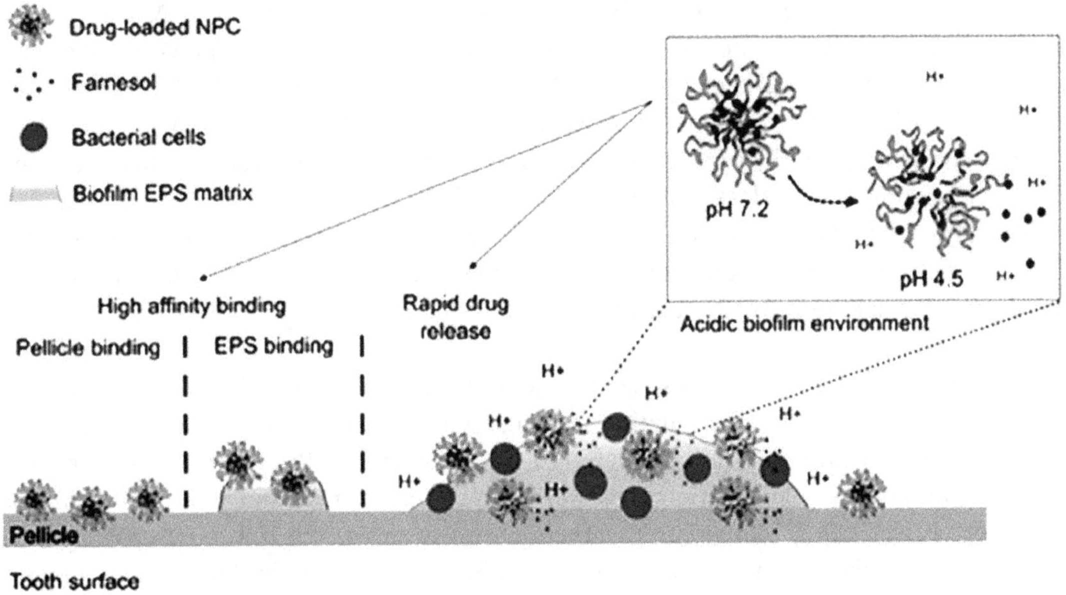

Haffajee, 1994). Different forms of periodontitis such as gingivitis, chronic or aggressive periodontitis prevail, based on the differences in clinical diagnosis (AlJehani, 2014). Bacterial adhesion and invasion of the gingival epithelium lays the foundation for pathogenesis of periodontitis (Colombo, Silva, Haffajee, & Colombo, 2006). The proximity of the subgingival biofilms to the underlying epithelial cells determines the extent to which the periodontal attachment may get affected, in order to illicit an inflammatory response (Lamont & Yilmaz, 2002). Periodontitis is often characterized by formation of periodontal pockets, resorption of alveolar bone and loss of periodontal support.

The moist, warm periodontal pockets provides a nutritious and anaerobic ambience conducive for microbial colonization and replication (Kinane, 2003; Williams, 1990). Antibiotic or antiseptic drugs loaded in biocompatible polymer micro and nano delivery systems enable the introduction of formulations directly into the root canal or inside the periodontal pocket with constant release of drugs for control of infections (Álvarez, Espinar, & Méndez, 2011). Minocycline (MIN), a tetracycline derivative, has been used in the treatment of periodontitis for a long time due to its anti-inflammatory and antibiotic activity, extended half-life, better absorption and reduced excretion rate (Ciancio, Mather, & McMullen, 1980). Considerable research has focused on using MIN loaded polymer nanoparticles for eliminating the bacteria associated to periodontitis. Minocycline-loaded PLGA microspheres (MIN-PLGA NPs), in the commercially successful form known as ARESTIN®, has demonstrated effective killing of the periodontal pathogens with their capacity to deliver MIN to periodontal tissues (Goodson et al., 2007; Kashi et al., 2012) as mentioned in Table 1. It has also been used as part of various oral health program including proper brushing, flossing and as an adjunct in scaling and root planing (Oringer et al., 2002). Their clinical efficacy and success in smokers with chronic periodontitis have also been discussed (Gopinath et al., 2009; Paquette et al., 2003). Moreover, the elimination of *Porphyromonas gingivalis* from the periodontal pocket with a potential to improve the clinical probable pocket depth, gingival and plaque index, in combination with surgery have also been proven (Hellstrom et al., 2008). Sustained release of MIN from alginate-core and chitosan-coated microcapsules have shown effective microfloral suppression for 1 week with their potential as an effective therapeutic modality (Park et al., 2005). An in vivo study conducted in beagle dogs has shown better anti-periodontitis activity of MIN-loaded PEG-PLA nanoparticles (MIN-NPs) when compared to that of commercial Periocline and MIN solution (Yao et al., 2014). Srirangarajan and workers have proved that the DOX-loaded PLGA/PCL microspheres can be in the treatment of refractory periodontal disease (Mundargi et al., 2007; Srirangarajan et al., 2011). Alginate coating of tetracycline hydrochloride-releasing PLGA microspheres have shown to enhance drug encapsulation and subsequent release following delivery in the periodontal pockets (Liu et al., 2005). PLGA microparticles containing chlorhexidine free base (Chx), chlorhexidine di gluconate (Chx-Dg) were effective against periodontal infections and delivered chlorhexidine salts in a targeted fashion (Yue et al., 2004). Hydroxyapatite and ofloxacin-loaded PLGA microspheres were able to eliminate *S. aureus* and *E. coli* (Jamal et al., 2012).

Natural polymers like gelatin have also been used in the treatment of periodontitis because they are mucoadhesive and are used for encapsulation of drugs with high toxicity or a short half-life (Gould, Westbury, & Tillman, 1982). A liquid crystalline phase modified with propolis-incorporated gelatin nanoparticles have shown stable retention in the periodontal pocket and their eventual controlled release thereof (Bruschi et al., 2008). Moulari and workers used flavonoid-rich Harungana madagascariensis leaf extract (HLE) and showed that its encapsulation in PLGA nanoparticles has not only increased the antibacterial efficiency but also implicated its potential use as an anticaries agent and in the prevention of gingivitis (Moulari et al., 2006). Rapid release of Triclosan (2,4,4′-trichloro-hydroxydiphenylether), an antimicrobial agent with anti-plaque properties, from PLGA nanoparticles were effective against induced periodontal defects and reduced the gingival inflammation with an ability to penetrate through the junctional epithelium (Pinon-Segundo, Ganem-Quintanar, Alonso-Perez, & Quintanar-Guerrero, 2005). When the periodontal defects in rat maxillae were filled with PDLLA-PLGA microparticles containing growth (PDGF, mitogen) and differentiation factors (simvastatin), acceleration of periodontal regeneration has been observed (Chang et al., 2013). Chitosan-based microspheres and nanoparticles have been used as a local therapeutic in periodontal diseases (Dung et al., 2007) and in vivo rat studies indicate enhanced implant absorption with potential applications in wound healing (L. C. Wang et al., 2008). Thrombin, an anticoagulant, when released in a sustained fashion, acts as a local bioactive coagulation device for use during anticoagulation therapy and periodontal surgical procedures (Smeets et al., 2011).

Endodontic Therapy

Endodontic disease is often biofilm-mediated and primarily aims at the elimination of root canal microorganisms by cleaning and sterilizing the root canals with irrigant antimicrobial agents followed by filling with gutta percha (Jaberi-Ansari, Ekrami, & Nojehdehian, 2013; Jhajharia, Parolia, Shetty, & Mehta, 2015). The presence of resistant microbes such as *Enterococcus faecalis, Staphylococcus aureus, Pseudomonas aeruginosa, Bacillus subtilis, Streptococcus spp., and Candida spp.* in the root canal is of particular concern (Molander, Reit, & Dahlén, 1999; Pinheiro et al., 2003; Portenier, Waltimo, & Haapasalo, 2003; Saleh, Ruyter, Haapasalo, & Ørstavik, 2004; Stuart, Schwartz, Beeson, & Owatz, 2006). The bacterial load present in the complex anatomy of root canal poses an important challenge for penetration of antibiotic medicaments, eventually causing endodontic failure (Graves, 2008; Lin, Skribner, & Gaengler, 1992). The difficulty in killing these persistent bacteria has led to the development of improvised formulations capable of prolonged release of antibiotics within the canal. Various studies have shown to benefit from using chitosan-based nanoparticles in the prevention and neutralization of root canal bacterial recolonization and biofilm formation (Anil Kishen et al., 2008; A. Kishen & Shrestha, 2013; Annie Shrestha, Fong, Khoo, & Kishen, 2009) as shown in Table 2. Their penetration inside dentinal tubules have been significantly enhanced by high intensity focused ultrasound and aided in the biofilm removal (Annie Shrestha et al., 2009). It has also shown to enhance the mechanical properties, improve the chemical stability of the connective tissues and/or the surface/interfacial integrity between filling materials and connective tissue when used as a carrier for photoactivatable antibacterial/antibiofilm compounds (A. Kishen & Shrestha, 2013). When used in combination with cationic ZnO nanoparticles, chitosan nanoparticles exhibit enhanced antibacterial action (Anil Kishen et al., 2008). PLGA nanoparticles loaded with endodontic antimicrobials have also shown potential activity against *E. faecalis* biofilms in the experimentally infected root canal (Pagonis et al., 2010; Sousa, Luzardo-Alvarez, Perez-Estevez, Seoane-Prado, & Blanco-Mendez, 2010). Polyethylene glycol coated maghemite nanoparticles have been used for dentinal tubule occlusion as a long-lasting remedy for dental hypersensitivity (Dabbagh et al., 2014).

Dentin Tissue Stabilization

The scope of micro and nanomaterials to impart the effect on biofilm elimination, hinder demineralization process and stimulate the process of tooth structure remineralization in order to restore the stability of previously affected or infected dentin matrix is promising. Nanoparticles made of natural bioactive polymers such as chitosan has shown the potential to intensify the mechanical and structural properties of dentin collagen. These nanoparticles are easy to functionalize due to the presence of highly reactive amino and hydroxyl groups on the surface. Cross-linking dentin with various agents has shown a considerable increase in the tensile properties, hardness, elastic modulus and toughness of demineralized dentin (Bedran-Russo, Pashley, Agee, Drummond, & Miescke, 2007; Bedran-Russo, Pereira, Duarte, Drummond, & Yamauchi, 2006; Bedran-Russo, Yoo, Ema, & Pashley, 2009; U. Daood, Iqbal, Nitisusanta, & Fawzy, 2012; Umer Daood, Swee Heng, Neo Chiew Lian, & Fawzy, 2015; Fawzy, Nitisusanta, Iqbal, Daood, Beng, et al., 2012; Fawzy, Nitisusanta, Iqbal, Daood, & Neo, 2012; A. Shrestha, Friedman, & Kishen, 2011; Annie Shrestha et al., 2014). Chitosan nanoparticles and their derivatives have shown to interact with endogenous MMPs and/or bacterial collagenase with a potential to neutralize them, inhibit collagen degradation and enhance the biodegradation resistance of dentin (M. M. Kim & Kim, 2006; Persadmehr et al., 2014). The inclusion of zinc-loaded polymeric nanocarriers into a dental adhesive system has shown to reduce the MMPs activity without affecting bond strength (Osorio, Osorio, Medina-Castillo, & Toledano, 2014). The use of poly (methylmethacrylate)-grafted nanoclay (PMMA-g-nanoclay) as a successful reinforcing filler has been investigated and shown to result in higher shear bond strength (Atai et al., 2009; Solhi, Atai, Nodehi, & Imani, 2012; Solhi, Atai, Nodehi, Imani, et al., 2012). Polymeric nanogels when reinforced in the experimental adhesives improve the short-term microtensile bond strength (Morães et al., 2012). Collagen fibrils present in dentin are the principal tensile stress–bearers and contribute a major part to the mechanical properties. Intermolecular cross-linking of collagen fibrils is one of the most commonly put forth mechanisms for developing resistance to proteolytic cleavage for improving the mechanical stability of dentin (Nakabayashi, 1982; N. Nakabayashi, Kojima, & Masuhara, 1982). The inclusion of water-soluble chitosan in the cross-linking procedure helped enhance the mechanical properties (A. Shrestha et al., 2011), use of Rose bengal-functionalized chitosan nanoparticles has achieved photodynamic cross-linking in a single step (Annie Shrestha et al., 2014). Bioactive polymeric nanoparticles disinfect the dentin with simultaneous tissue stabilization.

Regenerative Dentistry

Regenerative dentistry focus on tissue regeneration to compensate for lost tissues rather than replacement which is more beneficial and involves biology-based treatments (Galler & D'Souza, 2010; Rosa, Bona, Cavalcanti, & Nör, 2012). It is a well-known fact that small bone defects can spontaneously regenerate to their default anatomic configuration, however, regeneration of defects that exceed a certain size and degree of its severity, requires external augmentation using bone substitutes to accomplish this task (Schwartz-Arad & Chaushu, 1997; Zeren, 2006). For enhancement of bone regeneration, many research groups have attempted to incorporate bioactive agents and drugs into the bone substitutes (Boden, Martin Jr, Morone, Ugbo, & Moskovitz, 1999; Ginebra, Traykova, & Planell, 2006). In order to control the release profiles, studies have shown the encapsulation of these compounds in biodegradable polymers, attempting to prolong their pharmacological activity. PLGA microparticles are utilized frequently in this area of research as shown in Table 1. PDLLA-PLGA microparticles containing growth and differentiation factors induce osteogenesis, bone maturation and periodontal regeneration in rat maxillae (Chang et al., 2013). Estrogen-containing PLGA microparticles upregulates osteogenic differentiation of human bone marrow mesenchymal stromal cells (MSCs) (Hong et al., 2011). PLGA particles loaded with simvastatin (Naito et al., 2014; C.-Z. Wang et al., 2014), growth factors (F. Wang et al., 2010; Yonamine et al., 2010; Zou et al., 2012) and dexamethasone (Piao et al., 2014; Son et al., 2013) have significantly improved bone formation. Orchestrating the release of growth factors have shown improved osteointegration to titanium implants (F. Wang et al., 2010; Zou et al., 2012). Another study has shown that local delivery of biphosphonate PLGA microspheres as implants that can be an adjunct in the treatment of bone loss in the area of dental prostheses (Samdancioglu, Calis, Sumnu, & Atilla Hincal, 2006). Fulvastatin-releasing injectable PLGA microspheres prevents bone resorption during dental procedures and increases the mechanical stability of bone (Masuzaki et al., 2010) whereas insulin-containing PLGA microparticles improved the biomechanical retention of implants (Han et al., 2012). Arestin® and MIN-loaded PLGA have been used as an adjunct to mechanical methods for treatment of human peri-implantitis (Persson, Salvi, Heitz-Mayfield, & Lang, 2006; Stefan Renvert, Lessem, Dahlén, Lindahl, & Svensson, 2006; S. Renvert, Lessem, Dahlen, Renvert, & Lindahl, 2008). Heparin-conjugated PLGA nanoparticles loaded with bone morphogenetic protein-2 (BMP-2) has shown to regenerate bone in vivo (S. E. Kim et al., 2008). Collagen-conjugated polycaprolactone microparticles have shown controlled delivery of DOX as well as a potential to induce cell proliferation and tissue regeneration in the periodontal pockets (Aishwarya, Mahalakshmi, & Sehgal, 2008). Since regenerative dentistry is at its infancy, these procedures have great potential and applications in the future.

Prosthodontics

Prosthodontics is the branch of oral medicine that mainly deals with dental defects, treatments following tooth loss, such as crowns, and dentures, including the use of artificial prostheses for periodontal disease, maxillofacial tissue defects and mandibular joint disease (Mehra, Vahidi, & Berg, 2013; Saavedra et al., 2007). Dentures restore the dental functions and facial appearance of the wearer. Therefore, their composition and performance determines the long-term stability of these prostheses (Budtz-Jörgensen, 1996). Although polymethyl methacrylate (PMMA) has been used in the fabrication of denture teeth for various advantages such as lower susceptibility to fracture, chemical bond to denture base and reduced clicking (Adams, Jooste, Thomas, & Harris, 1996; Beall, 1943; Kawano, Ohguri, Ichikawa, Mizuno, & Hasegawa, 2002; Reis et al., 2008), its wear resistance when compared to ceramic teeth has been questioned (Ogle, David, & Ortman, 1985; Whitman, McKinney, Hinman, Hesby, & Pelleu, 1987). Cooper et al. showed that a PMMA matrix modified with carbon nanotubes (CNTs) or carbon nanofibrils significantly improved the strength of the composites (Cooper, Ravich, Lips, Mayer, & Wagner,

Table 1. Use of polymer microparticles in dentistry

Application	Polymer/Drug	Microparticle Characteristics	Key Findings	Citations
Cariostatic studies	Gelatin/NaF	Double-phase emulsified condensation polymerization Average dia: 11.33±5.56 μm NaF content: 8.80% Encapsulation efficiency: 76.73%	Gelatin/NaF prolongs fluoride release, delays demineralization and improves fluoride retention in dental plaque	(H. Wu et al., 2004)
Controlled delivery of fluoride	Chitosan/NaF	Spray drying Average dia: <6 μm NaF loading: 14% Encapsulation efficiency: 84.1%	Chitosan/NaF increases fluoride uptake that provides enhanced protection against dental caries	(Keegan et al., 2012)
Controlled delivery of fluoride	Ethylcellulose/NaF, MFP, AF	Emulsification/solvent evaporation Average dia: <145.35 μm Encapsulation efficiency: 137.45±0.00	Microparticles of Ethylcellulose and gelatin deliver fluoride ions in a controlled fashion that enhanced the protection against caries.	(de Francisco et al., 2012)
	Gelatin/NaF, MFP, AF	Dripping technique Average dia: <124.22 μm Encapsulation efficiency: 79.79±0.68%		
Dental caries vaccination	Chitosan-coated PLGA/rGbpD	Water/oil/water emulsification Average dia:<2 μm Loading efficiency: 1.21%	Chitosan coating of PLGA/ rGbpD enhanced protein loading and intranasal immunization demonstrated an effective vaccine delivery system	(Zhao et al., 2006)
Periodontal MIN delivery	PLGA/MIN (ARESTIN)	Average dia: 20 to 60 μm Arestin™ exhibits excellent adherence to the periodontal pocket and releases therapeutic doses of MIN for over 14 days	ARESTIN has proved to be a safe and efficient adjunct to scaling and root planing in the treatment of chronic periodontitis	(Gopinath et al., 2009)
Prolonged release of MIN	Alginate/MIN	Ionic gelation Average dia: 100μm Encapsulation efficiency: 74%	Alginate/MIN as an effective therapeutic modality for periodontitis	(Park et al., 2005)

continued on following page

Table 1. Continued

Application	Polymer/Drug	Microparticle Characteristics	Key Findings	Citations
Controlled delivery of DOX	PLGA-PCL blend/ DOX	Water/oil/water double emulsification Average dia: 90 to 200 μm Encapsulation efficiency: 9.00±0.20 to 24.7±0.53%	PLGA-PCL blend/ DOX can be effectively used in pocket therapy and treatment of refractory periodontal sites	(Mundargi et al., 2007)
Controlled delivery of Tc	Alginate-coated PLGA/Tetracycline	Double emulsion/solvent evaporation Average dia: 102.4±3.4 μm Encapsulation efficiency: 17.9±0.5%	Enhanced delivery of Tetracycline to periodontal pockets	(Liu et al., 2005)
Treatment of Periodontal Disease	Gelatin/Propolis (PM)	Spray drying Average dia: 2.48±0.81μm Drug loading: 6.41%	The rheological properties of Gelatin/Propolis have shown to be conducive for easy penetration into periodontal pockets and thereby its retention	(Bruschi et al., 2008)
Periodontal regeneration	PLGA-PDLLA/ PDGF and Simvastatin	Co-axial electrohydrodynamic atomization Average dia: ~15μm Encapsulation efficiency: Core-81.3±4.5 and Shell-72.6±2.4	Subsequent PGDF and Simvastatin delivery accelerates osteogenesis and bone maturation	(Chang et al., 2013)
Root canal disinfection	PLGA-zein/AMX	Spray drying Average dia: 5-38 μm Drug Loading: 2.1±0.8% to 5.8±0.8% Encapsulation efficiency: 38-51%	PLGA-zein/AMX demonstrated use as an effective antibacterial vehicles and showed efficacy against *E.faecalis*	(Sousa et al., 2010)
Osteogenic differentiation	PLGA/Estrogen	Emulsion/solvent evaporation Average dia: ~1.8μm Zeta Potential: +21±3.42 mV Encapsulation efficiency: 87.381%_2.97%	Intracellular delivery of estrogen to for effective regulation of MSCs	(Hong et al., 2011)
Bone defects	PLGA/Simvastatin	Emulsion/solvent evaporation Average dia: 21.07μm Drug loading: 91 ± 3.78%	Microspheres of PLGA/ Simvastatin can enhance bone formation in the defective areas of the rabbit calvaria	(Naito et al., 2014)
Osseointegration of dental implants	PLGA/rrIGF-1	Double emulsion/solvent evaporation Average dia: 1.25 ± 0.64μm Encapsulation efficiency: 78.3±2%	Osseointegration of dental implants in type 2 diabetes during the early post implantation healing phase and prolonged release of IGF-1 has resulted in new bone formation around the implants	(F. Wang et al., 2010)
Osseointegration of dental implants	PLGA/bFGF	Double emulsion/solvent evaporation Average dia: 1.138± 0.304μm	Early osseointegration observed in diabetic rats. Potential to stimulate bone formation in human patients.	(Zou et al., 2012)
Local delivery of dexamethasone (DEX)	PLGA/DEX	Emulsion/solvent evaporation Average dia: 0.8 to 4μm Zeta Potential: -24±2.1mV	PLGA/DEX showed osteoconductivity and proved to be an excellent platform for bone regeneration	(Son et al., 2013)
Implantation in Osteolysis	Chitosan/AS	Emulsion polymerization Average dia: 110.28±0.4μm Loading efficacy: 3.30%	Local delivery of these microspheres as implants may inhibit bone resorption during dental and orthopedic procedures	(Samdancioglu et al., 2006)
	PLGA/AS	Emulsion/solvent evaporation Average dia: 47.78± μm Loading efficacy: 7.70%		

Table 2. Use of polymer nanoparticles in dentistry

Application	Polymer/Drug	Nanoparticle Characteristics	Key Findings	Citations
Antimicrobial and antibiofilm activity	Chitosan	Ionic gelation Average dia: 20 to 1000 nm	LMW chitosan nanoparticles show uniform delivery of chitosan, affect the cell membrane integrity of entire *S. mutans* biofilm and therefore exhibits antibiofilm and antimicrobial activity	(Chávez de Paz et al., 2011)
Antibacterial/ biofilm activity	Chitosan/Rose Bengal (CSRBnp)	Ionic gelation Average dia: 60 ± 20 nm Zeta potential: +30 ± 0.8 mV	CSRBnp eliminates biofilm formation and restore mechanical integrity of infected dentin tissue	(Annie Shrestha et al., 2014)
Antibacterial/ biofilm activity	Chitosan (CS-NP)	Electrostatic layer-by-layer technique Average dia: ~70 nm Zeta potential: + 49 mV	Nanoparticles-treated dentin showed significant reduction in Enterococcus faecalis exhibiting a potential for root canal disinfection	(Anil Kishen et al., 2008)
		Electrostatic layer-by-layer technique Average dia: <100 nm		(Annie Shrestha et al., 2009)
Anti-plaque activity	PLGA/MB	Solvent displacement Average dia: <220nm Zeta Potential: -38.3 and +43.5 mV for anionic and cationic nanoparticles respectively	Cationic PLGA/MB nanoparticles in combination with PDT demonstrate effective elimination of biofilms	(Klepac-Ceraj et al., 2011)
Antibacterial nanoparticles incorporated in dental composites	Quatnery ammonium PEI	Crosslinking, alkylation and quaternarization Average dia: <100nm	Composite resin restorations when incorporated with antibacterial nanoparticles have potential in eliminating biofilm formation and secondary caries.	(Nurit Beyth et al., 2006)
Periodontal Minocycline delivery	PLGA/MIN	Emulsification, nanoprecipitation Average dia: < 500 nm Drug Loading: 0.26 ± 0.06% to 1.92 ± 0.19% Encapsulation efficiency: 0.81 ± 0.18% to 29.95 ± 2.47%	PLGA/MIN synthesized by ion pairing method showed highest drug loading and higher antibacterial activity against *Aggregatibacter actinomycetemcomitans*	(Kashi et al., 2012)
Local delivery of MIN	MPEG-PLA/ MIN	Emulsion/solvent evaporation Average dia: 98±12 nm Drug Loading: 1.92%±0.19% Encapsulation efficiency: 29.95%±2.47%	MPEG-PLA/MIN increased periodontal retention of MIN and showed anti-periodontitis effects	(Yao et al., 2014)
Antibacterial activity	PLGA/HSE	Interfacial polymer deposition/solvent diffusion Average dia: 255.09±31.1nm Encapsulation efficiency: 75% Zeta Potential: -31.1±0.4mV	PLGA/HSE demonstrated bactericidal activity against cariogenic bacteria and could be an effective anticaries agent	(Moulari et al., 2006)
Periodontal treatment	PLGA/Triclosan	Emulsification diffusion Average dia: <500nm Drug Loading: 0.84 ± 0.06% to 23.75 ± 0.06% Encapsulation efficiency: 63.88% to 85.12%	Preliminary in vivo study has shown that PLGA/Triclosan can reduce gingival inflammation but further experiments have to be conducted to confirm these results for periodontal treatment	(Pinon-Segundo et al., 2005)
Antimicrobial	PLGA/MB	Solvent displacement Average dia: ~150-200 nm Zeta Potential: -31.87 mV Bacterial cell wall toxicity: 34% to 58.5%	Synergistic action of light and PLGA/MB reduced the colony-forming units in planktonic phase and root canals to 2 and 1 log10, respectively	(Pagonis et al., 2010)

continued on following page

Table 2. Continued

Application	Polymer/Drug	Nanoparticle Characteristics	Key Findings	Citations
Treatment of dental hypersensitivity	PEG/Maghemite	"Graft-to" method Average dia: <25nm Dentin treatment of nanoparticles for 120min showed high occlusion of tubules	PEG/Maghemite can be used as potential biomedical carriers for dentin remineralization	(Dabbagh et al., 2014)
Dentin Adhesion	PolymP-nActive	Commercial PolymP-nActive from NanoMyP (Granada, Spain) Average dia: 350nm	Nanocarriers potentially inhibits MMP collagen degradation and enhances mineral growth	(Osorio et al., 2014)
Dentin Adhesion	Polymeric nanogels	Average dia: 10- to 100-nm	Nanogel-reinforcement of adhesives significantly improved the wet mechanical properties	(Morães et al., 2012)
Enhancing osteogenesis	BPPD/ simvastatin	Average dia: 231.5 nm, Zeta potential: -6.7 ± 2.8mV Encapsulation efficiency: $42.3 \pm 5.5\%$	BPPD/Simvastatin can be used as potential hydrophobic drug carriers to promote osteogenesis	(C.-Z. Wang et al., 2014)

2002). Such enhancement from using small amounts of single-wall nanotubes may be a considerable economic advantage (W. Wang et al., 2015). Since dentures come in direct contact with oral mucosa, their biocompatibility is very crucial for proper functioning. Incorporation of nanoparticles of TiO_2, Fe_2O_3 and silver in PMMA materials have shown to reduce bimolecular adherence in order to eliminate the plaque formation on PMMA based resins that eventually lead to oral cavity infections (L. S. Acosta-Torres, Mendieta, Nunez-Anita, Cajero-Juarez, & Castano, 2012; Laura S. Acosta-Torres et al., 2011; Monteiro et al., 2011). It has also shown to simultaneously improve the color of PMMA based materials (Fujishima, Rao, & Tryk, 2000; Hoffmann, Martin, Choi, & Bahnemann, 1995). Therefore, addition of metal oxides has shown to improve performance of PMMA formulations (Laura S. Acosta-Torres et al., 2011). Silver nanoparticles conjugated with polymers like PMMA and Polyamide-6 form nanocomposites that perform as effective antibacterial materials preventing the growth of infections involving the oral mucosal tissues in denture wearers (Damm, Münstedt, & Rösch, 2007; Magalh et al., 2012).

CONCLUSION

The use of adjunctive micro- and nanoparticle-based system has increased the effect of conventional dental therapies with clear clinical benefits. The preliminary preclinical studies in the various areas are rather exciting. As micro-and nano-particle can be easily functionalized, they can be combined with biomolecules or loaded with antibiotics and used as additives in several dental materials to improve their bioactivity, physical, chemical and mechanical properties The polymeric micro- and nano-particle maintain effective concentrations of therapeutic agents to reach the site of action namely the periodontal pocket, dental cavity, or surrounding bone. These encapsulation technologies may open up new directions in the field of dentistry.

Despite the excitement created by the promising capabilities of polymeric materials it exhibits some challenges which still need to be addressed before translating into clinical reality. Firstly, toxicity of the polymeric particle induced by release of degradation products and residual surfactant used during the synthesis process needs to be addressed. The efficacy of loaded drugs and antibiotics must be systematically evaluated in animal model studies and clinical trials. In addition to biosafety, there is also the need of gaining profound understanding of the mechanisms involved in polymeric material-mediated biological behavior at both cellular and tissue levels. Although these challenges remain open, the exciting findings presented here and beyond show that polymeric particle hold great potential for dental applications.

REFERENCES

Acosta-Torres, L. S., López-Marín, L. M., Núñez-Anita, R. E., Hernández-Padrón, G., & Castaño, V. M. (2011). Biocompatible Metal-Oxide Nanoparticles: Nanotechnology Improvement of Conventional Prosthetic Acrylic Resins. *Journal of Nanomaterials*, *2011*, 8. doi:10.1155/2011/941561

Acosta-Torres, L. S., Mendieta, I., Nunez-Anita, R. E., Cajero-Juarez, M., & Castano, V. M. (2012). Cytocompatible antifungal acrylic resin containing silver nanoparticles for dentures. *International Journal of Nanomedicine*, *7*, 4777–4786. PMID:22969297

Adams, L. P., Jooste, C. H., Thomas, C. J., & Harris, A. M. (1996). Biostereometric quantification of clinical denture tooth wear. *Journal of Oral Rehabilitation*, *23*(10), 667–674. doi:10.1046/j.1365-2842.1996.d01-178.x PMID:8933383

Aishwarya, S., Mahalakshmi, S., & Sehgal, P. K. (2008). Collagen-coated polycaprolactone microparticles as a controlled drug delivery system. *Journal of Microencapsulation*, *25*(5), 298–306. doi:10.1080/02652040801972004 PMID:18465301

AlJehani, Y. A. (2014). Risk factors of periodontal disease: Review of the literature. *International Journal of Dentistry*, *2014*, 182513. doi:10.1155/2014/182513 PMID:24963294

Álvarez, A. L., Espinar, F. O., & Méndez, J. B. (2011). The Application of Microencapsulation Techniques in the Treatment of Endodontic and Periodontal Disease. *Pharmaceutics*, *3*(3), 538–571. doi:10.3390/pharmaceutics3030538 PMID:24310596

Ambrosio, A., & Payne, J. (2013). Method of promoting new tissue growth and/or wound healing using bioresorbable dressing comprising microspheres or microparticles: Google Patents.

Armitage, G. C. (1999). Development of a classification system for periodontal diseases and conditions. *Annals of Periodontology*, *4*(1), 1–6. doi:10.1902/annals.1999.4.1.1 PMID:10863370

Atai, M., Solhi, L., Nodehi, A., Mirabedini, S. M., Kasraei, S., Akbari, K., & Babanzadeh, S. (2009). PMMA-grafted nanoclay as novel filler for dental adhesives. *Dental Materials*, *25*(3), 339–347. doi:10.1016/j.dental.2008.08.005 PMID:18829096

Avila, M., Ojcius, D. M., & Yilmaz, Ö. (2009). The Oral Microbiota: Living with a Permanent Guest. *DNA and Cell Biology*, *28*(8), 405–411. doi:10.1089/dna.2009.0874 PMID:19485767

Banfi, S., Caruso, E., Buccafurni, L., Battini, V., Zazzaron, S., Barbieri, P., & Orlandi, V. (2006). Antibacterial activity of tetraaryl-porphyrin photosensitizers: An in vitro study on Gram negative and Gram positive bacteria. *Journal of Photochemistry and Photobiology. B, Biology*, *85*(1), 28–38. doi:10.1016/j.jphotobiol.2006.04.003 PMID:16737820

Beall, J. R. (1943). Wear of Acrylic Resin Teeth (Progress Report). *The Journal of the American Dental Association, 30*(3), 252–256. doi:10.14219/jada.archive.1943.0043

Bedran-Russo, A. K., Pashley, D. H., Agee, K., Drummond, J. L., & Miescke, K. J. (2007). Changes in stiffness of demineralized dentin following application of collagen crosslinkers. *Journal of Biomedical Materials Research. Part B, Applied Biomaterials, 86*(2), 330–334. PMID:18161815

Bedran-Russo, A. K., Pereira, P. N., Duarte, W. R., Drummond, J. L., & Yamauchi, M. (2006). Application of crosslinkers to dentin collagen enhances the ultimate tensile strength. *Journal of Biomedical Materials Research. Part B, Applied Biomaterials, 80*(1), 268–272. PMID:16767722

Bedran-Russo, A. K., Yoo, K. J., Ema, K. C., & Pashley, D. H. (2009). Mechanical properties of tannic-acid-treated dentin matrix. *Journal of Dental Research, 88*(9), 807–811. doi:10.1177/0022034509342556 PMID:19767576

Besinis, A., De Peralta, T., Tredwin, C. J., & Handy, R. D. (2015). Review of Nanomaterials in Dentistry: Interactions with the Oral Microenvironment, Clinical Applications, Hazards, and Benefits. *ACS Nano, 9*(3), 2255–2289. doi:10.1021/nn505015e PMID:25625290

Beyth, N., Yudovin-Farber, I., Bahir, R., Domb, A. J., & Weiss, E. I. (2006). Antibacterial activity of dental composites containing quaternary ammonium polyethylenimine nanoparticles against Streptococcus mutans. *Biomaterials, 27*(21), 3995–4002. doi:10.1016/j.biomaterials.2006.03.003 PMID:16564083

Beyth, N., Yudovin-Farber, I., Perez-Davidi, M., Domb, A. J., & Weiss, E. I. (2010). Polyethyleneimine nanoparticles incorporated into resin composite cause cell death and trigger biofilm stress in vivo. *Proceedings of the National Academy of Sciences of the United States of America, 107*(51), 22038–22043. doi:10.1073/pnas.1010341107 PMID:21131569

Boden, S. D., Martin, G. J. Jr, Morone, M. A., Ugbo, J. L., & Moskovitz, P. A. (1999). Posterolateral lumbar intertransverse process spine arthrodesis with recombinant human bone morphogenetic protein 2/hydroxyapatite–tricalcium phosphate after laminectomy in the nonhuman primate. *Spine, 24*(12), 1179–1185. doi:10.1097/00007632-199906150-00002 PMID:10382242

Bruschi, M. L., de Freitas, O., Lara, E. H., Panzeri, H., Gremiao, M. P., & Jones, D. S. (2008). Precursor system of liquid crystalline phase containing propolis microparticles for the treatment of periodontal disease: Development and characterization. *Drug Development and Industrial Pharmacy, 34*(3), 267–278. doi:10.1080/03639040701655911 PMID:18363142

Budtz-Jörgensen, E. (1996). Restoration of the partially edentulous mouth — a comparison of overdentures, removable partial dentures, fixed partial dentures and implant treatment. *Journal of Dentistry, 24*(4), 237–244. doi:10.1016/0300-5712(95)00075-5 PMID:8783527

Campus, G., Lallai, M. R., & Carboni, R. (2003). Fluoride concentration in saliva after use of oral hygiene products. *Caries Research, 37*(1), 66–70. doi:10.1159/000068220 PMID:12566642

Chang, P. C., Dovban, A. S., Lim, L. P., Chong, L. Y., Kuo, M. Y., & Wang, C. H. (2013). Dual delivery of PDGF and simvastatin to accelerate periodontal regeneration in vivo. *Biomaterials, 34*(38), 9990–9997. doi:10.1016/j.biomaterials.2013.09.030 PMID:24079892

Chávez de Paz, L. E., Resin, A., Howard, K. A., Sutherland, D. S., & Wejse, P. L. (2011). Antimicrobial Effect of Chitosan Nanoparticles on Streptococcus mutans Biofilms. *Applied and Environmental Microbiology*, *77*(11), 3892–3895. doi:10.1128/AEM.02941-10 PMID:21498764

Ciancio, S. G., Mather, M. L., & McMullen, J. A. (1980). An Evaluation of Minocycline in Patients With Periodontal Disease*. *Journal of Periodontology*, *51*(9), 530–534. doi:10.1902/jop.1980.51.9.530 PMID:6999148

Colombo, A. V., Silva, C. M., Haffajee, A., & Colombo, A. P. (2006). Identification of oral bacteria associated with crevicular epithelial cells from chronic periodontitis lesions. *Journal of Medical Microbiology*, *55*(Pt 5), 609–615. doi:10.1099/jmm.0.46417-0 PMID:16585650

Cooper, C. A., Ravich, D., Lips, D., Mayer, J., & Wagner, H. D. (2002). Distribution and alignment of carbon nanotubes and nanofibrils in a polymer matrix. *Composites Science and Technology*, *62*(7–8), 1105–1112. doi:10.1016/S0266-3538(02)00056-8

Cristina Buzea, I. I. P. B., & Kevin, R. (2007). Nanomaterials and nanoparticles: Sources and toxicity. *Biointerphases*, *2*, MR17–MR172. PMID:20419892

Virlan, M. J. R., Miricescu, D., Totan, A., Greabu, M., Tanase, C., Sabliov, C. M.,... & Calenic, B. (2015). Current Uses of Poly(lactic-co-glycolic acid) in the Dental Field: A Comprehensive. *Review Journal of Chemistry*, 2015.

Dabbagh, A., Kasim, N. H. A., Bakri, M. M., Wakily, H., Ramasindarum, C., & Abdullah, B. J. J. (2014). Polyethylene-glycol coated maghemite nanoparticles for treatment of dental hypersensitivity. *Materials Letters*, *121*, 89–92. doi:10.1016/j.matlet.2014.01.120

Damm, C., Münstedt, H., & Rösch, A. (2007). Long-term antimicrobial polyamide 6/silver-nanocomposites. *Journal of Materials Science*, *42*(15), 6067–6073. doi:10.1007/s10853-006-1158-5

Daood, U., Iqbal, K., Nitisusanta, L. I., & Fawzy, A. S. (2012). Effect of chitosan/riboflavin modification on resin/dentin interface: Spectroscopic and microscopic investigations. *Journal of Biomedical Materials Research. Part A*, *101*(7), 1846–1856. PMID:23184366

Daood, U., Swee Heng, C., Neo Chiew Lian, J., & Fawzy, A. S. (2015). In vitro analysis of riboflavin-modified, experimental, two-step etch-and-rinse dentin adhesive: Fourier transform infrared spectroscopy and micro-Raman studies. *Journal of Oral Science*, *7*(2), 110–124. doi:10.1038/ijos.2014.49 PMID:25257880

de Francisco, L. M., Cerquetani, J. A., & Bruschi, M. L. (2012). Development and characterization of gelatin and ethylcellulose microparticles designed as platforms to delivery fluoride. *Drug Development and Industrial Pharmacy*, *39*(11), 1644–1650. doi:10.3109/03639045.2012.728610 PMID:23034061

Dhadse, P., Gattani, D., & Mishra, R. (2010). The link between periodontal disease and cardiovascular disease: How far we have come in last two decades? *Journal of Indian Society of Periodontology*, *14*(3), 148–154. doi:10.4103/0972-124X.75908 PMID:21760667

Diarra, M., Pourroy, G., Boymond, C., & Muster, D. (2003). Fluoride controlled release tablets for intrabuccal use. *Biomaterials*, *24*(7), 1293–1300. doi:10.1016/S0142-9612(02)00444-1 PMID:12527271

Dung, T. H., Lee, S. R., Han, S. D., Kim, S. J., Ju, Y. M., Kim, M. S., & Yoo, H. (2007). Chitosan-TPP nanoparticle as a release system of antisense oligonucleotide in the oral environment. *Journal of Nanoscience and Nanotechnology*, *7*(11), 3695–3699. doi:10.1166/jnn.2007.041 PMID:18047039

Fawzy, A. S., Nitisusanta, L. I., Iqbal, K., Daood, U., Beng, L. T., & Neo, J. (2012). Chitosan/Riboflavin-modified demineralized dentin as a potential substrate for bonding. *Journal of the Mechanical Behavior of Biomedical Materials*, *17*, 278–289. doi:10.1016/j.jmbbm.2012.09.008 PMID:23127636

Fawzy, A. S., Nitisusanta, L. I., Iqbal, K., Daood, U., & Neo, J. (2012). Riboflavin as a dentin cross-linking agent: Ultraviolet A versus blue light. *Dental Materials*, *28*(12), 1284–1291. doi:10.1016/j.dental.2012.09.009 PMID:23031483

Fujishima, A., Rao, T. N., & Tryk, D. A. (2000). Titanium dioxide photocatalysis. *Journal of Photochemistry and Photobiology C, Photochemistry Reviews*, *1*(1), 1–21. doi:10.1016/S1389-5567(00)00002-2

Galler, K. M., & D'Souza, R. N. (2010). Tissue engineering approaches for regenerative dentistry. *Regenerative Medicine*, *6*(1), 111–124. doi:10.2217/rme.10.86 PMID:21175291

Gibbons, R. J., & Houte, J. V. (1975). Dental Caries. *Annual Review of Medicine*, *26*(1), 121–136. doi:10.1146/annurev.me.26.020175.001005 PMID:1096752

Ginebra, M.-P., Traykova, T., & Planell, J. (2006). Calcium phosphate cements as bone drug delivery systems: A review. *Journal of Controlled Release*, *113*(2), 102–110. doi:10.1016/j.jconrel.2006.04.007 PMID:16740332

Goodson, J. M., Gunsolley, J. C., Grossi, S. G., Bland, P. S., Otomo-Corgel, J., Doherty, F., & Comiskey, J. (2007). Minocycline HCl microspheres reduce red-complex bacteria in periodontal disease therapy. *Journal of Periodontology*, *78*(8), 1568–1579. doi:10.1902/jop.2007.060488 PMID:17668977

Gopinath, V., Ramakrishnan, T., Emmadi, P., Ambalavanan, N., Mammen, B., & Vijayalakshmi,. (2009). Effect of a controlled release device containing minocycline microspheres on the treatment of chronic periodontitis: A comparative study. *Journal of Indian Society of Periodontology*, *13*(2), 79–84. doi:10.4103/0972-124X.55844 PMID:20407655

Gould, T., Westbury, L., & Tillman, J. (1982). Dentin matrix gelatin (DMG) as a possible "universal" grafting material in periodontics. *Journal of Periodontology*, *53*(1), 22–25. doi:10.1902/jop.1982.53.1.22 PMID:6948946

Graves, D. (2008). Cytokines that promote periodontal tissue destruction. *Journal of Periodontology*, *79*(8), 1585–1591. doi:10.1902/jop.2008.080183 PMID:18673014

Han, Y., Zeng, Q., Lingling, E., Wang, D., He, H., & Liu, H. (2012). Sustained Topical delivery of insulin from fibrin gel loaded with poly (lactic-co-glycolic acid) microspheres improves the biomechanical retention of titanium implants in type 1 diabetic rats. *Journal of Oral and Maxillofacial Surgery*, *70*(10), 2299–2308. doi:10.1016/j.joms.2012.05.028 PMID:22871310

Hannig, M., & Hannig, C. (2010). Nanomaterials in preventive dentistry. *Nature Nanotechnology*, *5*(8), 565–569. doi:10.1038/nnano.2010.83 PMID:20581832

He, J., Söderling, E., Vallittu, P. K., & Lassila, L. V. J. (2013). Preparation and Evaluation of Dental Resin with Antibacterial and Radio-Opaque Functions. *International Journal of Molecular Sciences*, *14*(3), 5445–5460. doi:10.3390/ijms14035445 PMID:23470923

Hellstrom, M. K., McClain, P. K., Schallhorn, R. G., Bellis, L., Hanlon, A. L., & Ramberg, P. (2008). Local minocycline as an adjunct to surgical therapy in moderate to severe, chronic periodontitis. *Journal of Clinical Periodontology*, *35*(6), 525–531. doi:10.1111/j.1600-051X.2008.01219.x PMID:18384391

Hoffmann, M. R., Martin, S. T., Choi, W., & Bahnemann, D. W. (1995). Environmental Applications of Semiconductor Photocatalysis. *Chemical Reviews*, *95*(1), 69–96. doi:10.1021/cr00033a004

Hong, L., Krishnamachari, Y., Seabold, D., Joshi, V., Schneider, G., & Salem, A. K. (2011). Intracellular Release of 17-β Estradiol from Cationic Polyamidoamine Dendrimer Surface-Modified Poly (Lactic-co-Glycolic Acid) Microparticles Improves Osteogenic Differentiation of Human Mesenchymal Stromal Cells. *Tissue Engineering. Part C, Methods*, *17*(3), 319–325. doi:10.1089/ten.tec.2010.0388 PMID:20883116

Horev, B., Klein, M. I., Hwang, G., Li, Y., Kim, D., Koo, H., & Benoit, D. S. W. (2015). pH-activated nanoparticles for controlled topical delivery of farnesol to disrupt oral biofilm virulence. *ACS Nano*, *9*(3), 2390–2404. doi:10.1021/nn507170s PMID:25661192

Howell, D. (2016). Tooth decay still on the rise among English children. from http://www.bbc.com/news/health-35672775

Hutter, E., & Maysinger, D. (2013). Gold-nanoparticle-based biosensors for detection of enzyme activity. *Trends in Pharmacological Sciences*, *34*(9), 497–507. doi:10.1016/j.tips.2013.07.002 PMID:23911158

Jaberi-Ansari, Z., Ekrami, M., & Nojehdehian, H. (2013). Controlled Release of Drugs for Management of Pulpitis. *Avicenna Journal of Dental Research, 6*(1).

Jamal, T., Rahman, M. A., Mirza, M. A., Panda, A. K., Talegaonkar, S., & Iqbal, Z. (2012). Formulation, antimicrobial and toxicity evaluation of bioceramic based ofloxacin loaded biodegradable microspheres for periodontal infection. *Current Drug Delivery*, *9*(5), 515–526. PMID:22758655

Jhajharia, K., Parolia, A., Shetty, K. V., & Mehta, L. K. (2015). Biofilm in endodontics: A review. *Journal of International Society of Preventive & Community Dentistry*, *5*(1), 1–12. doi:10.4103/2231-0762.151956 PMID:25767760

Jorgensen, J., Shariati, M., Shields, C. P., Durr, D. P., & Proskin, H. M. (1989). Fluoride uptake into demineralized primary enamel from fluoride-impregnated dental floss in vitro. *Pediatric Dentistry*, *11*(1), 17–20. PMID:2626334

Kashi, T. S., Eskandarion, S., Esfandyari-Manesh, M., Marashi, S. M., Samadi, N., & Fatemi, S. M. et al.. (2012). Improved drug loading and antibacterial activity of minocycline-loaded PLGA nanoparticles prepared by solid/oil/water ion pairing method. *International Journal of Nanomedicine*, *7*, 221–234. PMID:22275837

Kawaguchi, H. (2000). Functional polymer microspheres. *Progress in Polymer Science*, *25*(8), 1171–1210. doi:10.1016/S0079-6700(00)00024-1

Kawano, F., Ohguri, T., Ichikawa, T., Mizuno, I., & Hasegawa, A. (2002). Shock absorbability and hardness of commercially available denture teeth. *The International Journal of Prosthodontics*, *15*(3), 243–247. PMID:12066486

Keegan, G. M., Smart, J. D., Ingram, M. J., Barnes, L. M., Burnett, G. R., & Rees, G. D. (2012). Chitosan microparticles for the controlled delivery of fluoride. *Journal of Dentistry*, *40*(3), 229–240. doi:10.1016/j.jdent.2011.12.012 PMID:22212236

Khodashenas, B., & Ghorbani, H. R. Synthesis of silver nanoparticles with different shapes. *Arabian Journal of Chemistry*.

Kim, M. M., & Kim, S. K. (2006). Chitooligosaccharides inhibit activation and expression of matrix metalloproteinase-2 in human dermal fibroblasts. *FEBS Letters*, *580*(11), 2661–2666. doi:10.1016/j.febslet.2006.04.015 PMID:16647062

Kim, S. E., Jeon, O., Lee, J. B., Bae, M. S., Chun, H. J., Moon, S. H., & Kwon, I. K. (2008). Enhancement of ectopic bone formation by bone morphogenetic protein-2 delivery using heparin-conjugated PLGA nanoparticles with transplantation of bone marrow-derived mesenchymal stem cells. *Journal of Biomedical Science*, *15*(6), 771–777. doi:10.1007/s11373-008-9277-4 PMID:18773307

Kinane, D. L. J. (2003). Clinical Periodontology and Implant Dentistry (4 ed.). Copenhagen: Blackwell Munksgaard.

Kishen, A., Shi, Z., Shrestha, A., & Neoh, K. G. (2008). An investigation on the antibacterial and antibiofilm efficacy of cationic nanoparticulates for root canal disinfection. *Journal of Endodontics*, *34*(12), 1515–1520. doi:10.1016/j.joen.2008.08.035 PMID:19026885

Kishen, A., & Shrestha, A. (2013). Multi-functional micro and nanoparticles for use in root canal therapies: Google Patents.

Klepac-Ceraj, V., Patel, N., Song, X., Holewa, C., Patel, C., Kent, R., & Soukos, N. S. et al. (2011). Photodynamic effects of methylene blue-loaded polymeric nanoparticles on dental plaque bacteria. *Lasers in Surgery and Medicine*, *43*(7), 600–606. doi:10.1002/lsm.21069 PMID:22057487

Lamont, R. J., & Yilmaz, O. (2002). In or out: The invasiveness of oral bacteria. *Periodontology 2000*, *30*(1), 61–69. doi:10.1034/j.1600-0757.2002.03006.x PMID:12236896

Lin, L. M., Skribner, J. E., & Gaengler, P. (1992). Factors associated with endodontic treatment failures. *Journal of Endodontics*, *18*(12), 625–627. doi:10.1016/S0099-2399(06)81335-X PMID:1298804

Listgarten, M. A. (1987). Nature of periodontal diseases: Pathogenic mechanisms. *Journal of Periodontal Research*, *22*(3), 172–178. doi:10.1111/j.1600-0765.1987.tb01560.x PMID:2955092

Liu, D. Z., Chen, W. P., Lee, C. P., Wu, S. L., Wang, Y. C., & Chung, T. W. (2005). Effects of alginate coated on PLGA microspheres for delivery tetracycline hydrochloride to periodontal pockets. *Journal of Microencapsulation*, *21*(6), 643–652. doi:10.1080/02652040400000512 PMID:15762321

Longo, J. P. F., Leal, S. C., Simioni, A. R., Almeida-Santos, M. F. M., Tedesco, A. C., & Azevedo, R. B. (2012). Photodynamic therapy disinfection of carious tissue mediated by aluminum-chloride-phthalocyanine entrapped in cationic liposomes: An in vitro and clinical study. *Lasers in Medical Science*, *27*(3), 575–584. doi:10.1007/s10103-011-0962-6 PMID:21809069

Magalh, xe, es, A. P. R., Santos, L. B., Lopes, L. G., Estrela, C. R. d. A., et al. (2012). Nanosilver Application in Dental Cements. *ISRN Nanotechnology, 2012*, 6.

Mascarelli, A. (2011). Tooth decay is prevalent among poor children. Retrieved from http://articles.latimes.com/2011/jul/01/health/hk-he-dental-underserved-20110701

Masuzaki, T., Ayukawa, Y., Moriyama, Y., Jinno, Y., Atsuta, I., Ogino, Y., & Koyano, K. (2010). The effect of a single remote injection of statin-impregnated poly (lactic-co-glycolic acid) microspheres on osteogenesis around titanium implants in rat tibia. *Biomaterials*, *31*(12), 3327–3334. doi:10.1016/j.biomaterials.2010.01.016 PMID:20129662

Mehra, M., Vahidi, F., & Berg, R. W. (2013). A complete denture impression technique survey of postdoctoral prosthodontic programs in the United States. *Journal of Prosthodontics*, *23*(4), 320–327. doi:10.1111/jopr.12099 PMID:24118134

Melo, M. A. S., Guedes, S. F. F., Xu, H. H. K., & Rodrigues, L. K. A. (2013). Nanotechnology-based restorative materials for dental caries management. *Trends in Biotechnology*, *31*(8), 459–467. doi:10.1016/j.tibtech.2013.05.010 PMID:23810638

Molander, A., Reit, C., & Dahlén, G. (1999). The antimicrobial effect of calcium hydroxide in root canals pretreated with 5% iodine potassium iodide. *Dental Traumatology*, *15*(5), 205–209. doi:10.1111/j.1600-9657.1999.tb00775.x PMID:10825827

Monteiro, D. R., Gorup, L. F., Takamiya, A. S., de Camargo, E. R., Filho, A. C., & Barbosa, D. B. (2011). Silver distribution and release from an antimicrobial denture base resin containing silver colloidal nanoparticles. *Journal of Prosthodontics*, *21*(1), 7–15. doi:10.1111/j.1532-849X.2011.00772.x PMID:22050139

Morães, R. R., Garcia, J. W., Wilson, N. D., Lewis, S. H., Barros, M. D., Yang, B., & Stansbury, J. W. et al. (2012). Improved Dental Adhesive Formulations Based on Reactive Nanogel Additives. *Journal of Dental Research*, *91*(2), 179–184. doi:10.1177/0022034511426573 PMID:22019910

Moulari, B., Lboutounne, H., Chaumont, J.-P., Guillaume, Y., Millet, J., & Pellequer, Y. (2006). Potentiation of the bactericidal activity of Harungana madagascariensis Lam. ex Poir.(Hypericaceae) leaf extract against oral bacteria using poly (D, L-lactide-co-glycolide) nanoparticles: In vitro study. *Acta Odontologica Scandinavica*, *64*(3), 153–158. doi:10.1080/00016350500483152 PMID:16809192

Mundargi, R. C., Srirangarajan, S., Agnihotri, S. A., Patil, S. A., Ravindra, S., Setty, S. B., & Aminabhavi, T. M. (2007). Development and evaluation of novel biodegradable microspheres based on poly(d,l-lactide-co-glycolide) and poly(ε-caprolactone) for controlled delivery of doxycycline in the treatment of human periodontal pocket: In vitro and in vivo studies. *Journal of Controlled Release*, *119*(1), 59–68. doi:10.1016/j.jconrel.2007.01.008 PMID:17331611

Naito, Y., Terukina, T., Galli, S., Kozai, Y., Vandeweghe, S., Tagami, T., & Jimbo, R. et al. (2014). The effect of simvastatin-loaded polymeric microspheres in a critical size bone defect in the rabbit calvaria. *International Journal of Pharmaceutics*, *461*(1–2), 157–162. doi:10.1016/j.ijpharm.2013.11.046 PMID:24296045

Nakabayashi, N., Kojima, K., & Masuhara, E. (1982). The promotion of adhesion by the infiltration of monomers into tooth substrates. *Journal of Biomedical Materials Research*, *16*(3), 265–273. doi:10.1002/jbm.820160307 PMID:7085687

Nakabayashi. (1982). Bonding mechanism of resins and the tooth. *Kokubyo Gakkai Zasshi.*, *49*(410).

Ogle, R. E., David, L. J., & Ortman, H. R. (1985). Clinical wear study of a new tooth material: Part II. *The Journal of Prosthetic Dentistry*, *54*(1), 67–75. doi:10.1016/S0022-3913(85)80073-1 PMID:3894642

Oringer, R. J., Al-Shammari, K. F., Aldredge, W. A., Iacono, V. J., Eber, R. M., Wang, H. L., & Giannobile, W. V. et al. (2002). Effect of locally delivered minocycline microspheres on markers of bone resorption. *Journal of Periodontology*, *73*(8), 835–842. doi:10.1902/jop.2002.73.8.835 PMID:12211491

Osorio, R., Osorio, E., Medina-Castillo, A. L., & Toledano, M. (2014). Polymer Nanocarriers for Dentin Adhesion. *Journal of Dental Research*, *93*(12), 1258–1263. doi:10.1177/0022034514551608 PMID:25227634

Ozak, S. T., & Ozkan, P. (2013). Nanotechnology and dentistry. *European Journal of Dentistry*, *7*(1), 145–151. PMID:23408486

Pagonis, T. C., Chen, J., Fontana, C. R., Devalapally, H., Ruggiero, K., Song, X., & Yamazaki, H. et al. (2010). Nanoparticle-based endodontic antimicrobial photodynamic therapy. *Journal of Endodontics*, *36*(2), 322–328. doi:10.1016/j.joen.2009.10.011 PMID:20113801

Paquette, D., Oringer, R., Lessem, J., Offenbacher, S., Genco, R., Persson, G. R., & Williams, R. C. et al. (2003). Locally delivered minocycline microspheres for the treatment of periodontitis in smokers. *Journal of Clinical Periodontology*, *30*(9), 787–794. doi:10.1034/j.1600-051X.2003.00375.x PMID:12956654

Park, Y. J., Lee, J. Y., Yeom, H. R., Kim, K. H., Lee, S. C., Shim, I. K., & Lee, S. J. et al. (2005). Injectable polysaccharide microcapsules for prolonged release of minocycline for the treatment of periodontitis. *Biotechnology Letters*, *27*(22), 1761–1766. doi:10.1007/s10529-005-3550-7 PMID:16314967

Persadmehr, A., Torneck, C. D., Cvitkovitch, D. G., Pinto, V., Talior, I., Kazembe, M., & Kishen, A. et al. (2014). Bioactive chitosan nanoparticles and photodynamic therapy inhibit collagen degradation in vitro. *Journal of Endodontics*, *40*(5), 703–709. doi:10.1016/j.joen.2013.11.004 PMID:24767568

Persson, G. R., Salvi, G. E., Heitz-Mayfield, L. J., & Lang, N. P. (2006). Antimicrobial therapy using a local drug delivery system (Arestin®) in the treatment of peri-implantitis. I: Microbiological outcomes. *Clinical Oral Implants Research*, *17*(4), 386–393. doi:10.1111/j.1600-0501.2006.01269.x PMID:16907769

Piao, Z.-G., Kim, J.-S., Son, J.-S., Lee, S.-Y., Fang, X.-H., Oh, J.-S., & Kim, S.-G. et al. (2014). Osteogenic evaluation of collagen membrane containing drug-loaded polymeric microparticles in a rat calvarial defect model. *Tissue Engineering. Part A*, *20*(23-24), 3322–3331. doi:10.1089/ten.tea.2013.0717 PMID:24967649

Pinheiro, E., Gomes, B., Ferraz, C., Sousa, E., Teixeira, F., & Souza-Filho, F. (2003). Microorganisms from canals of root-filled teeth with periapical lesions. *International Endodontic Journal*, *36*(1), 1–11. doi:10.1046/j.1365-2591.2003.00603.x PMID:12656508

Pinon-Segundo, E., Ganem-Quintanar, A., Alonso-Perez, V., & Quintanar-Guerrero, D. (2005). Preparation and characterization of triclosan nanoparticles for periodontal treatment. *International Journal of Pharmaceutics*, *294*(1-2), 217–232. doi:10.1016/j.ijpharm.2004.11.010 PMID:15814246

Portenier, I., Waltimo, T. M., & Haapasalo, M. (2003). Enterococcus faecalis–the root canal survivor and 'star' in post-treatment disease. *Endodontic topics, 6*(1), 135-159.

Rai, M., Yadav, A., & Gade, A. (2009). Silver nanoparticles as a new generation of antimicrobials. *Biotechnology Advances*, *27*(1), 76–83. doi:10.1016/j.biotechadv.2008.09.002 PMID:18854209

Reis, K. R., Bonfante, G., Pegoraro, L. F., Conti, P. C. R., Oliveira, P. C. G., & Kaizer, O. B. (2008). In vitro wear resistance of three types of polymethyl methacrylate denture teeth. *Journal of Applied Oral Science*, *16*(3), 176–180. doi:10.1590/S1678-77572008000300003 PMID:19089214

Renvert, S., Lessem, J., Dahlén, G., Lindahl, C., & Svensson, M. (2006). Topical minocycline microspheres versus topical chlorhexidine gel as an adjunct to mechanical debridement of incipient peri-implant infections: A randomized clinical trial. *Journal of Clinical Periodontology*, *33*(5), 362–369. doi:10.1111/j.1600-051X.2006.00919.x PMID:16634959

Renvert, S., Lessem, J., Dahlen, G., Renvert, H., & Lindahl, C. (2008). Mechanical and repeated antimicrobial therapy using a local drug delivery system in the treatment of peri-implantitis: A randomized clinical trial. *Journal of Periodontology*, *79*(5), 836–844. doi:10.1902/jop.2008.070347 PMID:18454662

Rosa, V., Bona, A. D., Cavalcanti, B. N., & Nör, J. E. (2012). Tissue engineering: from research to dental clinics. *Dental materials: official publication of the Academy of Dental Materials, 28*(4), 341-348.

Saavedra, G., Valandro, L. F., Leite, F. P., Amaral, R., Ozcan, M., & Bottino, M. A. et al.. (2007). Bond strength of acrylic teeth to denture base resin after various surface conditioning methods before and after thermocycling. *The International Journal of Prosthodontics*, *20*(2), 199–201. PMID:17455445

Saleh, I., Ruyter, I., Haapasalo, M., & Ørstavik, D. (2004). Survival of Enterococcus faecalis in infected dentinal tubules after root canal filling with different root canal sealers in vitro. *International Endodontic Journal*, *37*(3), 193–198. doi:10.1111/j.0143-2885.2004.00785.x PMID:15009409

Samdancioglu, S., Calis, S., Sumnu, M., & Atilla Hincal, A. (2006). Formulation and in vitro evaluation of bisphosphonate loaded microspheres for implantation in osteolysis. *Drug Development and Industrial Pharmacy*, *32*(4), 473–481. doi:10.1080/03639040500528871 PMID:16638686

Scheifele, E., Studen-Pavlovich, D., & Markovic, N. (2002). Practitioner's guide to fluoride.[xi.]. *Dental Clinics of North America*, *46*(4), 831–846. doi:10.1016/S0011-8532(02)00019-8 PMID:12436834

Schwartz-Arad, D., & Chaushu, G. (1997). Placement of Implants Into Fresh Extraction Sites: 4 to 7 Years Retrospective Evaluation of 95 Immediate Implants. *Journal of Periodontology*, *68*(11), 1110–1116. doi:10.1902/jop.1997.68.11.1110 PMID:9407405

Selwitz, R. H., Ismail, A. I., & Pitts, N. B. (2007). Dental caries. *Lancet, 369*(9555), 51–59. doi:10.1016/S0140-6736(07)60031-2 PMID:17208642

Sharma, G., Puranik, M. P., & K.R, S. (2015). Approaches to Arresting Dental Caries: An Update. *Journal of Clinical and Diagnostic Research: JCDR, 9*(5), ZE08-ZE11.

Shrestha, A., Fong, S.-W., Khoo, B.-C., & Kishen, A. (2009). Delivery of Antibacterial Nanoparticles into Dentinal Tubules Using High-intensity Focused Ultrasound. *Journal of Endodontics, 35*(7), 1028–1033. doi:10.1016/j.joen.2009.04.015 PMID:19567328

Shrestha, A., Friedman, S., & Kishen, A. (2011). Photodynamically Crosslinked and Chitosan-incorporated Dentin Collagen. *Journal of Dental Research, 90*(11), 1346–1351. doi:10.1177/0022034511421928 PMID:21911787

Shrestha, A., Hamblin, M. R., & Kishen, A. (2014). Photoactivated rose bengal functionalized chitosan nanoparticles produce antibacterial/biofilm activity and stabilize dentin-collagen. *Nanomedicine; Nanotechnology, Biology, and Medicine, 10*(3), 491–501. doi:10.1016/j.nano.2013.10.010 PMID:24200522

Smeets, R., Gerhards, F., Stein, J., Pereira Paz, R. M., Vogt, S., Pautke, C., & Kolk, A. et al. (2011). A novel hemostatic delivery device for thrombin: Biodegradable poly(D,L-lactide-co-glycolide) 50:50 microspheres. *Journal of Biomedical Materials Research. Part A, 96A*(1), 177–185. doi:10.1002/jbm.a.32970 PMID:21105166

Socransky, S. S., & Haffajee, A. D. (1994). Evidence of bacterial etiology: A historical perspective. *Periodontology 2000, 5*(1), 7–25. doi:10.1111/j.1600-0757.1994.tb00016.x PMID:9673160

Solhi, L., Atai, M., Nodehi, A., & Imani, M. (2012). A novel dentin bonding system containing poly(methacrylic acid) grafted nanoclay: Synthesis, characterization and properties. *Dental Materials, 28*(10), 1041–1050. doi:10.1016/j.dental.2012.06.004 PMID:22795491

Solhi, L., Atai, M., Nodehi, A., Imani, M., Ghaemi, A., & Khosravi, K. (2012). Poly (acrylic acid) grafted montmorillonite as novel fillers for dental adhesives: Synthesis, characterization and properties of the adhesive. *Dental Materials, 28*(4), 369–377. doi:10.1016/j.dental.2011.11.010 PMID:22169675

Son, J. S., Choi, Y.-A., Park, E.-K., Kwon, T.-Y., Kim, K.-H., & Lee, K.-B. (2013). Drug delivery from hydroxyapatite-coated titanium surfaces using biodegradable particle carriers. *Journal of Biomedical Materials Research. Part B, Applied Biomaterials, 101B*(2), 247–257. doi:10.1002/jbm.b.32834 PMID:23143817

Sousa, F. F., Luzardo-Alvarez, A., Perez-Estevez, A., Seoane-Prado, R., & Blanco-Mendez, J. (2010). Development of a novel AMX-loaded PLGA/zein microsphere for root canal disinfection. *Biomedical Materials (Bristol, England), 5*(5), 055008. doi:10.1088/1748-6041/5/5/055008 PMID:20844319

Srirangarajan, S., Mundargi, R. C., Ravindra, S., Setty, S. B., Aminabhavi, T., & Thakur, S. (2011). Randomized, controlled, single-masked, clinical study to compare and evaluate the efficacy of microspheres and gel in periodontal pocket therapy. *Journal of Periodontology, 82*(1), 114–121. doi:10.1902/jop.2010.100324 PMID:20681818

Stuart, C. H., Schwartz, S. A., Beeson, T. J., & Owatz, C. B. (2006). Enterococcus faecalis: Its role in root canal treatment failure and current concepts in retreatment. *Journal of Endodontics*, *32*(2), 93–98. doi:10.1016/j.joen.2005.10.049 PMID:16427453

Sun, X. Z., Wang, N., Cao, D., Hu, Z. Y., Mao, P., Zhang, H. B., & Zhou, X. H. (2011). The antimicrobial activities of a series of bis-quaternary ammonium compounds. *Chinese Chemical Letters*, *22*(8), 887–890. doi:10.1016/j.cclet.2011.01.030

Tsukada, K., Goan, K., & Furusawa, N. (2008). Fluorescent semiconductor microparticle, method for production of the microparticle, fluorescent labeling agent for biological substance using the microparticle, and bioimaging method using the microparticle: Google Patents.

Upadya, M., Shrestha, A., & Kishen, A. (2011). Role of Efflux Pump Inhibitors on the Antibiofilm Efficacy of Calcium Hydroxide, Chitosan Nanoparticles, and Light-activated Disinfection. *Journal of Endodontics*, *37*(10), 1422–1426. doi:10.1016/j.joen.2011.06.017 PMID:21924195

Van Rijkom, H., Truin, G., & Van't Hof, M. (1998). A meta-analysis of clinical studies on the caries-inhibiting effect of fluoride gel treatment. *Caries Research*, *32*(2), 83–92. doi:10.1159/000016436 PMID:9544855

van Strijp, A., Buijs, M., & Ten Cate, J. (1999). In situ fluoride retention in enamel and dentine after the use of an amine fluoride dentifrice and amine fluoride/sodium fluoride mouthrinse. *Caries Research*, *33*(1), 61–65. doi:10.1159/000016496 PMID:9831781

Wang, C.-Z., Fu, Y.-C., Jian, S.-C., Wang, Y.-H., Liu, P.-L., Ho, M.-L., & Wang, C.-K. (2014). Synthesis and characterization of cationic polymeric nanoparticles as simvastatin carriers for enhancing the osteogenesis of bone marrow mesenchymal stem cells. *Journal of Colloid and Interface Science*, *432*, 190–199. doi:10.1016/j.jcis.2014.06.037 PMID:25086394

Wang, F., Song, Y. L., Li, C. X., Li, D. H., Zhang, H. P., Ma, A. J., & Zhou, W. et al. (2010). Sustained release of insulin-like growth factor-1 from poly(lactide-co-glycolide) microspheres improves osseointegration of dental implants in type 2 diabetic rats. *European Journal of Pharmacology*, *640*(1-3), 226–232. doi:10.1016/j.ejphar.2010.04.024 PMID:20438725

Wang, J. J., Zeng, Z. W., Xiao, R. Z., Xie, T., Zhou, G. L., & Zhan, X. R. et al.. (2011). Recent advances of chitosan nanoparticles as drug carriers. *International Journal of Nanomedicine*, *6*, 765–774. PMID:21589644

Wang, L. C., Wu, H., Chen, X. G., De Li, L., Ji, Q. X., & Liu, C. S. et al.. (2008). Biological evaluation of a novel chitosan-PVA-based local delivery system for treatment of periodontitis. *Journal of Biomedical Materials Research. Part A*, *91*(4), 1065–1076. PMID:19107793

Wang, W., Liao, S., Zhu, Y., Liu, M., Zhao, Q., & Fu, Y. (2015). Recent applications of nanomaterials in prosthodontics. *Journal of Nanomaterials*, *2015*, 3. doi:10.3390/nano6010003

Watson, P. S., Pontefract, H. A., Devine, D. A., Shore, R. C., Nattress, B. R., Kirkham, J., & Robinson, C. (2005). Penetration of fluoride into natural plaque biofilms. *Journal of Dental Research*, *84*(5), 451–455. doi:10.1177/154405910508400510 PMID:15840782

Whitman, D., McKinney, J., Hinman, R., Hesby, R., & Pelleu, G. Jr. (1987). In vitro wear rates of three types of commercial denture tooth materials. *The Journal of Prosthetic Dentistry*, *57*(2), 243–246. doi:10.1016/0022-3913(87)90154-5 PMID:3470516

Williams, R. C. (1990). Periodontal Disease. *The New England Journal of Medicine*, *322*(6), 373–382. doi:10.1056/NEJM199002083220606 PMID:2405268

Wilson, M. (1993). Photolysis of oral bacteria and its potential use in the treatment of caries and periodontal disease. *The Journal of Applied Bacteriology*, *75*(4), 299–306. doi:10.1111/j.1365-2672.1993.tb02780.x PMID:8226389

Wu, H., Zhang, Z., Zhao, H., Wu, D., Wu, B., & Cong, R. (2004). Preparation of sodium fluoride-loaded gelatin microspheres, characterization and cariostatic studies. *Journal of Microencapsulation*, *21*(8), 889–903. doi:10.1080/02652040400015445 PMID:15799544

Wu, S. Z., Hossainy, S. F., Harish, S., Sanders-Millare, D., & Mirzaee, D. (2003). Microparticle coated medical device: Google Patents.

Yao, W., Xu, P., Pang, Z., Zhao, J., Chai, Z., & Li, X. et al.. (2014). Local delivery of minocycline-loaded PEG-PLA nanoparticles for the enhanced treatment of periodontitis in dogs. *International Journal of Nanomedicine*, *9*, 3963–3970. PMID:25170266

Yonamine, Y., Matsuyama, T., Sonomura, T., Takeuchi, H., Furuichi, Y., Uemura, M., & Noguchi, K. et al. (2010). Effectable application of vascular endothelial growth factor to critical sized rat calvaria defects. *Oral Surgery, Oral Medicine, Oral Pathology, Oral Radiology, and Endodontology*, *109*(2), 225–231. doi:10.1016/j.tripleo.2009.09.010 PMID:20034820

Yong, C. W. (2014). Study of interactions between polymer nanoparticles and cell membranes at atomistic levels. *Philosophical Transactions of the Royal Society of London B: Biological Sciences, 370*(1661). Doi:10.1098/rstb.2014.0036

Yue, I. C., Poff, J., Cortes, M. E., Sinisterra, R. D., Faris, C. B., Hildgen, P., & Shastri, V. P. et al. (2004). A novel polymeric chlorhexidine delivery device for the treatment of periodontal disease. *Biomaterials*, *25*(17), 3743–3750. doi:10.1016/j.biomaterials.2003.09.113 PMID:15020150

Zeren, K. J. (2006). Minimally invasive extraction and immediate implant placement: The preservation of esthetics. *The International Journal of Periodontics & Restorative Dentistry*, *26*(2), 171–181. PMID:16642906

Zhao, H., Wu, B., Wu, H., Su, L., Pang, J., Yang, T., & Liu, Y. (2006). Protective immunity in rats by intranasal immunization with Streptococcus mutans glucan-binding protein D encapsulated into chitosan-coated poly(lactic-co-glycolic acid) microspheres. *Biotechnology Letters*, *28*(16), 1299–1304. doi:10.1007/s10529-006-9086-7 PMID:16804764

Zheng, Y., Chen, Y., Jin, L. W., Ye, H. Y., & Liu, G. (2016). Cytotoxicity and Genotoxicity in Human Embryonic Kidney Cells Exposed to Surface Modify Chitosan Nanoparticles Loaded with Curcumin. *AAPS PharmSciTech*. PMID:26718819

Zou, G.-K., Song, Y.-L., Zhou, W., Yu, M., Liang, L.-H., Sun, D.-C., et al. (2012). Effects of local delivery of bFGF from PLGA microspheres on osseointegration around implants in diabetic rats. *Oral surgery, oral medicine, oral pathology and oral radiology, 114*(3), 284-289.

This work was previously published in Advancing Medicine through Nanotechnology and Nanomechanics Applications edited by Keka Talukdar, Mayank Bhushan, and Anil Shantappa Malipatil, pages 44-77, copyright year 2017 by Medical Information Science Reference (an imprint of IGI Global).

Section 2
Diagnostics and Imaging

Chapter 6
Adding Technology to Diagnostic Methods

John C. Radke, BM, MBA
BioResearch Associates, USA

ABSTRACT

Adding technology to clinical diagnosis improves patient care, because objective measurements enhance the patient's report of symptoms and the observations made during an examination. The combination of multiple tests has universally been acknowledged to improve diagnostic sensitivity and specificity, as well as add value to treatment effectiveness monitoring and treatment outcomes. This chapter discusses four dental technologies that objectively measure differing masticatory functions: Surface Electromyography, Magnet-Based 3-Dimensional Electrognathography, Temporomandibular Joint Vibration Analysis, and T-Scan Computerized Occlusal Analysis. Each technology is presented with examples of its output data recorded from both an asymptomatic patient and one demonstrating masticatory system dysfunction. An included case report illustrates how combining these technologies can therapeutically improve a symptomatic Occluso-Muscle Disorder patient's diagnosis and treatment. Finally, recommendations are made that Dental Medicine accept these technologies as an indispensable part of modern clinical practice, so that resistance to their implementation will no longer inhibit their use.

INTRODUCTION

There are three types of data collection methods used in healthcare to gather information for research, for diagnostic purposes, or to monitor treatment outcomes. They are:

- Self Report (Patient History).
    - Type of data: Subjective
- Observation (Clinical Examination).
    - Type of data: Subjective/Objective
- Bio-Physiologic Measurement (BPM).
    - Type of data: Objective/Subjective (Interpretation)

DOI: 10.4018/978-1-5225-1903-4.ch006

Of the above three methods, Biophysiologic Measurement is the most quantifiable (e.g. blood pressure, heart rate, range of motion), since it incorporates modern measurement equipment, and currently takes full advantage of the latest advances in computer technology. Despite the advantages of incorporating digital technology in dental practice, resistance within the dental community discounts the application of technology to dental diagnosis and treatment monitoring (Reid and Greene, 2013; Greene, Klasser & Epstein, 2010; Greene, 2010a; Greene, 2010b). In the 21st century, this resistance is surprising especially considering that there exists a myriad of evidence -based information, published studies, and extensive dental literature, that demonstrate the efficacy of various technologies for specific dental applications.

However, a closer inspection of some published literature that appeared in1969, proposed a psycho-social and stress-related theoretical epidemiology of what was termed "Myofascial Pain Dysfunction Syndrome" (MPDS), that to date, has long fueled the debate as to the need, or lack thereof, to employ measurement technology when diagnosing Temporomandibular Disorders (TMD) (Greene, Lerman, Sutcher & Laskin, 1969). The biopsychosocial etiology minimizes the role that the breakdown of masticatory structures plays in the appearance of Temporomandibular Disorder symptoms, thereby eliminating the need to measure physical and structural function. This stress-related epidemiologic theory was further perpetuated into the early 1990s, when the so-called "Research Diagnostic Criteria" was first postulated as a valid method to diagnose TMD (Dworkin & LeResche, 1992). The ongoing belief within the dental profession that TMD is caused by emotional stress, explains why some clinicians and authors still resist using any bio-physiological measurements in clinical diagnosis. The "biopsychosocial" theorists' rejection of virtually all physical diagnostic measurement, is based in their (incorrect) assumption that TMD has no causative physical structural basis. It is interesting to note that resistance to technology-aided TMD diagnosis is maintained philosophically, despite there being a complete lack of reproducible physical data to support these biopsychosocial theories. Alternatively, the dental literature does contain many studies that detail the benefits that technology offers to patients who present with Temporomandibular Disorders, some of which will be described within this chapter. While scientific honesty requires acknowledging conflicting or competing theories, it can be a difficult pill to swallow.

Biophysiologic Measurements

In some cases BPM does require some interpretation (e.g. MRI Images), which adds a degree of subjectivity. However, *Observation* is far less quantifiable. For example there is no quantification obtained when stating, "you look sad and appear to have a rash", or when asking "are you just too warm?" (Carr, 1994; Pollack & Panacek, 2000) While some observations can be objective (e.g. a missing tooth), much of what is observed is highly subjective (e.g. muscle palpation). Thus, BPM is the most objective and *Observation* is the least objective, but BPM can also potentially be physically intrusive (e.g. ionizing radiation). Self-report falls somewhere in between, being less quantifiable, less objective, but also somewhat less intrusive than BPM. The analysis of a patient's history and/or examination data, due to the subjectivity of those methods, sometimes combines a number of variables into a scale or index in an attempt to mitigate this shortcoming (Helkimo, 1974).

Biophysiologic measurements are rarely applied in medicine or dentistry with the idea of arriving at a diagnosis in a vacuum (without an included history or clinical examination). Often, only a partial diagnosis is determined (e.g., an "arthritic condyle" is not a complete diagnosis for the typical TMD patient). It would be considered unusual to draw blood without taking a patient's oral disease history, examining the patient, and establishing a rationale for drawing the patient's blood. The objective measurements of physiologic parameters are routinely combined with the history and clinical findings to enhance the preliminary diagnosis, without eliminating their diagnostic need. Expecting technology to replace the need to evaluate a patient's history and/or examine the patient would be ludicrous. Yet, some authors have advocated, expected, or presumed, that technology is completely useless, if it cannot diagnose TMD in a vacuum, without any history, clinical examination, or radiographs (Greene, 1973; Lund, Widmer, & Feine, 1995).

Using Technology to Monitor the Progress and Outcome of Treatment

Implementing a technology can be a beneficial diagnostic tool in a modern day clinical practice to identify a specific type of dysfunction, such as muscle hyperactivity, joint structural breakdown, or occlusal forces, but technology also can be used to document the elimination of the dysfunction. In addition to relying on patient's subjective interpretation and feedback to questions such as, "can you chew better?", technology has offered means to obtain objective, quantifiable measurements of masticatory function. Diagnostic technology available today is useful for gathering essential, in-depth information during an initial patient examination, for the monitoring the progress of any rendered treatment, while providing an objective indicator of the extent of attained-improvement in function that can be observed during the course of treatment.

A Comparison of Data Quality

A number of factors are to be considered relevant when utilizing BPM methods to gather physiologic data:

- **Validity:** A measure of how well the method captures what is being measured. With BPM, it is possible to precisely measure the accuracy of the gathered measurements using accurate tools that are readily available and traceable to the National Institute of Standards and Technology (NIST). For example, the calibration of a jaw tracking device can be refined to within ± 0.1 mm, using a very accurate voltmeter. However, for Self-Report and Observation, "inter-rater reliability" and "repeat testing" are often used to estimate the accuracy, but no absolutely accurate "Gold Standard" is available.
- **Reliability:** The degree of consistency associated with the method. Again, BPM can be "bench tested" to a precise level, but *Observation* requires repeated testing of each new observer to establish even a reasonable estimate of reliability. While it is possible to sample a group of patients and estimate the reliability of the groups' reporting, there is no way to estimate the reliability of an individual patient's reporting. This requires that the clinician impart a degree of skepticism to a patient's uncorroborated reports, without offending the patient.
- **Stability:** The level of change over a time period. Self-Report has been shown to be rather unstable over time, especially with respect to grading pain (Sisk, Grover & Steflik, 1991; Eli, Baht, Kozlovsky & Simon, 2000; Salé, Hedman & Isberg, 2010; Yarnitsky, Sprecher, Zaslansky & Hemli, 1996). The stability of BPM is a function of the design of the specific instrument, but in healthcare applications, periodic re-calibration of the instrumentation is a routine requirement, which generally assures very consistent long-term stability.

Data Analysis

Subjective interpretation of the significance of data can be difficult in any clinical case, but the possibility of developing normal ranges of BPM data, is a distinct advantage of using technology to measure physiology. A commonly encountered error committed when analyzing subjective data, is the use of parametric statistics to analyze subjective data, without considering the assumptions that are inherent. It is always incorrect to treat subjective estimates, like a Visual Analog Scale (VAS), or the Beck Depression Inventory, as if they were precisely measured data (Freedman, 2000). While it can be useful in certain situations, using parametric statistics to evaluate subjective data requires a very thoughtful application (Dimitri, Wall & Oas, 1996). However, measured BPM data are real numbers, contain a zero value with interval or ratio scales, and can often be analyzed using parametric statistical methods. In general, categorical, rank, or nominal (subjective) data are limited to non-parametric methods. Small sample sizes where N values ≤ 6 that are common in dental research studies, also require the use of non-parametric statistics. The inappropriate use of parametric statistics can result in finding significance when it is not actually there (known as a Type II statistical error), but the use of non-parametric statistics also risks not finding significance when it is present (known as a Type I statistical error).

Normative Data Ranges

While medicine has normative ranges for all sorts of physiologic data (such as PSA, white blood cell counts, heart rate), dentistry has been rather skittish about accepting normative values, especially when related to bio-physiological measurements. The normal range of opening the mouth wide, which can be measured without any new technology, is reported to be between 40 to 70+ mm. While this is a rather broad range of values, a measurement of 27 mm is clearly not within the normal range. Thus, while normal ranges of values do not always identify a problem, they aid in establishing a diagnosis.

This chapter focuses on the individual advantages of the most popular masticatory system function technologies that are currently available to the clinician and can enhance their diagnostic capability. These technologies are capable of identifying various Stomatognathic system dysfunctions, and evaluating the overall quality of a patient's masticatory function.

BACKGROUND

Bio-physiological measurement, sometimes also referred to as "Biometrics," has been historically limited as research tools within the dental profession. Only forward-thinking clinicians have considered incorporating BPM into clinical protocols. An early recommendation for the use of Electromyography (EMG) for clinical diagnostic purposes occurred in the late 1940s (Thompson, 1949). He was perhaps, the first to recognize the significant affects that muscle function and dysfunction had on clinical orthodontic treatment. Minimal consideration was given to electromyography until the 1960s, when some clinicians more seriously began to study muscle function (Ahlgren & Posselt, 1963). During this period, occlusal equilibration was the most popular treatment for Occluso-muscle dysfunction (in1966, this condition was termed TMJ Dysfunction Syndrome), such that some clinicians were testing its efficacy (Liebman & Kussick, 1966). It was also during this time that TMJ Syndrome became a more broadly recognized condition within the dental profession (Weisengreen & Elliott, 1963; Franks, 1965). Additionally, other authors were beginning to consider the significance of the electromyographic silent period with respect to occlusal function (Brenman, Black, & Coslet, 1968).

During the 1970s, EMG was extensively studied, such that published research studies began to appear in the dental literature. Research was performed using animal models (dogs, cats, rabbits, rats, etc.), the research focused on revealing the workings of the neuromuscular system. The recording and analysis of the electromyographic silent period and neuromuscular reflexes, were an important part of that process (Fujii & Mitani, 1973). The power spectrum analysis of the EMG signal was hypothesized to be related to the level of fatigue within a muscle (Mitani, Yamashita, Fujii, Kato, & Koizumi, 1974). It was during the 1970s, that the argument between the TMJ oriented group (led by Dr. William Farrar), and the Myofascial Pain Dysfunction Syndrome (MPDS) oriented group (led by Dr. Dan Laskin) heightened. Farrar advocated differentiating specific physiological conditions within the, then named, "TMJ dysfunction syndrome" (Farrar, 1972), while Laskin advocated a mainly psychological and stress basis for the epidemiology of MPDS (Laskin, 1970).

While the MPDS theory became widely accepted during the 1970s, it later in the 1980s sustained a significant loss of support due to the popularity of the more physiological and TM Joint-based etiologic theories. Additionally, MPDS lacked valid research to substantiate it (McNeill, Danzig, Farrar, Gelb, Lerman, Moffett, Pertes, Solberg, & Weinberg, 1980). The concept that emotional stress could be the primary initiating factor in the development of the dysfunction, irrespective of the name, was contraindicated by the high prevalence of TM joint noises, TM joint pains, limitations in condylar translation, occlusal wear, chronic masticatory muscular pain and fatigue, and other non-emotional structural issues. Finally, a conference was organized to make some basic recommendations to the dental profession regarding the examination, diagnosis, and management of Temporomandibular Disorders (TMD) (American Dental Association, 1983). This report concluded that the dentist was well-suited to diagnose and treat TMD, using both the conservative physiological approach and patient counseling. However, the conference defined "TMD" as an umbrella term that encompassed the differing pain and dysfunctional symptoms that could occur in and around the TMJ region, which did not specify a definitive diagnosis (American Dental Association, 1983).

Beginning around 1990, a number of psychologists and psychiatrists became more vocal regarding TMD, and advocated to the dental profession that TMD should (always) be treated as a chronic pain condition, in which the patient was deemed to be overreacting emotionally to their pain. This approach allowed TMD to become a diagnosis such that TMD became synonymous with MPDS, and its diagnosis was based purely on the presence of reported orofacial pain. It was then, and still is a today, a "one size fits all" diagnosis where:

- The pain is the only concern,
- The underlying physiology or pathology is ignored, and not well understood
- Treatment is focused only on the psychological parameters of cognitive behavioral therapy

The Fallacy of Diagnosing "TMD"

The term "Temporomandibular Disorders" (TMD) was originally coined to replace earlier terminologies:

- **TMJ Dysfunction Syndrome (TMJ):** Terming TM disorders a syndrome, suggested that the cause of the condition was unknown, but (in this case) the condition often involved the joint.

Muscle involvement was considered to be a secondary concern. The term "TMJ Dysfunction Syndrome" replaced the earliest name given to the condition, that was based upon the name of the author who first reported observing this group of common dysfunctional symptoms; Costen's Syndrome (Costen, 1935).

- **Myofascial Pain Dysfunction Syndrome (MPDS):** This syndrome's etiology was also unknown, but was thought to result from emotional stress causing painful masticatory muscles. Any TM joint involvement was considered to be a secondary concern.

The term "Temporomandibular Disorders" was originally offered as a broad category that was supposed to cover any painful conditions affecting the TMJ, the muscles, the head, the neck, and the trigeminal nerves. However, TMD was never originally intended to be a diagnosis. If a clinician diagnosed a patient who presented with TMD, the patient could be suffering from one of the thirty-eight conditions that were deemed to fall under TMD, of which there are 13 categories of headaches, 6 boney disorders, 13 TMJ disorders, and 6 muscle disorders (Okeson, 1996). Thus, until a more specific diagnosis was achieved, an appropriate physiologic treatment could not be properly selected. However, *cognitive behavioral therapy* could be applied to virtually any physical or mental condition or circumstance. The purpose is to council the patient just to accept and learn to live with their condition.

The Research Diagnostic Criteria (RDC/TMD) was an attempt to diagnose specific joint, muscle and pain conditions, that fell under the TMD umbrella, using only subjective methods (Dworkin and LeResche, 1992). It was first published in 1992, two years after the same authors stated that the clinical diagnosis of TM joint conditions was unreliable (Dworkin, LeResche & Von Korff, 1990). They had previously claimed that "...clinical signs are themselves unreliable, changing spontaneously over time and making it difficult to find the same sign during successive examinations" (Dworkin, LeResche, DeRouen & Von Korff, 1990). However, these authors hypothesized that specific TMD conditions could be diagnosed reliably, from clinical subjective methods that graded the severity of chronic pain, and by calibrating examiners (Von Korff, Ormel, Keefe, & Dworkin, 1992). It was also theorized that "dysfunctional chronic pain was a subset of illness behaviors *inconsistent* with medically documented findings, while complaints of pain were prominent" (Dworkin, 1991). In other words, the author suggested that TMD patients have an exaggerated response to a chronic pain condition that most people learn to cope with. This theory suggested that *cognitive behavioral therapy* could effectively teach a TMD patient to "live with their condition" and to "stop acting so dysfunctional".

The RDC/TMD includes one set of rules that are supposed to help detect physical conditions (Axis I), and separate psychometric scales to evaluate the patient for mental disorders of pain-disability, depression, and somatization (Axis II).

Although vast efforts and resources have been expended in attempts to validate the RDC/TMD since 1992, the RDC/TMD has mostly eluded validation. (Schiffman, Truelove, Ohrbach, Gonzalez, Anderson, Jackson, Lenton, Pan & Look, 2007).

The Research Diagnostic Criteria for Temporomandibular Disorders (RDC/TMD)

Clinical TMD Conditions (Axis I)

The physical axis of the RDC/TMD recommended the use of subjective examination rules to distinguish between muscle and TM joint related conditions:

- **Group I:**
    a. Myofascial pain.
    b. Myofascial pain with limited opening.
- **Group II:**
    a. Disk displacement with reduction.
    b. Disk displacement without reduction with limited opening.
    c. Disk displacement without reduction, without limited opening (note: arthrography and MRI are mentioned as possible additional tests for type (c) conditions, but without defined specific criteria and guidelines.
- **Group III:**
    a. Arthralgia.
    b. Osteoarthritis of the TMJ.
    c. Osteoarthrosis of the TMJ.

Tomograms have also been mentioned as a possible additional test for Group III type b and c conditions, but the criteria are identical for:

- Erosion of normal cortical delineation,
- Sclerosis of parts or all of the condyle or the articular eminence, and
- Flattening of joint surfaces, with/without osteophyte formation.

Thus, it must be impossible to differentiate type b) from type c) conditions, tomographically.

The results of the official NIDCR funded validation studies presented at the 2007 IADR meeting in New Orleans (which included 683 subjects), revealed that within Group I, only the category I-b (muscle palpation with 2 pounds of applied load for myofascial pain, combined with a Range of Motion (ROM) limitation of $\leq$ 40 mm) satisfied the established validation requirements for adequate sensitivity and specificity. The other categories (Ia & Ic) in Group I, exhibited unacceptable sensitivities and/or specificities (Lenton, Garfinkel, Huggins, Jackson, Look, Pan, Ohrbach, Truelove & Schiffman, 2007).

Within the Group II of Axis I, no category met the established validation requirements for sensitivity and specificity (Look, Tai, Haugan & Schiffman, 2007).

Within the Group III of Axis I, no category met the established validation requirements for sensitivity and specificity (Truelove, Sommers, Huggins, Schiffman, Ohrbach, Look & Pan, 2007).

Pain-Related Disability and Psychological Status (Axis II)

The purpose of the Axis II was to provide a simple method to assess and classify the global severity of a pain condition, in terms of:

- Pain intensity,
- Pain-related disability,
- Depression, and
- Nonspecific physical symptoms (mainly pain).

Based on the understanding that the subjective report of pain (using a VAS scale) is not solely adequate to discriminate higher levels of pain, the RDC attempts to measure pain-related disability by assessing the extent to which the pain patient can carry out usual daily activities. In addition, self-report methods are employed to measure depression, specifically:

- Current Dysthynia/Depression (Major Depressive Episode, Not specific to TMD),
- Lifetime Dysthynia/Depression (Major Depressive Episode, Not Specific to TMD),
- Current Dysthynia/Depression (any Psychiatric Diagnosis, Not specific to TMD), and
- Lifetime Dysthynia/Depression (any Psychiatric Diagnosis, Not Specific to TMD).

Finally, while the term *somatization* describes a preoccupation with physical symptoms disproportionate to actual physical disease, it was not incorporated into the RDC. However, the SCL-90 somatization scale was included (perhaps just for research purposes), to facilitate the assessment of how subjects with and without diffuse physical symptoms, differ in terms of Axis I TMD status, psychological status, response to TMD pain, and disability" (Dworkin &LeResche, 1992). It is easy to imagine that a patient suffering from orofacial pain and dysfunction who had sought treatment and had been repeatedly been told that their condition is psychosomatic, might develop a dysthymia.

As described above, two aspects of somatization were considered:

- Current Somatization, and
- Lifetime Somatization.

The NIDCR funded RDC/TMD validation study presented at the 2007 IADR meeting in New Orleans did not demonstrate its validity with respect to any aspect of Axis II (Ohrbach, Sherman, Michalovic, Dworkin, Schiffman, Truelove & Turner, 2007). This author was in attendance at the session.

It was thought that adding some BPM to the RDC/TMD, in the form of imaging technology might help to validate it, but to date, no definitive RDC/TMD criteria have yet been proposed that established the indications for when imaging would be appropriate. A recent study determining the possibility of adding imaging to the RDC/TMD protocol, concluded that "it was not possible to select particular patient groups who would benefit more or less from a radiographic examination" (Wiese, Wenzel, Hintze, Petersson, Knutsson, Bakke, List, & Svensson, 2008). Presently, it appears that the use of strictly subjective methods to reliably diagnose specific TMD conditions has not yet been successfully accomplished.

The Research Diagnostic Criteria for Temporomandibular Disorders (Von Korff, Ormel, Keefe & Dworkin, 1992) has been a 20+ year attempt to diagnose a wide variety of orofacial pain conditions using simple clinical methods and avoiding most technological innovations. The vast and very costly efforts to validate this method have, to date, consistently failed such that since 1992, the RDC/TMD has mostly eluded validation. (Schiffman, Truelove, Ohrbach, Gonzalez, Anderson, Jackson, Lenton, Pan, & Look, 2007; Winocur, Reiter, Krichmer & Kaffe, 2010; Naeije, Kalaykova, Visscher & Lobbezoo, 2009). This body of work has made it clear that pain report by itself, or together with observation, cannot be relied upon to delineate a specific diagnosis. It is well past the time to acknowledge the failures associated with limiting the diagnostic protocol for TMD to only an oral history and a clinical examination. It should now be obvious that the addition of BPM to the TMD diagnostic protocol is needed, and in fact, long overdue. The numerous attempts to validate the RDC/TMD have definitively proven at least that much.

Adding Technology to Diagnosis

Combining Multiple Tests

The argument that a specific technology adds no value to the diagnosis of TMD unless it can diagnose TMD by itself, is generally invalid. However, it is somewhat true in the sense that no single test can diagnose all of the thirty-eight distinct categories within TMD. At the same time, it is also a fallacy because TMD is not considered to be a diagnosis.

It is a well-established principle that combining the indications of more than one test can improve the accuracy (sensitivity and/or specificity) of a diagnosis (Biller, Samuels, Zagar, Cook, Arafah, Bonert, Stavrou, Kleinberg, Chipman & Hartman, 2002). The common approach of combining a patient's history and clinical examination findings, is the universal example. Adding X-ray imaging is another way to improve the accuracy of the diagnosis. The concept behind incorporating technology in establishing a diagnosis is not to replace, but to augment the previously accepted methods. Multiple tests generally tend to clarify, rather than confound, the diagnosis.

The combining of tests does require some thought to establish a logical progression. Most diagnostic processes begin with the patient history, since it can be obtained prior to the doctor seeing the patient. The history can give clues about what the doctor should be specifically looking for during the examination. The examination often leads to recommendations of additional tests. Sometimes one diagnostic test will indicate the need for an additional test. This general process can be thought of as an escalation of diagnosis. There is absolutely no logical reason to exclude any part of this process. However, in some cases there may be an economical reason to limit the process.

An example of the contribution that technology can add to making a proper diagnosis is presented below:

A patient history indicated there was childhood trauma to the patient's face. This may, or may not have been the initiating factor for the patient's currently reported orofacial pain condition. The clinical examination revealed nothing obvious that would support a traumatic injury-related condition. A radiograph revealed that a previous fracture of the zygoma had completely healed. Occlusal indicating paper showed that the numbers of tooth contacts were evenly distributed around the arches. However, using available technology, the T-Scan Occlusal Analysis System (Tekscan, Inc. S. Boston, MA, USA), excessive occlusal force was detected between tooth #2 and tooth #31 (FDI #17 & #47). The excessive force was carefully reduced on that one contact. It was then verified that the excessive force had been properly reduced by reusing the computerized occlusal analysis technology after the initial occlusal adjustment procedure, which showed the force had been measurably lessened. This resulted in the elimination of the patient's initial complaint.

Applying Technology to Diagnosis and to Treatment Evaluation

In addition to toothache, dentists are often presented with patient complaints related to pain and dysfunction of the masticatory system. These complaints include, but are not limited to:

- The Temporomandibular joints,
- The masticatory and facial muscles,

- Seven of the 12 cranial nerves,
- The connective tissues,
- An existing malocclusion, and
- An uncomfortable maxillo-mandibular mal-relationship.

The two umbrella terms currently used to describe this broad category of patient complaints, are either Temporomandibular Disorders (TMD), or more recently, Temporomandibular Joint Disorders (TMJD), which was coined by the National Institute for Dental and Craniofacial Research (NIDCR). Neither of these two terms represents a diagnosis, nor do they elucidate the typical patient's condition. They refer to a basket full of conditions that usually interfere with masticatory function, but as defined, include orofacial pain as being the primary relevant symptom. However, pain is the least specific, most subjective symptom a patient can exhibit, and focusing exclusively on it, too often, leads to a narcotic prescriptive solution, which tends to create a new problem of addiction, rather than solving the patient's underlying condition. Addiction eventually leads to the necessity of a withdrawal of the pain medication, before it is possible to effectively treat the real physiologic basis for the condition.

No standard TMD treatment strategy has emerged (besides cognitive behavioral therapy), because TMD includes a heterogeneous variety of conditions. All current, future or previous efforts towards a one-size-fits-all treatment for TMD, is destined to be unsuccessful. The few randomized controlled clinical trials (RCCTs) that have applied various treatments to non-discriminately selected TMD patients, without first establishing a specific diagnosis for the subject group treated, have revealed equivocal results (Alencar Jr. & Becker, 2009; Hamata, Zuim & Garcia, 2009; Truelove, Huggins, Mancl & Dworkin, 2006). Applying the RCCT method to undiagnosed TMD patients guarantees randomly inappropriate treatment (RIT) and usually equivocal results. However, this has not inhibited some from attempting it, nor from publishing their results.

Available Biophysiologic Measurement Technologies

There are four bio-physiologic measurement technologies that can be applied in both the diagnosis, and the treatment monitoring procedures that involve dysfunctional masticatory conditions:

- Surface Electromyography (sEMG),
- Magnet-based Electrognathography (3-Dimensional Mandibular Tracking),
- Temporomandibular Joint Vibration Analysis (JVA), and
- T-Scan Computerized Occlusal Analysis.

Each of these technologies can provide valuable data for objectively assessing both the progress and outcome of treatment. Treatment evaluation and outcomes can be more objective when post-treatment measurements are compared to both normative and pre-treatment data

Electromyography

The relative level of a muscle's activity cannot be determined by palpation or visual means, but it can be determined for some muscles by using surface electromyography (sEMG), (BioEMG III, Bioresearch Associates, Inc., Milwaukee, WI, USA). Specifically, the superficial masseter, the anterior temporalis, the anterior belly of the digastric and the sternocleidomastoid muscles, can be recorded reliably and simultaneously (Christensen, 1989; Ferrario, Sforza, D'Addona, & Miani, 1991; Sforza, Rosati, De Menezes, Musto, & Toma, 2011). However, it should not be understated that the successful use of surface EMG requires proper technique.

Some, who are adamantly opposed to the diagnostic use of surface EMG, compared an undifferentiated group of TMD patients to a non-TMD group, and hypothesized that surface EMG, by itself in a vacuum, should be able to separate the two groups definitively (Manfredini, Cocilovo, Favero, Ferronato, Tonello, & Guarda-Nardini, 2011). However, this hypothesis approaches absurdity. Another longstanding argument against the use of diagnostic surface EMG states that fine wire electrodes embedded into the muscle should be used to measure EMG function, because they are thought to be superior to surface electrodes for EMG recording. However, that argument has been thoroughly disproven (Koole, 1998).

How Is EMG Used Clinically?

While a surface EMG signal is directly proportional to the level of force exerted by the muscle, it is not interchangeable with absolute force measurements. Thus, surface EMG is most useful for comparing several muscles' relative activity within a single individual. The most commonly recorded activities are:

- The residual activity when the mandible is at a resting posture,
- Hard clenching with and without cotton rolls,
- Swallowing activity, and
- During mastication.

An additional application is the use of EMG synchronized together with the T-Scan system, which can record both dynamic occlusal function and masticatory muscle activity levels simultaneously (Kerstein & Radke, 2012).

Due to the limitations of calibration, the analysis of surface EMG data is more qualitative than quantitative. For the most part, the relative values between muscles are usually more significant than the exact number of microvolts recorded per muscle. Since all of the muscles of mastication function together as one unit, their precise interaction is critical to normal function.

Residual Activity at Rest

The normal subject at rest exhibits little muscle activity, usually between 1 - 2 microvolts. This occurs because no "posturing" of the mandible is required for the patient to assume a normal rest position. Posturing is only needed when there is a malocclusion, or some type of skeletal problem exists that compromises a normal maxillo-mandibular relationship. Posturing of the mandible, however, does not require a lot of EMG activity, but when it is continuous, it fatigues the small motor units of hyperactive muscles. Figure 1 describes the relaxed muscle activity levels expected from a normal subject. While the activity level is not zero, it is at or below 2.0 microvolts (average). As the level increases above 2.0 microvolts, it is more likely to indicate problematic muscle physiology.

Hyperactivity at rest occurs when the patient must posture the mandible to compensate for an occlusal or skeletal mal-relationship. It is an auto adaptive mechanism that requires no patient conscious effort.

Figure 1. Relaxed muscles at rest with no evidence of posturing of the mandible[1]

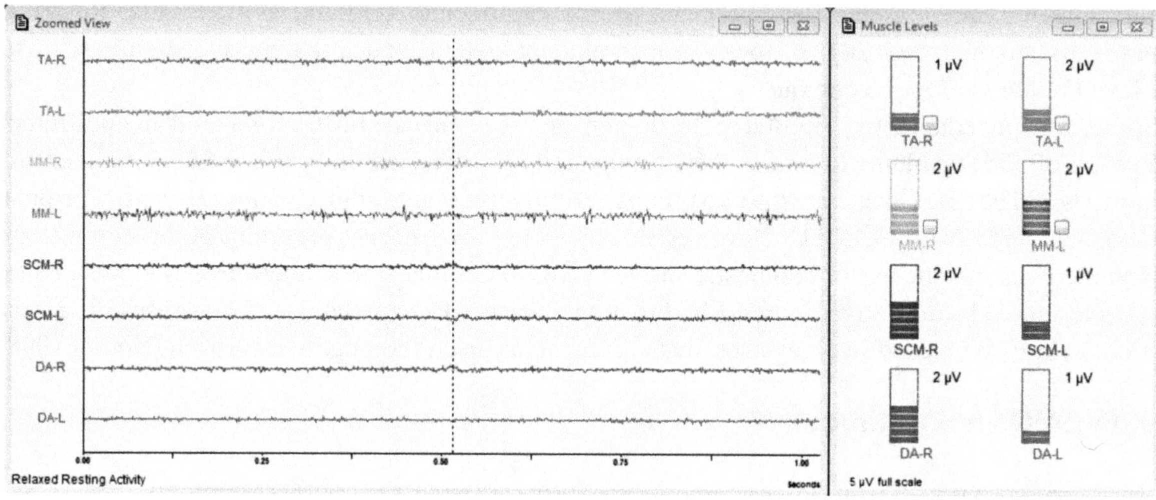

The smallest motor units are active in posturing, but when they fatigue, the next larger motor units are recruited, creating the appearance of "spiking" within the display (Figure 2).

The visible spiking in Figure 2 indicates that the smallest motor units have fatigued, and that the next larger motor units have taken over the posturing activity. The spiking rate is about 10 Hertz (Hz), which is at the slowest rate of firing for skeletal muscles. This rate would yield the lowest amount of force from a given motor unit.

Relaxing the muscles that have visible spiking can eliminate the hyperactivity, and the spiking activity will disappear. However, the spiking activity is a sign and correction of the underlying problem is necessary to maintain relaxation of the muscles at rest.

Figure 2. Hyperactive posturing activity with evidence of spiking with the smallest motor units indicating fatigue

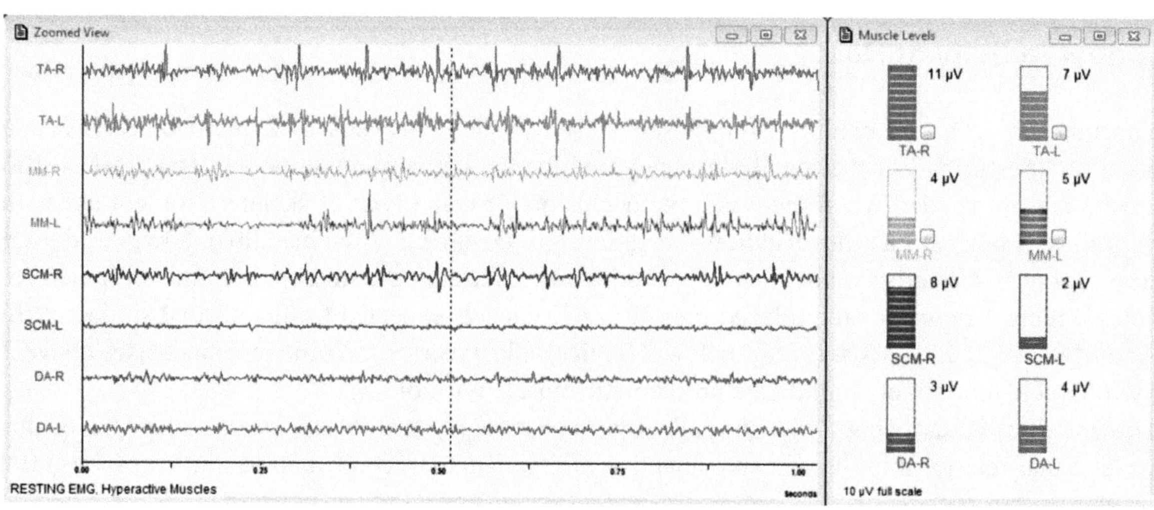

Hard Voluntary Clenching Activity

Clenching activity is usually recorded under one or more of these three conditions:

- A hard voluntary clench in the intercuspal position,
- A hard voluntary clench with cotton rolls between the molars and premolars bilaterally, and
- A hard voluntary clench with only the anterior teeth in contact.

Each clench action is recorded at least 3 times, to gauge its consistency. Clenching is mainly used to evaluate elevator muscles' contractile capability, especially the superficial masseter and anterior temporalis muscles (Figure 3).

When an asymptomatic subject produces a hard clench in the intercuspal position (ICP), the amount of activity will likely be uniform between their left and right side muscles. The levels should also be nearly as uniform between the masseter and temporalis on the same side of the head. Digastric and sternocleidomastoid activity during clenching should be at a minimal level.

When the alignment of the mandible to the maxilla is altered in such a way that the relative balance between these muscles is also altered, the musculature attempts to adjust to the condition by altering the distribution of muscle activity. This requires some muscles (one or two usually) to contract more than the others, while inhibiting the other muscles from contracting as much. Figure 4 shows a typically unbalanced clenching activity. The question then arises as to whether the low-firing muscles are either weak, or are being inhibited.

The cotton roll hard clench can be used to differentiate between muscle weakness and muscle inhibition from the Central Nervous System (CNS). If clenching on cotton rolls produces no change in the pattern towards improved muscular balance, the muscles that are low in output are considered to be weak and muscle strengthening exercises may be indicated. If the pattern improves, as seen in Figure 5, inhibition is responsible for the unbalanced pattern. Then correction of the occlusion or mal-alignment of the maxillomandibular relationship is indicated.

A hard clench with only anterior tooth contact will usually inhibit the elevator musculature overall from contracting. This is one simple way to test the effectiveness of an anterior "discluding" appliance,

Figure 3. An asymptomatic subject demonstrating 3 hard clenches in the intercuspal position. The muscle activity is evenly distributed between the four elevator muscles

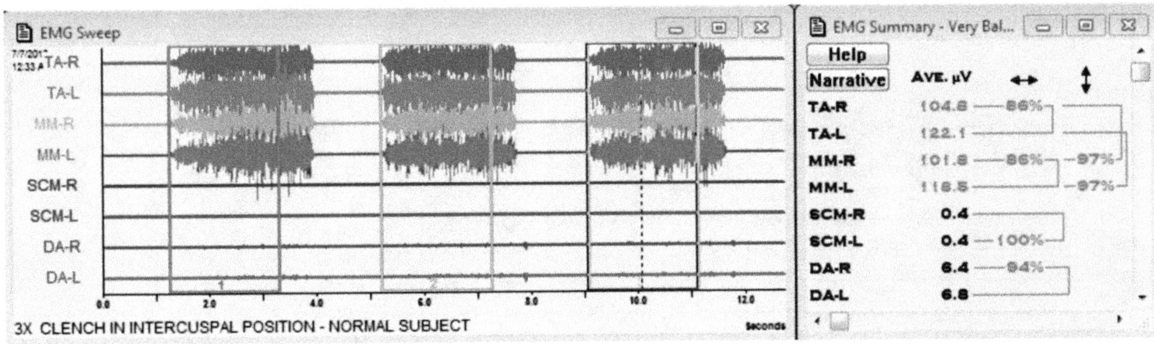

Figure 4. Hard clenching 3 times recorded from a patient with a mal-aligned maxillo-mandibular relationship

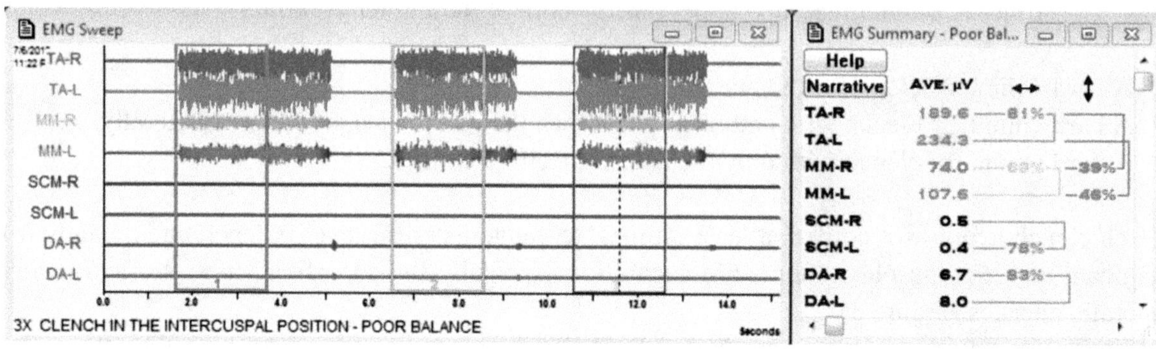

Figure 5. Two successive hard clenching cycles with cotton rolls placed between opposing molars and premolars bilaterally, shows improved balance between the muscles

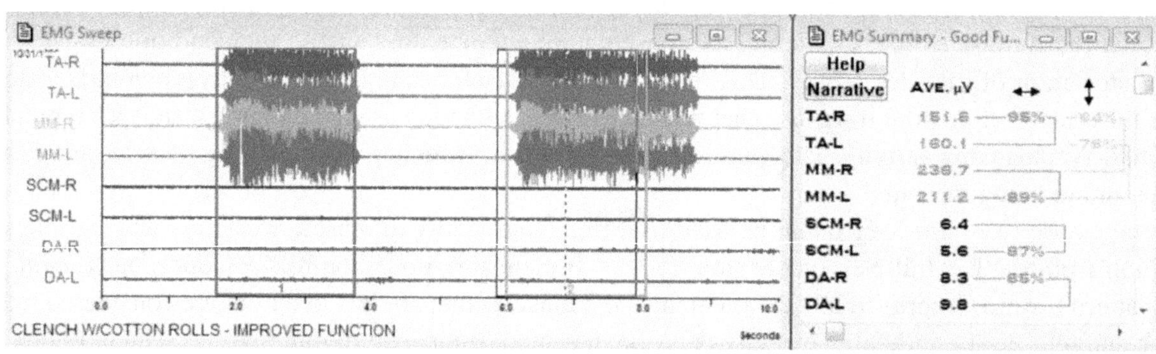

prior to its fabrication. Figure 6 illustrates significant reduction in muscle activity during the middle three clenches. This is not always the case, especially with Class I patients that have a Class III tendency. In most patients, the amount of contractile reduction is usually greater for the temporalis muscles than for the masseter muscles.

Figure 6. The sequence of 3 clenches into ICP, 3 clenches on 1 anterior cotton roll, and 3 clenches with posterior cotton rolls placed, bilaterally

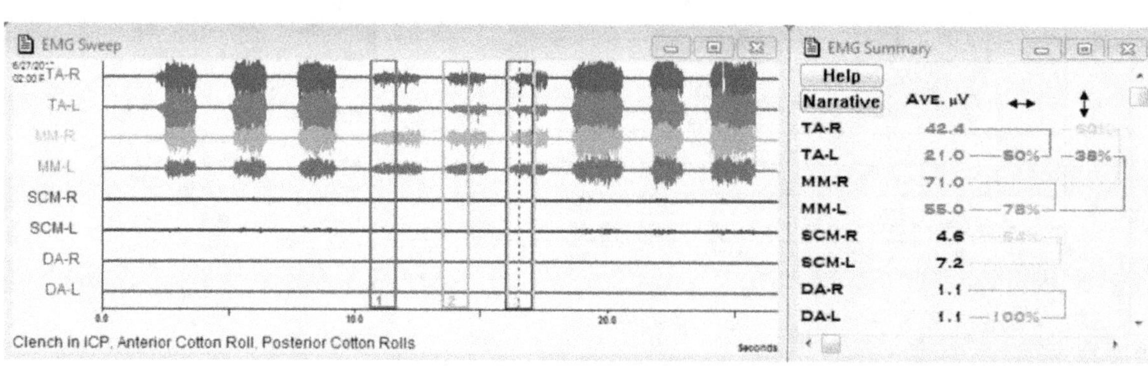

EMG During Mastication

One of the primary (survival) functions of the Stomatognathic system besides breathing and drinking, is the mastication of food. The masticatory system is the beginning of the gastrointestinal system. An efficient masticatory system facilitates the functions of the digestive system.

The relationship between TMD and Irritable Bowel Syndrome (IBS) has not been given significant consideration, although one study suggests a relationship exists. TMD patients exhibited a 46% higher rate of inpatient complaints of IBS, and a 61% higher rate of outpatient claims of IBS, than did non-TMD patients (Shimshak & DeFuria, 1998). However, the authors did not notice whether the reported differences were significant. More recently, another study showed no statistically significant difference in the neuropsychologic profile between a non-responding TMD group (n = 24), and an IBS group (n = 20) (Grossi, Goldberg, Locker & Tenenbaum, 2008). Despite the limited sample size studied, it appeared these two groups may share some common factors. This result suggests that there may be an overlooked connection between masticatory dysfunction and IBS.

These findings also demonstrate that Biometric measurements within the masticatory system may have significance with respect to other areas of the body. A similar study by Korszun et al., reported a 46% concurrence of IBS and TMD (Korszun, Papadopoulos, Demitrack, Engleberg, & Crofford, 1998). While IBS has mostly been dismissed as a stress-related or psychosomatic disorder, it may now be appropriate to evaluate and investigate this subject more thoroughly, to elucidate the relationship between masticatory dysfunction and Irritable Bowel Syndrome.

Evaluating Muscle Function During Mastication

The process of evaluating muscle function during mastication requires the recording of a sequence of muscle activity (EMG), and then averaging the activity across a chewing sequence of ten to twenty chewing cycles. Averaging is necessary to accommodate a changing bolus, since the nature of chewing is variable. To minimize the effect of changing bolus on muscle function during mastication, chewing gum can be used, which is soft and stable, and reproducible in its characteristics. Chewing gum is a bolus that poses a minimal challenge to the masticatory system. Thus, it can be effectively used to record even poor masticatory function. Gum can be considered as a base-line bolus, while food such as beef jerky is a tough bolus that challenges the entire masticatory system. Patients with substantial masticatory dysfunction usually cannot sufficiently masticate a tough bolus.

When the EMG activity is recorded during mastication, it appears as an alternating burst of activity with quiet spaces within the sequence (Figures 7, 8, and 9). The peak-to-peak Raw EMG data can give a qualitative impression of the chewing pattern, but to quantify the activity requires averaging a number of cycles (usually 10 – 15). The superficial masseter and anterior temporalis muscles can indicate chewing cycle closing activity, and the anterior belly of the digastric can indicate opening activity.

Averaging a single cycle can clarify the pattern of activity between muscles, but averaging an entire sequence provides a more accurate indication of muscular chewing capability. Figure 8 shows one right-sided gum chewing cycle from a "normal" subject. The normally expected pattern (mean pattern distribution $\pm$ 2 standard deviations) would have the working masseter (R) as the most active, followed by the working temporalis (R), the non-working temporalis (L) and the non-working masseter (L). That is approximately what we see in the Figure 8. However, each muscle has a unique pattern of activity with significant overlap between the muscles during both elevation and depression. Considering that ad-

Figure 7. The Raw EMG activity of six muscles while chewing gum. The top two channels are the temporalis muscles, the next two below are masseter muscles, and the bottom two are from the anterior belly of the digastric/suprahyoid area musculature

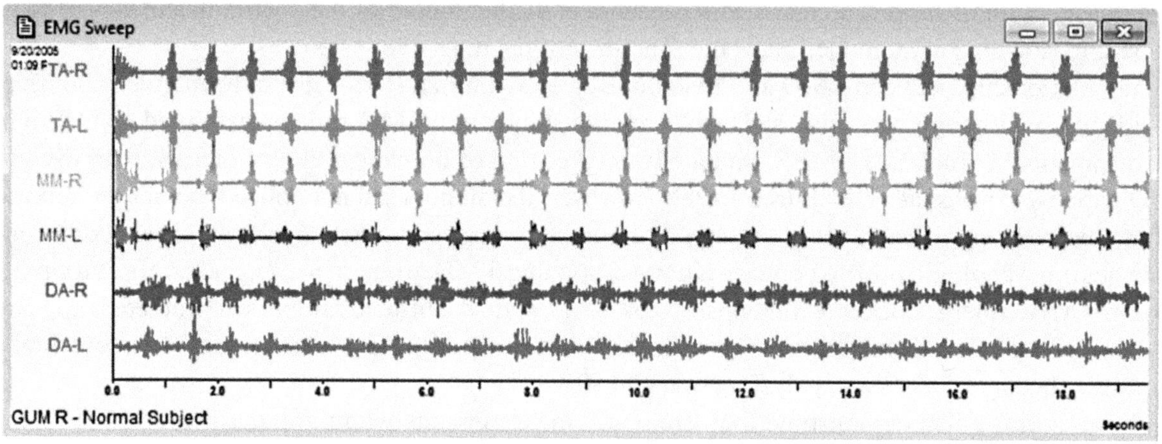

Figure 8. The averaged EMG of one right side chewing cycle with gum as the bolus. The activity of this "normal" subject is distributed non-uniformly between the muscles with considerable overlap and unique timing for each muscle

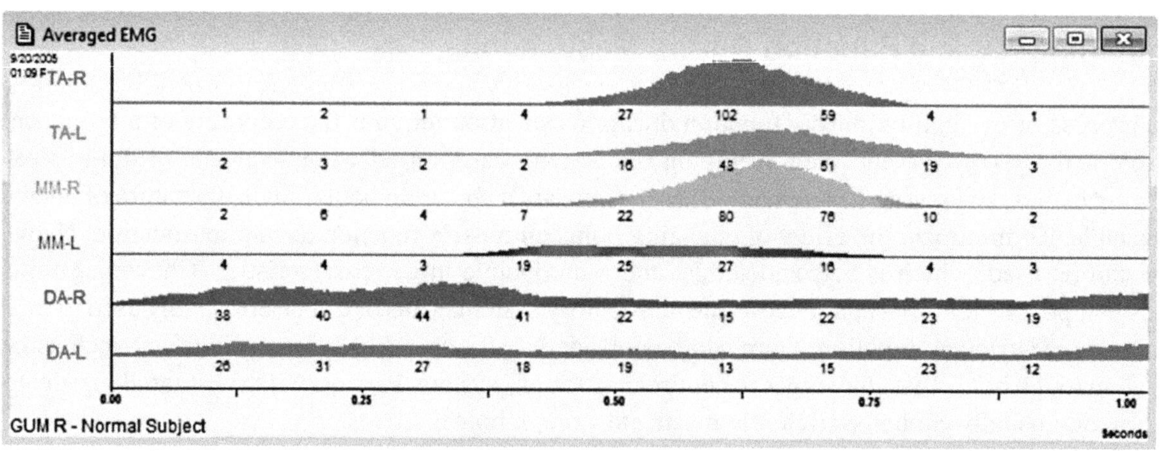

ditional muscles are also contracting, even in this limited example, it is clear that mastication is a group muscle function, such that no one muscle by itself can provide masticatory function.

By averaging 10 - 15 chewing cycles, it is possible to quantify the amount of activity each muscle is contributing to the mastication process. In Figure 9, the activity of an asymptomatic Class I subject is graphed and displayed quantitatively. In terms of both the peak muscle activity, and the average (mean) area under the functional curve (integrated muscle activity), the pattern nicely follows the expected distribution of activity.

Note in Figure 9 that the working masseter is the most active, followed by the working temporalis, then the non-working temporalis, with the least active being the non-working masseter. It is also apparent

Figure 9. The averaged graph and quantitative values of a full sequence of 15 cycles of left-sided gum chewing in an asymptomatic Class I subject

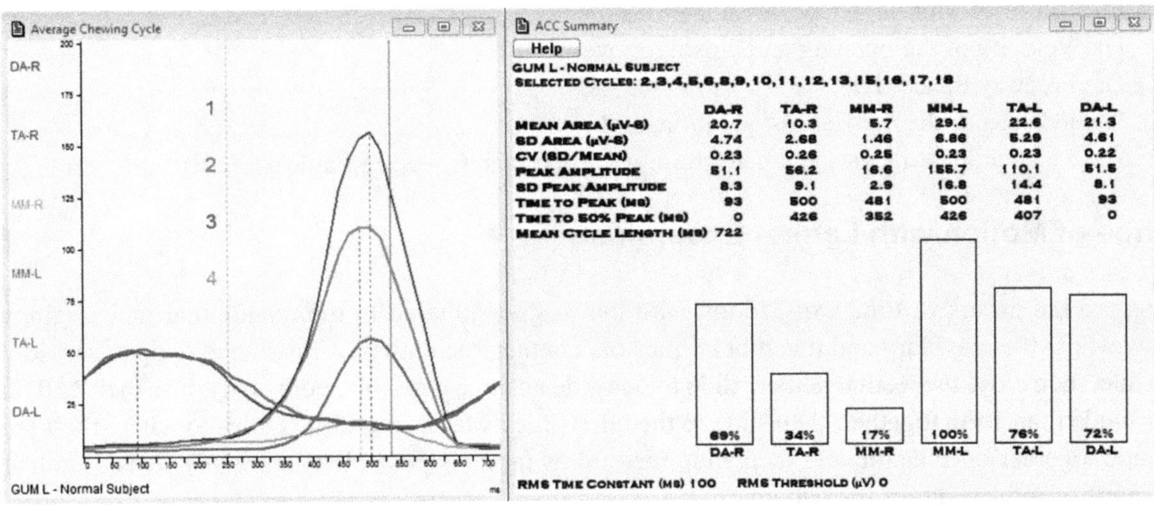

in the graph that the digastric is most active during opening, but that it remains active throughout the complete cycle. Within the data, it is also possible to note the timing of the chewing activity.

In general, malocclusion has three main effects on the muscle activity in mastication:

- A reduced speed of the activity,
- An increase in the variability of the activity, and
- An increase in the overall amount of work that is necessary to perform the activity.

Often, there is also a change in the hierarchy of activity, compared to the ideal relationship shown in Figure 9. In a worst case, the non-working side may be more active than the working side. Thus, correcting a malocclusion accelerates the process of mastication, reduces the variability of the muscle activity and/or reduces the amount of effort required from the muscles. This affect has been demonstrated clearly in a group of 30 malocclusion patients (Kerstein and Radke, in Press).

Magnet-Based Incisor-Point 3-Dimensional Mandibular Electrognathography

The mandibular range of motion (ROM) and lateral excursions can be reasonably assessed manually using a millimeter ruler. These are important measurements that are routinely performed during a clinical examination. However, the significant advantages of magnet-based incisor-point mandibular Electrognathography, with 3 degrees of freedom (EGN, Bioresearch Associates, Brown Deer, WI, USA), includes the ability to record the freeway space, to locate the relaxed mandibular rest position, and record free mandibular movements during mastication, with a minimum of interference to the recording of natural function. All existing 6-degree jaw trackers, which can also record condylar movements, require the patient to wear clutches adhered to their teeth, that can interfere with the natural muscular processes of masticatory function. The efficient quick set-up of the magnetic system facilitates clinical convenience and acts as a cost containment feature.

The most common measurements made using magnet-based incisor-point Electrognathography include:

- The Range of Motion (ROM) with lateral excursions,
- The Velocity of the opening and closing movements,
- The Freeway Space (FS),
- The location of the relaxed rest position, and
- The Mastication Analysis and determining the Average Chewing Pattern (ACP).

Range of Motion with Lateral Excursions

To record the excursive Range of Motion with the magnet adhered to the mandibular incisal gingiva below where the maxillary and mandibular incisors contact, the patient is instructed to open as wide as possible, then close the teeth together, slide to one side as far as possible, come back into their MIP and re-occlude their teeth together, then slide to the other side as far as possible, return to where their teeth occlude together once again, and then slide forward as far as is possible (Figure 10). This establishes the limits of movement for the patient.

There are a number of factors that are to be considered with respect to Figure 10:

- The 47.4 mm measurement is equivalent to the ROM with the overbite added in.
- The 7.8 mm right and 9.3 mm left are the lateral excursive range.
- The 1.9 mm below the frontal view, is the opening deflection to the left.
- The 7.4 mm in the antero-posterior direction is the range of protrusion.

In Figure 10, any overbite or overjet is automatically included in the ROM measurement. There is also a 1.9 mm deflection to the left at maximum opening (the red line = Opening in the frontal view). All of the movements in Figure 10 fall within normal limits (ROM = 40 to 70+ mm, lateral excursions = 7 to 12+ mm, deflections and/or deviations less than 3 mm).

When a disk displaces without reducing, referred to as a "closed lock," there is an immediate reduction in the range of motion, which usually accompanies a painful joint. Over time, the joint will begin to adapt, the pain in the joint will likely dissipate, and the patient will re-gain a portion of the original range of motion, often up to about 80% with successful adaptation.

A typical acute closed lock will limit the comfortable opening range to approximately 27 mm. As the condition progresses, the joint begins to adapt by pushing the disk further forward over time, which increases the range of opening. With a completely successful adaptation, the posterior attachment tissue denervates and devascularizes, and then forms a pseudo-disk, consisting primarily of scar tissue.

Figure 11 shows a partially adapted TM joint, with a 31.2 mm ROM. Pain had subsided and the ROM is beginning to increase towards a normal range. This is a (confirmed by MRI) bilateral condition as indicated by:

- The lack of any deflection at maximum opening
- The symmetrical left (5.8 mm) and right (5.4 mm) lateral ranges
- A straight protrusion (4.9 mm).

Figure 10. A typical normal Range of Motion (ROM) recorded with lateral excursions and protrusion

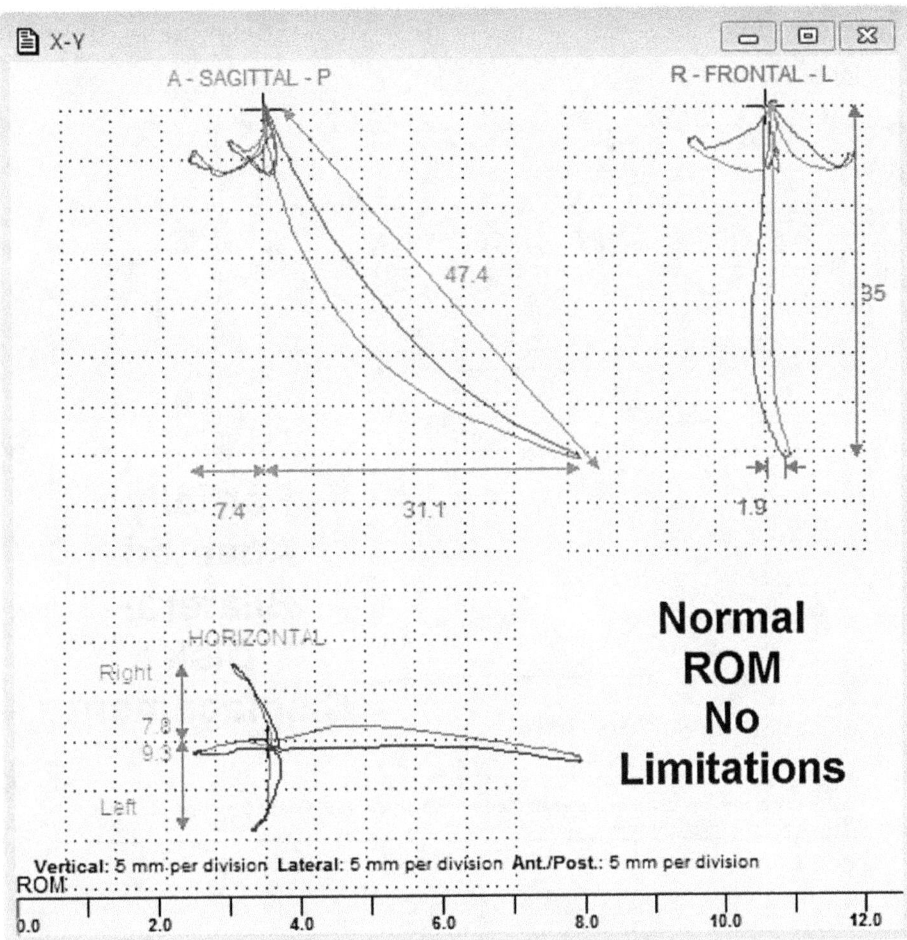

Unilateral acute disk displacement without reduction appears with a lateral deflection to the affected side during opening, unequal lateral ranges, and a protrusive guidance path that veers off toward the affected side. A deflection at maximum opening, that is less than 3 mm, is considered to be within normal limits.

Velocity Pattern

The velocity graph of the opening and closing jaw movements is primarily concerned with the speed and smoothness of the movement. Any type of dysfunction, whether initiated by the Temporomandibular joint or the musculature, will change the velocity profile. In Figure 12, the difference is very apparent. A normal subject produces a very smooth, fast and consistent velocity profile. A dysfunctional patient produces a slow and erratic velocity profile. As a patient adapts successfully to a disk displacement, the velocity profile improves towards a more nearly normal appearance.

Figure 11. A ROM recording of a patient with partially adapted bilateral Disk Displacement without reduction (DD)

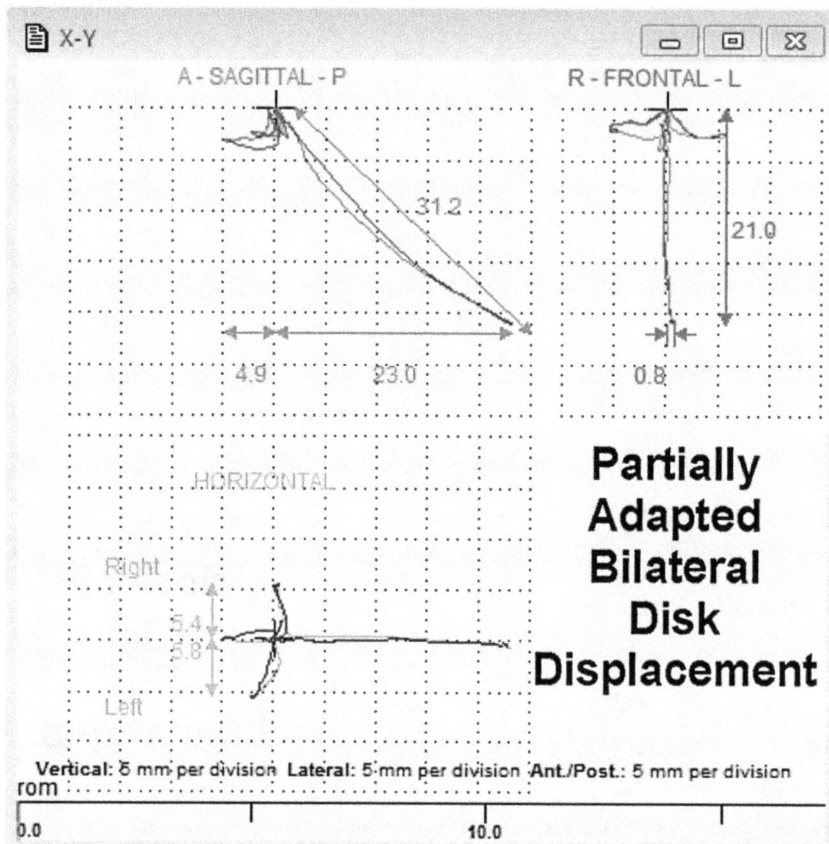

Freeway Space and the Location of Rest Position

The Freeway Space is the distance between the rest position, where all of the masticatory muscles are relaxed, and the intercuspal position (ICP). Using a magnetic Electrognathograph (EGN), the recording is made by having the patient relax their jaw muscles and remain passive at rest for a short period of time, while the incisal position is continuously recorded for a few moments. With a relaxed musculature, the rest position is stable so the trace overlaps itself. The patient is then instructed to close on their back teeth and tap their teeth together 3 times, then to keep their teeth in light contact, and slide their mandible forward. This produces the trace seen in Figure 13, which indicates there is slightly more than a 2 mm closure distance from the rest position into ICP.

The rest position, the tapping trajectory, and the protrusive guidance are all visible when this trace is displayed in an X – Y view (Figure 14). In this example, the rest position is about 1 mm anterior to the tapping trajectory, which indicates that the intercuspal position is slightly retruded with respect to an ideal muscular relationship (the ideal occurs when the tapping passes through the rest position). The protrusive guidance is visible, and not too severe.

Figure 12. The 3-Dimensional velocity plotted against the vertical dimension. The left plot is normal and the right plot shows an erratic velocity due to the presence of a disk displacement with reduction

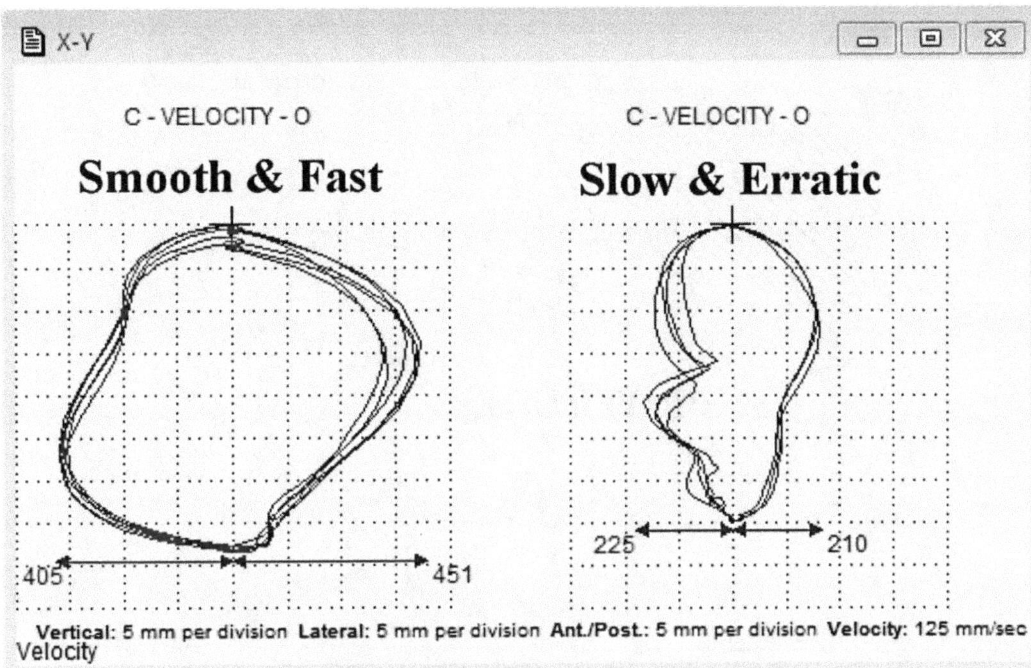

Figure 13. A normal freeway space equals 1–3 mm. To record the freeway space, the trace starts with the patient at rest, after which they are instructed to close on their back teeth, tap their teeth together 3 times, then to keep their teeth in light contact, and slide their mandible forward

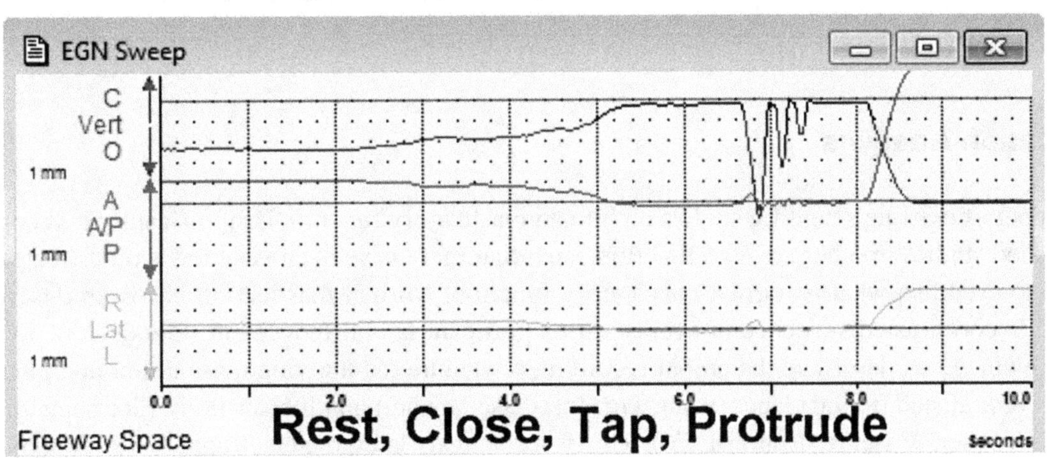

In Figure 14, the rest position is slightly to the right of ICP (about 0.4 mm), which indicates a YAW exists, that can sometimes cause a problem within the occlusion, usually only when it is greater than 0.5 mm. The overbite of 5 mm (1 mm per square), is not steep enough to interfere with normal function. Although a protrusive deflection of 2mm is observed, it is well within reported normal limits.

Figure 14. An X – Y view of the freeway space, tapping trajectory and protrusive guidance in three planes; sagittal, frontal, and horizontal. The grid is in 1 mm divisions

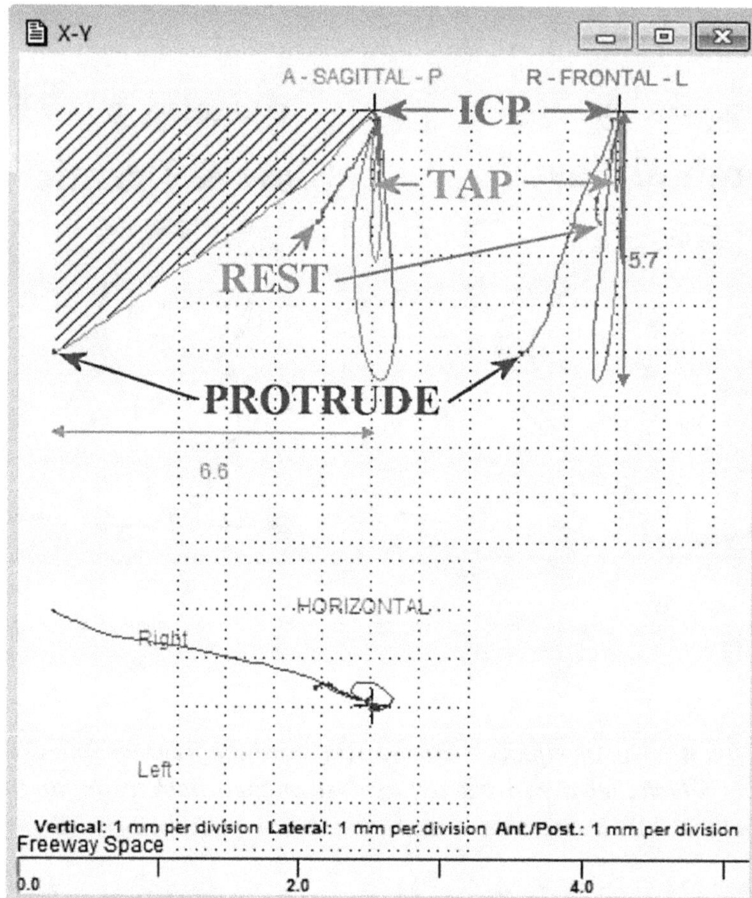

Mastication Analysis

The number of existing scientific studies on human masticatory function is significantly less compared to published studies in other areas of function, such that there have been very few studies that have attempted to establish what is normal masticatory function. Normal mastication has been described as a smoothly coordinated sequence of events with significant lateral movement (Goodson & Johansen, 1975). Lewin et. al., described the proper recording procedure for studying mastication in 3 planes (the sagittal, coronal, and frontal planes) using a magnet-based mandibular incisor-point Electrognathograph (Lewin, Lemmer, & van Rensburg, 1976). Thirty-seven years later, the electrognathographic recording of masticatory function is still a rare event in both clinical diagnostic testing, and occlusion research protocols. Is that because dentistry is considered only cosmetic?

A small number of chewing efficiency studies have used the *Sieve Method* to evaluate the ability of subjects to masticate a natural or artificial bolus (Toro, Buschang, Throckmorton, & Roldán, 2006; Woda, Nicolas, Mishellany-Dutour, Hennequin, Mazille, Veyrune, & Peyron, 2010; Witter, Woda, Bronkhorst & Creugers, 2013). The most recent of these studies concluded that a food particle size of 3.68 mm or less, should be expected to result from fully dentate masticating patients, while patients who masticated with dental prostheses, swallowed larger particles.(Witter, Woda, Bronkhorst, & Creugers, 2013). It should be noted that there are various limitations and drawbacks associated with performing particle measurement studies. Some of these include the excessive consumption of time required for particle size analysis, study design standardization, and study messiness. Another limitation is that this method is not likely to reveal any factors that may be contributory when poor efficiency is detected.

The Average Chewing Pattern (ACP)

Some authors have attempted to compare mastication movement patterns in asymptomatic subjects with chewing movement patterns observed in Temporomandibular joint dysfunction patients (Kuwahara, Miyauchi & Maruyama, 1990). The same authors developed both a system for analyzing the Average Chewing Pattern (ACP), and a system for identifying different types of chewing patterns (Kuwahara, Miyauchi and Maruyama, 1992):

- [F1] normal TM joint function (or well adapted),
- [F2] disk displacement with reduction,
- [F3] acute disk displacement without reduction, and
- [F4] chronic-adapted disk displacement without reduction.

A recently published study suggested that the presence of reverse chewing cycle sequencing observed in children was not an indication of abnormal function, but is more likely a natural process of adaptation to a continuously changing dentition (Saitoh, Yamada, Hayasaki, Maruyama, Iwase, & Yamasaki, 2010).

The process of determining the Average Chewing Pattern is accomplished by recording a 15 – 20 cycle gum chewing sequence. One full stick of gum is chewed by the patient for about 30 seconds before testing, to soften the gum into a very stable consistency, after which 25 or more chewing cycles are recorded. The first cycle is automatically ignored as it usually is not typical of the rest of the trace, because the bolus is usually excessively manipulated into position between the teeth before the first closure, to properly position it for the continuous chewing that will follow.

Figure 15. shows the Mastication Sweep View of a left-sided gum chewing sequence, from cycles numbered two through sixteen. This automatic process segmented the trace into fifteen individual cycles, which can then be averaged to create the ACP. In Figure 15, the green vertical line marks the beginning of opening in each individual cycle (0.3 mm open from the previous maximum bolus crush). The dashed cyan vertical line indicates the "Turning Point" in each cycle where the opening transitions to closing. The red vertical line represents the end of closure, which is set at 0.3 mm prior to the next maximum bolus crush.

A Normal ACP

The ACP is calculated by averaging the 15 cycles into one mean (average) cycle. By averaging the 15 cycles, the random variations in each cycle tend to cancel each other out of the total pattern, which reveals the underlying movement pattern. The black lines in the frontal, sagittal, and horizontal views represent the mean movement patterns of 500 asymptomatic subjects. The mean normal pattern is scaled to match

Figure 15. Mastication Sweep view of left-sided gum chewing. The cycles are automatically detected, and each one is divided into three parts; an opening phase, a closing phase, and an occlusal phase

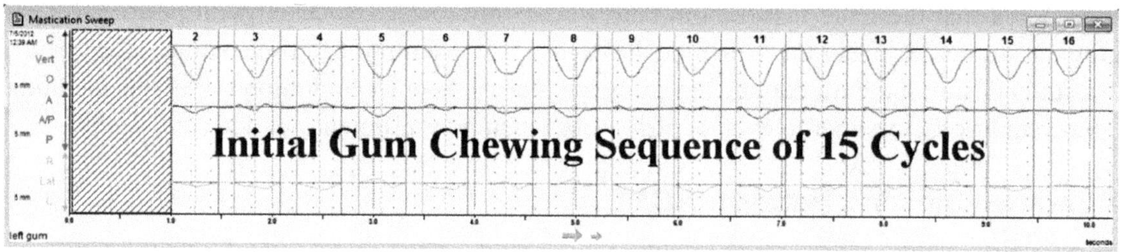

the size of each individual patient's ACP. The sample trace in Figure 16 appears broader in the frontal view, but maintains the same general shape as the mean pattern. Despite the variations seen in the sizes and structures of the human mouth, the general F1 shape of a normal chewing pattern remains consistent.

A Dysfunctional ACP

Masticatory dysfunctions are likely to occur due to a variety of pathologic conditions. Consequently, it is not rational to expect a single treatment option to be applicable for every dysfunctional case. However, it is possible to objectively evaluate a patient's function and measure the degree of improvement during the course of treatment, irrespective of the treatment option employed.

Masticatory dysfunction tends to exhibit three main effects upon masticatory movements:

- A reduction in the size of the activity,
- A reduction in the speed of the activity, and
- An increase in the variability of the activity.

The left side gum chewing pattern of a dysfunctional patient can be seen in Figure 17. This ACP is typically seen in patients who demonstrate a non-reducing chronic right disk displacement. The dysfunctional pattern is distorted towards the affected side (the right side), due to the limited translation of the right condyle. The wide areas of the red and cyan lines in the frontal and horizontal views indicate that those portions of the pathways are more than 2 standard deviations away from the mean normal pathway (the black pattern). The red vertical bar under the sagittal view indicates that the total vertical height of this chewing pattern that has been affected by the non-reducing right disk displacement. It is more than 2 standard deviations smaller than the mean normal vertical chewing amplitude.

The Significance of the ACP

A normal appearing ACP ($\pm$ 2 standard deviations from the mean pattern) is usually seen in asymptomatic subjects and in those patients with some dysfunction who have successfully adapted. The chewing patterns of most asymptomatic patients are not perfectly matched to the mean pattern. However, due to an adequate level of adaptability, they are able to function near normally so that they chew pain free and symptom free, generating relatively normal chewing motion patterns. An adaptive muscle pattern and

Figure 16. A typical "normal" average chewing pattern (ACP) is smooth, and demonstrates a frontal plane "tear-drop" configuration that is easy to identify

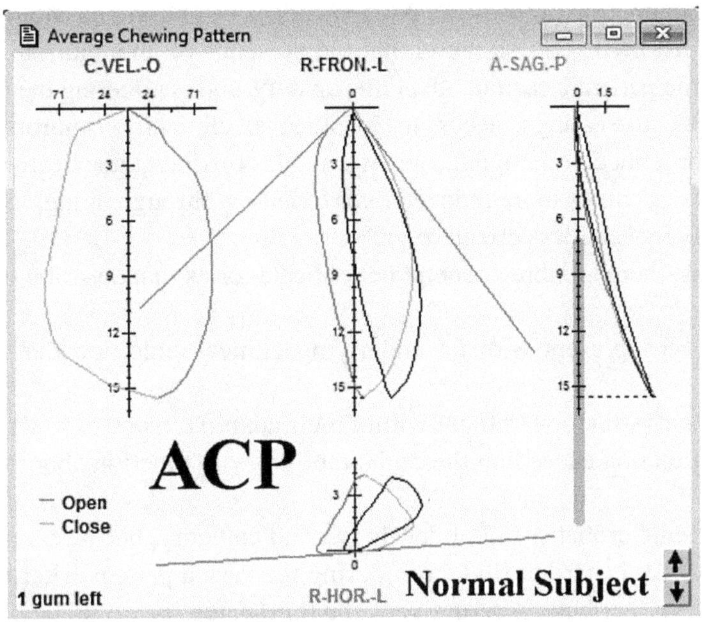

Figure 17. An ACP from a patient with a non-reducing disk displacement in the right TMJ, showing a chewing pattern that is more than two standard deviations from the mean normal pattern, in both opening and closing. The vertical dimension of the movement is also more than two standard deviations smaller than the mean normal chewing pattern

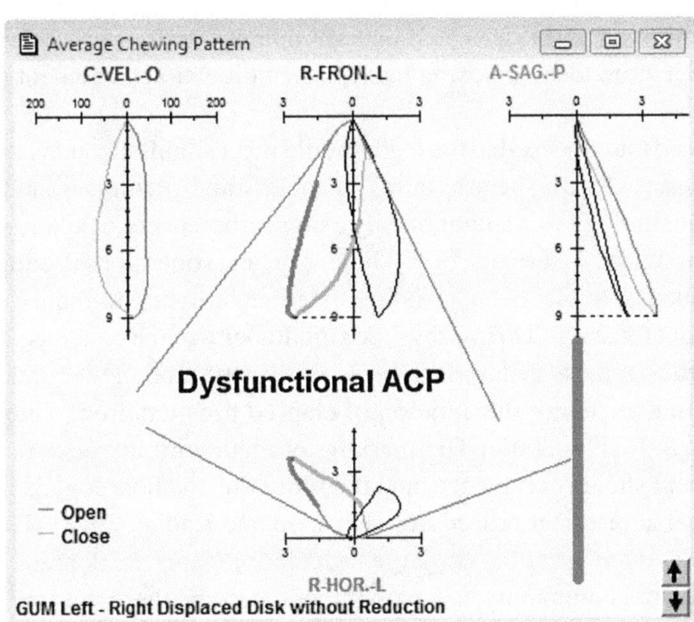

in some cases, successfully adapted Temporomandibular joints, can allow the moderately dysfunctional patient to function as if the entire system were anatomically, structurally, and physiologically normal.

When the level of dysfunction exceeds the patient's adaptive or compensatory ability, then the ACP becomes abnormal or distorted. This suggests that the presence of an abnormal ACP, means the dysfunction has exceeded the patient's current adaptive capacity, and is affecting the quality of the patient's masticatory function. Because eating is necessary for survival, clinically compromised patients still continue to eat, despite their reduced functional capacity, and less efficient masticatory system. However, if their functional capacity becomes more reduced over time (e.g. through aging, loss of teeth, etc.), their mastication can become less and less effective.

In the simplest terms, there are three general patient categories that describe mastication capability:

- Healthy subjects who present with no underlying clinical condition that affects their chewing capacity.
- Patients with some dysfunction, but are within their adaptive range to function near-normally
- Patients with dysfunction exceeding their adaptability, who function abnormally

The majority of patients probably fall under the second category, because a perfectly healthy in all respects masticatory system is hard to find, considering the varied patient criteria required of a patient to be denoted as relatively "perfect." Alternatively, the third category would be limited to patients with varying symptoms of Stomatognathic dysfunction who are definitely in need of treatment.

Technology as It Applies to Occlusion

Traditional occlusal adjustment procedures are comprised of:

- Grinding on the teeth to make them fit together better,
- Restoring teeth with crowns, bridges, and dental implants, and
- Moving teeth into a more ideal opposing maxillo-mandibular arrangement (Angle's Class I).

Gnathology introduced the concept that the teeth should meet simultaneously, with the contacts spread evenly around the arches, and with specific cusps of molars and premolars landing neatly in specific fossae (Stuart, 1973). Gnathology was taught mainly using carbon paper or silk ribbon, to mark the tooth contact points (Gazit, Fitzig, & Lieberman, 1986). In theory (and sometimes in clinical practice), occlusal adjustments are performed by subjectively grinding off tooth structure to reduce the area of contact, to lessen the occlusal contact forces, and to improve the simultaneity of the contacts. The limitation of using paper or silk is that neither of these materials indicates either the amount of contact force, or the timing sequence of the contacting teeth, nor the duration of elapsed time required to close into intercuspation (Kerstein, Lowe, Harty & Radke, 2006). The marking of teeth with ink does not sufficiently indicate where occlusal adjustment should commence, and therefore this methodology is inadequate for predictably performing occlusal adjustment procedures (Kerstein and Radke, 2013). Thus, while the concept of adjusting teeth by selectively grinding off large articulation paper mark areas visible on the tooth is widely accepted in the dental community as a proper methodology, there is a lack of scientific evidence that substantiates this method as being reliable (Torii & Chiwata, 2010).

Published studies about articulation paper, and Shim-stock foil are analyses of their physical properties themselves, describing thickness, composition, ink substrate and plastic deformity (Schelb & Kaiser, 1985; Carey, Craig, Kerstein & Radke, 2007). Studies show that articulation paper marks do not quantify occlusal force or contact sequence, and that the ink substrate left on the teeth is not a reliable indicator to accurately judge occlusal contact force levels (Qadeer et. al., 2012; Carey et. al., 2007; Saad, et. al, 2008). A few authors have suggested that traditional occlusal adjustment is no longer an acceptable treatment approach (Koh & Robinson, 2004). However, digital occlusal analysis technology (T-Scan III, Version 8, Tekscan, Inc., S. Boston, MA, USA) offers the clinician performing an occlusal adjustment procedure, precise occlusal contact timing sequence data, and relative occlusal force data, which can be used to guide the occlusal reshaping, thereby limiting the corrections made solely to the occlusal contacts that display measured time and force aberrancies. In this way, the clinician can rely on precise, repeatable data for occlusal equilibration and adjustment procedures, which cannot be obtained using conventional methods such as silk ribbon or articulation paper markings.

How Much Does the T-Scan Itself Affect Occlusal Measurement?

There exists a principle of Physics that states; "one cannot measure something without affecting it." However, an inexact measurement can be very helpful, especially when an inexact measurement is compared to making no measurement, at all. The amount that the T-Scan sensor affects the measurement is well within clinical feasibility. That is, if all the errors were somehow reduced to zero, no clinician would therefore be able to more precisely adjust an occlusion. This is because the precision of adjusting the teeth is already less than the precision of a properly accomplished T-Scan measurement.

This author measured twenty T-Scan intraoral recording sensors at two hundred locations (ten locations per sensor). The mean thickness uncompressed was 99.86 microns (± 1.72 microns). Thus, the sensor locations appear to be very uniform in thickness throughout the occluding area. Although there is some variation in the overall thickness of individual sensors from batch to batch, the uniformity of each sensor throughout its occluding area is remarkable. This uniformity is intentional because a constant thickness of the occluding area is far more important for precise measurement, than is the actual thickness of the sensor.

It is critical that the opposing arches are covered equally and in total, when the patient occludes with uniform occlusal force into the recording sensor. Uneven arch coverage could lead to mandibular closure path distortions that can alter the muscular response during the performed closure (Christensen & Rassouli, 1995). Because the masticatory system has numerous periodontal ligament and pulpal mechanoreceptors that can detect extremely small objects that fit between two opposing teeth, the slightest lack of uniformity in a sensor's thickness could create false positive indications of high force contacts, or false negative indications of no occlusal contact.

One group of authors inadvertently demonstrated the absolute necessity of fully covering the arches with the T-Scan sensors by not doing so purposefully, within their study (Forrester, Pain, Presswood, & Toy, 2009; Forrester, Presswood, Toy, & Pain, 2011). The same study was published twice, where the authors cut the T-Scan sensor in half, and placed it between opposing teeth unilaterally. The results demonstrated an altered muscular response was observed in the masseter muscle, compared to when the same patient clenched into the complete natural dentition (Forrester et al., 2011). Their findings reinforced the necessity of using a complete T-Scan recording sensor, and to not using one that has been cut in half. Employing a completely intact sensor limits any altered muscle contractile patterns that could occur during the recording of occlusal contact force and timing data. This would also apply equally to silk ribbon that is much thicker than the T-Scan sensor.

Although the mandible both rotates and translates during wide opening and closing, the amount of rotation occurring as the mandible approaches occlusal contact, appears to be minimal (Torii, 1989). If the mandible approaches the maxilla approximately perpendicular to the occlusal plane, then the exact thickness of the T-Scan sensor is insignificant, as long as all of the occlusal surfaces are fully covered by a sensor of uniform thickness. Routinely, when the T-Scan III High Density sensor (HD Sensor, Tekscan Inc. S. Boston, MA, USA) is occluded into by asymptomatic subjects, there have been no subject reports of there being a sensation of occlusal unevenness brought on by the sensor, itself.

What Is Measured With the T-Scan III?

When a patient occludes into a T-Scan sensor, the system records a movie of the onsets, and relative amplitudes of the occlusal forces that are applied to the individual teeth. The elapsed time of closure from the first tooth contact until the completion of intercuspation is referred to as the Occlusion Time, which ideally requires only about 0.2 seconds or less to complete (Kerstein & Grundset, 2001). The movie quantifies the amount of relative force applied at each contact point during the elapsed time required to close into MIP. This allows the operator to focus attention on the reduction of early and/or excessively forceful contacts. Figure 18 illustrates T-Scan data with excessively high occlusal forces being shared between teeth numbers15 & 18.

Another advantage of using measurements from the T-Scan technology is to bring about the delayed loading for an implant-supported prosthesis (Kerstein, 1999). Because implants do not have periodontal ligaments to act as shock absorbers as do natural teeth, the simultaneous loading on an implant prosthesis could risk overloading the implant prosthesis. Adjusting the implant-supported contacts so they occlude slightly after most of the natural teeth come into low to moderate force contact, prevents overloading an implant prosthesis. However, the clinician must be precise about making these time-delayed correc-

Figure 18. A T-Scan screen capture showing imbalanced occlusal forces, with nearly double the force on left side (65.6% left vs. 35.4% right). This is partially by intent in order to reduce the occlusal load on the implant prosthesis represented in RED on the right side of the arch[2]

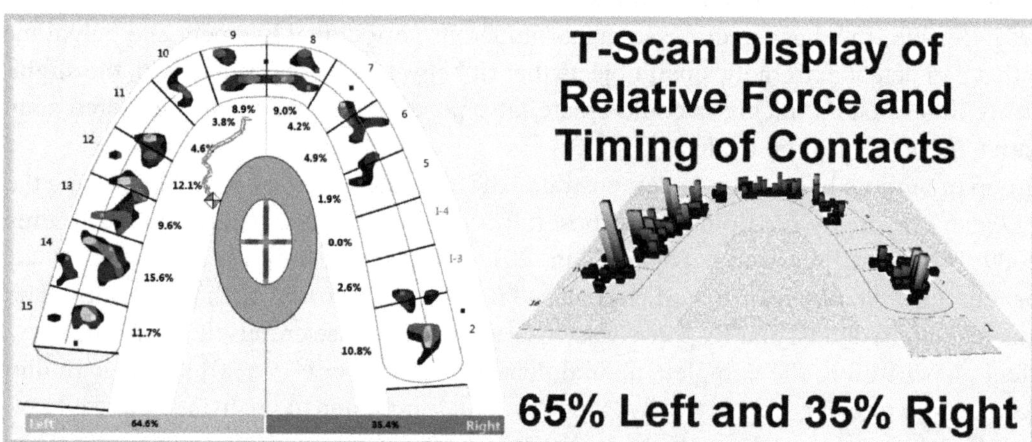

tions, otherwise, the implant supported prostheses can be over adjusted to where the prosthesis is taken completely out of occlusal contact (as seen in Figure 18).

The T-Scan can also be used to record a patient's excursive movements made from the intercuspal position, into their left and right lateral excursions. These recordings measure the elapsed time required to completely disclude the posterior teeth during excursions, which is known as the Disclusion Time. It is considered ideal when it less than 0.5 seconds per excursion (Kerstein & Wright, 1991). These two lateral measurements (left and right) can reveal occlusal interferences that elevate masseter and temporalis activity levels (Kerstein & Wright, 1991; Kerstein and Radke, 2012). Although these movements are in the reverse direction to the movements associated with mastication, they allow the operator to limit the time-duration of both working and non-working interfering contacts. Lessening the duration of the lateral excursive interferences can reduce the amount of effort required by the muscles to perform mastication. This muscle activity affect can be further verified by simultaneously recording masticatory muscle activity using synchronized electromyography (EMG) (Figure 19).

In Figure 19, muscle hyperactivity can be seen during the lateral excursion (after line C) where the duration of the posterior occlusal contacts present within the excursion exceeded 2.0 seconds. Using the Immediate Complete Anterior Guidance Development (ICAGD) coronoplasty (Kerstein & Wright 1991; Kerstein, 1992; Kerstein, 1993), a patient's Disclusion Time can typically be reduced to less than 0.5 seconds. Resultant from the reduced time of posterior tooth excursive engagement, the elevated muscle activity can be significantly reduced (Figure 20) (Kerstein & Wright 1991; Kerstein & Radke, 2012).

Figure 20 illustrates the combined T-Scan/BioEMG recording after ICAGD had been performed. Note the reduced EMG activity in the area of the right lateral excursion, and the much faster completion of the excursive event (from C to D). The contralateral activity is especially reduced. This lowered muscle activity represents an ongoing cumulative muscle activity reduction that allows the patient to function for the long-term (over months and years) with reduced functional effort.

The T-Scan computerized occlusal analysis technology has the ability to accurately pinpoint areas of excessively forceful occlusal contacts, so the clinician can make precise adjustments that are based upon

Figure 19. The simultaneous recording and analysis of occlusal force and timing can be recorded when the T-Scan program is "linked" to the BioPAK EMG program. This is an example of pre-treatment excessive muscle activity of the left masseter and right temporalis muscles, during a right excursion

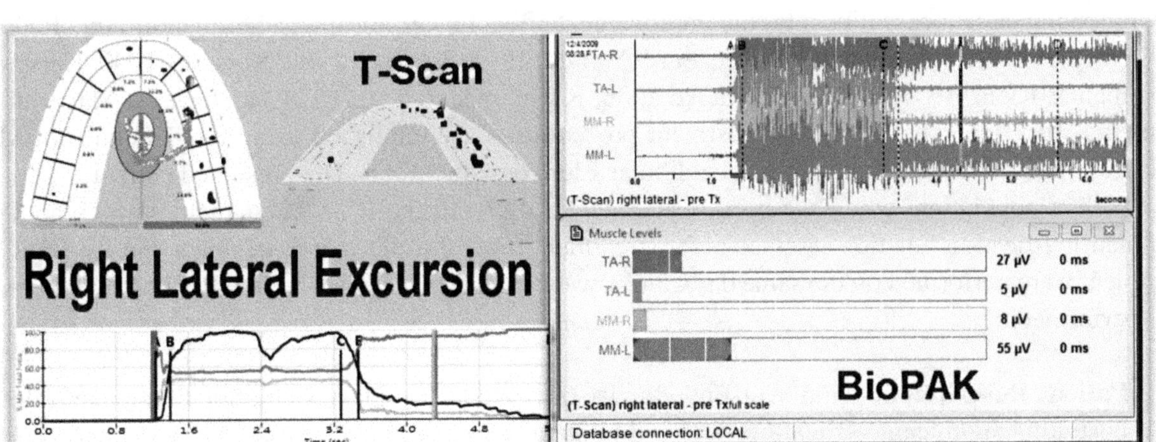

Figure 20. A simultaneous T-Scan/ BioEMG recording made after the ICAGD treatment. The amount of EMG activity during the excursion is obviously reduced compared to Figure 19, resultant from the shorter Disclusion Time (represented by the C-D period seen in the T-Scan window). Post ICAGD treatment, there is a much shorter duration of excursive posterior tooth contact

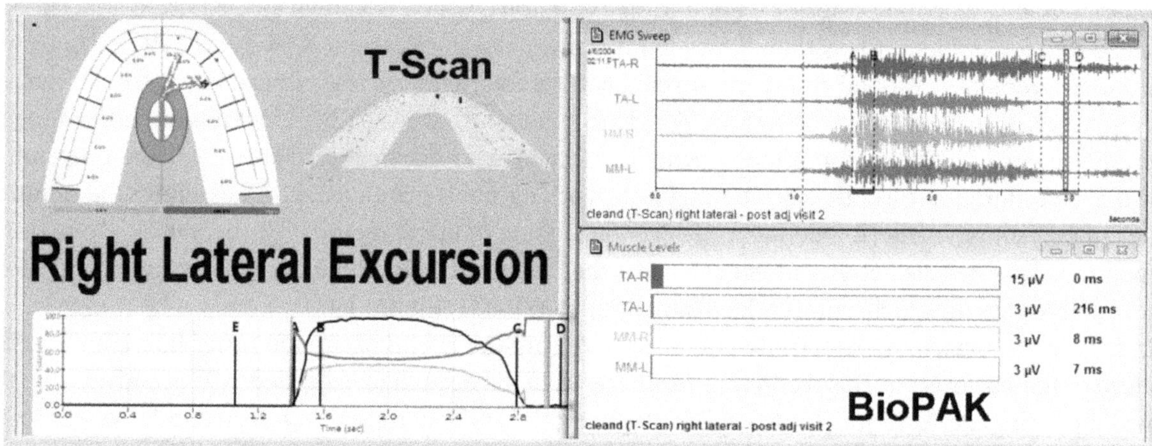

objective data. Therefore, when occlusal adjustments are performed using this technology, only the occlusal contact points that require adjustment are treated, making this computer-guided procedure far less invasive than conventional methods that are guided by the clinician's Subjective Interpretation of paper marks (Kerstein & Radke, 2013). In this way, only the teeth that are measured as "high" or frictionally prolonged are the ones that will undergo adjustment. Additionally, the T-Scan's quantifiable data can effectively demonstrate whether or not the desired "end point" goal of a bilaterally balanced occlusion has, or has not yet, been achieved. Therefore, the T-Scan represents to the clinician a definitive method of knowing when the procedure has been successfully completed.-

A Clinical Case Report: Documenting the Effect Disclusion Time Reduction Treatment Can Have on the Superficial Masseter and Anterior Temporalis Muscles During Mastication

The following patient case illustrates the improvement affect that performing a Disclusion Time Reduction with the ICAGD enameloplasty (Kerstein & Wright, 1991; Kerstein, 1992; Kerstein, 1993; Kerstein, Chapman & Klein, 1997; Kerstein & Radke 2006; Kerstein & Radke, 2012), can have on Mastication (chewing) function. This occlusal adjustment procedure is accomplished using the T-Scan/BioEMG synchronization module, and the 3-D Mandibular Electrognathograph. The presented patient is part of a 27-patient population, who have been treated occlusally with the ICAGD enameloplasty, who also had their mastication function assessed before treatment (both the chewing assessment and the ICAGD treatment were performed on the same day), and 1 week after the Disclusion Time Reduction treatment was performed.

- **Patient Description:** A 65 year-Endodontist presented as a Class I anterior relationship demonstrating significant vertical overbite and bilateral concave lingual canine contours that were in contact with the opposing dentition in maximum intercuspation (MIP) (Figure 21). The posterior right quadrant presented with 2 gold crowns installed years prior, on teeth #s 3 and 4. The left posterior quadrant presented in cross-bite, where teeth #s 13, 14, and 15 lied lingual to teeth #s 18, 19, and 20. Both posterior quadrants showed poor vertical tooth alignment, with the left side alignment significantly more non-vertical than the right side. All 3rd molars had been previously extracted.

- **History and Presentation of Occlusal Disease:** For over 20+ years prior to consultation, the patient had experienced chronic bilateral masseter tension, with regular morning jaw soreness that worsened during stressful periods. The patient reported clenching during the day while working on patients, and bruxing to some degree during the nighttime. Additionally, his chewing function at times was problematic, where his mandible would fatigue when challenged with difficult foods. Lastly, although he reported that most of his discomforts were in the masseter muscles bilaterally, he also reported experiencing frequent temporal headaches that could become severe.
- **Previous Unsuccessful Treatments:** The patient reported wearing an oral appliance for most of those 20+ years nightly, but as the years had passed, the appliance became less and less effective at controlling chronic discomforts. As such, he reduced his wearing of the appliance, but still wore it at times when symptoms were at their worst.
- **Temporomandibular Joint Status:** The patient was able to open 51 mm, with 1 mm deviation to the left. The patient had infrequent clicking and popping, but no locking, dislocation, or avascular necrosis. Joint Vibration Analysis (JVA) did not show the presence of any significant internal derangements.

Figure 21. Facial retracted view of a 65 year-old Endodontist, who presented as a Class I with significant vertical overbite, and concave canine lingual contours. The left posterior quadrant presented in cross-bite, where teeth #s 13, 14, and 15 lied lingual to teeth #s 18, 19 and 20. Both posterior quadrants showed poor vertical tooth alignment

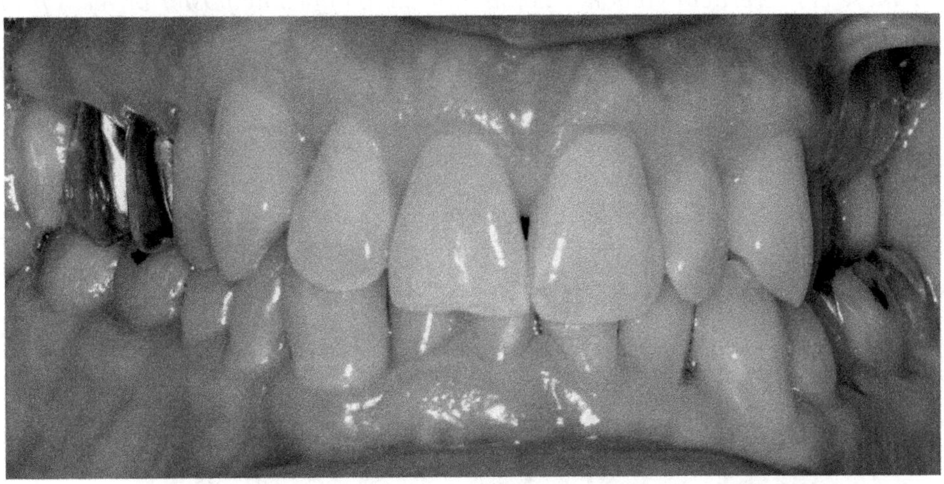

Patient Functional Clinical Presentation

The left buccal view of the left excursion (Figure 22a) showed the presence of crossbite in the posterior quadrant, and the presence of a canine concavity on #11's lingual surface, both of which contribute to the visible excursive friction. The right buccal view (Figure 22b) of the right excursion shows complete buccal posterior group function and excursive friction visible because of the #6 canine lingual guidance surface concavity.

Figures 23a and 23b detail the preoperative right and left excursive T-Scan/EMG data.

Figures 23c, 23d, and 23e are clinical photographs of the maxillary right, and left, and the mandibular right articulating paper markings, prior to the teeth undergoing the ICAGD enameloplasty.

The maxillary left paper markings (Figure 23e) show the friction visible on the buccal and lingual aspects of tooth #15, that is detailed in the pre-treatment left excursive T-Scan data (Figure 23a).

Protrusive excursions were analyzed and recorded but not presented here for brevity, as the protrusive Disclusion Time was short due to the significant vertical overlap of the maxillary anterior teeth.

Mastication Functional Analysis Method

The Bipolar EMG electrodes were left in place bilaterally over the anterior portion of the temporalis muscle and the mid-point of the superficial masseter (four channels) such that the chewing movements and muscle activity were simultaneously recorded with JT-3D Mandibular Electrognathograph and the BioEMG III electromyograph (Figure 24).

Figure 22a. 1 mm into the left excursion as the canine teeth begin to engage. Note the complete crossbite buccal posterior group function and the excursive friction visible. The concave canine surface allows the mandible to move laterally a few millimeters before the canine guidance can lift the posterior teeth apart. Because there is no vertical guidance contact present, opposing posterior teeth frictionally engage very early in the movement both buccally and lingually (unseen). The friction is worsened by the crossbite and the very poor vertical tooth orientation

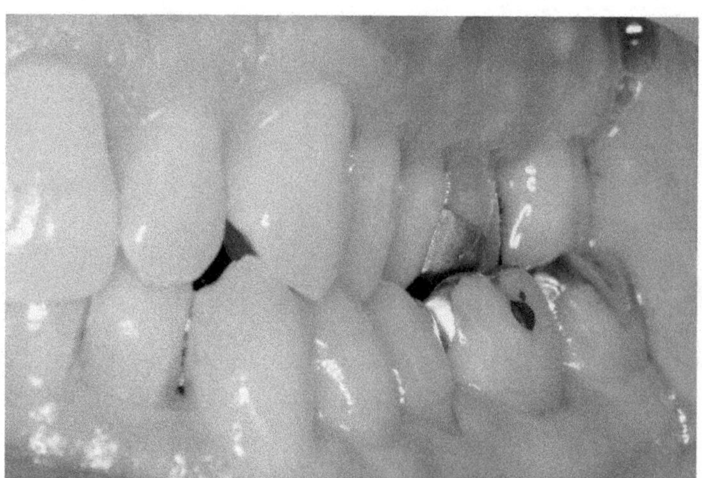

Figure 22b. 1 mm into the right excursion, the distal aspect of tooth #6 canines begin to engage tooth #28. Note the complete buccal posterior group function and excursive friction visible because of the canine concavity

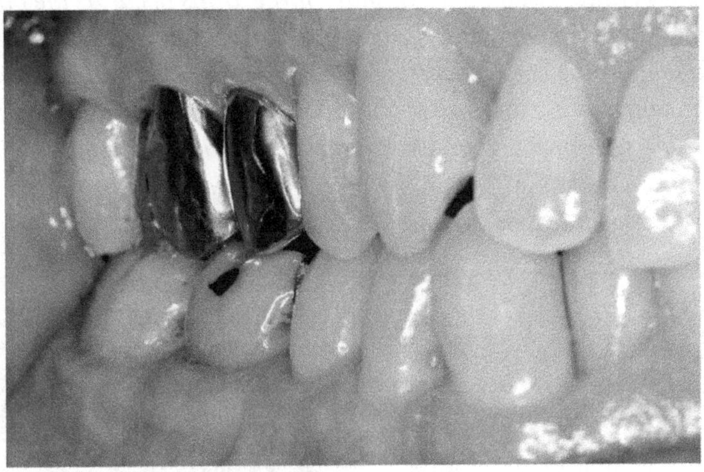

Figure 23a. Pre operative left excursive T-Scan/BioEMG data showing (in the T-Scan) prolonged left Disclusion Time (C-D = 1.82 seconds), with working and balancing excursive frictional occlusal contacts present in the 2D and 3D ForceViews, that make the Total Force Line "step down." Within the EMG data, there is extensive excursive hyperactivity visible in the left temporalis and the right masseter muscles (to the right of D). The left temporalis exhibits very prolonged and sizeable excursive hyperactivity that lasts nearly until the end of the recording. This would be contributory to the patient's chronic temporal headache condition. Note that after D the hyperactivity lessens, somewhat

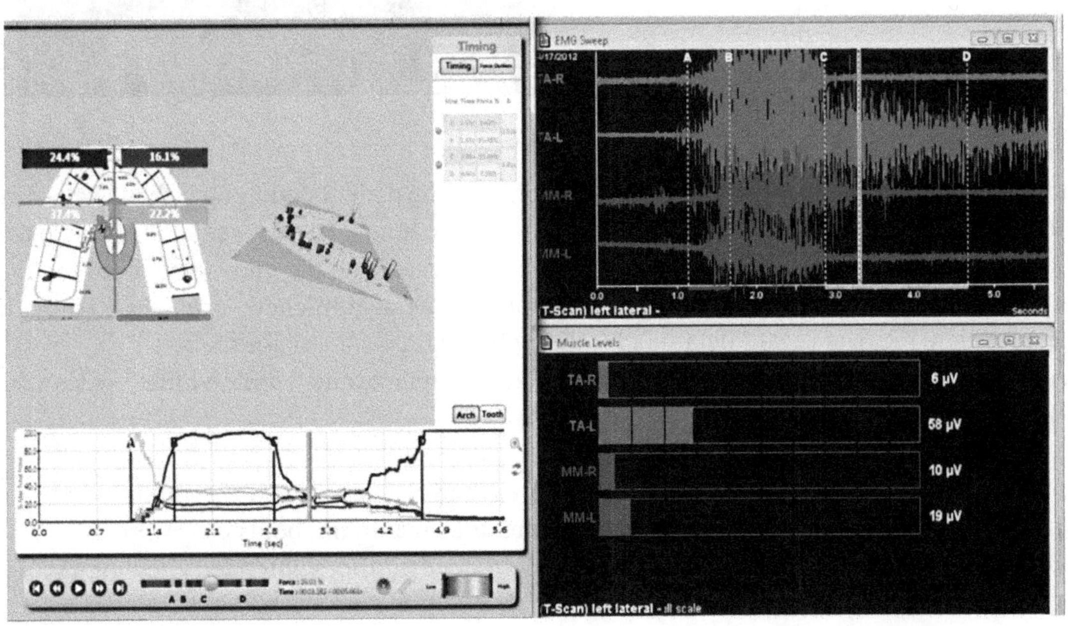

Figure 23b. Pre operative right excursive T-Scan/BioEMG data showing (in the T-Scan) prolonged right Disclusion Time (C-D = 4.29 seconds), and significant 2nd molar lingual-to-lingual working excursive frictional occlusal contact forces (see Figure 23c and d). There are steep Total Force Line "step downs" visible early in the excursion (after C), indicating sharp force drops occur as the patient's posterior teeth frequently "stop" the mandible from moving easily across each other, as the excursion evolves. Within the EMG data, the right temporalis and left masseter muscles exhibit prolonged and elevated contractile levels. After C, the right temporalis exhibits very high levels of prolonged contractions, which would be a contributor to his chronic temporal headache condition. The right masseter demonstrates spasm during the movement, illustrated in the EMG data, by the successive and repeating higher and lower EMG waves. The right masseter spasm lessens in amplitude and frequency later in the excursion nearing D

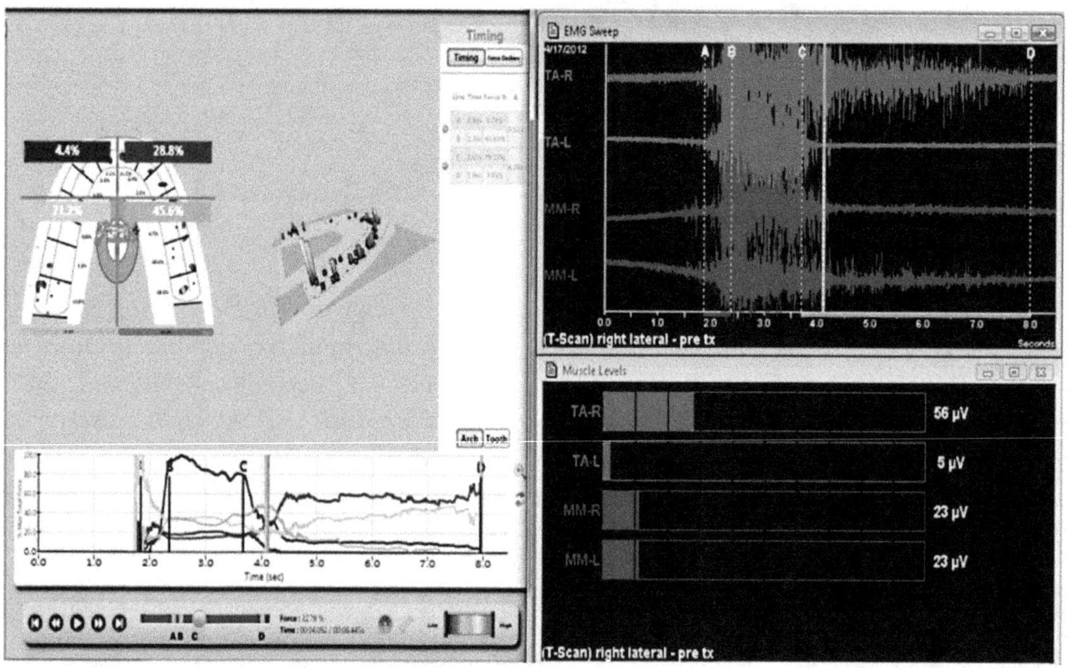

Following the above T-Scan/EMG analysis, and prior to the patient undergoing the Disclusion Time Reduction treatment, the patient was asked to chew softened gum solely between the left side teeth for more than 15 cycles, and then to do the same 15 chewing cycles with the gum solely between the right side teeth. The patient was then asked to re-perform both unilateral gum-chewing cycles, to provide four, 15-cycle gum chewing data sets (2 data sets for the right side; 2 data sets for the left).

After saving the data, each chewing sequence was segmented into 15 individual cycles using the following movement criterion:

- The time marking the beginning of opening for each cycle recorded, was established at a vertical dimension 0.3 mm open from the point of the previous maximum bolus crush (Figure 25a).
- The activity levels of each muscle from the 15 left-sided and 15 right-sided chewing cycles, were rectified and averaged separately (Figure 26).

Figure 23c. Maxillary right articulating paper markings illustrating the 2nd molar, lingual-to-lingual contact markings visible, as very high force contacts in Figure 23b. Note how misleading the paper mark appearance on the lingual of tooth #2 can be, as it is a small thin line that "looks' to not be very forceful, but is actually a high force, lingual-to-lingual, interfering contact

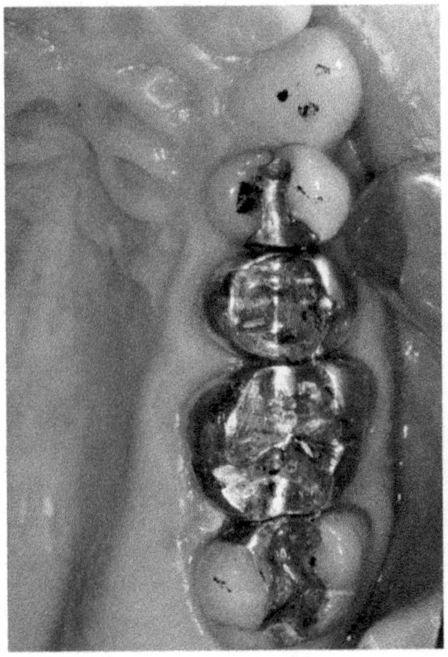

Figure 23d. Mandibular right paper markings illustrating the forceful lingual-to-lingual contact present on the distolingual of tooth #31, which is the counterpart of the palatal black paper mark present on tooth #2 (Figure 23c)

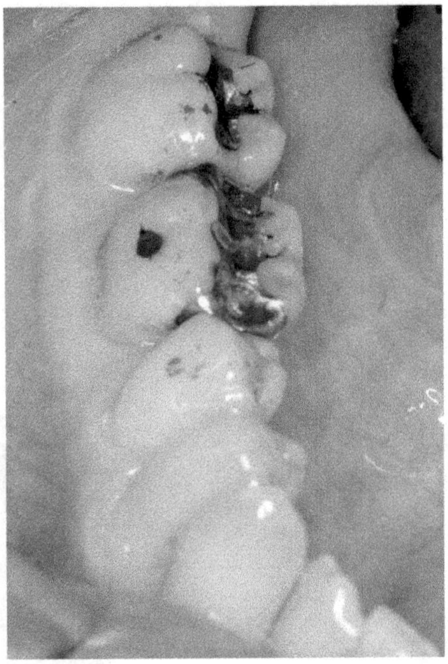

Figure 23e. The maxillary left paper markings show the friction visible on the buccal and lingual aspects of tooth #15, which is detailed in the pre-treatment left excursive T-Scan data (Figure 23a)

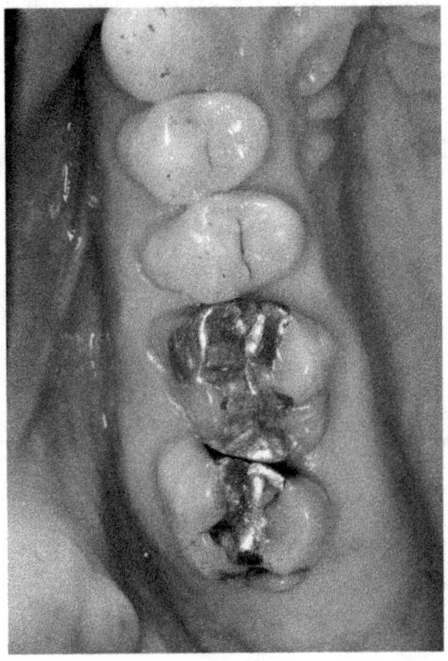

Figure 24. The 3-D Mandibular Electrognathograph and the BioEMG III electromyograph in place on a different (female) patient's head, ready for mastication analysis where all 8 possible channels will be recorded. In the presented case example, only 4 channels were recorded (the bilateral masseter and temporalis muscles). These combined technologies record mandibular motion and muscle activity simultaneously, during gum chewing

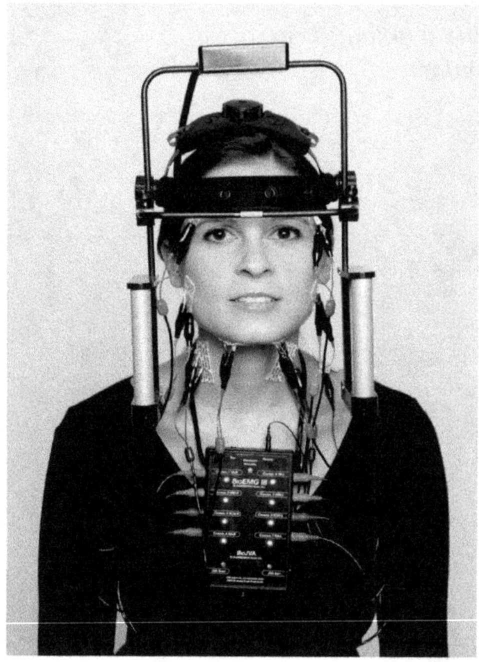

Figure 25a. Pre and post-treatment muscle activity level data of the four measured muscles recorded during 15 individual chewing cycles. The 15 cycles were superimposed to contrast the variability of the muscle activity from pre to post-treatment. The patterns shows higher peak muscle activity and less variability in the post-treatment data than in the preoperative data

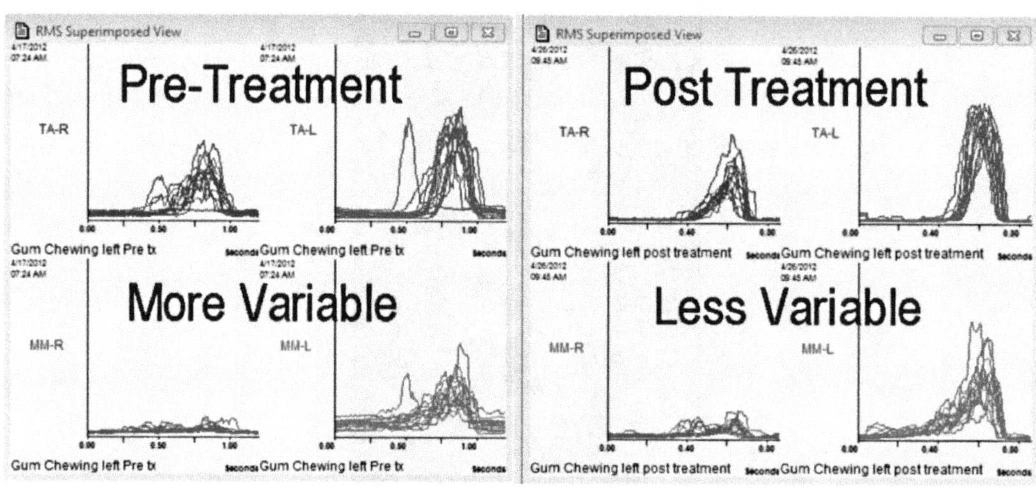

It is important to note that normal subjects reach peak EMG before, or right at the end of closure (Figure 25b), whereas dysfunctional subjects that are more tentative in their chewing action, often wait until they are secure in the intercuspal position before applying maximum force. Therefore, their peak muscle activity occurs after they finish making the closure into intercuspation (Figure 26; left pane, red vertical line is end of closure).

Following the mastication data capture, the patient underwent the ICAGD enameloplasty (described in detail, in Chapter 7).

The same unilateral gum chewing data capture would be repeated 1 week later, following the initial ICAGD procedure (1 week earlier), and prior to any further occlusal refinement that might be performed at the 1 week, follow up appointment.

T-Scan/EMG Results of the ICAGD Treatment

The excursive function muscular affects of the ICAGD procedure can be seen in Figures 27a and 27b. With the pre-treatment prolonged Disclusion Times bilaterally now drastically shortened, much of the pre-treatment muscular excursive hyperactivity seen in Figures 23a and 23b (to the right of C), has been greatly lessened.

Figure 25b. Normal subjects reach peak EMG and apply maximum force before, or right at the end of closing into the intercuspal position (red vertical line)

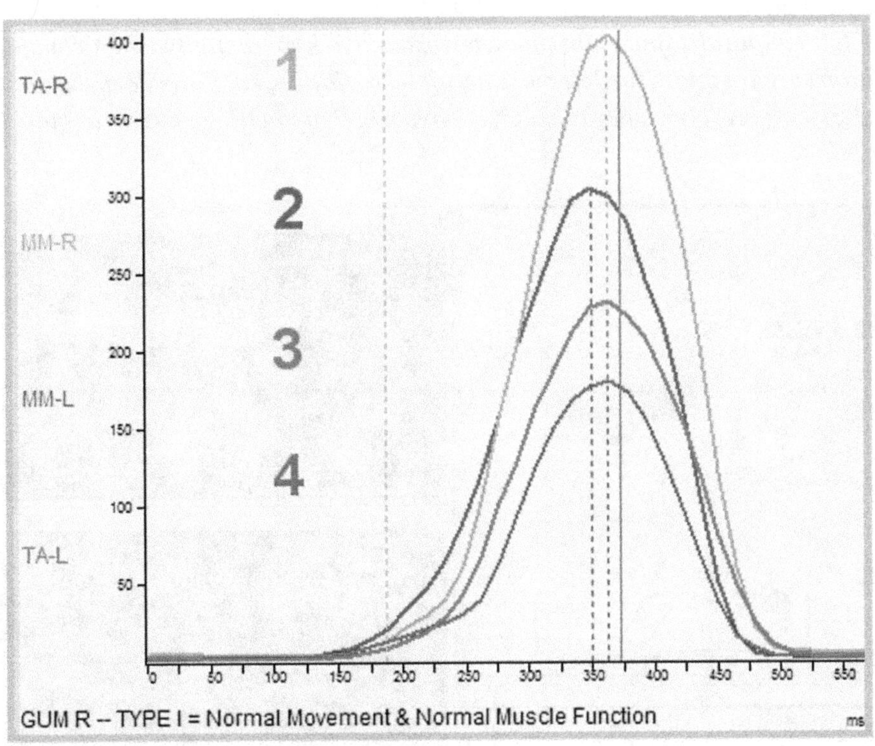

Figure 26. The rectified and averaged muscle activity levels of each muscle from the 15 left-sided and 15 right-sided chewing cycles. Note the higher peak and narrower base of each muscle trace post-treatment (similar to the normal pattern shown in Figure 25b). The 15 cycles averaged, showed the change in the muscle firing pattern from pre-treatment to post ICAGD treatment, where the pattern is taller (more force) and narrower (chewing happens quicker) in the post-treatment data. The red vertical line marks the end of closure, where the mandible is 0.3 mm short of maximum bolus compression

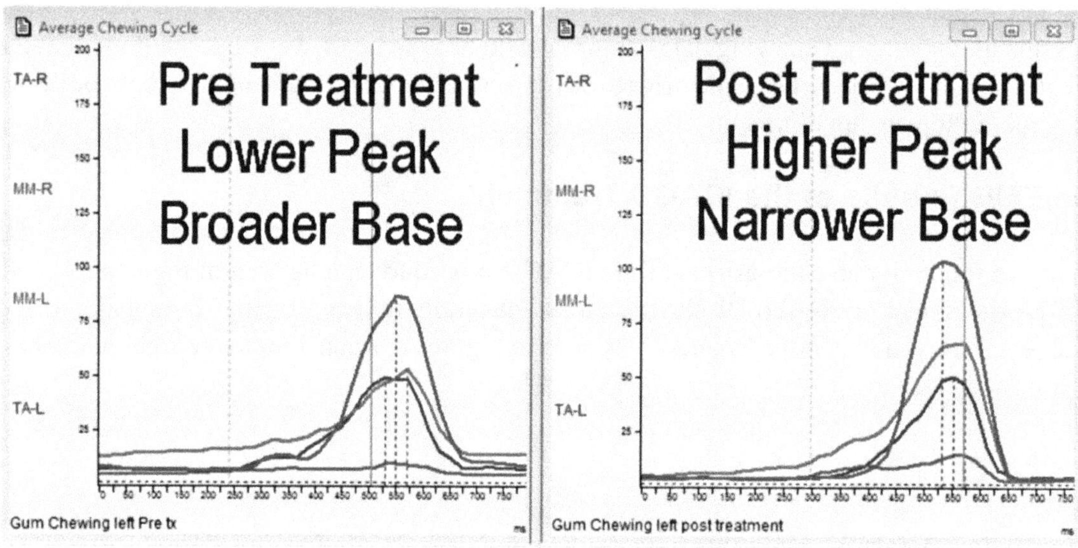

Figure 27a. The left excursion 1 week after ICAGD. The Disclusion Time = 0.71 seconds duration, which is slightly elongated from the desired norm of < 0.5 seconds per excursion. ICAGD treatment had reduced the left temporalis and right masseter excursive hyperactivity when compared to the pre-treatment condition (Figure 23a). The left masseter quickly flatlines at C, as does the non-working right temporalis. The left temporalis maintains excursive hyperactivity between C-D, but quickly lessens after C, to flatline at D

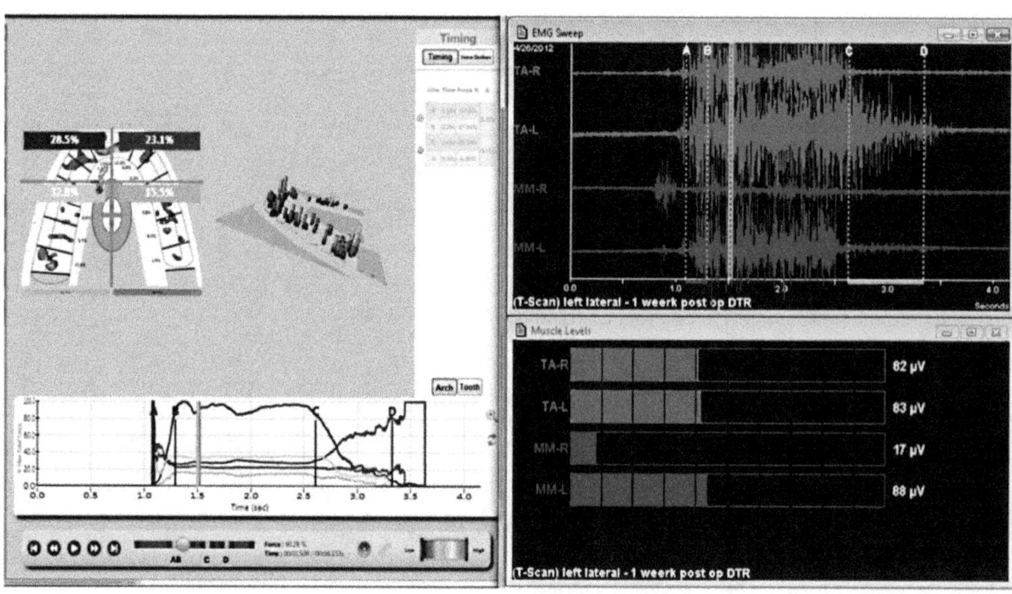

Figure 27b. 1-week right excursive EMG improvements from ICAGD where there is less excursive hyperactivity visible with a Disclusion Time of 0.57 seconds duration, compared to Figure 23b. The right temporalis maintains excursive hyperactivity between C- D, but quickly lessens to where shortly after D, the contractions cease and flatline. The left masseter quickly reduces contractions after C, until just before D

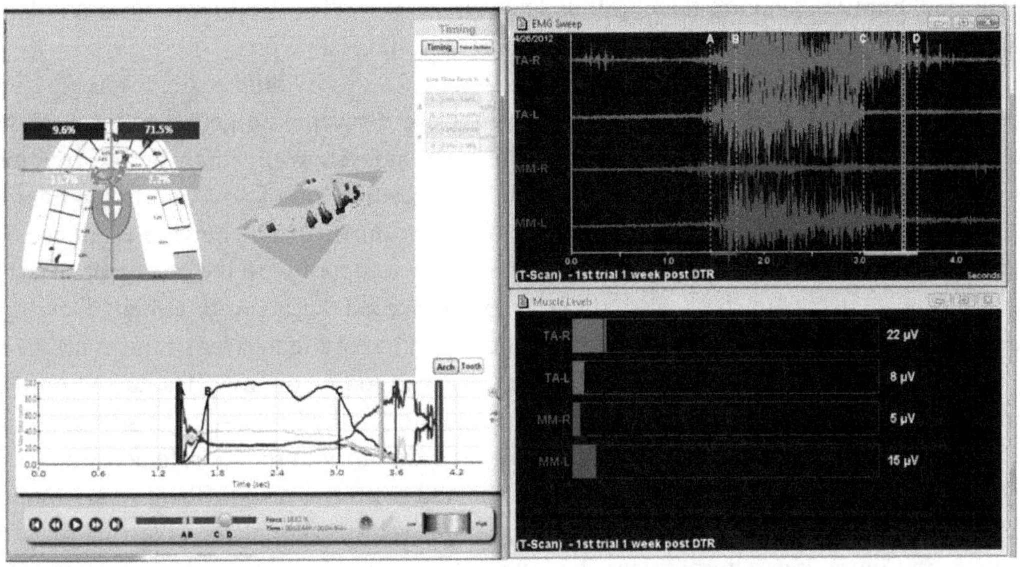

Mastication Function Changes Resultant from ICAGD Treatment

Seven numerical parameters were compared between the pre-treatment chewing electromyographic activity to the post-treatment chewing activity, both individually, and as a total group, using the Student's Paired t-test ($p< 0.05$). The seven parameters listed below were employed to detect any significant change in overall muscle activity during masticatory function, resultant from the rendered ICAGD occlusal treatment.

The seven computed mastication parameters were:

- **The Mean Area:** Measured by calculating the area under the rectified and averaged EMG activity of chewing gum.
- **The SD Area (The Standard Deviation of the Mean Area):** Calculated to describe the amount of change from cycle to cycle, or to illustrate the variability of the muscle activity visible from cycle to cycle.
- **The Coefficient of Variation (SD Area/Mean Area):** Calculated to measure the relative muscle variability, independent of the amplitude of the muscle activity.
- **The Peak Amplitude:** Showed the highest rectified average amplitude, which indicated the highest muscle activity level each muscle demonstrated, at any time during the chewing cycle.
- **The SD Amplitude:** Calculated as the standard deviation of the *Peak Amplitude*.
- **The Time to Peak:** Showed the time (in milliseconds) measured from the beginning of mandibular opening to when the peak closing muscle activity was observed.

- **The Time to 50% of Peak:** Showed the time (in milliseconds) measured from the beginning of mandibular opening to when 50% of peak activity levels were observed.

It was considered possible that the ICAGD occlusal adjustment might alter individual muscles, without changing the overall system muscle activity levels, thereby shifting some of the activity from one muscle to a different one, but not changing the combined activity levels. This would represent a redistribution of activity rather than a change in the overall muscle activity levels.

To address this possibility, the four muscle's activities of an individual patient making15 chewing cycles (n = 4 muscles x 15 cycles = 60 chewing events), were summed together to produce the seven combined parameters (listed above) for left-side and right-side chewing, both before treatment, and seven days post-treatment (Figure 28). This allowed for the evaluation of any significant change in the combined muscle activity levels of the four muscles recorded during each chewing sequence.

The left-sided post-treatment muscular chewing data (the arch half with the posterior crossbite), observed nine days post Disclusion Time Reduction, when compared to the pre-treatment chewing muscle activity levels, disclosed that a significant reduction occurred in the Mean Area of the combined muscle activity. This finding suggested that less overall effort was exerted by the muscles during gum chewing post-treatment ($p < 0.024$). The SD Area (the standard deviation of the Mean Area) also was significantly reduced after treatment ($p < 0.030$), indicating a reduced variability in the muscle activity. In addition, the coefficient of variation ($p < 0.039$), which also indicated there was a significant reduction in overall muscular function variability. This can be seen in the improved overlap of the post-treatment chewing muscular traces in Figure 25a. Alternatively, there was observed a significant increase in the Peak Amplitude ($p < 0.043$), with discernible trends towards both a shorter Time to Peak ($p > 0.055$) and shorter Time to 50% of Peak ($p > 0.065$). The overall left-sided muscular changes resultant from treatment, il-

Figure 28. Statistical analysis of muscle activity pre and post ICAGD occlusal adjustment, showed significant changes occurred between pre-treatment and post treatment. There were more significant changes found on the left (crossbite) side than on the right (normal bite) side (ns = not significant).

	Sum of 4 muscles	Pre Tx	Post Tx	p	
Chewing Gum Left Side	Mean Area	53	44.6	< 0.024	
	SD Area	24.7	13.9	< 0.030	
	CV	1.84	1.26	< 0.039	
	Peak Amplitude	181	239	< 0.043	
	SD Amplitude	44.6	50.1	> 0.320	ns
	Time to Peak	2431	2185	> 0.055	ns
	Time to 50% Peak	1927	1714	> 0.065	ns
	Combined	**4663.14**	**4247.86**	**< 0.024**	

	Sum of 4 muscles	Pre Tx	Post Tx	p	
Chewing Gum Right Side	Mean Area	55.6	51.2	> 0.340	ns
	SD Area	26.8	32.8	> 0.148	ns
	CV	1.94	2.46	< 0.010	
	Peak Amplitude	184	271	> 0.058	ns
	SD Amplitude	46.6	47.1	> 0.483	ns
	Time to Peak	2416	2091	< 0.0002	
	Time to 50% Peak	1741	1722	> 0.452	ns
	Combined	**4471.94**	**4217.56**	**< 0.122**	**ns**

lustrated that the patient used shorter duration chewing strokes, more quickly applied increased crushing force, with less overall effort expended. When all seven individual parameters were considered together, the combined treatment changes in muscular activity, were also significant ($p < 0.024$) (Figure 28).

The right side occlusal alignment was not in crossbite, and in retrospect, appeared to have been functioning better pre-treatment, than was the left side. The most dramatic change in the right-sided chewing activity was a significant decrease in the Time to Peak ($p < 0.0002$). There was also a trend towards an increase in the Peak Amplitude ($p > 0.058$), suggesting that the same type of change (although less dramatic than on the left side) was affected on the right side, where there were observed post treatment, faster and more forceful closing strokes, with less overall muscular effort required (Figure 28). Perhaps, because the chewing function on the right arch half was better prior to the ICAGD treatment, the amount of change of the right parameters post-treatment, were not statistically significant, despite the right side trending toward marked improvement from treatment ($p > 0.122$).

Additional Evidence of How Changes to the Disclusion Time Improved Mastication Patterns

It has been shown in a number of previously published studies that tooth contacts that occur during mastication, can produce exteroceptive suppression of the masseter and temporalis muscles (Atkinson, 1976; Mushimoto, 1981; Takada, et. al., 1992), which when observed within an EMG trace, are referred to as *Silent Periods* (SP). This suppression of muscle contraction typically lasts for 10-25 milliseconds duration (Iino, et. al., 1989). It has been suggested that silent periods within EMG data, could be a simple way to identify the presence of excessive and/or pre-mature occlusal contacts (McNamara, 1977; Sohn, Miyawaki, Noguchi, & Takada, 1997).

To date, the prevalence of Silent Periods during gum chewing in a normal population has not been published. In an ongoing study involving 78 asymptomatic subjects (44 female and 34 male), where masseter and temporalis activity was recorded during left and right-sided gum chewing (156 total recordings), when observed for the presence or absence of Silent Periods (SPs), the mean number of SP occurrences observed within 15 chewing cycles was 0.55 ($\pm$ 0.882), which ranged from 0 - 3 SPs per recording. Unlike foods that are more difficult to chew than gum, it is likely that the chewing of gum did not often trigger any occlusally activated nociceptive reflex within this asymptomatic group. The lack of Silent Periods seen in the above asymptomatic group likely reflected that gum is a soft bolus that does not fragment, nor change in size or texture, and therefore represents a very predictable bolus.

In the presented case above, the pre and post-treatment recordings were both reviewed for the presence of SPs, as another method to determine masticatory functional improvements from the ICAGD treatment. The pre-treatment left side gum chewing sequence exhibited 9 SPs between cycles 2 and 16 while the right side pre-treatment gum chewing data exhibited 12 SPs between cycles 2 and 16 (Figure 29). In contrast, the post-treatment left side gum chewing sequence exhibited 0 SPs from cycles 2 through 16 while the right side gum chewing post-treatment, exhibited only 1 SP from cycles 2 through 16 (Figure 30). It was clear in this case, that the ICAGD treatment rendered reduced numbers of SP incidences to well within the range of the studied asymptomatic group, with in a very short period of time, post-treatment.

Correcting the occlusion in the presented case did not require correcting the crossbite, only removing the prolonged excursive frictional interferences present within the existing occlusion, that affected the efficiency of the patient's masticatory function. While posterior crossbite should not be considered to be a normal occlusal relationship, some patients are able to adapt to this malrelation, quite well. It is

Figure 29. Exteroceptive suppression (the EMG Silent Period) within a pre-ICAGD treatment right gum-chewing burst. The activity of the masseter and anterior temporalis muscles cease typically for 10 – 25 milliseconds, and then re-start. In this example, the duration of the Silent Period is 21 milliseconds long

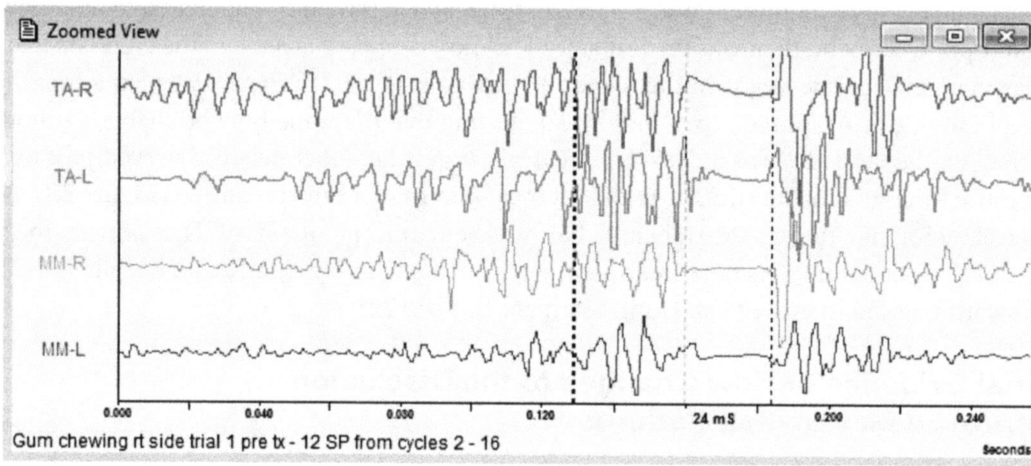

Figure 30. A post ICAGD treatment right gum chewing burst, showing no evidence of a visible silent period

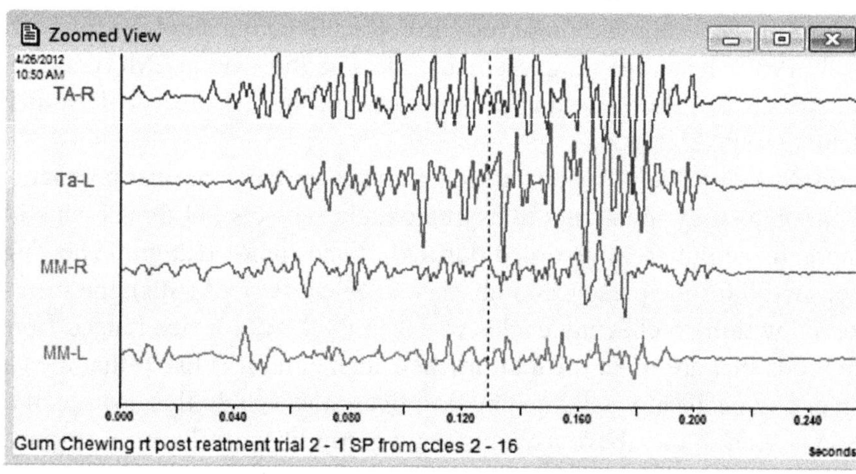

this author's opinion that chronic conditions that have undergone successful long-term adaptation do not require restoring the patient to a completely ideal condition, because function may be improved without doing so. However, it can be presumed that this patient was non-adapted, as he exhibited longstanding chronic Occluso-muscle Disorder symptoms that were not adequately quelled despite long-term appliance use. Through his lifetime with his left-sided crossbite, the repeated prolonged excursive frictional contacts added on excess muscle contractions to the baseline contractions that were required by the patient's musculature to move the mandible during chewing. Throughout his adult years, these prolonged posterior contacts created lactic acid build-up followed by ischemia, and the chronic appearance of his Occluso-muscle Disorder symptoms.

The ICAGD treatment reduced the excursive contact frictional durations to be measurably immediate, such that the pre-treatment excursive elevated levels of muscle activity were significantly reduced (Figures 27a and 27b compared to pre-treatment Figures 23a and 23b). This reduced excursive muscle activity resulted in reduced lactic acid accumulation and less ischemia, that ultimately led to statistically significant increases in muscular chewing capacity (Figures 25 and 26). The chewing improvements were accompanied by this patient exhibiting rapid Occluso-muscle Disorder symptom resolution, such that he no longer required an appliance.

The treatment effect and chewing function improvements observed with the presented patient are similar to those experienced by the group of 27 treated subjects who have been involved in an ongoing study assessing Disclusion Time Reduction's affect on Mastication.

Average Chewing Pattern (ACP)

Within the process of recording EMG activity during mastication, is it also necessary to record the movement of the mandibular incisor-point, for the purpose of segmenting and analyzing individual chewing cycles. A large amount of data has previously been reported upon, that established the mean normal chewing pattern and its consistency (Kuwahara, Miyauchi, & Maruyama, 1992; Ferrario, et. al., 2006). Poorer chewing performers chew more slowly, and demonstrate more variability within an altered chewing cycle shape, than do more normal chewers (Lepley, Throckmorton, Parker, & Buschang, 2010). In particular, a convex shape of the closing path has been associated with better chewing performance (Watanabe, Shiga, & Kobayashi, 2011). It has also been shown that better chewing performance is related to both a wider lateral closure movement, and to the smoothness of the motion (Wilding, & Lewin, 1994). Figure 31 shows the general frontal mandibular incisor point Average Chewing Pattern (ACP) shape when left and right gum-chewing is performed by a subject that is considered to be normal or relatively ideal Class I.

Figure 31. The general shape of the normal frontal ACP F1 chewing patterns, when left and right gum-chewing is performed by a normal subject

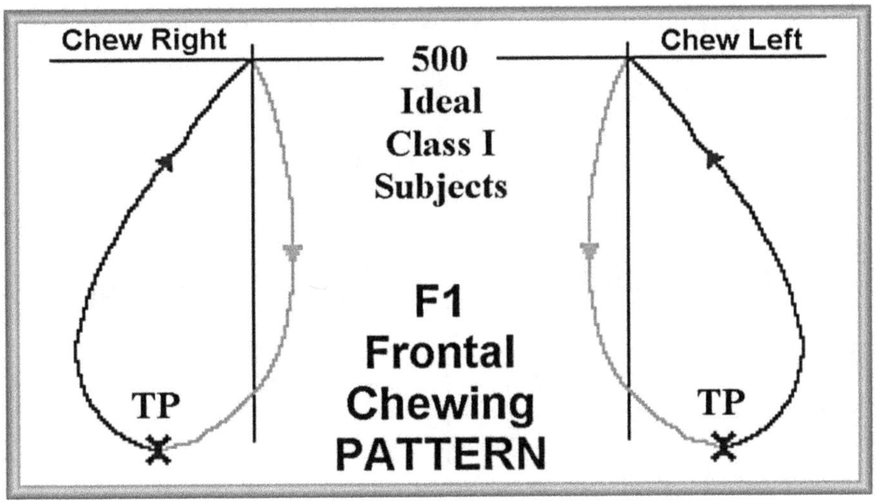

Figure 32a represents the pre and post ICAGD treatment, right-sided gum chewing patterns of the patient presented in Figure 21. The ACP visible within the left pane of Figure 32a appears very different from the normal chewing pattern seen in Figure 30. Due to the presence of the left posterior crossbite and the patient's adaptation to it, both the pre and post-treatment ACP patterns had been dramatically affected. However, the lateral dimension of the post-treatment frontal pattern of the right-sided chewing pattern (Figure 32a, right pane) has significantly changed as a result of the ICAGD occlusal treatment rendered. The pre-treatment reversed sequence (Figure 32a, left pane), in which the closure motion was medial to the opening motion, post-treatment appears more normal, with the closure now lateral to the opening (Figure 32a, right pane). This right-sided ACP change was a statistically significant improvement to the chewing pattern ($p < 0.0136$).

Figure 32b represents the pre and post-treatment left-sided gum chewing patterns of the patient presented in Figure 1 (Figure 32b, left pane), which also appears very different from the normal chewing pattern shown in Figure 31. Post ICAGD occlusal treatment, the left sided chewing ACP pattern remained reversed as mandated by the posterior crossbite, but the ACP actually opened up, appearing smoother, faster and somewhat closer to a normal ACP (Figure 32b, right pane). These observed changes to the complete ACP were not significantly different from pre to post-treatment for the vertical dimension ($p > 0.150$), although it did increase, however, the lateral component of the ACP did change significantly ($p < 0.00001$). Treatment that increases the size, increases the velocity and/or reduces the variability of the ACP generally improves function.

It should be noted that this case result may not be typical for patients with posterior crossbite that are much younger than this 65 year-old patient, who likely demonstrated long-term adaptation to the left-

Figure 32a. The pretreatment (left pane) and post ICAGD treatment (right pane), right-sided gum chewing patterns of the patient presented in Figure 21. The pre-treatment ACP (left pane) demonstrates a reversed sequence where the closure motion is medial to the opening motion. The post ICAGD ACP (right pane) demonstrates a more normal pattern where the closure motion has changed to be lateral to the opening motion. Although the vertical dimension did not change significantly ($p > 0.141$), it did increase and the lateral dimension did change significantly ($p < 0.0136$)

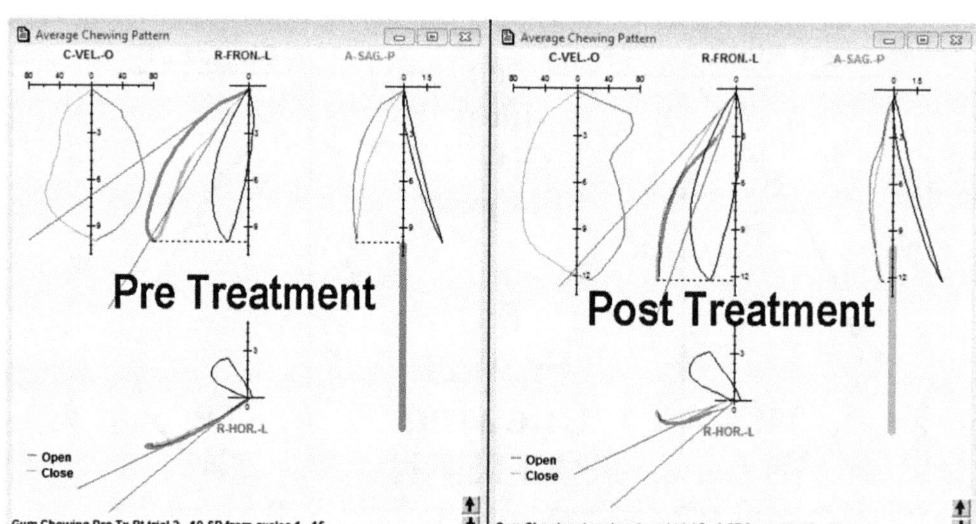

Figure 32b. The pre (left pane) and post ICAGD treatment (right pane), left-sided gum chewing patterns of the patient presented in Figure 21. The pre-treatment ACP (left pane) demonstrates a reversed sequence due to the crossbite. The post ICAGD ACP (right pane) opened up, appearing smoother and closer to a normal ACP. A significant change was found only in the lateral dimension of the ACP (p < 0.00001)

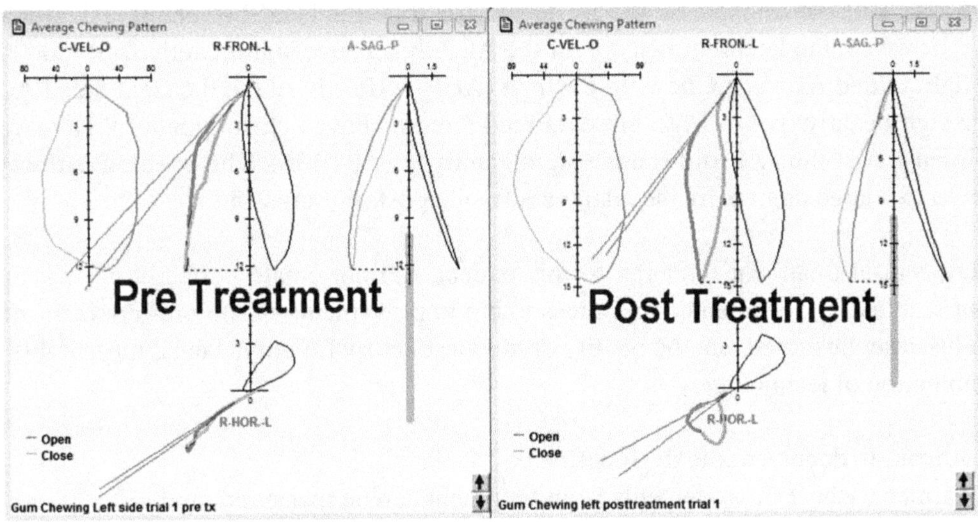

sided posterior crossbite condition. As was discussed earlier in this chapter, while the posterior crossbite is not considered to be a normal interocclusal relationship, some patients are likely able to adapt to the condition well-enough, to function despite their dental malrelation.

It has been observed that completely correcting, or removing a crossbite malrelation in an older patient, can actually interfere with their adapted function, because it forces the patient to learn a new chewing pattern that they may not necessarily readily accommodate. It may be simpler to just open up the existing chewing pattern so the affected patient can make a smoother chewing action (as was observed in this presented case). Alternatively, in young patients correcting a crossbite appears to be a positive interocclusal relationship improvement. Young patients that have not yet adapted thoroughly to the crossbite can easily change to more normal pattern of movement, after crossbite correction (Takeda, Nakamura, Handa, Ishii, Hamada, & Seto, 2009).

Summary of the Presented Patient's Mastication Statistical Results

- **Left-Sided Chewing Gum:** After ICAGD treatment, the overall muscle activity was reduced ($p < 0.024$), the variability was reduced ($p < 0.039$), and the peak muscle activity increased ($p < 0.043$). There were trends towards faster ($p > 0.055$) and less variable ($p > 0.065$) chewing.
- **Right-Sided Chewing Gum:** After ICAGD treatment, the rate of chewing increased most dramatically ($p < 0.0002$), the overall muscle activity remained constant, but with a reduction in variability ($p < 0.010$). The patient demonstrated a trend towards higher peak muscle activity ($p > 0.058$), as well.
- **For Both the Left-Sided and Right-Sided Chewing Gum:** The number of EMG Silent Periods observed within the chewing sequence was dramatically reduced from 9 - 12 Silent Periods per

sequence before ICAGD treatment, to 0 - 1 Silent Periods per sequence after ICAGD treatment. This change indicated there was a large reduction in the number of unavoidable tooth contacts present during the chewing of gum.

- **The Left-Sided Average Chewing Pattern (ACP):** After ICAGD treatment, the left-sided ACP pattern was still constrained by the posterior crossbite, and did not change significantly ($p > 0.154$). However, the lateral dimension of the ACP did change significantly ($p < 0.00001$).
- **The Right-Sided Average Chewing Pattern (ACP):** After ICAGD, the right-sided ACP did not change significantly ($p < 0.147$), but exhibited a more convex closing pattern. However, the lateral dimension of the ACP did change significantly ($p < 0.0136$). The opening pathway was still restricted to a large degree, by the adapted left-side posterior crossbite.

The ICAGD occlusal treatment rendered to this patient, did not create perfectly normal masticatory function, but resulted in documented and measurable improvements in the pre-treatment masticatory condition. This case illustrated that the quality of the masticatory function can be measurably evaluated using a combination of technologies:

- Pretreatment, to document the dysfunction;
- Post treatment, where improvements from treatment can be measured; and
- Where functional measurements can be recorded from a very compromised level of masticatory function prior to commencing any occlusal treatment.

Although it is an unrealistic expectation that all patient conditions can be made to function perfectly from undergoing treatment, it is particularly valuable for both researchers and clinicians alike to be able to quantify whether a rendered treatment has been effective. As such, the modern occlusal technologies presented within this chapter make measuring treatment effectiveness a clinical reality, and practicing without their use, makes measuring treatment effectiveness a clinical impossibility.

SOLUTIONS AND RECOMMENDATIONS

Technology has influenced every aspect of society, with new innovative developments that are rapidly replacing conventional methods. This has brought about a definitive paradigm shift. The medical profession has adapted to latest technologies and advancements, many of which have changed the diagnostic approach, and treatment modalities that were commonly employed over the last 50 years. Technology for diagnosis and treatment monitoring is routinely used in everyday medicine, yet unfortunately, the digital approach to diagnosis and treatment planning seems to have faced significantly more resistance within the dental community.

The available advanced dental technologies (T-Scan, Electromyography (EMG), Temporomandibular Joint Vibration Analysis (JVA), and Electrognathography EGN), can be used to enhance the sensitivity and the specificity of a diagnosis, to objectively monitor the progress of treatment, to evaluate the treatment outcome, and to quantify the effect a treatment has made upon the patient's function, and general dental well-being. Every case can be fully documented to detect the presence of masticatory dysfunction that is occurring within the Temporomandibular joints (JVA), within the musculature (EMG), within the overall masticatory function (EGN) and within a malocclusion (T-Scan). Subsequent to rendered treatment, the functional performance can be thoroughly re-tested, to reveal the extent of masticatory system improvements.

Digital diagnostic technologies have been repeatedly shown to be:

- Non-invasive
- Inexpensive to implement
- Reliable indicators of masticatory function and dysfunction
- Valuable guides to successfully evaluate improvements in masticatory function.

A few educational institutions, such as Tufts University School of Dental Medicine, in Boston, Massachusetts, and the University of Tennessee Dental School, in Memphis, Tennessee, as well as other dental schools in thirty countries around the globe, have introduced digital technology and biometric measurement into their curriculum (primarily at the graduate level), where young students are more receptive to the latest technologies and advancements. It appears that the older generations of clinicians are more indoctrinated to resist change. With persistent efforts to emphasize the value, efficiency, and adequacy of digital diagnostic technology, modern authors and researchers should strive to bring about a much needed change amongst the dental community, where technology is embraced into daily practice

FUTURE DIRECTIONS OF DIAGNOSTIC TECHNOLOGY

With the advent of the communication whirlwind that was marked by technologies like the iPhone, and iPad (Apple, Cupertino, CA, USA), this new era of portability and miniaturization will undoubtedly create a new paradigm, wherein diagnosis will be enhanced not only by technology, but by instant access to expert, and on-line systems. Instead of practicing in isolation, as has been the previous model, dentists in the future will network and share knowledge and capabilities, as never before.

Perhaps the largest barrier to the use of technology is the learning curve. The process of educating the profession in new technology has not yet fully penetrated the dental schools. Dental education has readily adopted replacement treatment technologies (such as dental implants, high-speed hand-pieces, machined ceramic crowns) and replacement diagnostic technologies (such as MRI, and CBCT), that upgrade the previous methods, but do not involve any new concepts. Therefore, the dental educators are still teaching many of the same manual diagnostic methods that they learned as students, and that their teachers' teachers learned before them. It seems that changing the curriculum in a dental school has been described as something akin to the *Impossible Dream*.

Learning to use new technology requires more than just understanding how to operate it. It requires an educational commitment to learning what the technology does and how to employ the valuable information it can provide. It also requires comprehension of how and when to use the new information appropriately. This could appear to be a daunting task for those established older clinicians who have not grown up with technology.

The solution to this rapidly changing scenario will be to establish on-line expert consultant capabilities, where the clinician will be required to gather the data based on validated protocols. The data will be transmitted to a central processing area for on-line analysis. Something similar to a lab report will be returned to the clinician, along with treatment recommendations. This will greatly reduce the technological learning curve and make it faster and simpler for a motivated clinician to implement these new technologies.

CONCLUSION

The new diagnostic and treatment evaluation technologies that are available today can add, in-depth value and quantifiable information, to assist a clinician in making a more accurate diagnosis, and enhance the evaluation of the success of a patient's treatment outcome. Resistance to applying digital technology as a diagnostic tool has not resulted from its cost or its complexity, but because of the steep learning curve required, and a general prejudice by some against all new methods, or concepts. These technological breakthroughs will hopefully persist and increase in usage among the more technology-savvy, present day trained clinicians. With time and persistent efforts, despite the ongoing current resistance, diagnostic and treatment monitoring technologies will continue to expand in dentistry.

REFERENCES

Ahlgren, J., & Posselt, U. (1963). Need of functional analysis and selective grinding in orthodontics: A clinical and electromyographic study. *Acta Odontologica Scandinavica*, *21*(6), 187–226. doi:10.3109/00016356308993958 PMID:14042471

Alencar, F. Jr, & Becker, A. (2009). Evaluation of different occlusal splints and counseling in the management of myofascial pain dysfunction. *Journal of Oral Rehabilitation*, *36*(2), 79–85. doi:10.1111/j.1365-2842.2008.01913.x PMID:18976268

American Dental Association. (1983). Report of the president's conference on the examination, diagnosis, and management of temporomandibular disorders. *The Journal of the American Dental Association*, *106*(1), 75–77. PMID:6574170

Atkinson, H. F. (1976). Research into mastication. *Australian Dental Journal*, *21*(1), 23–29. doi:10.1111/j.1834-7819.1976.tb04413.x PMID:1065270

Biller, B. M., Samuels, M. H., Zagar, A., Cook, D. M., Arafah, B. M., & Bonert, V. et al. (2002). Sensitivity and specificity of six tests for the diagnosis of adult GH deficiency. *The Journal of Clinical Endocrinology and Metabolism*, *87*(5), 2067–2079. doi:10.1210/jcem.87.5.8509 PMID:11994342

Brenman, H. S., Black, M. A., & Coslet, J. G. (1968). Interrelationship between the electromyographic silent period and dental occlusion. *Journal of Dental Research*, *47*(3), 502. doi:10.1177/00220345680470033301 PMID:5240811

Carey, J. P., Craig, M., Kerstein, R. B., & Radke, J. (2007). Determining a relationship between applied occlusal load and articulation paper mark area. *The Open Dental Journal*, *1*(1), 1–7. doi:10.2174/1874210600701010001 PMID:19088874

Carr, L. T. (1994). The strengths and weaknesses of quantitative and qualitative research: What method for nursing? *Journal of Advanced Nursing*, *20*(4), 716–721. doi:10.1046/j.1365-2648.1994.20040716.x PMID:7822608

Christensen, L. V. (1989). Reliability of maximum static work efforts by the human masseter muscle. *American Journal of Orthodontics and Dentofacial Orthopedics*, *95*(1), 42–45. doi:10.1016/0889-5406(89)90134-0 PMID:2910025

Christensen, L. V., & Rassouli, N. M. (1995). Experimental occlusal interferences. Part I. A review. *Journal of Oral Rehabilitation*, *22*(7), 515–520. doi:10.1111/j.1365-2842.1995.tb01197.x PMID:7562217

Dimitri, P. S., Wall, C. III, & Oas, J. G. (1996). Classification of human rotation test results using parametric modeling and multivariate statistics. *Acta Oto-Laryngologica*, *116*(4), 497–506. doi:10.3109/00016489609137880 PMID:8831833

Dworkin, S. F. (1991). Illness behavior and dysfunction: Review of concepts and application to chronic pain. *Canadian Journal of Physiology and Pharmacology*, *69*(5), 662–671. doi:10.1139/y91-099 PMID:1863918

Dworkin, S. F., & LeResche, L. (1992). Research diagnostic criteria for temporomandibular disorders: Review, criteria, examinations and specifications, critique. *Journal of Craniomandibular Disorders*, *6*(4), 301–355. PMID:1298767

Dworkin, S. F., LeResche, L., DeRouen, T., & Von Korff, M. (1990). Assessing clinical signs of temporomandibular disorders: Reliability of clinical examiners. *The Journal of Prosthetic Dentistry*, *63*(5), 574–579. doi:10.1016/0022-3913(90)90079-R PMID:2338670

Dworkin, S. F., LeResche, L., & Von Korff, M. R. (1990). Diagnostic studies of temporomandibular disorders: Challenges from an epidemiologic perspective. *Anesthesia Progress*, *37*(2-3), 147–154. PMID:2085194

Eli, I., Baht, R., Kozlovsky, A., & Simon, H. (2000). Effect of gender on acute pain prediction and memory in periodontal surgery. *European Journal of Oral Sciences*, *108*(2), 99–103. doi:10.1034/j.1600-0722.2000.00777.x PMID:10768721

Farrar, W. B. (1972). Differentiation of temporomandibular joint dysfunction to simplify treatment. *The Journal of Prosthetic Dentistry*, *28*(6), 629–636. doi:10.1016/0022-3913(72)90113-8 PMID:4508486

Ferrario, V. F., Sforza, C., D'Addona, A., & Miani, A. Jr. (1991). Reproducibility of electromyographic measures: A statistical analysis. *Journal of Oral Rehabilitation*, *18*(6), 513–521. doi:10.1111/j.1365-2842.1991.tb00074.x PMID:1845607

Forrester, S. E., Pain, M. T., Presswood, R., & Toy, A. (2009). Do the physical properties of occlusal-indicating media affect muscle activity (EMG) during use? *Texas Dental Journal*, *126*(6), 516–525. PMID:19639919

Forrester, S. E., Presswood, R. G., Toy, A. C., & Pain, M. T. (2011). Occlusal measurement method can affect SEMG activity during occlusion. *Journal of Oral Rehabilitation*, *38*(9), 655–660. doi:10.1111/j.1365-2842.2011.02205.x PMID:21314708

Franks, A. S. (1965). The role of electromyography in the diagnosis of complaints about the temporomandibular joint. *Nederlands Tijdschrift voor Tandheelkunde*, *72*(1), 1–11. PMID:14277620

Freedman, D. (2000). *Statistical Models: Theory and Practice*. Cambridge, MA: Cambridge University Press.

Fujii, H., & Mitani, H. (1973). Reflex responses of the masseter and temporal muscles in man. *Journal of Dental Research*, *52*(5), 1046–1050. doi:10.1177/00220345730520050801 PMID:4517741

Gazit, E., Fitzig, S., & Lieberman, M. A. (1986). Reproducibility of occlusal marking techniques. *The Journal of Prosthetic Dentistry*, *55*(4), 505–509. doi:10.1016/0022-3913(86)90188-5 PMID:3457184

Goodson, J.M., & Johansen, E. (1975). Analysis of human mandibular movement. *Monographs in Oral Science*, 5(1)-80.

Greene, C. S. (1973). A survey of current professional concepts and opinions about the myofascial pain-dysfunction (MPD) syndrome. *The Journal of the American Dental Association*, *86*(1), 128–136. PMID:4508871

Greene, C. S. (2010a). Managing the care of patients with temporomandibular disorders: A new guideline for care. *The Journal of the American Dental Association*, *141*(9), 1086–1088. doi:10.14219/jada.archive.2010.0337 PMID:20807907

Greene, C. S. (2010b). Diagnosis and treatment of temporomandibular disorders: Emergence of a new "standard of care". *Quintessence International*, *41*(8), 623–624. PMID:20677398

Greene, C.S., Klasser, G.D., & Epstein, J.B. (2010). Revision of the American Association of Dental Research's Science Information Statement about Temporomandibular Disorders.*Journal of the Canadian Dental Association, 76*(a), 115.

Greene, C. S., Lerman, M. D., Sutcher, H. D., & Laskin, D. M. (1969). The TMJ pain-dysfunction syndrome: Heterogeneity of the patient population. *The Journal of the American Dental Association*, *79*(5), 1168–1172. PMID:5259143

Grossi, M. L., Goldberg, M. B., Locker, D., & Tenenbaum, H. C. (2008). Irritable bowel syndrome patients versus responding and non-responding temporomandibular disorder patients: A neuro-psychologic profile comparative study. *The International Journal of Prosthodontics*, *21*(3), 201–209. PMID:18548956

Hamata, M. M., Zuim, P. R., & Garcia, A. R. (2009). Comparative evaluation of the efficacy of occlusal splints fabricated in centric relation or maximum intercuspation in temporomandibular disorders patients. *Journal of Applied Oral Science*, *17*(1), 32–38. doi:10.1590/S1678-77572009000100007 PMID:19148403

Helkimo, M. (1974). Studies on function and dysfunction of the masticatory system. II. Index for anamnestic and clinical dysfunction and occlusal state. *Svensk Tandlakare Tidskrift. Swedish Dental Journal*, *67*(2), 101–121. PMID:4524733

Iino, M., Takamatsu, T., Mizukami, Y., Bando, S., Kato, Y., & Nakagawa, H. et al. (1989). Silent period and initial occlusal sliding time in patients with premature contacts. *Nippon Shishubyo Gakkai Kaishi*, *31*(4), 1130–1137. doi:10.2329/perio.31.1130 PMID:2489547

Kerstein, R., & Radke, J. (2014). Analysis of masticatory muscle activity pre and post immediate complete anterior guidance development. *Journal of Craniomandibular and Sleep Practice.*

Kerstein, R. B. (1992). Disclusion time reduction therapy with immediate complete anterior guidance development, the technique. *Quintessence International, 23*, 735–747. PMID:1305288

Kerstein, R. B. (1999). Computerized occlusal management of a fixed/detachable implant prosthesis. *Practical Periodontics and Aesthetic Dentistry, 11*(9), 1093–1102. PMID:10853592

Kerstein, R. B., & Grundset, K. (2001). Obtaining Bilateral Simultaneous Occlusal Contacts With Computer Analyzed and Guided Occlusal Adjustments. *Quintessence International, 32*, 7–18.

Kerstein, R. B., Lowe, M., Harty, M., & Radke, J. (2006). A force reproduction analysis of two recording sensors of a computerized occlusal analysis system. *The Journal of Cranio-Mandibular Practice, 24*(1), 15–24. PMID:16541841

Kerstein, R. B., & Radke, J. (2013). Clinician accuracy when subjectively interpreting articulating paper markings. *The Journal of Craniomandibular & Sleep Practice, 32*(1), 13–23. PMID:24660642

Koh, H., & Robinson, P. G. (2004). Occlusal adjustment for treating and preventing temporomandibular joint disorders. *Journal of Oral Rehabilitation, 31*(4), 287–292. doi:10.1046/j.1365-2842.2003.01257.x PMID:15089931

Koole, P. (1998). *Masticatory muscle function: A multichannel electromyographic investigation.* Groningin, Netherlands: Self Published.

Korszun, A., Papadopoulos, E., Demitrack, M., Engleberg, C., & Crofford, L. (1998). The relationship between temporomandibular disorders and stress-associated syndromes. *Oral Surgery, Oral Medicine, Oral Pathology, Oral Radiology, and Endodontics, 864*(4), 416–420. doi:10.1016/S1079-2104(98)90366-3 PMID:9798224

Kuwahara, T., Miyauchi, S., & Maruyama, T. (1990). Characteristics of condylar movements during mastication in stomatognathic dysfunction. *The International Journal of Prosthodontics, 3*(6), 555–566. PMID:2083024

Kuwahara, T., Miyauchi, S., & Maruyama, T. (1992). Clinical classification of the patterns of mandibular movements during mastication in subjects with TMJ disorders. *The International Journal of Prosthodontics, 5*(2), 122–129. PMID:1524632

Laskin, D. M. (1970). Etiology of the myofascial pain-dysfunction syndrome. *Journal of the Massachusetts Dental Society, 19*(4), 227–228. PMID:5277795

Lenton, P., Garfinkel, L., Huggins, K. H., Jackson, A., Look, J., Pan, W., et al. (2007, March). *Examiner reliability for the RDC/TMD group I myofascial pain diagnoses.* Paper presented at the Meeting of the International Association for Dental Research. New Orleans, LA.

Lewin, A., Lemmer, J., & van Rensburg, L. B. (1976). The measurement of jaw movement. Part II. *The Journal of Prosthetic Dentistry, 36*(3), 312–318. doi:10.1016/0022-3913(76)90189-X PMID:1066485

Liebman, F. M., & Kussick, L. (1966). Relationship between force, velocity, and integrated electrical activity in the masticatory muscles of man: Normal and abnormal occlusions. *Journal of Dental Research*, *45*(6), 1752–1761. doi:10.1177/00220345660450062801 PMID:5226541

Look, J. O., Tai, F., Haugan, M., & Schiffman, E. (2007, March). *A prediction model for detection of TMJ intra-articular disorders.* Paper presented at the meeting of the International Association for Dental Research. New Orleans, LA.

Lund, J. P., Widmer, C. G., & Feine, J. S. (1995). Validity of diagnostic and monitoring tests used for temporomandibular disorders. *Journal of Dental Research*, *74*(4), 1133–1143. doi:10.1177/00220345950740041501 PMID:7782545

Manfredini, D., Cocilovo, F., Favero, L., Ferronato, G., Tonello, S., & Guarda-Nardini, L. (2011). Surface electromyography of jaw muscles and kinesiographic recordings: Diagnostic accuracy for myofascial pain. *Journal of Oral Rehabilitation*, *38*(11), 791–799. doi:10.1111/j.1365-2842.2011.02218.x PMID:21480942

McNamara, D. C. (1977). Occlusal adjustment for a physiologically balanced occlusion. *The Journal of Prosthetic Dentistry*, *38*(3), 284–293. doi:10.1016/0022-3913(77)90305-5 PMID:269270

McNeill, C., Danzig, W. M., Farrar, W. B., Gelb, H., Lerman, M. D., & Moffett, B. C. et al. (1980). Position paper of the American Academy of Craniomandibular Disorders: Craniomandibular (TMJ) disorders--the state of the art. *The Journal of Prosthetic Dentistry*, *44*(4), 434–437. doi:10.1016/0022-3913(80)90104-3 PMID:6997473

Mitani, H., Yamashita, A., Fujii, H., Kato, H., & Koizumi, T. (1974). On the power-spectra of the surface electromyograms of masticatory muscles. *Journal of Osaka Dental University*, *8*(1-2), 8–18. PMID:4535008

Mushimoto, E. (1981). The role in masseter muscle activities of functionally elicited periodontal afferents from abutment teeth under overdentures. *Journal of Oral Rehabilitation*, *8*(5), 441–455. doi:10.1111/j.1365-2842.1981.tb00518.x PMID:7028928

Naeije, M., Kalaykova, S., Visscher, C. M., & Lobbezoo, F. (2009). Evaluation of the Research Diagnostic Criteria for Temporomandibular Disorders for the recognition of an anterior disc displacement with reduction. *Journal of Orofacial Pain*, *23*(4), 303–311. PMID:19888478

Ohrbach, R., Sherman, J., Michalovic, S., Dworkin, S. F., Schiffman, E., Truelove, E., & Turner, J. (2007, March). *Validity of RDC/TMD Axis II: Identifying psychiatric morbidity.* Paper presented at the Meeting of the International Association for Dental Research. New Orleans, LA.

Okeson, J. P. (Ed.), *Orofacial Pain: Guidelines for assessment, diagnosis and management.* Chicago, IL: Quintessence, Inc.

Pollack, C. V., & Panacek, E. A. (2000). Basics of Research – Part 4B: Sample size, data collection and bias. *Hong Kong Journal of Emergency Medicine*, *7*(1), 51–56.

Qadeer, S., Kerstein, R. B., Kim, R. J. Y., Huh, J. B., & Shin, S. W. (2012). Relationship between articulation paper mark size and percentage of force measured with computerized occlusal analysis. *Journal of Advanced Prosthodontics*, *4*(1), 7–12. doi:10.4047/jap.2012.4.1.7 PMID:22439094

Reid, K. I., & Greene, C. S. (2013). Diagnosis and treatment of temporomandibular disorders: An ethical analysis of current practices. *Journal of Oral Rehabilitation*, *40*(7), 546–561. doi:10.1111/joor.12067 PMID:23691977

Saad, M. N., Weiner, G., Ehrenberg, D., & Weiner, S. (2008). Effects of load and indicator type upon occlusal contact markings. *Journal of Biomedical Materials Research Part B*, *85*(1), 18–22. doi:10.1002/jbm.b.30910 PMID:17618516

Saitoh, I., Yamada, C., Hayasaki, H., Maruyama, T., Iwase, Y., & Yamasaki, Y. (2010). Is the reverse cycle during chewing abnormal in children with primary dentition? *Journal of Oral Rehabilitation*, *37*(1), 26–33. doi:10.1111/j.1365-2842.2009.02006.x PMID:19874450

Salé, H., Hedman, L., & Isberg, A. (2010). Accuracy of patients' recall of temporomandibular joint pain and dysfunction after experiencing whiplash trauma: A prospective study. *The Journal of the American Dental Association*, *141*(7), 879–886. doi:10.14219/jada.archive.2010.0287 PMID:20592409

Schelb, E., Kaiser, D. A., & Brukl, C. E. (1985). Thickness and marking characteristics of occlusal registration strips. *The Journal of Prosthetic Dentistry*, *54*(1), 122–126. doi:10.1016/S0022-3913(85)80086-X PMID:3860648

Schiffman, E., Truelove, E., Ohrbach, R., Gonzalez, Y., Anderson, G., Jackson, A., et al. (2007, March). *Diagnostic validity of current and revised RDC/TMD myofascial pain diagnoses.* Paper presented at the Meeting of the International Association for Dental Research. New Orleans, LA.

Sforza, C., Rosati, R., De Menezes, M., Musto, F., & Toma, M. (2011). EMG analysis of trapezius and masticatory muscles: Experimental protocol and data reproducibility. *Journal of Oral Rehabilitation*, *38*(9), 648–654. doi:10.1111/j.1365-2842.2011.02208.x PMID:21332571

Shimshak, D. G., & DeFuria, M. S. (1998). Health care utilization by patients with temporomandibular disorders. *The Journal of Cranio-Mandibular Practice*, *16*(3), 185–193. PMID:9852811

Sisk, A. L., Grover, B., & Steflik, D. E. (1991). Long-term memory of acute postsurgical pain. *Journal of Oral and Maxillofacial Surgery*, *49*(4), 353–358. doi:10.1016/0278-2391(91)90369-W PMID:2005492

Sohn, B. W., Miyawaki, S., Noguchi, H., & Takada, K. (1997). Changes in jaw movement and jaw closing muscle activity after orthodontic correction of incisor crossbite. *American Journal of Orthodontics and Dentofacial Orthopedics*, *112*(4), 403–409. doi:10.1016/S0889-5406(97)70048-9 PMID:9345152

Stuart, C.E. (1973). The contributions of gnathology to prosthodontics. *Journal of Prosthetic Dentistry*, *30*(4), 607-608.

Takada, K., Nagata, M., Miyawaki, S., Kuriyama, R., Yasuda, Y., & Sakuda, M. (1992). Automatic detection and measurement of EMG silent periods in masticatory muscles during chewing in man. *Electromyography and Clinical Neurophysiology*, *32*(10-11), 499–505. PMID:1446582

Thompson, J. R., & Graddock, F. W. (1949). Functional analysis of occlusion. *The Journal of the American Dental Association*, *39*(4), 404–406. PMID:18147468

Torii, K. (1989). Analysis of rotation centers of various mandibular closures. *The Journal of Prosthetic Dentistry*, *61*(3), 285–291. doi:10.1016/0022-3913(89)90129-7 PMID:2921746

Torii, K., & Chiwata, I. (2010). Occlusal adjustment using the bite plate-induced occlusal position as a reference position for temporomandibular disorders: A pilot study. *Head & Face Medicine*, *6*(1), 5. doi:10.1186/1746-160X-6-5 PMID:20346167

Toro, A., Buschang, P. H., Throckmorton, G., & Roldán, S. (2006). Masticatory performance in children and adolescents with Class I and II malocclusions. *European Journal of Orthodontics*, *28*(2), 112–119. doi:10.1093/ejo/cji080 PMID:16272209

Truelove, E., Huggins, K. H., Mancl, L., & Dworkin, S. F. (2006). The efficacy of traditional, low-cost and non-splint therapies for temporomandibular disorder: A randomized controlled trial. *The Journal of the American Dental Association*, *137*(8), 1099–1107. doi:10.14219/jada.archive.2006.0348 PMID:16873325

Truelove, E., Sommers, E., Huggins, K. H., Schiffman, E., Ohrbach, R., Look, J. O., & Pan, W. (2007, March). *Diagnostic validity of current and revised RDC/TMD protocols for arthralgia.* Paper presented at the Meeting of the International Association for Dental Research. New Orleans, LA.

Von Korff, M., Ormel, J., Keefe, F. J., & Dworkin, S. F. (1992). Grading the severity of chronic pain. *Pain*, *50*(2), 133–149. doi:10.1016/0304-3959(92)90154-4 PMID:1408309

Wahlund, K., List, T., & Dworkin, S. F. (1998). Temporomandibular disorders in children and adolescents: Reliability of a questionnaire, clinical examination, and diagnosis. *Journal of Orofacial Pain*, *12*(1), 42–51. PMID:9656898

Weisengreen, H., & Elliott, H. W. (1963). Electromyography in patients with orofacial pain. *The Journal of the American Dental Association*, *67*(12), 798–804. PMID:14063214

Wiese, M., Wenzel, A., Hintze, H., Petersson, A., Knutsson, K., & Bakke, M. et al. (2008). Osseous changes and condyle position in TMJ tomograms: Impact of RDC/TMD clinical diagnoses on agreement between expected and actual findings. *Oral Surgery, Oral Medicine, Oral Pathology, Oral Radiology, and Endodontics*, *106*(2), e52–e63. doi:10.1016/j.tripleo.2008.03.021 PMID:18547834

Winocur, E., Reiter, S., Krichmer, M., & Kaffe, I. (2010). Classifying degenerative joint disease by the RDC/TMD and by panoramic imaging: A retrospective analysis. *Journal of Oral Rehabilitation*, *37*(3), 171–177. doi:10.1111/j.1365-2842.2009.02035.x PMID:20002532

Witter, D. J., Woda, A., Bronkhorst, E. M., & Creugers, N. H. (2013). Clinical interpretation of a masticatory normative indicator analysis of masticatory function in subjects with different occlusal and prosthodontic status. *Journal of Dentistry*, *41*(5), 443–448. doi:10.1016/j.jdent.2013.02.004 PMID:23438416

Woda, A., Nicolas, E., Mishellany-Dutour, A., Hennequin, M., Mazille, M. N., Veyrune, J. L., & Peyron, M. A. (2010). The masticatory normative indicator. *Journal of Dental Research*, *89*(3), 281–285. doi:10.1177/0022034509357022 PMID:20118433

Yarnitsky, D., Sprecher, E., Zaslansky, R., & Hemli, J. A. (1996). Multiple session experimental pain measurement. *Pain*, *67*(2-3), 327–333. doi:10.1016/0304-3959(96)03110-7 PMID:8951926

ADDITIONAL READING

Abrão, A. F., Paiva, G., Weffort, S. Y., & de Fantini, S. M. (2011). Clinical exam and electrovibratography detecting articular disk displacement: A comparative study. *The Journal of Cranio-Mandibular Practice*, *29*(4), 270–275. PMID:22128666

Acosta-Ortiz, R., Schulte, J. K., Sparks, B., & Marsh, W. (2004). Prediction of different mandibular activities by EMG signal levels. *Journal of Oral Rehabilitation*, *31*(5), 399–405. doi:10.1111/j.1365-2842.2004.01251.x PMID:15140163

Alarcón, J. A., Martín, C., Palma, J. C., & Menéndez-Núñez, M. (2009). Activity of jaw muscles in unilateral cross-bite without mandibular shift. *Archives of Oral Biology*, *54*(2), 108–114. doi:10.1016/j.archoralbio.2008.10.001 PMID:19019348

Anderson, K., Throckmorton, G. S., Buschang, P. H., & Hayasaki, H. (2002). The effects of bolus hardness on masticatory kinematics. *Journal of Oral Rehabilitation*, *29*(7), 689–696. doi:10.1046/j.1365-2842.2002.00862.x PMID:12153460

Ardizone, I., Celemin, A., Aneiros, F., del Rio, J., Sanchez, T., & Moreno, I. (2010). Electromyographic study of activity of the masseter and anterior temporalis muscles in patients with temporomandibular joint (TMJ) dysfunction: comparison with the clinical dysfunction index. *Medicina Oral Patologia Oral Cirugia Bucal, 1*(15), 1, e14-19.

Baad-Hansen, L., Jadidi, F., Castrillon, E., Thomsen, P. B., & Svensson, P. (2007). Effect of a nociceptive trigeminal inhibitory splint on electromyographic activity in jaw closing muscles during sleep. *Journal of Oral Rehabilitation*, *34*(2), 105–111. doi:10.1111/j.1365-2842.2006.01717.x PMID:17244232

Bakke, M., Møller, E., Thomsen, C. E., Dalager, T., & Werdelin, L. M. (2007). Chewing in patients with severe neurological impairment. *Archives of Oral Biology*, *52*(4), 399–403. doi:10.1016/j.archoralbio.2007.01.003 PMID:17275777

Botelho, A. L., Silva, B. C., Gentil, F. H., Sforza, C., & da Silva, M. A. (2010). Immediate effect of the resilient splint evaluated using surface electromyography in patients with TMD. *The Journal of Cranio-Mandibular Practice*, *28*(4), 266–273. PMID:21032981

Burnett, C. A., & Clifford, T. J. (1999). The mandibular speech envelope in subjects with and without incisal tooth wear. *The International Journal of Prosthodontics*, *12*(6), 514–518. PMID:10815604

Carlson, C. R., Okeson, J. P., Falace, D. A., Nitz, A. J., & Lindroth, J. E. (1993). Reduction of pain and EMG activity in the masseter region by trapezius trigger point injection. *Pain*, *55*(3), 397–400. doi:10.1016/0304-3959(93)90018-K PMID:8121703

Castroflorio, T., Icardi, K., Torsello, F., Deregibus, A., Debernardi, C., & Bracco, P. (2005). Reproducibility of surface EMG in the human masseter and anterior temporalis muscle areas. *The Journal of Cranio-Mandibular Practice*, *23*(2), 130–137. PMID:15898569

Cecere, F., Ruf, S., & Pancherz, H. (1996). Is quantitative electromyography reliable? *Journal of Orofacial Pain*, *10*(1), 38–47. PMID:8995915

Celebic, A., Alajbeg, Z. I., Kraljevic-Simunkovic, S., & Valentic-Peruzovic, M. (2007). Influence of different condylar and incisal guidance ratios to the activity of anterior and posterior temporal muscle. *Archives of Oral Biology*, *52*(2), 142–148. doi:10.1016/j.archoralbio.2006.08.005 PMID:17052681

Ciavarella, D., Mastrovincenzo, M., Sabatucci, A., Parziale, V., Granatelli, F., Violante, F., & Chimenti, C. (2010). Clinical and computerized evaluation in study of temporomandibular joint intracapsular disease. *Minerva Stomatologica*, *59*(3), 89–101. PMID:20357736

Combadazou, J. C., Combelles, R., & Cadenat, H. (1990). The value of mandibular kinesiography and of T-Scanning in the diagnosis and treatment of algo-dysfunctional syndrome of the temporomandibular joint. *Revue de Stomatologie et de Chirurgie Maxillo-Faciale*, *91*(2), 86–91. PMID:2309097

De Felício, C. M., Sidequersky, F. V., Tartaglia, G. M., & Sforza, C. (2009). Electromyographic standardized indices in healthy Brazilian young adults and data reproducibility. *Journal of Oral Rehabilitation*, *36*(8), 577–583. doi:10.1111/j.1365-2842.2009.01970.x PMID:19548958

De Oliveira Serrano, P., Cavalcante, L. M., Del Bel Cury, A. D., Bovi Ambrosano, G. M., & Rodrigues Garcia, R. C. (2008). Effect of incisal tooth wear and restoration on interocclusal distance during Brazilian Portuguese language speech. *Minerva Stomatologica*, *57*(6), 301–308. PMID:18617878

De Rossi, M., De Rossi, A., Hallak, J. E., Vitti, M., & Regalo, S. C. (2009). Electromyographic evaluation in children having rapid maxillary expansion. *American Journal of Orthodontics and Dentofacial Orthopedics*, *136*(3), 355–360. doi:10.1016/j.ajodo.2007.08.027 PMID:19732669

de Souza, R. F., & Compagnoni, M. A. (2004). Relation between speaking space of the /s/ sound and freeway space in dentate and edentatc subjects. *Brazilian Oral Research*, *18*(4), 333–337. doi:10.1590/S1806-83242004000400011 PMID:16089266

Farias Gomes, S. G., Custodio, W., Moura Jufer, J. S., Del Bel Cury, A. A., & Rodrigues Garcia, R. C. (2010). Correlation of mastication and masticatory movements and effect of chewing side preference. *Brazilian Dental Journal*, *21*(4), 351–355. doi:10.1590/S0103-64402010000400011 PMID:20976387

Ferrario, V. F., Piancino, M. G., Dellavia, C., Castroflorio, T., Sforza, C., & Bracco, P. (2006). Quantitative analysis of the variability of unilateral chewing movements in young adults. *The Journal of Cranio-Mandibular Practice*, *24*(4), 274–782. doi:10.1179/crn.2006.043 PMID:17086857

Ferrario, V. F., Sforza, C., Colombo, A., & Ciusa, V. (2000). An electromyographic investigation of masticatory muscles symmetry in normo-occlusion subjects. *Journal of Oral Rehabilitation*, *27*(1), 33–40. doi:10.1046/j.1365-2842.2000.00490.x PMID:10632841

Ferrario, V. F., Sforza, C., Miani, A., & Serrao, G. (1992). Kinesiographic three-dimensional evaluation of mandibular border movements: A statistical study in a normal young non-patient group. *The Journal of Prosthetic Dentistry*, *68*(4), 672–676. doi:10.1016/0022-3913(92)90385-N PMID:1403948

Ferrario, V. F., Sforza, C., Miani, A. Jr, Serrao, G., & Tartaglia, G. (1996). Open-close movements in the human temporomandibular joint: Does a pure rotation around the intercondylar hinge axis exist? *Journal of Oral Rehabilitation*, *23*(6), 401–408. doi:10.1111/j.1365-2842.1996.tb00871.x PMID:8809695

Fresno, M. J., Miralles, R., Valdivia, J., Fuentes, A., Valenzuela, S., Ravera, M. J., & Santander, H. (2007). Electromyographic evaluation of anterior temporal and suprahyoid muscles using habitual methods to determine clinical rest position. *The Journal of Cranio-Mandibular Practice*, *25*(4), 257–263. PMID:17983125

Garcia, A. R., Folli, S., Zuim, P. R., & de Sousa, V. (2008). Mandible protrusion and decrease of TMJ sounds: An electrovibratographic examination. *Brazilian Dental Journal*, *19*(1), 77–82. doi:10.1590/S0103-64402008000100014 PMID:18438565

Garcia, A. R., Madeira, M. C., Paiva, G., & Olivieri, K. A. (2000). Joint vibration analysis in patients with articular inflammation. *The Journal of Cranio-Mandibular Practice*, *18*(4), 272–279. PMID:11202847

Goiato, M. C., Garcia, A. R., dos Santos, D. M., & Pesqueira, A. A. (2010). TMJ vibrations in asymptomatic patients using old and new complete dentures. *Journal of Prosthodontics*, *19*(6), 438–442. doi:10.1111/j.1532-849X.2010.00614.x PMID:20546491

Goodson, J. M., & Johansen, E. (1975). Analysis of human mandibular movement. *Monographs in Oral Science*, *5*, 1–80. PMID:1058999

Hashii, K., Tomida, M., & Yamashita, S. (2009). Influence of changing the chewing region on mandibular movement. *Australian Dental Journal*, *54*(1), 38–44. doi:10.1111/j.1834-7819.2008.01086.x PMID:19228131

Honda, K., Natsumi, Y., & Urade, M. (2008). Correlation between MRI evidence of degenerative condylar surface changes, induction of articular disc displacement and pathological joint sounds in the temporomandibular joint. *Gerodontology*, *25*(4), 251–257. doi:10.1111/j.1741-2358.2008.00219.x PMID:18312371

Huang, Z. S., Lin, X. F., & Li, X. L. (2011). Characteristics of temporomandibular joint vibrations in anterior disk displacement with reduction in adults. *The Journal of Cranio-Mandibular Practice*, *29*(4), 276–283. PMID:22128667

Hwang, I. T., Jung, D. U., Lee, J. H., & Kang, D. W. (2009). Evaluation of TMJ sound on the subject with TMJ disorder by Joint Vibration Analysis. *Journal of Advanced Prosthodontics*, *1*(1), 26–30. doi:10.4047/jap.2009.1.1.26 PMID:21165251

Ishigaki, S., Bessette, R. W., & Maruyama, T. (1993). Vibration analysis of the temporomandibular joints with degenerative joint disease. *The Journal of Cranio-Mandibular Practice*, *11*(4), 276–283. PMID:8118898

Ishigaki, S., Bessette, R. W., & Maruyama, T. (1993). Vibration analysis of the temporomandibular joints with meniscal displacement with and without reduction. *The Journal of Cranio-Mandibular Practice*, *11*(3), 192–201. PMID:8242781

Ishigaki, S., Bessette, R. W., & Maruyama, T. (1993). Vibration of the temporomandibular joints with normal radiographic imagings: Comparison between asymptomatic volunteers and symptomatic patients. *The Journal of Cranio-Mandibular Practice*, *11*(2), 88–94. PMID:8495512

Ishigaki, S., Bessette, R. W., & Maruyama, T. (1994). Diagnostic accuracy of TMJ vibration analysis for internal derangement and/or degenerative joint disease. *The Journal of Cranio-Mandibular Practice*, *12*(4), 241–245. PMID:7828206

Ishigaki, S., Kurozumi, T., Morishige, E., & Yatani, H. (2006). Occlusal interference during mastication can cause pathological tooth mobility. *Journal of Periodontal Research*, *41*(3), 189–192. doi:10.1111/j.1600-0765.2005.00856.x PMID:16677287

Ishigaki, S., Nakamura, T., Akanishi, M., & Maruyama, T. (1989). Clinical classification of maximal opening and closing movements. *The International Journal of Prosthodontics*, *2*(2), 148–154. PMID:2597300

Kamyszek, G., Ketcham, R., Garcia, R. Jr, & Radke, J. (2001). Electromyographic evidence of reduced muscle activity when ULF-TENS is applied to the Vth and VIIth cranial nerves. *The Journal of Cranio-Mandibular Practice*, *19*(3), 162–168. PMID:11482827

Katase-Akiyama, S., Kato, T., Yamashita, S., Masuda, Y., & Morimoto, T. (2009). Specific increase in non-functional masseter bursts in subjects aware of tooth-clenching during wakefulness. *Journal of Oral Rehabilitation*, *36*(2), 93–101. doi:10.1111/j.1365-2842.2008.01911.x PMID:18976275

Kecik, D., Kocadereli, I., & Saatci, I. (2005). Condylar disc relationships and vibration energy in asymptomatic class I 9- to 12-year olds. *The Angle Orthodontist*, *75*(1), 54–62. PMID:15747816

Kerstein, R. B. (2004). Combining technologies: A computerized occlusal analysis system synchronized with a computerized electromyography system. *The Journal of Cranio-Mandibular Practice*, *22*(2), 96–109. doi:10.1179/crn.2004.013 PMID:15134409

Kerstein, R. B. (2010). Reducing chronic masseter and temporalis muscular hyperactivity with computer-guided occlusal adjustments. *The Compendium of Continuing Education in Dentistry*, *31*(7), 530–534, 536, 538 passim. PMID:20879206

Kerstein, R. B., & Radke, J. (2012). Masseter and temporalis excursive hyperactivity decreased by measured anterior guidance development. *The Journal of Cranio-Mandibular Practice*, *30*(4), 243–254. PMID:23156965

Kerstein, R. B., & Wright, N. R. (1991). Electromyographic and computer analyses of patients suffering from chronic myofascial pain-dysfunction syndrome: Before and after treatment with immediate complete anterior guidance development. *The Journal of Prosthetic Dentistry*, *66*(5), 677–686. doi:10.1016/0022-3913(91)90453-4 PMID:1805009

Kim, S. K., Kim, K. N., Chang, I. T., & Heo, S. J. (2001). A study of the effects of chewing patterns on occlusal wear. *Journal of Oral Rehabilitation*, *28*(11), 1048–1055. doi:10.1046/j.1365-2842.2001.00761.x PMID:11722722

Kimoto, K., Fushima, K., Tamaki, K., Toyoda, M., Sato, S., & Uchimura, N. (2000). Asymmetry of masticatory muscle activity during the closing phase of mastication. *The Journal of Cranio-Mandibular Practice*, *18*(4), 257–263. PMID:11202845

Kobayashi, Y., Shiga, H., Yokoyama, M., Arakawa, I., & Nakajima, K. (2009). Differences in masticatory function of subjects with different closing path. *Journal of Prosthodontic Research, 53*(3), 142–145. doi:10.1016/j.jpor.2009.04.001 PMID:19464981

Komiyama, O., Wang, K., Svensson, P., Arendt-Nielsen, L., & De Laat, A. (2006). Reproducibility of the masseteric exteroceptive suppression period using stimulus-response curves. *Journal of Oral Rehabilitation, 33*(10), 741–748. doi:10.1111/j.1365-2842.2006.01624.x PMID:16938102

Kubota, N., Hayasaki, H., Saitoh, I., Iwase, Y., Maruyama, T., Inada, E., & Yamasaki, Y. (2010). Jaw motion during gum-chewing in children with primary dentition. *The Journal of Cranio-Mandibular Practice, 28*(1), 19–29. PMID:20158006

Kuwahara, T., Bessette, R. W., & Maruyama, T. (1995). Chewing pattern analysis in TMD patients with and without internal derangement: Part I. *The Journal of Cranio-Mandibular Practice, 13*(1), 8–14. PMID:7586007

Kuwahara, T., Bessette, R. W., & Maruyama, T. (1995). Chewing pattern analysis in TMD patients with and without internal derangement: Part II. *The Journal of Cranio-Mandibular Practice, 13*(2), 93–98. PMID:8697506

Kuwahara, T., Bessette, R. W., & Maruyama, T. (1995). Chewing pattern analysis in TMD patients with unilateral and bilateral internal derangement. *The Journal of Cranio-Mandibular Practice, 13*(3), 167–172. PMID:8949856

Kuwahara, T., Bessette, R. W., & Maruyama, T. (1996). Characteristic chewing parameters for specific types of temporomandibular joint internal derangements. *The Journal of Cranio-Mandibular Practice, 14*(1), 12–22. PMID:9086871

Kuwahara, T., Miyauchi, S., & Maruyama, T. (1992). Clinical classification of the patterns of mandibular movements during mastication in subjects with TMJ disorders. *The International Journal of Prosthodontics, 5*(2), 122–129. PMID:1524632

Kuwahara, T., Yoshioka, C., Ogawa, H., & Maruyama, T. (1994). Effect of malocclusion on mandibular movement during speech. *The International Journal of Prosthodontics, 7*(3), 264–270. PMID:7916893

Learreta, J. A., Beas, J., Bono, A. E., & Durst, A. (2007). Muscular activity disorders in relation to intentional occlusal interferences. *The Journal of Cranio-Mandibular Practice, 25*(3), 193–199. PMID:17696036

Lepley, C., Throckmorton, G., Parker, S., & Buschang, P. H. (2010). Masticatory performance and chewing cycle kinematics-are they related? *The Angle Orthodontist, 80*(2), 295–301. doi:10.2319/061109-333.1 PMID:19905854

Li, X., Lin, X., & Wang, Y. (2009). Temporomandibular joint vibration in bruxers. *The Journal of Cranio-Mandibular Practice, 27*(3), 167–173. PMID:19697644

Lin, X. F., Li, S. H., Huang, Z. S., & Wu, X. Y. (2010). Relationship between occlusal plane and masticatory path in youth with individual normal occlusion. *Zhonghua Kou Qiang Yi Xue Za Zhi, 45*(6), 370–375. PMID:21163016

Liu, Z. J., Yamagata, K., Kasahara, Y., & Ito, G. (1999). Electromyographic examination of jaw muscles in relation to symptoms and occlusion of patients with temporomandibular joint disorders. *Journal of Oral Rehabilitation*, *26*(1), 33–47. doi:10.1046/j.1365-2842.1999.00356.x PMID:10080323

Mazzeto, M. O., Hotta, T. H., & Mazzetto, R. G. (2009). Analysis of TMJ vibration sounds before and after use of two types of occlusal splints. *Brazilian Dental Journal*, *20*(4), 325–330. doi:10.1590/S0103-64402009000400011 PMID:20069257

Mazzetto, M. O., Hotta, T. H., Carrasco, T. G., & Mazzetto, R. G. (2008). Characteristics of TMD noise analyzed by electrovibratography. *The Journal of Cranio-Mandibular Practice*, *26*(3), 222–228. PMID:18686500

Mioche, L., Bourdiol, P., Martin, J. F., & Noël, Y. (1999). Variations in human masseter and temporalis muscle activity related to food texture during free and side-imposed mastication. *Archives of Oral Biology*, *44*(12), 1005–1012. doi:10.1016/S0003-9969(99)00103-X PMID:10669078

Montgomery, M. W., Shuman, L., & Morgan, A. (2010). Joint vibration analysis in routine restorative dentistry. *Dentistry Today*, *29*(9), 94, 96–97. PMID:20973423

Murakami, T., Harada, T., Abe, K., & Tanaka, T. (2000). Masticatory movement in two cases with unusual alignment of the maxillary canine. *Journal of Oral Rehabilitation*, *27*(4), 317–331. doi:10.1046/j.1365-2842.2000.00565.x PMID:10792593

Ohrbach, R., Markiewicz, M. R., & McCall, W. D. Jr. (2008, October). Waking-state oral parafunctional behaviors: Specificity and validity as assessed by electromyography. *European Journal of Oral Sciences*, *116*(5), 438–444. doi:10.1111/j.1600-0722.2008.00560.x PMID:18821986

Olivieri, K. A., Garcia, A. R., Paiva, G., & Stevens, C. (1999). Joint vibrations analysis in asymptomatic volunteers and symptomatic patients. *The Journal of Cranio-Mandibular Practice*, *17*(3), 176–183. PMID:10650404

Ono, T., Iwata, H., Hori, K., Tamine, K., Kondoh, J., Hamanaka, S., & Maeda, Y. (2009). Evaluation of tongue-, jaw-, and swallowing-related muscle coordination during voluntarily triggered swallowing. *The International Journal of Prosthodontics*, *22*(4), 493–498. PMID:20095201

Piancino, M. G., Farina, D., Talpone, F., Merlo, A., & Bracco, P. (2009). Muscular activation during reverse and non-reverse chewing cycles in unilateral posterior crossbite. *European Journal of Oral Sciences*, *117*(2), 122–128. doi:10.1111/j.1600-0722.2008.00601.x PMID:19320720

Pinho, J. C., Caldas, F. M., Mora, M. J., & Santana-Penín, U. (2000). Electromyographic activity in patients with temporomandibular disorders. *Journal of Oral Rehabilitation*, *27*(11), 985–990. doi:10.1046/j.1365-2842.2000.00571.x PMID:11106990

Radke, J., Garcia, R. Jr, & Ketcham, R. (2001). Wavelet transforms of TM joint vibrations: A feature extraction tool for detecting reducing displaced disks. *The Journal of Cranio-Mandibular Practice*, *19*(2), 84–90. PMID:11842869

Radke, J. C., Ketcham, R., Glassman, B., & Kull, R. (2003). Artificial neural network learns to differentiate normal TMJs and non-reducing displaced disks after training on incisor-point chewing movements. *The Journal of Cranio-Mandibular Practice*, *21*(4), 259–264. PMID:14620698

Radke, J. C., & Kull, R. S. (2012). Distribution of temporomandibular joint vibration transfer to the opposite side. *The Journal of Cranio-Mandibular Practice*, *30*(3), 194–200. PMID:22916672

Ries, L. G., Alves, M. C., & Bérzin, F. (2008). Asymmetric activation of temporalis, masseter, and sternocleidomastoid muscles in temporomandibular disorder patients. *The Journal of Cranio-Mandibular Practice*, *26*(1), 59–64. PMID:18290526

Rodrigues Garcia, R. C., Oliveira, V. M., & Del Bel Cury, A. A. (2003). Effect of new dentures on inter-occlusal distance during speech. *The International Journal of Prosthodontics*, *16*(5), 533–537. PMID:14651241

Rohida, N. S., & Bhad, W. (2010). A Clinical, MRI, And EMG Analysis Comparing The Efficacy Of Twin Blocks And Flat Occlusal Splints In The Management Of Disc Displacements With Reduction. *World Journal of Orthodontics*, *11*(3), 236–244. PMID:20877732

Rossetti, L. M., Pereira de Araujo Cdos, R., Rossetti, P. H., & Conti, P. C. (1986). Association between rhythmic masticatory muscle activity during sleep and masticatory myofascial pain: A polysomnographic study. *Journal of Orofacial Pain*, *22*(3), 190–200. PMID:18780532

Savabi, O., Nejatidanesh, F., & Khosravi, S. (2007). Effect of occlusal splints on the electromyographic activities of masseter and temporal muscles during maximum clenching. *Quintessence International*, *38*(2), e129–e132. PMID:17510715

Serrano Pde, O., Faot, F., Del Bel Cury, A. A., & Rodrigues Garcia, R. C. (2008). Effect of dental wear, stabilization appliance and anterior tooth reconstruction on mandibular movements during speech. *Brazilian Dental Journal*, *19*(2), 151–158. doi:10.1590/S0103-64402008000200012 PMID:18568231

Sforza, C., Peretta, R., Grandi, G., Ferronato, G., & Ferrario, V. F. (2008). Soft tissue facial planes and masticatory muscle function in skeletal Class III patients before and after orthognathic surgery treatment. *Journal of Oral and Maxillofacial Surgery*, *66*(4), 691–698. doi:10.1016/j.joms.2007.06.645 PMID:18355592

Sforza, C., Zanotti, G., Mantovani, E., & Ferrario, V. F. (2007). Fatigue in the masseter and temporalis muscles at constant load. *The Journal of Cranio-Mandibular Practice*, *25*(1), 30–36. PMID:17304915

Sierpińska, T., Gołebiewska, M., & Długosz, J. W. (2006). The relationship between masticatory efficiency and the state of dentition at patients with non-rehabilitated partial loss of teeth. *Advances in Medical Sciences*, *51*(Suppl 1), 196–199. PMID:17458090

Sierpinska, T., Golebiewska, M., & Lapuc, M. (2008). The effect of mastication on occlusal parameters in healthy volunteers. *Advances in Medical Sciences*, *53*(2), 316–320. doi:10.2478/v10039-008-0049-1 PMID:19095582

Suzuki, E., Ishigaki, S., Yatani, H., Morishige, E., & Uchida, M. (2010). Mean power frequency during speech in myalgia patients. *Journal of Oral Rehabilitation*, *37*(9), 692–697. doi:10.1111/j.1365-2842.2010.02101.x PMID:20492433

Tartaglia, G. M., Barozzi, S., Marin, F., Cesarani, A., & Ferrario, V. F. (2008). Electromyographic activity of sternocleidomastoid and masticatory muscles in patients with vestibular lesions. *Journal of Applied Oral Science*, *16*(6), 391–396. doi:10.1590/S1678-77572008000600007 PMID:19082397

Tartaglia, G. M., Testori, T., Pallavera, A., Marelli, B., & Sforza, C. (2008). Electromyographic analysis of masticatory and neck muscles in subjects with natural dentition, teeth-supported and implant-supported prostheses. *Clinical Oral Implants Research*, *19*(10), 1081–1088. doi:10.1111/j.1600-0501.2008.01574.x PMID:18828826

Tecco, S., Epifania, E., & Festa, F. (2008). An electromyographic evaluation of bilateral symmetry of masticatory, neck and trunk muscles activity in patients wearing a positioner. *Journal of Oral Rehabilitation*, *35*(6), 433–439. doi:10.1111/j.1365-2842.2007.01788.x PMID:18318706

Tecco, S., Tetè, S., D'Attilio, M., Perillo, L., & Festa, F. (2008). Surface electromyographic patterns of masticatory, neck, and trunk muscles in temporomandibular joint dysfunction patients undergoing anterior repositioning splint therapy. *European Journal of Orthodontics*, *30*(6), 592–597. doi:10.1093/ejo/cjn052 PMID:18990679

Tsolka, P., Fenlon, M. R., McCullock, A. J., & Preiskel, H. W. (1994). A controlled clinical, electromyographic, and kinesiographic assessment of craniomandibular disorders in women. *Journal of Orofacial Pain*, *8*(1), 80–89. PMID:8032335

Vaiman, M., & Eviatar, E. (2009). Surface electromyography as a screening method for evaluation of dysphagia and odynophagia. *Head & Face Medicine*, *20*(5), 9. doi:10.1186/1746-160X-5-9 PMID:19232090

van der Kaaij, N. C., Maillou, P., van der Weijden, J. J., Naeije, M., & Lobbezoo, F. (2009). Reproducible effects of subjectively assessed muscle fatigue on an inhibitory jaw reflex in humans. *Archives of Oral Biology*, *54*(9), 879–883. doi:10.1016/j.archoralbio.2009.06.001 PMID:19555924

Wang, M. Q., He, J. J., Wang, K., & Svensson, P. (2009). Influence of changing occlusal support on jaw-closing muscle electromyographic activity in healthy men and women. *Acta Odontologica Scandinavica*, *67*(3), 187–192. doi:10.1080/00016350902794800 PMID:19291503

Wang, X. R., Zhang, Y., Xing, N., Xu, Y. F., & Wang, M. Q. (2013). Stable tooth contacts in intercuspal occlusion makes for utilities of the jaw elevators during maximal voluntary clenching. *Journal of Oral Rehabilitation*, *40*(5), 319–328. doi:10.1111/joor.12044 PMID:23480460

Wilding, R. J., & Lewin, A. (1991). A model for optimum functional human jaw movements based on values associated with preferred chewing patterns. *Archives of Oral Biology*, *36*(7), 519–523. doi:10.1016/0003-9969(91)90145-K PMID:1776926

Wilding, R. J., & Lewin, A. (1994). The determination of optimal human jaw movements based on their association with chewing performance. *Archives of Oral Biology*, *39*(4), 333–343. doi:10.1016/0003-9969(94)90125-2 PMID:8024498

Wilding, R. J., & Shaikh, M. (1997). Jaw movement tremor as a predictor of chewing performance. *Journal of Orofacial Pain, 11*(2), 101–114. PMID:10332316

Wilding, R. J., & Shaikh, M. (1997). Muscle activity and jaw movements as predictors of chewing performance. *Journal of Orofacial Pain, 11*(1), 24–36. PMID:10332308

Wilson, E. M., & Green, J. R. (2009). The development of jaw motion for mastication. *Early Human Development, 85*(5), 303–311. doi:10.1016/j.earlhumdev.2008.12.003 PMID:19185434

Wintergerst, A. M., Throckmorton, G. S., & Buschang, P. H. (2008). Effects of bolus size and hardness on within-subject variability of chewing cycle kinematics. *Archives of Oral Biology, 53*(4), 369–375. doi:10.1016/j.archoralbio.2007.10.012 PMID:18093571

Yashiro, K., Miyawaki, S., & Takada, K. (2004). Stabilization of jaw-closing movements during chewing after correction of incisor crossbite. *Journal of Oral Rehabilitation, 31*(10), 949–956. doi:10.1111/j.1365-2842.2004.01326.x PMID:15387833

Yashiro, K., & Takada, K. (2004). Validity of measurements for cycle-by-cycle variability of jaw movements: Variability of chewing cycles in cases of prognathism. *Physiological Measurement, 25*(5), 1125–1137. doi:10.1088/0967-3334/25/5/004 PMID:15535179

Yoshioka, C., Ogawa, H., Kuwahara, T., Takashima, F., & Maruyama, T. (1993). The relationship between the mandibular movements during speech and specific types of malocclusions. *The Journal of Osaka University Dental School, 33*, 39–44. PMID:8935081

KEY TERMS AND DEFINITIONS

Average Chewing Pattern (ACP): The mean frontal, coronal and sagittal patterns of a patient's chewing movements, calculated from a complete mastication sequence.

Bio-Physiologic Measurement: The measurement of any physiologic processes, usually for the purpose of evaluating its function. Also referred to as, Biometrics.

Dysthymia: A neurotic, chronic depression. A mood disorder with the same cognitive and physical symptoms as depression, but less severe with longer-lasting symptoms.

Electrognathograph: A magnet-based incisor-point jaw movement recording technology. It records in 3-Dimensions (frontal, coronal and sagittal planes), the path and speed of the lower incisors during various mandibular movements.

Electromyograph: A device for measuring the electrical activity associated with skeletal muscle contractions. The unit of measure is the microvolt, one millionth of a volt.

Immediate Complete Anterior Guidance Development: A method of coronoplasty utilizing the T-Scan, to detect and remove excursive friction present in all excursive movements.

Irritable Bowel Syndrome (IBS): A condition of unknown etiology causing disruption of lower intestinal function and discomfort, but without evidence of inflammation.

Joint Vibration Analysis System: A device for recording and analyzing vibrations emanating from the Temporomandibular joints during movements. The recorded vibrations are described by a unit of pressure, equivalent to loudness known as the Pascal, which is defined as 101.97 grams of force, spread over a one meter area.

Myofascial Pain Dysfunction Syndrome (MPDS): A term coined in 1970 under the theory that painful conditions of the masticatory system are primarily due to emotional stresses rather than physiologic causes.

Research Diagnostic Criteria: A scheme designed to diagnose all TMD conditions as if they were somatized pain conditions irrespective of actual etiology. Introduced in 1992 and extensively studied, it has never been successfully validated.

Temporomandibular Disorders (TMD or TMJD): An umbrella term referring to one or more of at least, 38 distinct pathologic conditions within the head and neck area. It is always a plural term and never represents a diagnosis.

ENDNOTES

1. The Figures 1–20 are all captured from the BioPAK™ computer program, © 2013 BioResearch Associates, Inc. Milwaukee, WI 53223.
2. The Figures 18 and 19 are captured from the T-Scan® Program, © 2013 Tekscan, Inc., South Boston, MA.

This work was previously published in the Handbook of Research on Computerized Occlusal Analysis Technology Applications in Dental Medicine edited by Robert B. Kerstein, DMD, pages 153-214, copyright year 2015 by Medical Information Science Reference (an imprint of IGI Global).

Chapter 7
Dental Diagnosis From X-Ray Images Using Fuzzy Rule-Based Systems

Tran Manh Tuan
Thai Nguyen University, Vietnam

Nguyen Thanh Duc
Hanoi University of Science and Technology, Vietnam

Pham Van Hai
Hanoi University of Science and Technology, Vietnam

Le Hoang Son
VNU University of Science, Vietnam

ABSTRACT

In practical dentistry, dentists use their experience to examine dental X-ray images and to derive symptoms from patients for concluding possible diseases. This method is based solely on the own dentists' experience. Dental diagnosis from X-Ray images is proposed to support for dentists in their decision making. This paper presents an application of consultant system for dental diagnosis from X-Ray images based on fuzzy rule. Fuzzy rule was applied in many applications and has important role in computational intelligence, data mining, machine learning, etc. Based on a dental X-ray image dataset, we use Fuzzy C-Means to classify them into clusters and construct the rule set. Fuzzy Inference System is then used to evaluate the rules by three validity indices. These rules accompanied with symptoms from patients help dentists in diagnosing dental diseases. This method is implemented and experimentally validated on the real dataset of Hanoi Medical University Hospital, Vietnam against the related algorithms.

1. INTRODUCTION

In the modern world, the health of human gets a special caring. Scientists try to find out the way for supporting clinicians in diagnosing disease. In 2012, Support Vector Machine (SVM) was used in diagnosis of osteoporosis from dental panoramic images by Kavitha, et al. (2012). Chattopadhyay et al. (2012) presented an application of Bayesian classifier for diagnosis of dental pain. Oad, DeZhi and Butt (2014) proposed a fuzzy rule-based approach to predict risk level of heart disease. Ramírez, Castillo and Soria (2010) used Fuzzy K-Nearest Neighbor (FKNN) algorithm for various medical problems

DOI: 10.4018/978-1-5225-1903-4.ch007

including dental diagnosis. However, dentists use their experiences to diagnose diseases from dental X-ray images of a patient. Such the experts' experience varies by different dentists. Thus, it is necessary to predict dental diseases from X-ray images and to support the dentists in diagnosing dental diseases. Computerized medical diagnosis systems are of great interest to clinicians for accurate decision making of possible diseases and treatments (Doi, 2014). One of the most typical approaches is *fuzzy inference system* (FIS) which determines a projection from a given input data set to an output data set using fuzzy logic (Guillaume, 2001 and Oad, DeZhi and Butt (2014)). However, forming such the rules requires much experience from experts in order to guarantee accurate diagnosis and avoid duplicate, conflict and meaningless rules (Grabisch, Nguyen and Walker, 2013). Another rule-based technique proposed (Hühn and Hüllermeier, 2009) is FURIA (Fuzzy Unordered Rule Induction Algorithm) which deals with uncovered examples by making use of an efficient rule stretching method. FURIA applies pruning modifications for optimizing the rule sets represented in a specific form and fuzzified by a greedy algorithm. A classifier output is given by using this method.

Fuzzy inference (Guillaume, 2001) is a process that determines exactly a projection from a given input data set to an output data set using fuzzy logic. This projection provides a basic in which we can make decisions or visual models. Fuzzy inference progress consists of three main parts: membership function, logic operators and rules in the form of "If.... then..." and works through five periods: 1) Fuzzification input variables; 2) Apply fuzzy operators (AND or OR) to these variables; 3) Infer results from given input; 4) Summary obtained results; and 5) Defuzzification. Fuzzy inference system (FIS) has been applied successfully in many different fields such as automatic control (Hosseini and Etemadi, 2008 and Lee, 1990), data classification (Wang and Lee, 2002), expert system (Togai and Watanabe, 1986) and computer vision (Ho et al., 2002), and stock market (Boyacioglu and Avci, 2010). FIS is also called as a fuzzy rule based system, a fuzzy expert system, a fuzzy model, a fuzzy combination memory, a fuzzy logic control set and a fuzzy system. There are three kinds of FIS: Mamdani FIS, Sugeno FIS and Tsukamoto FIS. The idea of applying FIS for the dental diagnosis problem is demonstrated as follows. FIS is a rule-based system, so that, it needs a rule set. At the beginning, we extract dental features from the training dataset to create a dental database. Fuzzy rules are then generated by the Fuzzy C-Means (FCM) method (Bezdek, Ehrlich and Full, 1984). Those rules are used to predict the diseases in the testing set by an inference mechanism of FIS.

The new contributions of this paper are: 1) Building a dental feature database from dental X-ray images of Hanoi Medical University; 2) Proposing a new FIS-based model to support diagnosing dental diseases via the obtained database; 3) Implementing this model and validating its performance by different criteria in comparison with FKNN. Such the contributions prove the roles of fuzzy systems to dental diagnosis problem.

The rests of this paper are organized as follow. Section 2 presents some background knowledge including the FCM method, an overview of FIS, and details of FKNN. Section 3 describes the new contributions namely mechanism of fuzzy control system, feature extraction methods and the rule generation progress. Section 4 shows experimental results and discussions. Finally, some conclusions and future works are drawn in Section 5.

2. BACKGROUND

In this section, we firstly overview about the Fuzzy C-Means (FCM), and then describes background knowledge of Fuzzy Inference System (FIS). Lastly, details of Fuzzy K-Nearest Neighbor (FKNN) are given.

2.1. Fuzzy C-Means (FCM)

Fuzzy C-Means (Bezdek, Ehrlich and Full, 1984) is based on an iteration process to optimize the membership matrix and the cluster centers. The objective function of FCM is:

$$J = \sum_{k=1}^{N} \sum_{j=1}^{C} u_{kj} \times \left\| X_k - V_j \right\| \to \min \tag{1}$$

$$\begin{cases} u_{kj} \in [0,1] \\ \sum_{j=1}^{C} u_{kj} = 1 \\ k = \overline{1,N};\ j = \overline{1,C} \end{cases} \tag{2}$$

where m is fuzzier, C is the number of clusters, N is the number of data elements, r is the dimensionality of the data, u_{kj} is the membership degree of data elements X_k to cluster j, $X_k \in R^r$ is the kth element of $X = \{X_1, X_2, \ldots, X_N\}$, and V_j is the center of cluster j. Using the Lagrange multiplier method for problem (1-2), the cluster centers and the membership matrix are determined in the Equations (3-4), respectively:

$$V_j = \frac{\sum_{k=1}^{C} u_{kj}^m X_k}{\sum_{k=1}^{C} u_{kj}^m} \tag{3}$$

$$u_{kj} = \frac{1}{\sum_{i=1}^{C} \left(\frac{\left\| X_k - V_j \right\|}{\left\| X_k - V_i \right\|} \right)^{\frac{1}{m-1}}} \tag{4}$$

2.2. Fuzzy Inference Systems

Fuzzy inference system (FIS) is a popular computing framework based on the concept of fuzzy set theory which has been applied successfully in many fields such as control, decision support, system identifica-

Figure 1. General diagram of FIS

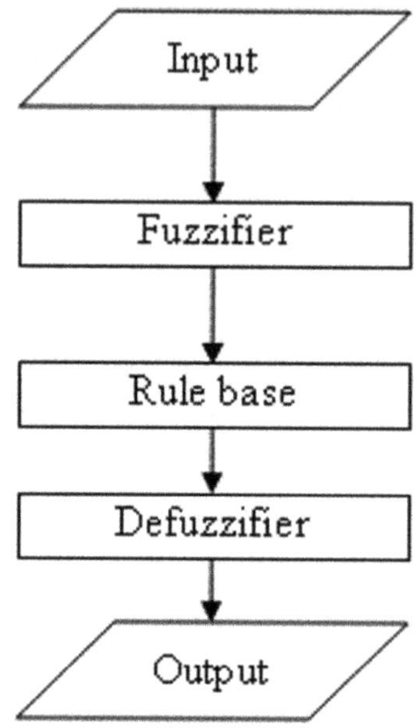

tion, etc. (Chaudhari, Patil, and Bambhori, 2014). General diagram of a FIS includes three main parts: a fuzzifier, a rule base and a defuzzifier (see Figure 1).

There are three types of FIS (Sun, 1994): Mamdani fuzzy inference, Sugeno (or Takagi-Sugeno) fuzzy inference, Tsukamoto fuzzy inference. In this paper, Sugeno FIS is mentioned and used. A *Sugeno fuzzy inference system* has R rules, each of them is:

$$K\text{: If } x \text{ is } A^k_i \text{ and } y \text{ is } B^k_j \text{ then } z^k = f(x,y) \tag{5}$$

Similar to Mamdani, $k = 1, \ldots, R$, $i = 1, \ldots, N$ and $j = 1 \ldots M$ where N and M are the numbers of membership functions for inputs. The defuzzification of this system uses the weighted average operator. Because a Sugeno system is a more compact and computationally efficient representation than a Mamdani system, it lends itself to the use of adaptive techniques for constructing fuzzy models. These adaptive techniques can be used to customize the membership functions so that the fuzzy system best models the data. The advantages of Sugeno are computationally efficient, working well with linear techniques and optimization and adaptive techniques, guaranteed continuity of the output surface and lastly well suited to mathematical analysis. One of the large problems with the Sugeno FIS is that there is no good intuitive method for determining the coefficients, p, q, and r. Also, the Sugeno has only crisp outputs. We also can see the structure of ANFIS implementing Sugeno as in Figure 2.

In the recent studies, there are several results providing the comparison among FIS models (Mamdani, Sugeno and ANFIS). Nayak, Narayanan, and Paramasivam (2013) showed that these models used different methods (namely grid partitioning, fuzzy c-means, and subtractive clustering) to get the membership function during the fuzzification of inputs which is the first step in the creation of FIS. Based on the comparison table that has been prepared to list out the efficiencies in terms of accuracy for the different techniques used, the results showed that among the Mamdani-type FIS, grid partitioning method

Figure 2. Architecture of ANFIS implementing Tsukamoto FIS

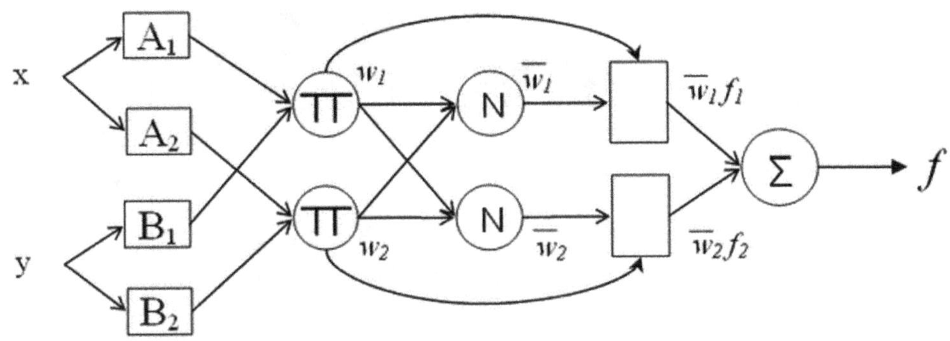

gave better accuracy than subtractive and fuzzy c-means clustering techniques. In the works of Nayak, Narayanan and Paramasivam (2013), fuzzy inference systems (Mamdani, Sugeno and ANFIS fuzzy models) are used to predict the weekly prices of Fund for the Egyptian Market. The results of the three fuzzy inference systems (FIS) are compared based on MAE index with the different sample size (from minimum 30 to maximum 862) and T-test between Actual values and predicted values as well. For this typical application, the performance of ANFIS method is better than that of Sugeno and Mamdani for the same fuzzy technique.

2.3. Fuzzy K-Nearest Neighbor

FKNN is called as nonparametric lazy algorithm because it does not make any assumptions on the underlying data distribution and does not use the training data points to do any generalization used for classification and regression (Ramírez, Castillo and Soria, 2010). The input consists of k closest training examples in the feature space. In FKNN, the output is a class membership. An object is classified by a majority vote of its neighbors, with the object being assigned to the class most common among its k nearest neighbors (k is a positive integer, typically small). If $k = 1$, then the object is simply assigned to the class of that single nearest neighbor. The best choice of k depends upon the data; generally, larger values of k reduce the effect of noise on the classification but it is difficult to determine the common boundary.

3. PROPOSED FIS BASED SYSTEM FOR DENTAL DIAGNOSIS

In this section, we firstly propose a general diagram for inference mechanism in Section 3.1. Then, in Section 3.2, feature extraction of dental X-ray images in order to build a dental feature database is described. Section 3.3 describes the methods for generating rules from this database. Finally, Section 3.4 gives inference mechanism for dental diagnosis problem.

3.1. The Main Mechanism

Figure 3 presents the general diagram for inference mechanism. In this figure, the features of dental images are determined to build a dental feature database (see Section 3.2). After that, this database is

Figure 3. Main mechanism

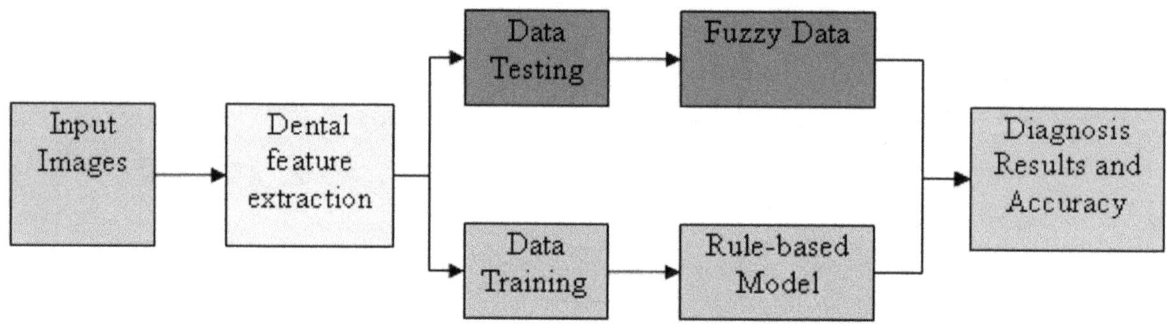

divided into 2 parts: training and testing sets. The former is used for generating fuzzy rules (see Section 3.3), and the latter is used for inference (see Section 3.4).

3.2. Dental Feature Extraction

In this section, we present 5 dental image features and the methods used to extract them as follows. The output of these processes is a dental feature database.

3.2.1. Entropy, Edge-Value and Intensity

1. **Entropy:** A measure for the randomness level of achieved information within a certain extent (Lai and Lin, 2008) and is calculated by Equation (6):

$$r(x,y) = -\sum_{i=1}^{L} p(z_i)\log_2 p(z_i) \tag{6}$$

where z is a random variable, $p(z_i)$ is probability of ith pixel, i = 1,2,..., L (L being the number of pixels):

$$R(x,y) = \frac{r(x,y)}{\max\{r(x,y)\}} \tag{7}$$

2. **Edge-Value and Intensity:** Measure the numbers of changes of pixel values in a region (Lai and Lin, 2008):

$$e(x,y) = \sum_{p=-\lfloor w/2 \rfloor}^{\lfloor w/2 \rfloor} \sum_{q=-\lfloor w/2 \rfloor}^{\lfloor w/2 \rfloor} b(x,y) \tag{8}$$

$$b(x,y)=\begin{cases}1, & \nabla f(x,y)\geq T_1\\ 0, & \nabla f(x,y)<T_1\end{cases} \tag{9}$$

$$\nabla f(x,y)=\sqrt{\left(\frac{\partial g(x,y)}{\partial x}\right)^2+\left(\frac{\partial g(x,y)}{\partial y}\right)^2} \tag{10}$$

where $\nabla f(x,y)$ is the length of gradient vector, $b(x,y)$ and $e(x,y)$ are a binary image and intensity of the X-ray image respectively. T_1 is a threshold. These features are normalized in the forms:

$$E(x,y)=\frac{e(x,y)}{\max\{e(x,y)\}} \tag{11}$$

$$G(x,y)=\frac{g(x,y)}{\max\{g(x,y)\}} \tag{12}$$

3.2.2. Local Binary Patterns - LBP

This feature is invariant to any light intensity transformation and ensures the order of pixel density in a given area (see Figure 4). Dental X-ray image includes light-sensitive part and scalenus part. The bone and teeth belong to the first part and the others belong to the second one which is invariant with the changing of light. LBP value is determined under following steps (Ahonen, Hadid, and Pietikainen, 2006):

1. Select a 3 x 3 window template from a given central pixel;
2. Compare its value with those of pixels in the window. If greater then mark as 1; otherwise mark as 0;
3. Put all binary values from the top-left pixel to the end pixel by clock-wise direction into a 8-bit string. Convert it to decimal system:

$$LBP(x_c,y_c)=\sum_{n=0}^{7}s(g_n-g_c)2^n \tag{13}$$

$$s(x)=\begin{cases}1 & x\geq 0\\ 0 & otherwise\end{cases} \tag{14}$$

where g_c is value of the central pixel (x_c,y_c) and g_n is value of nth pixel in the window.

Figure 4. LBP value

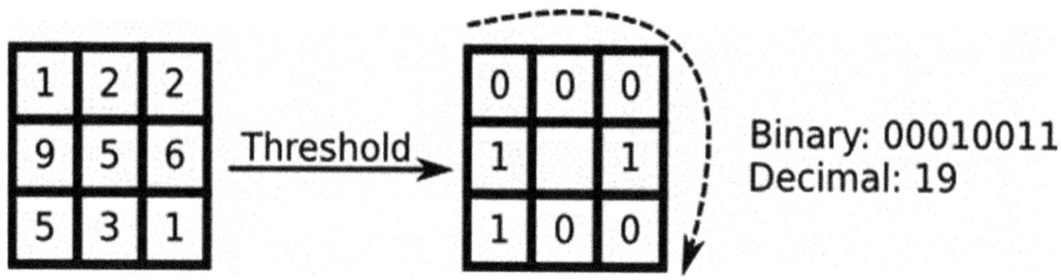

3.2.3. Red-Green-Blue - RGB

This characterizes the color of an X-ray image according to Red-Green-Blue values. For a 24 bit image, the RGB feature is computed as follows (N is the number of pixels):

$$h_{R,G,B}[r,g,b] = N * Prob\{R=r, G=g, B=b\} \tag{15}$$

There is another way to calculate the RGB feature that is isolating three matrices $h_R[]$, $h_G[]$ and $h_B[]$ with values being specified from the equivalent color band in the image.

3.2.4. Gradient Feature

This feature is used to differentiate various tiny teeth's parts such as enamel, cementum, gum, root canal, etc (Ghazali et al., 2007). The following steps calculate the Gradient value. Firstly, we apply Gaussian filter to the X-ray image to reduce the background noises. After that Difference of Gaussian (DoG) filter is applied to calculate gradient of the image according to x and y axes. Each pixel is the characterized by a gradient vector. Lastly, we get normalization form of the gradient vector and receive a 2D vector for each pixel as follows:

$$\theta(z) = [\sin \alpha, \cos \alpha] \tag{16}$$

where α is direction of the gradient vector. For instance, length and direction of a pixel are calculated as follows. For instance, length and direction of a pixel are calculated as follows:

$$m(x,y) = \sqrt{\left(L(x+1,y)-L(x-1,y)\right)^2 + \left(L(x,y+1)-L(x,y-1)\right)^2} \tag{17}$$

$$\theta(x,y) = \tan^{-1}\left(\left(L(x+1,y+1)-L(x-1,y-1)\right)/\left(L(x+1,y)-L(x-1,y)\right)\right) \tag{18}$$

$$L(x,y) = G(x,y) * I(x,y) \tag{19}$$

$$G(x,y)=\frac{1}{\sqrt{2\pi\sigma^2}}e^{-(x^2+y^2)/(2\sigma^2)} \tag{20}$$

where I(x,y) is a pixel vector, G(x,y) is a Gaussian function of (x,y), σ is a constant, operator '*' is the convolution operation between x and y, θ_1 is a threshold.

3.2.5. Patch Level Feature

This feature was used to calculate all gradient vectors of pixels in a patch P, denoted by δ(*z*) (Oad, DeZhi and Butt, 2014):

$$F_h(P)=\sum_{z\in P}\tilde{m}(z)\delta(z) \tag{21}$$

$$\tilde{m}(z)=\frac{m(z)}{\sqrt{\sum_{z\in P}m(z)^2+\varepsilon_g}} \tag{22}$$

where *m*(*z*) is the gradient amplitude at pixel z, $\tilde{m}(z)$ is the normalization value of *m*(*z*) and ε_g is a small constant. δ(*z*) is often specified by Hard Binning method as follows:

$$\delta_i(z)=\begin{cases}1, & \left\lfloor \frac{d\theta(z)}{2\pi} \right\rfloor = i-1 \\ 0, & otherwise\end{cases} \tag{23}$$

3.3. Rule Generation from the Dental Feature Database

There are two methods for generating fuzzy rules (Bezdek, Ehrlich and Full, 1984). The first one is partition and the second is clustering. In our proposed model, we use the FCM clustering algorithm for making this kind of rule set. The Input contains Entropy – Edge – Intensity (EEI), LBP, RGB, Gradient, and Patch variables. The Output variable is the Disease consisting of 5 classes. Linguistic labels are set up as follows:

EEI, LBP, RGB, Gradient and Patch: {"High", "Medium", "Low"} (C=3)

Disease: {"Cracked", "Hidden", "Cavities", "Missing", "Periodontitis"} (C=5)

As presented in Table 1, the statement of the first rule is written as below:

"If *EEI is Medium* **and** *LBP is High* **and** *RGB is Medium* **and** *Gradient is High* **and** *Patch is Low* **then** *Label is Cracked"*.

Similarity to other rules, we can write each of them as the first one.

The result of rule generation process is a set of rules including duplicate and conflict rules. Gauss functions are used to remove these unexpected kinds of rules. These functions are used also for FIS in Section 3.4. The weight of each rule is calculated. For duplicate or conflict rules, only rules with high weights are kept, others are rejected. The final results are noted as in Table 1.

In order to perform the inference progress, the dental diseases are labeled by 1, 2, 3, 4 and 5, respectively. They are used as parameters for defuzzification in fuzzy inference progress. The symmetric Gauss function is formulated by the equation below:

$$y = \exp\left(-\frac{(x-c)^2}{2\sigma^2}\right) \tag{24}$$

Table 1. Fuzzy rules

Rule No.	EEI	LBP	RGB	Gradient	Patch	Label
1	Medium	High	Medium	Medium	Low	Cracked
2	Medium	Medium	Medium	High	Low	Cracked
3	High	Low	High	High	Low	Cracked
4	Medium	Low	Medium	High	Low	Cracked
5	High	Medium	High	Medium	Low	Hidden
6	Low	Low	Low	High	Medium	Hidden
7	Low	High	Low	Medium	Medium	Hidden
8	Medium	Medium	Medium	High	Medium	Cavities
9	Medium	Low	Medium	High	Medium	Cavities
10	High	Low	High	High	Medium	Missing
11	High	Medium	High	High	Medium	Missing
12	Medium	High	Medium	Medium	Medium	Missing
13	Medium	Medium	Medium	Low	Medium	Missing
14	Low	Medium	Low	High	High	Periodontitis
15	Low	High	Low	Medium	High	Periodontitis
16	High	Low	High	High	High	Periodontitis
17	Medium	Low	Medium	High	High	Periodontitis
18	Low	Medium	Medium	High	High	Periodontitis
19	Medium	Medium	Medium	High	High	Periodontitis
20	High	Medium	High	High	High	Periodontitis
21	Medium	High	Medium	Medium	High	Periodontitis

Figure 5. Gaussian functions of the inputs and output

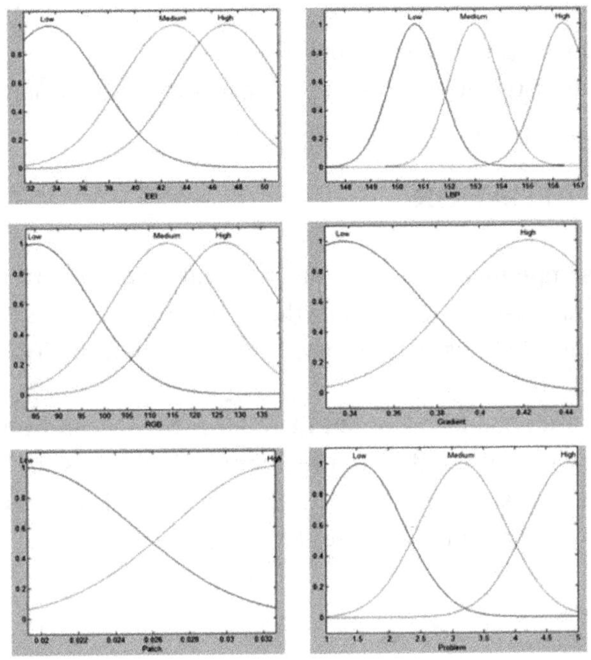

This function depends on two parameters σ and *c* where *c* is retrieved from one of the FCM output in the previous step and σ can be calculated as:

$$\sigma = \frac{d}{2\sqrt{2\ln(2)}} \tag{25}$$

where *d* is the Euclidean distance between two centers of a clustered feature. Gauss membership functions are plotted in Figure 5.

3.4. Inference Mechanism

A FIS can be classified based on formalization of fuzzy rules. There are two types of fuzzy inference systems that can be implemented in the Fuzzy Logic Toolbox: Mamdani-type and Sugeno-type. This paper only focuses on the Mamdani-type. Mamdani's fuzzy inference method is the most commonly fuzzy inference methodology. Mamdani's method was proposed in 1975 by Ebrahim Mamdani based on fuzzy algorithms for complex systems and decision processes. From given inputs, to compute the output of this FIS, we must go through six steps:

1. Determining a set of fuzzy rules;
2. Fuzzifying the inputs using the input membership functions. The purpose of this step is to map the inputs from a set of sensors to values from 0 to 1;
3. Combining the fuzzified inputs according to the fuzzy rules to establish the rule strength;

4. Finding the consequence of the rule by combining the rule strength and the output membership function;
5. Combining the consequences to get an output distribution;
6. Defuzzifying the output distribution (this step is necessary as if a crisp output (class) is needed).

4. EXPERIMENTAL EVALUATION

The proposed algorithm was implemented on Matlab 2014 and executed on a PC VAIO laptop with Core i3 processor. The experimental results are taken as the average values after 20 runs. The experimental datasets were taken from Hanoi Medical University, Vietnam including 56 dental images in the period 2014 – 2015 (see Figure 6).

In order to evaluate performance of proposed method, MSE (Mean Squared Error), MAE (Mean Absolute Error) and Accuracy were used. If $\hat{Y}$ is a vector of n predictions, and Y is the vector of observed values corresponding to the inputs of the function which generated the predictions, then MSE of the predictor can be estimated by (Lehmann and Casella, 1998):

$$MSE = \frac{1}{n}\sum_{i=1}^{n}\left(\hat{Y}_i - Y_i\right)^2 = \frac{1}{n}\sum_{i=1}^{n}\left|e_i\right| \tag{26}$$

It means that the MSE is the mean of the square of the errors. This is an easily computable quantity for a particular sample. The best value of MSE index is the smallest one. MAE is a common measure of forecast error in time series analysis. In statistics, it is a quantity used to measure how close forecasts or predictions are to the eventual outcomes. The mean absolute error is given by (Hyndman and Koehler, 2006):

$$MAE = \frac{1}{n}\sum_{i=1}^{n}\left|f_i - y_i\right| = \frac{1}{n}\sum_{i=1}^{n}\left|e_i\right| \tag{27}$$

where f_i: the prediction and y_i: the true value. Note that alternative formulations may include relative frequencies as weight factors. The best value of MAE index is also the smallest one. The Accuracy index is the simplest measure of diagnostic decision. It is calculated by following formula (Hyndman and Koehler, 2006) where a is the result of diagnostic of the disease that is True Positive; b is the result of diagnostic of the disease that is False Positive; c is the result of diagnostic of the disease that is False Negative; d is the result of diagnostic of the disease that is True Negative. The larger the Accuracy value is, the better the algorithm is:

$$Accuracy = \frac{a+d}{A+b+c+d} \tag{28}$$

In Table 2, by using MSE, MAE and Accuracy indexes, the comparison among graph-based clustering methods and other related methods (FKNN and Furia) with the proposed method (FIS) is presented.

Figure 6. Some dental X-ray images

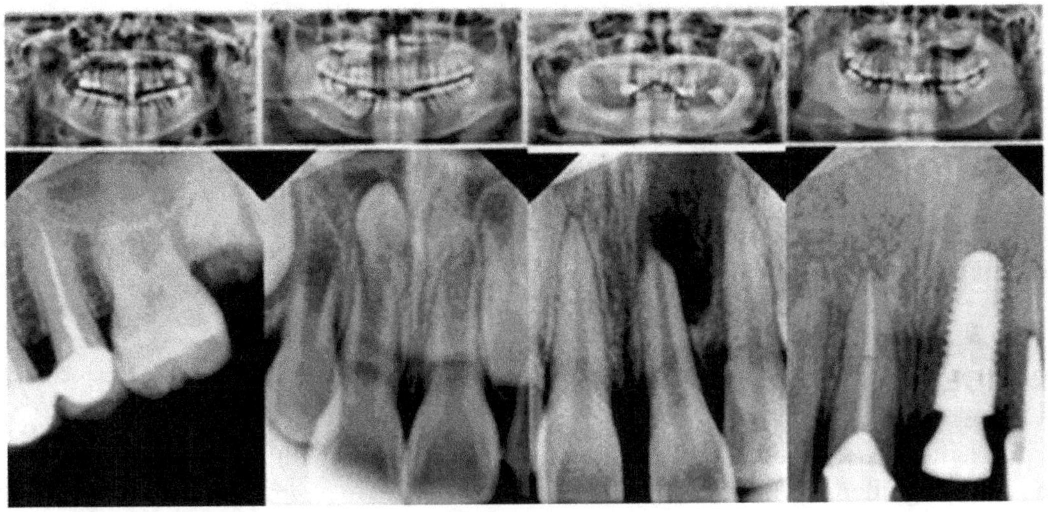

Table 2. Evaluation performance of all methods

	GCP	GCK	APC	FKNN	FURIA	FIS
MSE	2.0830	2.0840	0.8210	0.2727	0.1822	0.2445
MAE	0.9170	0.9160	0.7010	0.2273	0.0700	0.1264
Accuracy (%)	58.30	58.30	89.10	79.55	88.24	90.29

Graph-based clustering methods include Prim spanning tree - GCP, Kruskal spanning tree - GCK, and Affinity Propagation Clustering - APC (Vathy-Fogarassy and Abonyi, 2013).

It has been observed from the results in Table 2 that our proposed method is not good as FURIA in MSE and MAE indexes but it has higher value than the other methods especially in Accuracy. In these experiment results, FURIA was performed via WEKA package so that we do not consider the comparison of computational time between algorithms.

5. CONCLUSION

In this paper, we concentrated on problem of dental diagnosis and proposed a new diagram to solve it. Specifically, the feature extraction methods were used to create a dental feature database from dental X-ray images. The FCM algorithm was then used to classify these features into clusters and from that, a rule base was generated. Based on the fuzzy rules, Mamdani FIS based method was applied to infer consequences from given inputs. The proposed work supports dentists in diagnosing dental diseases. The new method has been implemented and compared with the FKNN algorithm in term of accuracy. The results showed that the new method has better performance than FKNN.

In the future, this research can be continued with some following ideas: i) Using other clustering methods to improve clustering quality; ii) Increasing the number of dental features to get more accurate prediction results; ii) Improving FIS to get higher performance.

ACKNOWLEDGMENT

The authors are greatly indebted to the editor-in-chief, Prof. Deng-Feng Li and anonymous reviewers for their comments and their valuable suggestions that improved the quality and clarity of paper.

REFERENCES

Ahonen, T., Hadid, A., & Pietikainen, M. (2006). Face description with local binary patterns: Application to face recognition. *IEEE Transactions on Pattern Analysis and Machine Intelligence*, *28*(12), 2037–2041. doi:10.1109/TPAMI.2006.244 PMID:17108377

Bezdek, J. C., Ehrlich, R., & Full, W. (1984). FCM: The fuzzy c-means clustering algorithm. *Computers & Geosciences*, *10*(2), 191–203. doi:10.1016/0098-3004(84)90020-7

Boyacioglu, M. A., & Avci, D. (2010). An adaptive network-based fuzzy inference system (ANFIS) for the prediction of stock market return: The case of the Istanbul stock exchange. *Expert Systems with Applications*, *37*(12), 7908–7912. doi:10.1016/j.eswa.2010.04.045

Chattopadhyay, S., Davis, R. M., Menezes, D. D., Singh, G., Acharya, R. U., & Tamura, T. (2012). Application of Bayesian classifier for the diagnosis of dental pain. *Journal of Medical Systems*, *36*(3), 1425–1439. doi:10.1007/s10916-010-9604-y PMID:20945154

Chaudhari, S., Patil, M., & Bambhori, J. (2014). Study and review of fuzzy inference systems for decision making and control. *AIJRSTEM*, *5*(1), 88–92.

Doi, K. (2014). Current status and future potential of computer-aided diagnosis in medical imaging. *The British Journal of Radiology*, 78(Suppl. 1), s3–s19

Fahmy, R., Zaher, H., & Kandil, A. E. (2015). A Comparison between Fuzzy Inference Systems for Prediction (with Application to Prices of Fund in Egypt). *International Journal of Computers and Applications*, *109*(13), 6–11. doi:10.5120/19246-0604

Ghazali, K. H., Mustafa, M. M., Hussain, A., Bandar, M. E. C., & Kuantan, G. (2007). Feature Extraction technique using SIFT keypoints descriptors.*Proceedings of the International Conference on Electrical and Engineering and Informatics Institute technology* (pp. 17-19).

Grabisch, M., Nguyen, H. T., & Walker, E. A. (2013). *Fundamentals of uncertainty calculi with applications to fuzzy inference* (Vol. 30). Springer Science & Business Media.

Guillaume, S. (2001). Designing fuzzy inference systems from data: An interpretability-oriented review. *IEEE Transactions on Fuzzy Systems*, *9*(3), 426–443. doi:10.1109/91.928739

Ho, S. Y., Lee, K. C., Chen, S. S., & Ho, S. J. (2002). Accurate modeling and prediction of surface roughness by computer vision in turning operations using an adaptive neuro-fuzzy inference system. *International Journal of Machine Tools & Manufacture*, *42*(13), 1441–1446. doi:10.1016/S0890-6955(02)00078-0

Hosseini, S. H., & Etemadi, A. H. (2008). Adaptive neuro-fuzzy inference system based automatic generation control. *Electric Power Systems Research*, *78*(7), 1230–1239. doi:10.1016/j.epsr.2007.10.007

Hühn, J., & Hüllermeier, E. (2009). FURIA: An algorithm for unordered fuzzy rule induction. *Data Mining and Knowledge Discovery*, *19*(3), 293–319. doi:10.1007/s10618-009-0131-8

Hyndman, R. J., & Koehler, A. B. (2006). Another look at measures of forecast accuracy. *International Journal of Forecasting*, *22*(4), 679–688. doi:10.1016/j.ijforecast.2006.03.001

Kavitha, M. S., Asano, A., Taguchi, A., Kurita, T., & Sanada, M. (2012). Diagnosis of osteoporosis from dental panoramic radiographs using the support vector machine method in a computer-aided system. *BMC Medical Imaging*, *12*(1), 2–11. PMID:22248480

Lai, Y. H., & Lin, P. L. (2008). Effective segmentation for dental X-ray images using texture-based fuzzy inference system. In *Advanced Concepts for Intelligent Vision Systems* (pp. 936–947). Springer Berlin Heidelberg. doi:10.1007/978-3-540-88458-3_85

Lee, C. C. (1990). Fuzzy logic in control systems: Fuzzy logic controller. *IEEE Transactions on Systems, Man, and Cybernetics*, *20*(2), 419–435. doi:10.1109/21.52552

Lehmann, E. L., & Casella, G. (1998). *Theory of point estimation* (Vol. 31). Springer Science & Business Media.

Nayak, G. K., Narayanan, S. J., & Paramasivam, I. (2013). Development and comparative analysis of fuzzy inference systems for predicting customer buying behavior. *IACSIT International Journal of Engineering and Technology*, *5*(5), 4093–4108.

Oad, K. K., DeZhi, X., & Butt, P. K. (2014). A Fuzzy Rule Based Approach to Predict Risk Level of Heart Disease. *Global Journal of Computer Science and Technology*, *14*(3), 16–22.

Ramírez, E., Castillo, O., & Soria, J. (2010). Hybrid System for Cardiac Arrhythmia Classification with Fuzzy K-Nearest Neighbors and Neural Networks Combined by a Fuzzy Inference System. In *Soft Computing for Recognition Based on Biometrics* (pp. 37–55). Springer Berlin Heidelberg. doi:10.1007/978-3-642-15111-8_3

Sun, C. T. (1994). Rule-base structure identification in an adaptive-network-based fuzzy inference system. *IEEE Transactions on Fuzzy Systems*, *2*(1), 64–73. doi:10.1109/91.273127

Togai, M., & Watanabe, H. (1986). A VLSI implementation of a fuzzy-inference engine: Toward an expert system on a chip. *Information Sciences*, *38*(2), 147–163. doi:10.1016/0020-0255(86)90017-4

Vathy-Fogarassy, Á., & Abonyi, J. (2013). *Graph-Based Clustering and Data Visualization Algorithms*. Springer. doi:10.1007/978-1-4471-5158-6

Wang, J. S., & Lee, C. G. (2002). Self-adaptive neuro-fuzzy inference systems for classification applications. *IEEE Transactions on Fuzzy Systems*, *10*(6), 790–802. doi:10.1109/TFUZZ.2002.805880

APPENDIX

Matlab source codes of all algorithms and experimental data can be found at the URL: https://www.mathworks.com/matlabcentral/fileexchange/52993-dental-using-fuzzy-rule-based-systems.

This work was previously published in the International Journal of Fuzzy System Applications (IJFSA), 6(1); edited by Deng-Feng Li, pages 1-16, copyright year 2017 by IGI Publishing (an imprint of IGI Global).

Chapter 8
Thermal Evaluation of Myogenous Temporomandibular Disorders and Myofascial Trigger Points in the Masticatory Muscles

Denise Sabbagh Haddad
University of São Paulo, Brazil

Marcos Leal Brioschi
University of São Paulo, Brazil

Emiko Saito Arita
University of São Paulo, Brazil

ABSTRACT

It is known that the myofascial trigger points (MTP) and myogenous temporomandibular disorders (TMDs) cause regional sympathetic hyperactivity in local temperature due to the cutaneous vasomotor activity and, for detection of functional changes, thermography is used as a complementary diagnostic imaging method. This chapter intends to study two masticatory muscles, masseter and anterior temporalis, in measurement of the cutaneous temperature of volunteers with and without myogenous TMD and MTP. Results: The temperature levels measured at both muscles regions in myogenous TMD volunteers were significantly lower than those measured in controls. Infrared imaging indicated differences between referred and local pain in MTPs of 0.5°C. Conclusions: Infrared imaging measurements seem to indicate that it can be used as an aid in complimentary diagnosing of TMDs and MTPs in masticatory muscles.

DOI: 10.4018/978-1-5225-1903-4.ch008

INTRODUCTION

Temperature is a long established as a diagnostic sign and thus an indicator of health. In 400 B.C., Hippocrates wrote "In whatever part of the body excess of heat or cold is felt, the disease is there to be discovered" (Brioschi et al., 2010). The beginning of the infrared temperature measurement started, in 1800, with the discovery of the infrared radiation by Sir William Herschel (Brioschi et al., 2010; Haddad, 2001).

During the World War II, military research in monitoring infrared systems allowed the beginning of a new era in thermal diagnosis. In the 50s was developed the first generation of infrared tracking for military applications, named FLIR (Forward Looking InfraRed) (Sanches, 2009). However, the first medical publication using infrared thermography was in 1956, by Dr. Ray N. Lawson of McGill University (Montreal, Canada) (Lawson, 1956). The first dental research using infrared thermography was done by Crandell and Hill in 1966 (Crandell & Hill, 1966). Since that time, many researches were done in Dentistry (Haddad, Brioschi & Arita, 2012; Haddad et al., 2014; Canavan & Gratt, 1995; Johansson, Kopp & Haraldson, 1985; Gratt et al., 1989; Gratt & Sickles, 1993; Gratt & Sickles, 1995; Gratt & Anbar, 1998; Dworkin et al., 1990; Fillingim et al., 1996; Pogrel et al., 1989; Christensen, Vaeth & Wenzel, 2012; Kawano et al., 1993; Gratt et al., 1994; Leonardi et al., 1991; Anbar, Gratt & Hong, 1998; Weinstein et al., 1991; Biagioni et al., 1996; Berry & Yemm, 1971; Berry & Yemm, 1974; Mongini et al., 1990; Gratt et al., 1996; Dibai-Filho et al., 2014; Dibai-Filho et al., 2015].

Medical infrared thermography is a nonionizing and noninvasive imaging technique that allows the real-time representation of the skin surface thermal distribution into images (Brioschi et al., 2010; Haddad, Brioschi & Arita, 2012; Haddad et al., 2014). The skin temperature distribution depends on the heat exchange processes between skin tissue, local vasculature and metabolic activity (Brioschi et al., 2010; Haddad, Brioschi & Arita, 2012; Haddad et al., 2014; Merla & Romani, 2008). Natural vascular heat emissions that present on the human face can provide physiologic indicators of underlying health or disease. All of these processes are mediated and regulated by the autonomous nervous system to maintain the thermal homeostasis (Brioschi et al., 2010; Haddad, Brioschi & Arita, 2012; Haddad et al., 2014; Merla & Romani, 2008). The resultant thermal image indicates the amount of heat given off by blood flowing within and beneath the skin and muscles. As the amount of blood circulating within and beneath the skin layers varies, so does the skin temperature. Only the body surface and a superficial layer 6 to 10 mm in depth is surveyed and recorded using thermography

The literature clearly documents that, in a normal situation, blood flow through the skin of most body parts produces a nearly symmetrical thermal pattern (Haddad, Brioschi & Arita, 2012; Canavan & Gratt, 1995; Gratt & Sickles, 1993; Gratt & Sickles, 1995; Gratt & Anbar, 1998; Vardasca et al., 2012). The presence of biological dysfunctions can affect the heat balance or exchange processes, resulting in an increase or a decrease of the local skin temperature. Quantitative and qualitative changes in infrared heat emission by the skin have been reported to occur in a variety of diseases. These changes include conditions involving facial structures, such as temporomandibular joint (TMJ) disorders, atypical facial pain (atypical odontalgia), nerve damage and repair following oral surgery, headache, inflammation of the lacrimal drainage system, and psychogenic facial pain (Merla & Romani, 2008).

Anatomical and functional information of the structures of interest are the basis of radiology interpretation. For recognizing diseases it is necessary to understand and identify the anatomical structures and its variations. Many diagnosis of some facial diseases (e.g.: bone alterations, caries, temporomandibular joint disorders, etc) may be done through medical imaging techniques, however the most conventional present lack of information in analyzing physiological functional aspects such as microcirculation and autonomous nervous system. The measurements of facial skin temperature may be used to investigate and assess lesions of peripheral branches of cranial nerves supplying the face.

The literature reports different methods of evaluating skin facial surface but all authors affirm that infrared thermography is a promising imaging method in Dentistry (Haddad, Brioschi & Arita, 2012; Haddad et al., 2014; Gratt & Sickles, 1995; Merla & Romani, 2008). This method can provide new complementary information on the anatomy of the vasculature, neuronal systemic and local control of vascular blood flow and perfusion of the capillary bed (Anbar, 2008) and therefore it can be correlated with the patient complains (e.g.: pain in the area of masticatory muscles, headaches, athypical odontalgias, etc).

Temporomandibular disorders are characterized by pain and mobility dysfunction in the temporomandibular joint area, masticatory muscles and associated musculoskeletal structures in the head and neck (Dworkin et al., 1990). The aetiology and pathogenesis of TMD have been suggested as indicative of a psychophysiological disorder involving changes in regulatory pain pathways, resulting in maladaptive emotional, physiological and neuroendocrine responses to physical and psychological stressors (Fillingim et al., 1996).

Numerous complementary diagnostic methods have been proposed for TMDs. The current diagnostic imaging methods for the assessment of the TMDs include plain film radiography, panoramic radiography, tomography, arthrotomography, arthroscopy, computerized tomography and magnetic resonance imaging. Most of these techniques require ionizing radiation, are invasive, or are costly.

The research diagnostic criteria for TMDs (RDC/TMD) (Dworkin & LeResche, 1992) are the gold standard available for TMD diagnostic system and are empirically based. It uses operationally defined measurement criteria to generate computer-derived diagnostic algorithms for the most common TMD forms (Dworkin & LeResche, 1992) and provides specifications for conducting a standardized clinical physical examination (John, Dworkin & Mancl, 2005).

Physical disorders that are related to the TMDs and have been reported to produce abnormal facial thermograms include (but are not limited to) myofascial pain syndromes, myositis, musculoligamentous injury, temporomandibular joint disorders, motor and sensory radiculopathy, and the inflammation of arthritis and bursitis. Hence, the TMD can be evaluated morphologically and dynamically through medical imaging techniques; however, the most conventional present lack of information in analyzing physiological functional aspects such as microcirculation and autonomous nervous system. This information would be of major importance for clinical conditions such as trigeminal neuralgia and facial musculoskeletal pain.

Myofascial pain syndrome (MPS) is characterized by diffuse muscle pain and the presence of myofascial trigger points (MTPs) (de Leeuw, 2008). MPS is much more common than is generally recognized (Simons, Travell & Simons, 1999), affecting the quality of life of patients with this condition. Simons (Simons, 1988) found that 85% of patients admitted to a chronic pain center were suffering primarily from MPS. Early identification of the disease, using precise diagnostic methods, improves the effectiveness of treatment and, consequently, leads to a reduction in the cost of public health.

MPS is not limited to the masticatory muscles. It can occur anywhere in the body, most commonly involving muscles in the neck and back.

Clinically, an MTP can be defined as a hyperirritable nodule of spot tenderness in a palpable taut band of skeletal muscle. The spot is a site of exquisite tenderness to palpation, from which a local twitch response can be elicited when appropriately stimulated, which refers pain to a distance. That response can cause distant motor and autonomic effects (Simons, Travell & Simons, 1999; Simons, 2004). Algometry, or the measurement of the pressure threshold meter (PTM), is a diagnostic method used to document the sensitivity of MTPs quantitatively. The pressure pain threshold (PPT) for the examination of MTPs is the minimal force that induces pain (Fischer, 1983; Fischer & Chang, 1986; Jaeger & Reeves, 1986; Fischer, 1987).

This chapter intends to summarize significant studies in measurement of the cutaneous temperature not just in asymptomatic masticatory muscles, but also in myogenous temporomandibular disorder (TMD) and myofascial trigger points (MTP). In addition, the authors proposed a new facial protocol evaluation of the superficial facial anatomy (facial thermoanatomy) and how the medical infrared imaging can be used.

FACIAL THERMOANATOMY

It is essential to know the pattern of facial skin temperatures in normal subjects to be able to objectively assess differences in cases of illness. It is widely accepted that injuries of the peripheral nervous system result in disturbance of sympathetic innervation, causing changes in cutaneous blood flow, surface temperature, sweat secretion and piloerection.

Two types of thermographic projections can be done for analyzing the face: frontal and lateral views. In the assessment of asymptomatic volunteers for orofacial pain, some regions are considered colder than others, for example, nose, chin and cheek (Figure 1). It depends on the regional vasculature anatomy. On the other hand, hottest areas can be detected over superficial arteries regions as temporal, frontal, lips, temporomandibular joint and eyelid medial and lateral commissure (Figure 1).

Due to the lack of facial protocol in the dental literature, the authors proposed three different methods to explore the facial skin temperature surface based on the vascular and nervous systems.

Figure 1. Facial thermograms (frontal and lateral views) showing the superficial vasculature regions, which hottest areas can be detected over temporal, frontal, lips, temporomandibular joint, eyelid medial and lateral commissure regions. Cold regions can be seeing over the nose, chin and cheek regions.

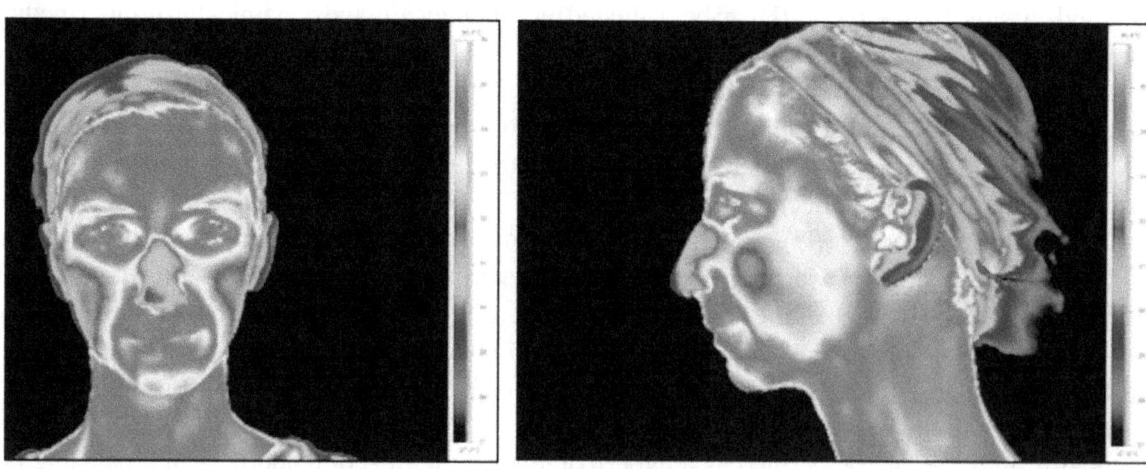

Vascular Division

The vascular division was based on the facial vascular regions. The Figure 2 shows all the regions of interest (ROIs):

1. Supratrochlear;
2. Supraorbital;
3. Frontal;
4. Temporal;
5. Superior eyelid;
6. Eyelid medial commissure;
7. Dorsal nose;
8. Infraorbital;
9. Lateral palpebral commissure;
10. Superior-anterior buccal;
11. Superior-posterior buccal;
12. Parotid-masseteric;
13. Upper lip;
14. Oral rhyme;
15. Lower lip;
16. Mental;
17. Inferior buccal;
18. Temporomandibular Joint.

Figure 2. Facial thermograms (frontal and lateral views) with the vascular ROIs proposed by the authors: 1- Supratrochlear; 2- Supraorbital; 3- Frontal; 4- Temporal; 5- Superior eyelid; 6- Eyelid medial commissure ; 7- Dorsal nose; 8- Infraorbital; 9- Lateral palpebral commissure; 10- Superior-anterior buccal; 11- Superior-posterior buccal; 12- Parotid-masseteric; 13- Upper lip; 14- Oral rhyme; 15- Lower lip; 16- Mental; 17- Inferior buccal; 18- Temporomandibular Joint.

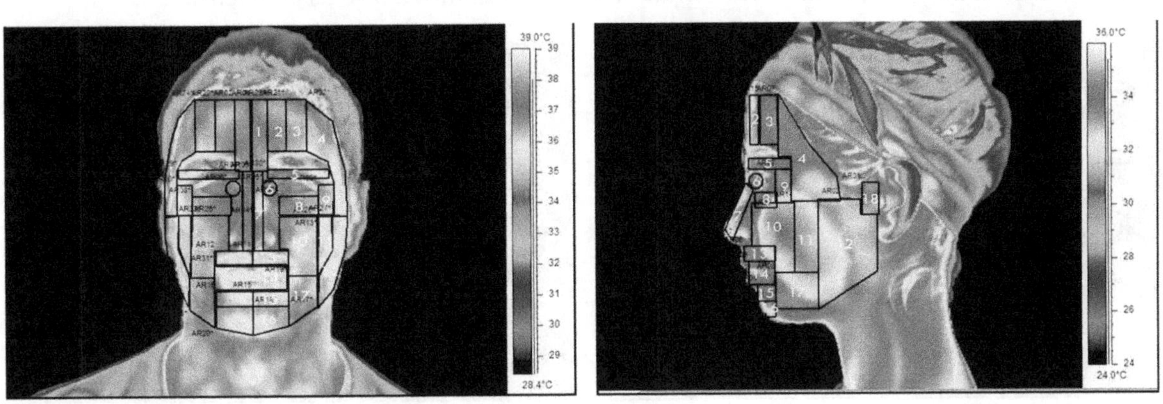

Trigeminal Nerve Division

The proposed of the trigeminal nerve division was based on the trigeminal nerve branches and the Figure 3 shows all ROIs:

1. Ophthalmic;
2. Maxillary;
3. Mandibular.

Facial Nerve Division

The proposed of the facial nerve division was based on the facial nerve branches and the Figure 4 shows all ROIs:

1. Temporal;
2. Zygomatic;
3. Buccal;
4. Marginal mandibular.

METHODS AND MATERIALS

This diagnostic study was lead in 2013 after approved by the Research Ethics Committee, School of Dentistry, University of São Paulo, São Paulo, Brazil. The Standards for Reporting of Diagnostic Accuracy (STARD) guidelines were followed in this investigation. All volunteers gave their signed informed consent (Haddad, 2001; Haddad, Brioschi & Arita, 2012; Haddad et al., 2014).

Figure 3. Facial thermograms (frontal and lateral views) with the trigeminal ROIs proposed by the authors: 1- Ophthalmic; 2- Maxillary; 3- Mandibular (trigeminal nerve assessment).

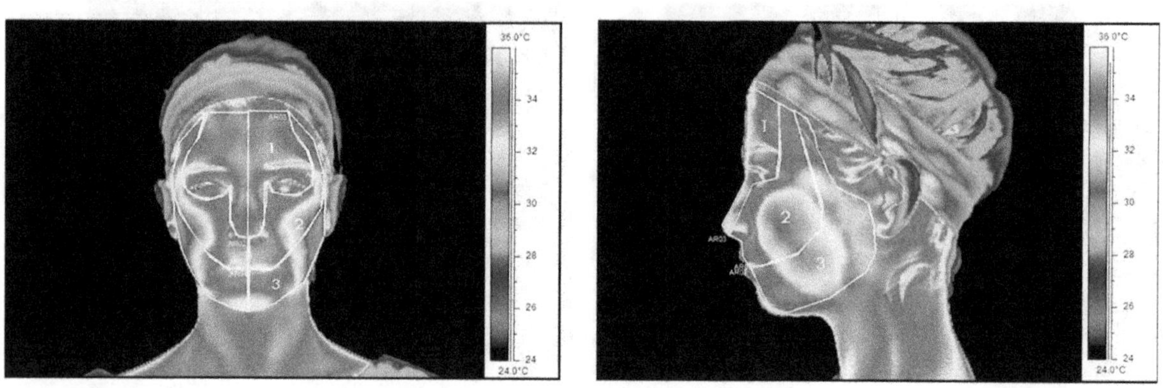

Figure 4. Facial thermograms (frontal and lateral views) with the facial ROIs proposed by the authors: 1- Temporal; 2- Zygomatic; 3- Buccal; 4- Marginal mandibular (facial nerve assessment).

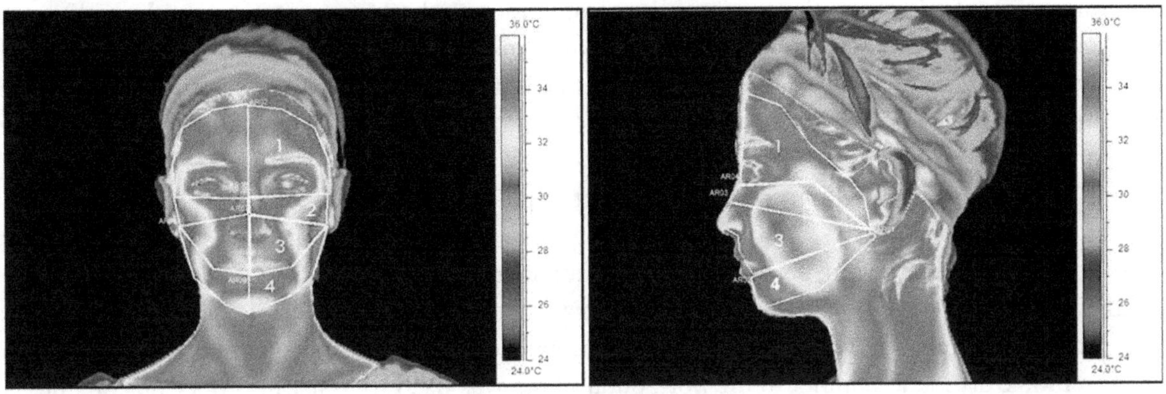

Volunteers

The volunteers were recruited at the clinic of Dentistry Faculty, University of São Paulo, São Paulo, Brazil. Patients with and without TMD and MPS were recruited during a period of 2 months.

Only adult females were investigated in this study because masticatory pain disorders are more prevalent in females than in males (de Leeuw, 2008). Twenty-six volunteers, with a mean age of 41 years, were included in the MTP study and 23 volunteers were included in the TMD study. All subjects underwent clinical and dental examinations. The selection criteria for this research included a negative history for systemic problems (e.g. hypothyroidism, diabetes, hypertension, fibromyalgia), headaches, toothache pain, history of eye surgery, impaired vision, contact lenses, hearing aids, facial blemishes, arthritis, sinusitis, rhinitis, dry mouth, sensitivity to cosmetics, wisdom tooth extraction, or previous use of orthodontic appliances (braces), scars or wheals on the face, articular temporomandibular disorders (TMDs), premenopausal females should be in the second phase of the menstrual cycle and the menopause females were absent of hot flushes (Keith, Thomas & Ferganson, 1973).

In order to detect the presence of TMDs, Research Diagnostic Criteria for Temporomandibular Disorders (RDC/TMD) were applied (Dworkin & LeResche, 1992). The subjects were instructed in the use of a visual analogue scale (VAS).

Facial Thermography: Measurement Procedure

Thermographic images were recorded following a standard protocol, recommended by the Brazilian Association of Medical Thermology and Academy of Neuro-Muscular Thermography (Schwartz, 2006). The subjects were instructed not to apply any lotion, makeup or powder to the skin; not to use a dryer or flat iron on the hair; and not to smoke for 2 h before the recording. Also, they were instructed to avoid skeletal manipulation, acupuncture, physical therapy, the use of transcutaneous neural stimulation units or electrodiagnostic testing for 12 h prior to the test and for at least 24 h after the test; not to drink coffee or alcoholic drinks; and not to use nasal decongestants, analgesics, anti-inflammatory drugs or any substance that alters sympathetic function.

Patients were acclimatized in a room with a mean temperature of 23 °C and a relative humidity of 80% for 15 min. They were instructed not to palpate, press, rub or scratch the facial skin at any time up to the completion of the entire thermographic examination. Ambient temperature and humidity were controlled in a draught-free environment. Air flow was maintained at less than $0.2ms^{-1}$, to avoid loss of heat through forced convection. Ambient temperature was measured using a reliable digital thermohygrometer that was visible and easy to read. Thermographic images were taken by an experienced physician who also evaluated them.

To facilitate image acquisition, the hair was held in place with a head band and a disposable head covering.

The examiner had the patient sit on the examination chair. A cephalostat (Figure 5) (Haddad, 2001; Haddad, Brioschi & Arita, 2012; Haddad et al., 2014), constructed specifically for these studies, was used in order to standardize the positioning of the patients during the thermal and photographic acquisitions. The Frankfurt plane parallel to the horizontal plane was used to assist in proper placement. The subject was asked to relax the muscles with the teeth apart. In a randomized order, two series of colour thermograms were taken, from the right and left perpendicular projections.

Skin temperature of all muscles (masseter and anterior temporalis muscles) was registered using a computer assisted infrared thermograph (ThermaCAM® T400, FLIR Systems, Inc., Wilsonville, OR). The infrared detector has a thermal sensitivity of 0.05 °C at 30 °C; spectral range between 7.5 μm – 13 μm; and the built-in digital video with 320x240 pixels resolution. Data were obtained using high-speed (30 Hz) analysis and recording systems coupled to a desktop computer. This equipment allows images with spatial resolution (IFOV) of 1.4 mrad to be obtained for the visualization of hot spots of 1.4 mm at 1 m distance, using a standard lens of 25° with no additional lenses.

The infrared camera produces a high definition matrix of temperature values. Each pixel represents a correct calibrated temperature in the picture measured.

Figure 5. The cephalostat constructed specifically for these studies A- Frontal view, B- Lateral view
Source: Haddad, 2001; Haddad, Brioschi, & Arita, 2012; Haddad et al., 2014

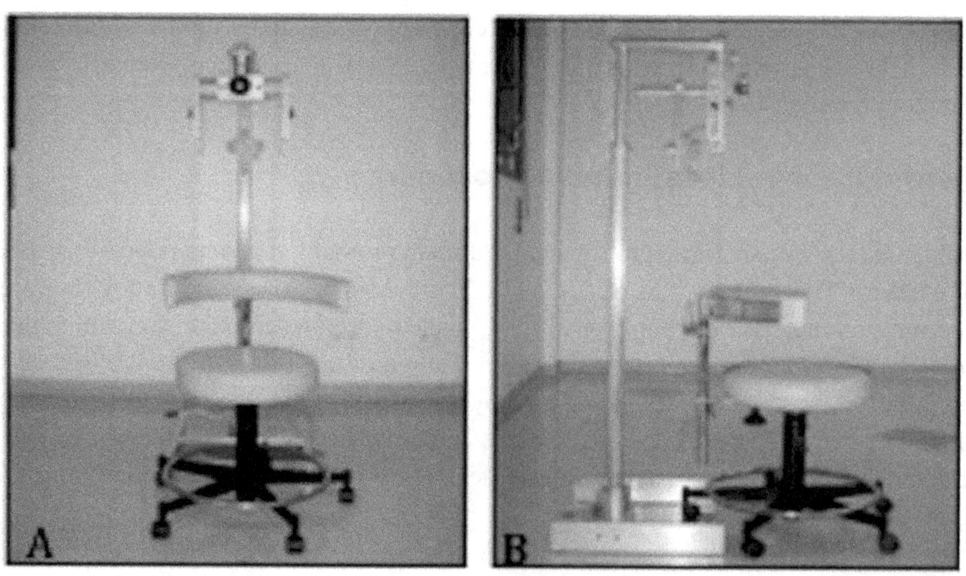

The thermograph allows quantitative and qualitative mapping of superficial temperature, which can be related to different pathological conditions and blood flow. It was possible to show the images in greyscale or in colour scales available within the software. All images were analysed and showed at least one palette of 256 colours, with a 0.15 °C thermal window for each colour. Thermal sensitivity of 0.51°C per colour tone was used, based on a rainbow-type colorimetric scale (colour palette), in which the colours were, from hottest to coldest: white, pink, red, orange, yellow, light green, dark green, light blue, dark blue, purple and black (FLIR QuickReport® v. 1.2 and FLIR Reporter® v. 8.5, FLIR Systems, Inc.). The colours indirectly indicated the degree of distribution of local cutaneous blood perfusion. All images were displayed with the palette beside the image, for reference.

The distance between the camera and the lateral face measured was adjusted to 0.75 m, at an angle of 90°, with the lens of the camera parallel to the assessed region. The emissivity value of the skin considered for this study was 0.987.

The core body temperatures of volunteers were measured using an infrared, digital thermometer ThermoScan® Instant Ear Thermometer IRT 1020 (Braun®; BraunAG, Frankfurt am Main, Germany). This thermometer measures temperature values of the eardrum and the surrounding tissues, the location most frequently indicated for measuring body temperature owing to its proximity to the hypothalamus and the perfusion of the arterial labyrinth (Vargas et al., 2009).

Clinical Examination and Algometry (MTP Study)

A trained specialist in TMD management area divided the surface facial area over the masseter and anterior temporalis muscles into 15 ROIs (Figure 6) on each side (n=780), with an area of approximately 1 cm^2 (Haddad, 2001; Haddad, Brioschi & Arita, 2012). This marking was based on Pogrel et al. study (Pogrel et al., 1989). The reference for defining regions of the masseter muscle was the zygomatic arch

Figure 6. Schematic design of the ROI (MTP study), restricted to the masseter and anterior part of the temporalis muscles, on both sides
Source: Haddad, Brioschi, & Arita, 2012

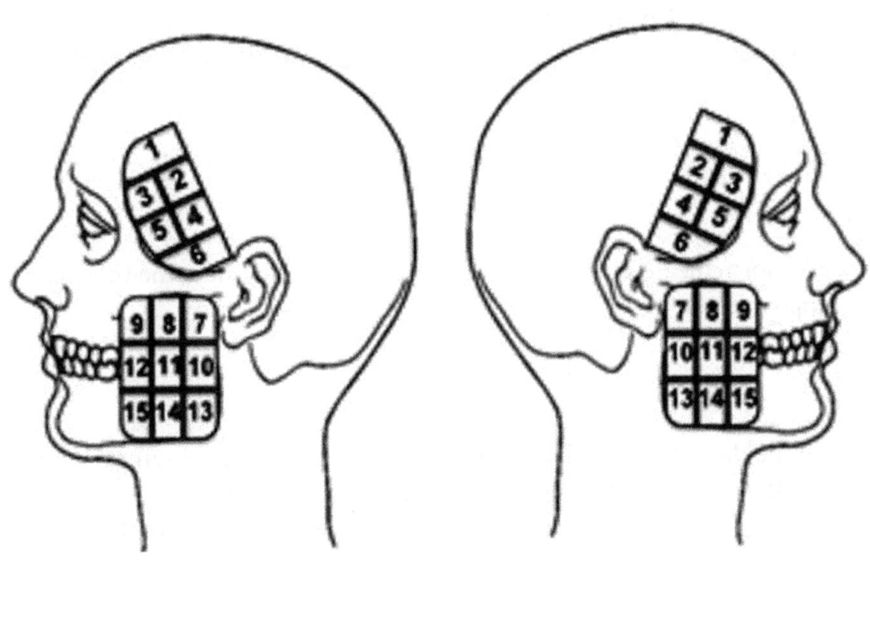

(proximal insertion) and the lateral surface of the mandibular angle (distal insertion). The temporalis muscle was evaluated only in its exposed anterior part not hidden by hair. Examination of MTPs was performed according to the Fischer protocol (Fischer, 1983; Fischer & Chang, 1986; Jaeger & Reeves, 1986), which uses the PPT to evaluate the minimal force that induces pain, expressed in kilograms of pressure. PTM is a hand force gauge calibrated to 10x0.01kgf and the area of the algometer tip was 1 cm^2. Before the test, the subject was instructed to relax the masticatory muscles with the teeth apart. First, the presence and location of the MTP was confirmed via palpation and was marked using a coloured pencil. Next, the pressure threshold was measured. The PTM was applied directly onto the location of tenderness, with the axis of the shaft maintained at 90° to the examining surface. The subject was instructed to inform verbally when pain or discomfort was initially felt. At this moment, the compression lasted for 5 seconds in the same location, with the same pressure maintained. The patient was asked if the pain was felt only in this location, or if it extended to another region. Finally, digital photographs (Nikon Coolpix S51® 8.1 megapixels; Nikon, Sendai, Japan) of the lateral face with the head in the same position as the infrared thermography examination were taken (Haddad, 2001; Haddad, Brioschi & Arita, 2012).

In order to correlate the PPT values with the values obtained from the thermographs of the ROI, the thermographs were superimposed on the digital photographs using dedicated infrared imaging software (Reporter 8.5—SP3 Professional Edition and QuickReport 1.2). The standardized reference points of the superimposition were:

1. Midpoint of the median sagittal plane between the chin and the hyoid bone;
2. Lowest portion of the earlobe; and
3. The apex of the nasal pyramid (Haddad, 2001; Haddad, Brioschi & Arita, 2012).

The averages of the temperature of the ROI of the muscles were calculated individually (T), and thermal asymmetry between the corresponding opposite sides, also called the conjugated gradient of the absolute temperature (xT).

In order to normalize the temperature results, it was used an adimensional variable (θ) proposed by Vargas and Brioschi for quantitative thermography analysis (Vargas et al., 2009).

Thus, the interpretation of the infrared camera readings was done using an adimensional temperature (θ) which combines the measured local skin temperature with the core body (T_b) and ambient temperatures (T_∞) during the infrared imaging caption, according to the following equation 1 (Vargas et al., 2009):

$$\theta = \frac{T - T_\infty}{T_b - T_\infty} \quad (1)$$

The gradient of the normalized temperature was also used to calculate the thermal asymmetry with the corresponding opposite ROIs:

$$x\theta = |\theta_{right} - \theta_{left}| \quad (2)$$

After obtaining all the data (PPT, T, θ) and calculating the gradients of temperature and normalized temperature (xT and xθ), the assessed points were divided into three groups: no MTP, MTP with local pain and MTP with referred pain (Haddad, 2001; Haddad, Brioschi & Arita, 2012).

Clinical Examination (TMD Study)

The RDC/TMD is an instrument widely used in research and clinical practice for identifying TMDs and was applied to detect the presence of TMD in this study (Dworkin & LeResche, 1992). After that, a trained specialist in TMD management divided the facial surface area over the anterior temporalis and masseter muscles into four regions to facilitate the palpation (Figure 7) (Haddad et al., 2014). The temporalis muscle region was defined as the anterior portion, not covered by hair, whereas the reference points used to define the masseter muscle region were the zygomatic arch (proximal insertion) and the lateral surface of the mandibular angle (distal insertion).

The ROIs were marked with a dermatographic pencil on the patient's skin after the thermal images and before the palpation examination. Digital photographs of the lateral face were taken after the thermal images in the same position as that used for the infrared thermographic examination. The positioning of the volunteer during the thermal and photographic images was standardized by the same cephalostat (Haddad, Brioschi & Arita, 2012) as used in the MTP study.

For precise evaluation of the ROIs, the same technique of thermograms and digital photographs superimposition was done (Haddad, 2001; Haddad, Brioschi & Arita, 2012; Haddad et al., 2014).

The mean absolute temperatures (T) were averaged according to the landmarks (ROIs) recorded on photographic images, and the normalized temperature (θ) (Vargas et al., 2009) of each ROI was calculated individually. During the data analysis, all volunteers were separated into two groups: symptomatic and asymptomatic for myogenous TMD.

Figure 7. Regions of interest (ROI) of the TMD study, restricted to the masseter and anterior part of the temporalis muscles, on left (L) and right (R) sides (ROI 1- anterior temporalis, ROI 2- superior masseter, ROI 3- middle masseter, ROI 4- inferior masseter, ROI 5- masseter)
Source: Haddad et al., 2014

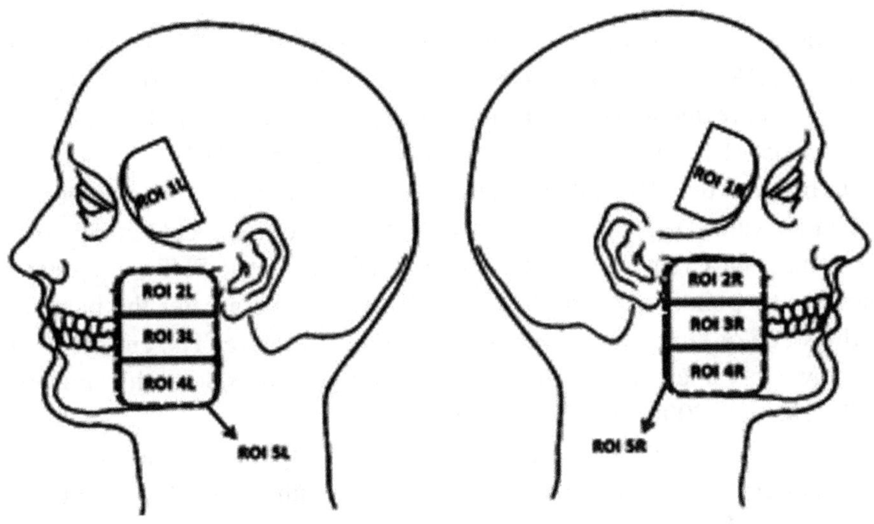

Statistical Analyses

The data were tabulated using Microsoft Excel (Microsoft Corporation, Redmond, WA). The analyses were performed using SPSS® 19 (IBM Corporation, Armonk, NY). Pearson's x^2 test and the non-parametric Kruskal–Wallis test with Bonferroni correction were used when necessary.

The sensitivity and specificity of the ratings were calculated using receiver operating characteristic (ROC) curve analysis. The receiver operating characteristic curve is a plot of the true-positive rate (sensitivity) against the false-positive rate (specificity) for the different possible cut-off points of a diagnostic test. It shows the trade-off between sensitivity and specificity. A level of $p<0.05$ was considered to be statistically significant. The correlation coefficient for the entire sample was calculated using Spearman's non-parametric method.

RESULTS

MTP Study

The sample consisted of 26 female volunteers (mean age 41±15 years, range 22–82 years). Of the 780 ROIs assessed over the masseter and anterior temporalis muscles (15 ROI on each side), MTPs were found in 395 ROIs (50.6%). All volunteers were asymptomatic on the day of the examination (VAS=0) (Haddad, 2001; Haddad, Brioschi & Arita, 2012).

Of the entire sample of 395 MTPs, physical examination findings characterized 264 as points of local pain, consisting of 74 (18.7%) anterior temporalis and 190 (48.1%) masseter muscles, and 131 were points of referred pain, consisting of 35 (8.9%) anterior temporalis and 96 (24.3%) masseter muscles (Haddad, 2001; Haddad, Brioschi & Arita, 2012).

When the right ($T = 33.71 \pm 1.21$ °C; $\theta = 0.805 \pm 0.087$) and left ($T = 33.76 \pm 1.13$ °C; $\theta = 0.803 \pm 0.082$) hemifacials were compared, no thermal predominance was found for either side, either for T or for θ ($p>0.05$) (Haddad, 2001; Haddad, Brioschi & Arita, 2012).

The temporalis muscle showed higher temperature ($T = 34.63 \pm 0.73$ °C; $\theta = 0.861 \pm 0.768$) than the masseter muscle ($T = 33.18 \pm 1.05$ °C; $\theta = 0.768 \pm 0.078$), for all subjects ($p<0.05$). The masseter muscle (1.54±0.58 kgf) showed greater sensitivity to pain sensations of the PPT than the temporalis muscle (1.67±0.62 kgf) ($p<0.05$) (Haddad, 2001; Haddad, Brioschi & Arita, 2012).

The correlations between the PPT (kgf) and temperature (T) were positive and moderate ($0.4 \leq r < 0.7$), with the higher the PPT value (kgf) applied to the ROI, the higher the local temperature.

The values for temperature (T), normalized temperature (θ) and the PPT were greater for the points of local pain than for the points of referred pain ($p<0.05$), i.e. the greater the pain sensitivity of the point, the lower the value of temperature and normalized temperature. The cut-off points found for T, θ, xT and xT are shown in Table 1; the gradient temperature in all muscles, with and without MTP, was greater than 0.3 °C (Haddad, 2001; Haddad, Brioschi & Arita, 2012).

The area under the ROC curve is interpreted as the probability that the individual with MTPs has a diagnostic test result of greater magnitude than the individual without MTPs. A test that can distinguish them has an area under the ROC curve above 0.5 and is described in Table 2. For both T and θ, the sensitivity of the method to identify MTPs with referred pain was average (50%), although the specificity was low (17%). By evaluation of the cut-off points, the value of the conjugated gradient (xT) was higher

Table 1. Cutoff points found for temperature (T), normalized temperature (θ), gradient temperature (xT) and gradient of the normalized temperature (xθ)

	T (°C)	*θ*	*xT (°C)**	*xθ*
Without MTP	*>34*	*>0.810*	*<0.3*	*<0.036*
Local Pain	*34-33.3*	*0.810-0.756*	*0.4*	*0.037*
Referred Pain	*<33.3*	*<0.756*	*0.5*	*0.048*

MTP: Myofascial Trigger Points
* values considered only when the contralateral side showed no MTP
** in the situation in which local pain exists on one side, and referred pain on the other side, the observed values were xT=0.5 °C and xθ=0.045

Table 2. Areas under the ROC curve (AUC) and the confidence interval (CI) of the myofascial trigger points (MTP)

MTP - Local Pain x Referred Pain	**AUC**	**CI95%**	
T	**0.564**	**0.504**	**0.623**
xθ	**0.578**	**0.041**	**0.743**
xT	**0.609**	**0.451**	**0.766**
θ	**0.617**	**0.559**	**0.674**
PPT	**0.737**	**0.685**	**0.789**

T: temperature; xθ: gradient of the normalized temperature; xT: gradient temperature; θ: normalized temperature; PPT: Pressure Pain Threshold; CI: confidence interval.

than 0.3 °C and the normalized temperature value (xθ) was greater than 0.036. Regarding the presence of MTPs, sensitivity and specificity for both xT and xθ were 62.5% and 71.31%, respectively (Haddad, 2001; Haddad, Brioschi & Arita, 2012).

TMD Study

The sample consisted of 23 female volunteers (mean age, 41 years; range, 33–49 years). They were divided into two groups according to the RDC/TMD: asymptomatic and symptomatic (Haddad, 2001; Haddad et al., 2014).

On the day of the examination, all volunteers had no pain (visual analogue scale = 0). For all ROIs used, it can be seen that there was no statistical evidence ($p>0.05$) of dependence between the asymptomatic and symptomatic groups of participants considering the bilateral mean temperature differences.

Absolute mean temperatures (Table 3) and normalized mean temperatures (Table 4) for asymptomatic and symptomatic participants were calculated for all muscle ROIs ($p<0.05$). The absolute mean temperature (Table 3) and the normalized mean temperature over the temporalis muscle (Table 4) was higher than that over the masseter muscle for all participants ($p<0.05$). The absolute (Table 3) and normalized (Table 4) mean temperatures of the muscle ROIs of asymptomatic and symptomatic subjects were compared (Haddad, 2001; Haddad et al., 2014).

The absolute mean temperature in symptomatic participants was lower than that in the control group ($p<0.05$). In the assessment of the absolute mean temperature of the anterior temporalis ROI, it showed

Table 3. Analysis of absolute mean temperature (°C) for asymptomatic and symptomatic participants

Muscle ROIs	Asymptomatic (n = 26)		Symptomatic (n = 20)		*p*-value
	xT (°C)	s.d.	xT (°C)	s.d.	
Anterior Temporalis (ROI 1)	34.78	0.44	34.37	0.64	0.0016
Superior Masseter (ROI 2)	33.49	1.00	32.81	0.83	0.0116
Middle Masseter (ROI 3)	33.54	0.92	32.91	0.85	0.0093
Inferior Masseter (ROI 4)	33.45	0.89	32.82	0.94	0.0050
Masseter (ROI 5)	33.49	0.92	32.85	0.86	0.0067

xT: absolute mean temperature; s.d.: standard deviation

Table 4. Analysis of normalized mean temperature (θ) for asymptomatic and symptomatic participants

Muscle ROIs	Asymptomatic (n = 26)		Symptomatic (n = 20)		*p*-value
	xθ	s.d.	xθ	s.d.	
Anterior Temporalis (ROI 1)	0.877	0.04	0.831	0.04	0.0001
Superior Masseter (ROI 2)	0.795	0.08	0.732	0.05	0.0014
Middle Masseter (ROI 3)	0.798	0.07	0.738	0.05	0.0008
Inferior Masseter (ROI 4)	0.791	0.06	0.733	0.06	0.0004
Masseter (ROI 5)	0.795	0.07	0.734	0.05	0.0006

xθ: normalized mean temperature; s.d.: standard deviation

higher sensitivity and lower specificity (respectively, 80% and 62%), when compared with the sensitivity and specificity observed for the masseter ROI (70% and 73%, respectively). Assessing the normalized muscle mean temperature for the anterior temporalis and the masseter ROI showed almost the same sensitivity and specificity when compared with the absolute mean temperature (Haddad, 2001; Haddad et al., 2014).

DISCUSSION

Solutions and Recommendations

Only adult females were investigated in these studies because masticatory pain disorders are more prevalent in females than in males (de Leeuw, 2008).

Medical infrared thermography is a non-invasive and non-ionizing bidimensional imaging technique that maps the distribution of body surface thermal radiation into images. It is based on the capture and transformation of infrared radiation emitted by the human skin to form images that reflect the local vasomotor response. Although it is not standardized at all, qualitative and quantitative changes in symmetrical thermal patterns have been reported as indicators of changes in metabolism, hemodynamics or neuronal thermoregulatory processes in the ROI [Haddad, Brioschi & Arita, 2012; Gratt et al., 1989; Gratt & Sickles, 1993; Gratt & Sickles, 1995; Christensen, Vaeth & Wenzel, 2012; Kawano et al., 1993; Vardasca et al., 2012; Vargas et al., 2009).

Different results about temperature values in skin facial surface were present in the literature. This can be owing to the usage of distinct capture methodologies (Gratt & Anbar, 1998; Gratt et al., 1994; Leonardi et al., 1991). Despite numerous articles addressing infrared thermography as a promising method in the diagnosis of TMD (Haddad, Brioschi & Arita, 2012; Canavan & Gratt, 1995; Gratt et al., 1989; Gratt & Sickles, 1993; Gratt & Sickles, 1995; Gratt & Anbar, 1998; Pogrel et al., 1989; Anbar, Gratt & Hong, 1998; Weinstein et al., 1991; Biagioni et al., 1996), so far, no study has specifically used superimposition of ROI images, as performed in these studies.

MTPs are one of the diagnostic criteria of MPS. However, they are commonly overlooked as sources of pain because the sensory experience may be local or widespread, owing to pain referral mechanisms being not yet fully understood. MTPs are thought to be initiated by a muscle or connective tissue change that sets up positive feedback with the central nervous system, resulting in sensory, motor and autonomic changes (Kruse & Christiansen, 1992).

Algometry provides us with a means to gauge the pain sensitivity of trigger points quantitatively. The results of many studies confirm that MTPs are more sensitive than contralateral, MTP-free muscle areas (Simons, 1988; Fischer & Chang, 1986; Kruse & Christiansen, 1992). The MTP study confirms those findings, and the pressure threshold for MTPs was lower in points of referred pain (1.28 kg cm^{-2}) than in points of local pain (1.73 kg cm^{-2}), i.e. the greater the pain sensitivity of the point, the lower the value of PPT (Haddad, 2001; Haddad, Brioschi & Arita, 2012).

When right–left sensitivity to pain was compared with the PPT no statistically significant difference was found between the temporalis muscles, only between the masseter muscles ($p<0.05$). Visscher et al (Visscher, Lobbezoo & Naeije, 2004) demonstrated that the PPT test result was greater on the right side of the face than on the left. According to them, a possible explanation for this fact is that the side with the greater value is related to the dominant side of the body. However, in this study, a statistical difference ($p<0.05$) was found when the sensitivity to pain between the temporalis and masseter muscles on the same side was compared. The masseter muscle was more sensitive than the temporalis muscle. These results are also in agreement with those found by Visscher et al (Visscher, Lobbezoo & Naeije, 2004).

The sensitivity and specificity to the PPT in the assessment of referred muscle pain were 0.66 and 0.73, respectively (Haddad, 2001; Haddad, Brioschi & Arita, 2012). Farella et al (Farella et al., 2000) found the sensitivity of the temporalis and masseter muscles to be 0.85 and 0.67, respectively, and the specificity to be 0.87 and 0.77, respectively. Similar results for sensitivity and specificity were observed by Visscher et al (Visscher, Lobbezoo & Naeije, 2004), respectively, for groups both without temporomandibular disorders (0.64 and 0.68), and with temporomandibular disorders (0.7 and 0.72).

Thermal symmetry is present in many parts of the body in a normal population. Skin temperature is a function of blood flow, controlled by the autonomic nervous system. This affects both sides of the body uniformly and simultaneously, resulting in near symmetry of thermal patterns (Gratt et al., 1989; Gratt et al., 1994; Weinstein et al., 1991; Berry & Yemm, 1971; Berry & Yemm, 1974; Mongini et al., 1990).

The literature describes the infrared hyper-radiation presence in the regions of muscle tension when compared with the unaffected opposing muscle (Kawano et al., 1993; Berry & Yemm, 1971; Berry & Yemm, 1974; Fischer & Chang, 1986; Fischer, 1988; Fischer, 1991). However, all authors evaluated large ROIs. Owing to its size and functionality, a single masticatory muscle can have more than one MTP. When calculating the average temperature of the entire muscle, without individualizing the MTP, a false thermal symmetry of the face might be observed because the values obtained may be dissipated by calculating the average temperature. However, when evaluating smaller areas corresponding to the size of an MTP this tends not to occur. This makes the results of thermal studies of smaller ROIs much more reliable, in relation to the study of a single ROI corresponding to an entire muscle. In addition, the higher the image resolution of the infrared sensor (in this case, 76 000 pixels), the more precise will be the thermal assessment of smaller ROIs. It is important to take into consideration that the thermal assessment protocol is very important to assist in the conclusion of the exam. So, using this methodology based on Pogrel et al's study (Pogrel et al., 1989), it was possible to observe the thermal behavior of the cutaneous region exactly at the location of the area of muscular tension.

In these studies, infrared imaging revealed a difference of 1.4 ºC between mean anterior temporalis and masseter muscle temperatures and a difference of 0.09 between the corresponding normalized temperatures in asymptomatic subjects for TMD, indicating that the temporalis muscle was significantly more hyper-radiant than the masseter ($p<0.05$) (Haddad et al., 2014). Similar results were found in the literature [Pogrel et al., 1989; Kawano et al., 1993; Weinstein et al., 1991; Berry & Yemm, 1971). This difference in temperature between these muscles is explained on the basis of anatomy: the temporalis muscle, in addition to being thinner than the masseter, is influenced by the superficial path of the temporal artery, which makes the region more hyper-radiant. In the thermal comparison (xT; xθ) between the opposing sides, the temporalis and masseter muscles showed no significant difference.

Although the PPT and thermographic examinations serve totally different purposes, in which the first assesses tenderness to compression and the second evaluates the local vasomotor response, moderately significant correlations were observed between the PPT values (kgf) and the temperature (T and θ), suggesting that the greater the force applied, the greater the local temperature recorded. Also, the temperatures (T, θ) at the points of local pain were higher than those at areas of referred pain ($p<0.05$). Therefore, the temperature decreases according to the severity of myofascial dysfunction. Similar results of the chronicity of myogenous TMD changes the skin temperature over the anterior temporalis muscle was found in the literature (Dibai-Filho et al., 2014; Dibai-Filho et al., 2015).

The most heated areas of the face were correlated with regions without MTP, seen in the ROC curve as cut-off points with T above 34 °C and θ above 0.810, between the corresponding ROIs. At the same time, PPT values below 1.35 kgf, T below 33 °C, and θ under 0.756 were related to MTPs with referred pain. In a middle range, values of T between 34 °C and 33.3 °C and θ between 0.810 and 0.756 were present in cases of MTPs with local pain (Haddad, 2001; Haddad, Brioschi & Arita, 2012). These results are apparently different from those found in the literature, which state that an MTP is always hotter than the unaffected side (Simons, Travell & Simons, 1999; Simons, 1988; Fischer & Chang, 1986; Kruse & Christiansen, 1992; Fischer, 1988; Diakow, 1992; Fischer, 1991a). A single study also found no relationship between hyper-radiant points and active MTPs when studying the upper trapezius muscle (Swerdlow & Dieter, 1992). In the present studies, an inverse behavior of the vasomotor response was observed in the ROIs, corresponding to the MTP and myogenous temporomandibular disorder of the masseter and temporalis muscles. That is, they were cooler than the corresponding contralateral asymptomatic region.

The explanation formulated for this result is given on the basis of studies conducted by Simons (Simons, 1988) elucidating on autonomic disorders in myofascial dysfunction. Cutaneous temperature is a function of blood flow, controlled by the autonomic sympathetic small nervous fibers. In the presence of a sarcomeric contraction of the muscle fiber, there can be a response of reduced blood flow, thus reducing local muscle oxygenation (hypoxia) (Berry & Yemm, 1974; Simons, Travell & Simons, 1999; Simons, 2004; Gerwin, Dommerholt & Shah, 2004; Shah et al., 2008). This hypoxia can trigger a regional sympathetic hyperactivity in the cutaneous projection area of the muscle, also decreasing the local temperature through skin vasoconstrictive activity sometimes as a referred pain (Haddad, 2001;

Haddad, Brioschi & Arita, 2012). Pogrel et al (Pogrel et al., 1989) also described that ischemic areas and areas of increased sympathetic tone would show as cold areas on a thermogram, thus myogenic facial pain may in part be attributed to muscle ischemia.

The parameter most used in the evaluation of infrared thermography is thermal asymmetry, also known as the conjugated gradient (xT) between the corresponding opposite sides. According to the literature, right–left thermal differences greater than 0.3 °C can define a myofascial dysfunction (Canavan & Gratt, 1995; Gratt & Sickles, 1993; Kawano et al., 1993; Gratt et al., 1994; Weinstein et al., 1991; Gratt et al., 1996; Vargas et al., 2009; Gerwin, Dommerholt & Shah, 2004). By the evaluation of the cut-off points, the value of the conjugated gradient (xT) was higher than 0.3 °C and the normalized temperature value (xθ) was greater than 0.036. When the MTPs were separated into local and referred pain, the values of xT = 0.4 °C and xθ = 0.037 were found to detect the point of local pain, and xT = 0.5 °C and xθ = 0.048 to detect ROIs with referred pain. In cases in which there was local pain on one side and referred pain on the other, the values recorded were xT = 0.5 °C and xθ = 0.045. Except for Fischer and Chang (Fischer & Chang, 1986), who described MTPs with xT much higher, ranging from 0.5 °C to 1 °C, all other authors agree with the variations between 0.3 °C and 0.5 °C. However, they all agree in saying that the thermal image formed in the projection region of the MTP is a local vasomotor response (Haddad, 2001; Haddad, Brioschi & Arita, 2012).

In this study, the presence of an MTP in the ROI showed progressive positive predictive values of T, θ and the PPT as 36.8%, 39.3% and 53.4%, respectively. For both T and θ, the sensitivity of the method to identify an MTP with referred pain was average (50%), although the specificity was low (17%). Regarding the presence of an MTP, sensitivity and specificity for both xT and xθ were 62.5% and 71.31%, respectively. These results suggest greater diagnostic accuracy when different temperatures (xT; xθ), rather than absolute temperature (T), are used, even when corrected for each individual core temperature (θ) for the identification of MTPs. The results of sensitivity and specificity of the thermographic assessment for masticatory muscle regions suggest greater diagnostic accuracy when absolute mean temperature (T) is used, even when converted to dimensionless temperature (θ) (Haddad, 2001; Haddad, Brioschi & Arita, 2012).

These results suggest that thermal values, if used in conjunction with physical assessment, can serve as a means of screening and improved diagnostic accuracy in myogenous TMDs and MTP.

FUTURE RESEARCH DIRECTIONS

The literature reports different methods of evaluating facial skin surface but there is not a consensus. Due to this fact, the authors proposed a new facial protocol to facilitate the thermal evaluation of the vascular and nervous systems. Further investigations is needed for testing this proposed, which this protocol may prove helpful in the objective evaluation of diseases that could occur or refer to the facial region.

Further investigation is needed of MTPs and myogenous TMD in masticatory muscles, but these findings suggest that thermography may prove helpful in the objective evaluation of MTPs and temporomandibular disorders, especially if it is used in conjunction with physical assessment, as a means of screening and of improved diagnostic accuracy in clinical practice. In order to highlight the findings of this research, the use of a stimulus (thermal, mechanical and chemical) with dynamic thermal imaging is advised. It will provide important and new pathophysiological information characterization for TMD patients, myofascial pain syndrome and healthy individuals.

CONCLUSION

In conclusion, there is a statistically significant and directly proportional correlation between algometry and thermography in the assessment of MTPs, in which the greater the force applied, the greater the local temperature recorded. Thus, the temperature of facial cutaneous areas over the masseter and anterior temporalis muscles decreases in the presence of myogenous TMD and MTP.

The facial protocol proposed also can provide new information on the anatomy of the vasculature, on systemic changes in blood flow, or neuronal systemic changes.

These findings suggest that infrared thermography is helpful in evaluating myogenous TMD and MTP. It could be used as a complementary diagnostic imaging method and improved diagnostic accuracy in clinical practice.

REFERENCES

Anbar, M. (2008). Dynamic Thermal Assessment. In N. A. Diakides & J. D. Bronzino (Eds.), *Medical infrared imaging* (pp. 8.1–8.17). Boca Raton, FL: CRC Press.

Anbar, M., Gratt, B. M., & Hong, D. (1998). Thermology and facial telethermography. Part I: History and technical review. *Dento Maxillo Facial Radiology*, *27*(2), 61–67. doi:10.1038/sj.dmfr.4600314 PMID:9656868

Berry, D. C., & Yemm, R. (1971). Variations in skin temperature of the face in normal subjects and in patients with temporomandibular dysfunction. *The British Journal of Oral Surgery*, *8*(3), 242–247. doi:10.1016/S0007-117X(70)80086-5 PMID:5282910

Berry, D. C., & Yemm, R. (1974). A further study of facial skin temperature in patients withmandibular dysfunction. *Journal of Oral Rehabilitation*, *1*(3), 255–264. doi:10.1111/j.1365-2842.1974.tb01437.x PMID:4530064

Biagioni, P. A., Longmore, R. B., McGimpsey, J. G., & Lamey, P. J. (1996). Its role in dental research with particular reference to craniomandibular disorders. *Dento Maxillo Facial Radiology*, *25*(3), 119–124. doi:10.1259/dmfr.25.3.9084259 PMID:9084259

Brioschi, M. L., Teixeira, M. J., Silva, F. M., & Colman, D. (2010). *Princípios e Indicações da Termografia Médica*. São Paulo: Andreoli.

Canavan, D., & Gratt, B. M. (1995). Electronic thermography for the assessment of mild and moderate temporomandibular joint dysfunction. *Oral Surgery, Oral Medicine, Oral Pathology, Oral Radiology, and Endodontics*, *79*(6), 778–786. doi:10.1016/S1079-2104(05)80316-6 PMID:7621039

Christensen, J., Vaeth, M., & Wenzel, A. (2012). Thermographic imaging of facial skin-gender differences and temperature changes over time in healthy subjects. *Dento Maxillo Facial Radiology*, *41*(8), 662–667. doi:10.1259/dmfr/55922484 PMID:22554986

Crandell, C. E., & Hill, R. P. (1966). Thermography in dentistry: A pilot study. *Oral Surgery, Oral Medicine, and Oral Pathology*, *21*(3), 316–320. doi:10.1016/0030-4220(66)90064-8 PMID:5216735 de Leeuw, R. (2008). *Orofacial pain: guidelines for assessment, diagnosis and management. The American Academy of Orofacial Pain* (4th ed.). Chicago, IL: Quintessence.

Diakow, P. R. (1992). Differentiation of active and latent trigger points by thermography. *Journal of Manipulative and Physiological Therapeutics*, *15*(7), 439–441. PMID:1431631

Dibai-Filho, A. V., Packer, A. C., Costa, A. C., & Rodrigues-Bigaton, D. (2014). The chronicity of myogenous temporomandibular disorder changes the skin temperature over the anterior temporalis muscle. *Journal of Bodywork and Movement Therapies*, *18*(3), 430–434. doi:10.1016/j.jbmt.2013.11.001 PMID:25042314

Dibai-Filho, A. V., Packer, A. C., Costa, A. C., & Rodrigues-Bigaton, D. (2015). Women with more severe degrees of temporomandibular disorder exhibit an increase in temperature over the temporomandibular joint. *The Saudi Dental Journal*, *27*(1), 44–49. doi:10.1016/j.sdentj.2014.10.002 PMID:25544814

Dworkin, S. F., Huggins, K. H., LeResche, L., Von Korff, M., Howard, J., Truelove, E., & Sommers, E. (1990). Epidemiology of signs and symptoms in temporomandibular disorders: Clinical signs in cases and controls. *The Journal of the American Dental Association*, *120*(3), 273–281. doi:10.14219/jada.archive.1990.0043 PMID:2312947

Dworkin, S. F., & LeResche, L. (1992). Research diagnostic criteria for temporomandibular disorders: Review, criteria, examinations and specifications, critique. *Journal of Craniomandibular Disorders*, *6*(4), 301–355. PMID:1298767

Farella, M., Michelotti, A., Steenks, M. H., Romeo, R., Cimino, R., & Bosman, F. (2000). The diagnostic value of pressure algometry in myofascial pain of the jaw muscles. *Journal of Oral Rehabilitation*, *27*(1), 9–14. doi:10.1046/j.1365-2842.2000.00526.x PMID:10632838

Fillingim, R. B., Maixner, W., Kincaid, S., Sigurdsson, A., & Harris, M. B. (1996). Pain sensitivity in patients with temporomandibular disorders: Relationship to clinical and psychosocial factors. *The Clinical Journal of Pain*, *12*(4), 260–269. doi:10.1097/00002508-199612000-00005 PMID:8969871

Fischer, A.A. (1983). Advances in documentation of pain and soft tissue pathology. *J Fam Med*, 24–31.

Fischer, A. A. (1987). Pressure algometry over normal muscles. Standard values, validity and reproducibility of pressure threshold. *Pain*, *30*(1), 115–126. doi:10.1016/0304-3959(87)90089-3 PMID:3614975

Fischer, A. A. (1988). Documentation of myofascial trigger points. *Archives of Physical Medicine and Rehabilitation*, *69*(4), 286–291. PMID:3281631

Fischer, A. A. (1991). Muscle spasm: Documentation by thermography and by clinical methods. *Thermology*, *3*, 276.

Fischer, A. A. (1991a). Trigger points: Visualization by thermography. *Thermology*, *3*, 276.

Fischer, A. A., & Chang, C. H. (1986). Temperature and pressure threshold measurements in trigger points. *Thermology*, *1*, 212–215.

Gerwin, R. D., Dommerholt, J., & Shah, J. P. (2004). An expansion of Simons integrated hypothesis of trigger point formation. *Current Pain and Headache Reports*, *8*(6), 468–475. doi:10.1007/s11916-004-0069-x PMID:15509461

Gratt, B. M., & Anbar, M. (1998). Thermology and facial telethermography: Part II. Current and future clinical applications in dentistry. *Dento Maxillo Facial Radiology*, *27*(2), 68–74. doi:10.1038/sj.dmfr.4600324 PMID:9656869

Gratt, B. M., Graff-Radford, S. B., Shetty, V., Solberg, W. K., & Sickles, E. A. (1996). A 6-year clinical assessment of electronic facial thermography. *Dento Maxillo Facial Radiology*, *25*(5), 247–255. doi:10.1259/dmfr.25.5.9161178 PMID:9161178

Gratt, B. M., Pullinger, A., Sickles, E. A., & Lee, J. J. (1989). Electronic thermography of normal facial structures: A pilot study. *Oral Surgery, Oral Medicine, and Oral Pathology*, *68*(3), 346–351. doi:10.1016/0030-4220(89)90222-3 PMID:2771378

Gratt, B. M., & Sickles, E. A. (1993). Thermographic characterization of the asymptomatic temporomandibular joint. *Journal of Orofacial Pain*, *7*(1), 7–14. PMID:8467300

Gratt, B. M., & Sickles, E. A. (1995). Electronic facial thermography: An analysis of asymptomatic adult subjects. *Journal of Orofacial Pain*, *9*(3), 255–265. PMID:8995925

Gratt, B. M., Sickles, E. A., Ross, J. B., Wexler, C. E., & Gornbein, J. A. (1994). Thermographic assessment of craniomandibular disorders: Diagnostic interpretation versus temperature measurement analysis. *Journal of Orofacial Pain*, *8*(3), 278–288. PMID:7812225

Haddad, D. S. (2001). *Correlação clínica e termográfica do ponto-gatilho miofascial nos músculos da mastigação* (dissertação). São Paulo: Universidade de São Paulo, Faculdade de Odontologia.

Haddad, D. S., Brioschi, M. L., & Arita, E. S. (2012). Thermographic and clinical correlation of myofascial trigger points in the masticatory muscles. *Dento Maxillo Facial Radiology*, *41*(8), 621–629. doi:10.1259/dmfr/98504520 PMID:23166359

Haddad, D. S., Brioschi, M. L., Vardasca, R., Weber, M., Crosato, E. M., & Arita, E. S. (2014). Thermographic characterization of masticatory muscle regions in volunteers with and without myogenous temporomandibular disorder: Preliminary results. *Dento Maxillo Facial Radiology*, *43*(8), 20130440. doi:10.1259/dmfr.20130440 PMID:25144605

Jaeger, B., & Reeves, J. L. (1986). Quantification of changes in myofascial trigger point sensitivity with the pressure algometer following passive stretch. *Pain*, *27*(2), 203–210. doi:10.1016/0304-3959(86)90211-3 PMID:3797015

Johansson, A., Kopp, S., & Haraldson, T. (1985). Reproducibility and variation of skin surface temperature over the temporomandibular joint and masseter muscle in normal individuals. *Acta Odontologica Scandinavica*, *43*(5), 309–313. doi:10.3109/00016358509046513 PMID:3866482

John, M. T., Dworkin, S. F., & Mancl, L. A. (2005). Reliability of clinical temporomandibular disorder diagnoses. *Pain*, *118*(1-2), 61–69. doi:10.1016/j.pain.2005.07.018 PMID:16154702

Kawano, W., Kawazoe, T., Tanaka, M., & Hikida, Y. (1993). Deep thermometry of temporomandibular joint and masticatory muscle regions. *The Journal of Prosthetic Dentistry*, *69*(2), 216–221. doi:10.1016/0022-3913(93)90143-C PMID:8429516

Keith, L. E., Thomas, W. D., & Ferganson, J. L. (1973). Effects of activity, alcohol, smoking, and the menstrual cycle on liquid crystal breast thermography. *The Ohio Journal of Science*, *73*, 55–58.

Kruse, R. A., & Christiansen, J. A. (1992). Thermographic imaging of myofascial trigger points: A follow-up study. *Archives of Physical Medicine and Rehabilitation*, *73*(9), 819–823. PMID:1514891

Lawson, R. N. (1956). Implications of surface temperatures in the diagnosis of breast cancer. *Canadian Medical Association Journal*, *75*(4), 309–311. PMID:13343098

Leonardi, R., Zaborra, G., Li Pera, A. M., & Tripi, T. R. (1991). Comparison of telethermography and electromyography in instrumental symptomologic evaluation of the anterior temporalis and the masseter. [In Italian.]. *Stomatologia Mediterranea*, *11*(1), 5–10. PMID:1871658

Merla, A., & Romani, G. L. (2008). Biomedical appplications of functional infrared imaging. In N. A. Diakides & J. D. Bronzino (Eds.), *Medical infrared imaging* (pp. 15.1–15.20). Boca Raton, FL: CRC Press.

Mongini, F., Caselli, C., Macri, V., & Tetti, C. (1990). Thermographic findings in cranio-facial pain. *Headache*, *30*(8), 497–504. doi:10.1111/j.1526-4610.1990.hed3008497.x PMID:2228600

Pogrel, M. A., Erbez, G., Taylor, R. C., & Dodson, T. B. (1989). Liquid crystal thermography as a diagnostic aid and objective monitor for TMJ dysfunction and myogenic facial pain. *Journal of Craniomandibular Disorders*, *3*(2), 65–70. PMID:2606998

Sanches, I. J. (2009). *Sobreposição de Imagens de Termografia e Ressonância Magnética: uma nova modalidade de imagem médica tridimensional*. Curitiba: Universidade Tecnológica Federal do Paraná, Engenharia Elétrica e Informática Industrial.

Schwartz, R. G. (2006). Guidelines for Neuromusculoskeletal Thermography. Wheeling. *Thermol Int*, *16*(1), 5–9.

Shah, J. P., Danoff, J. V., Desai, M. J., Parikh, S., Nakamura, L. Y., Phillips, T. M., & Gerber, L. H. (2008). Biochemicals associated with pain and Inflammation are elevated in sites near to and remote from active myofascial trigger points. *Archives of Physical Medicine and Rehabilitation*, *89*(1), 16–23. doi:10.1016/j.apmr.2007.10.018 PMID:18164325

Simons, D. G. (1988). Myofascial pain syndromes: Where are we? Where are we going? *Archives of Physical Medicine and Rehabilitation*, *69*(3 Pt 1), 207–212. PMID:3279935

Simons, D. G. (2004). Review of enigmatic MTP as a common cause of enigmatic musculoskeletal pain and dysfunction. *Journal of Electromyography and Kinesiology*, *14*(1), 95–107. doi:10.1016/j.jelekin.2003.09.018 PMID:14759755

Simons, D. G., Travell, J. G., & Simons, L. S. (1999). *Travell & Simons' myofascial pain and dysfunction: the trigger point manual* (2nd ed.; Vol. 1). Baltimore, MD: Williams & Wilkins.

Swerdlow, B., & Dieter, J. N. I. (1992). An evaluation of the sensitivity and specificity of medical thermography for the documentation of myofascial trigger points. *Pain*, *48*(2), 205–213. doi:10.1016/0304-3959(92)90060-O PMID:1589239

Vardasca, R., Ring, E. F. J., Plassmann, P., & Jones, C. D. (2012). Thermal symmetry of the upper and lower extremities in healthy subjects. *Thermol Int*, *22*(3), 53–60.

Vargas, J. V. C., Brioschi, M. L., Dias, F. G., Parolin, M. B., Mulinari-Brenner, F. A., Ordonez, J. C., & Colman, D. (2009). Normalized methodology for medical infrared imaging. *Infrared Physics & Technology*, *52*(1), 42–47. doi:10.1016/j.infrared.2008.11.003

Visscher, C. M., Lobbezoo, F., & Naeije, M. (2004). Comparison of algometry an palpation in the recognition of temporomandibular disorder pain complaints. *Journal of Orofacial Pain*, *18*(3), 214–219. PMID:15509000

Weinstein, S. A., Weinstein, G., Weinstein, E. L., & Gelb, M. (1991). Facial thermography, basis, protocol, and clinical value. *Cranio*, *9*(3), 201–211. doi:10.1080/08869634.1991.11678368 PMID:1810666

KEY TERMS AND DEFINITIONS

Algometer: It is an instrument for measuring the degree of pain caused by pressure.

Masticatory Muscles: They are responsible for the mastication. They are characterized by four muscles: temporalis, masseter, lateral pterygoid and medial pterygoid.

Medical Infrared Thermography: It is a noninvasive and nonionizing imaging technique that allows the real-time representation of the thermal skin surface distribution into thermograms.

Myofascial Pain Syndrome (MPS): It is characterized by diffuse muscle pain and the presence of myofascial trigger points (MTPs).

Myofascial Trigger Point (MTP): It is a hyperirritable nodule of spot tenderness in a palpable taut band of skeletal muscle. The spot is a site of exquisite tenderness to palpation, from which a local twitch response can be elicited when appropriately stimulated, which refers pain to a distance.

Temporomandibular Disorder (TMD): They are characterized by orofacial pain and mobility dysfunction of the masticatory structures.

Thermology: It is the medical science that derives diagnostic indications from highly detailed and sensitive infrared images of the human body.

This work was previously published in Innovative Research in Thermal Imaging for Biology and Medicine edited by Ricardo Vardasca and Joaquim Gabriel Mendes, pages 119-140, copyright year 2017 by Medical Information Science Reference (an imprint of IGI Global).

Chapter 9
Computerized Occlusal Analysis in Occlusal Splint Therapy

Roger Solow, DDS
The Pankey Institute, USA

ABSTRACT

Occlusal splints are used to protect teeth, relieve orofacial pain, and preview the patient response to a simulated occlusal correction. This chapter outlines proper occlusal splint fabrication that employs T-Scan analysis to verify a therapeutic occlusion. The T-Scan provides objective relative occlusal force and timing data that guides the refinement of a splint's occlusal scheme. Therefore, this chapter explains adjusting an occlusal splint's contact pattern with ink ribbon followed by the T-Scan. It also addresses the controversy regarding the existence of, or lack thereof, a relationship between occlusal interferences and masticatory muscle dysfunction. The author postulates that the research studies that argue against the existence of a relationship are absent of occlusal measurement and lack a scientific basis to deny a relationship exists. Lastly, recommendations are made to include the T-Scan in Temporomandibular Disorder treatment studies with both occlusal splints and natural teeth, so that researchers might resolve this controversy for dental clinicians.

INTRODUCTION

Optimal dental care is based on making a thorough diagnosis, followed by patient education detailing all of the patient's problems and their solutions, prior to determining an individualized, and appropriate treatment plan. Occlusal analysis is an integral part of the comprehensive dental examination. Mounted diagnostic casts show the size and location of occlusal interferences. T-Scan 8 (Tekscan, Inc. S. Boston, MA, USA) computerized occlusal analysis specifies the location, timing, and the relative force of differing occlusal contacts. This digital diagnostic modality accurately identifies the locations of problematic occlusal contacts that are not always visualized by direct clinical observation, or with ink ribbon markings.

Occlusal splint (OS) therapy is a conservative and reversible modality to verify a diagnosis, and treat occlusal problems. OS therapy is commonly used in the protection from bruxism-related attrition, the preservation of porcelain restorations, and in the treatment of myogenous orofacial pain (Okeson,

DOI: 10.4018/978-1-5225-1903-4.ch009

Kemper, & Moody, 1982; Clark, 1984a). Proper fabrication of the OS that fulfills all the requirements of stability and comfort to both the teeth and soft tissues, while establishing an optimum occlusion, is essential to obtain a predictable, therapeutic result. By using a properly designed OS, the clinician and patient can then assess the physiologic effects of a corrected occlusion, that could be later attained with occlusal adjustment (OA), orthodontics, or comprehensive restoration.

The recommended OS physical design features should provide for full arch coverage, made from a hard methylmethacrylate resin. The occlusal requirements are to develop even, bilateral posterior tooth contacts coincident with physiologic condylar seating, smooth anterior guidance contacts whereby the anterior portion of the appliance immediately discludes the opposing posterior teeth, and no anterior teeth contact heavier than the posterior teeth (Barker, 2004).

After all the details of a conventional OS delivery are completed, the T-Scan can be used to guide the refinement of the splint's occlusion. Scans can be recorded in maximum intercuspation (MIP), during guided centric relation closures (CR), and during all mandibular excursions, in the same way as can be accomplished on natural teeth. This author's clinical experience with splint occlusal refinement using the T-Scan system, consistently shows there is a lack of optimal occlusion design achieved when adjustments are performed with ink ribbon marking combined with patient occlusal "feel" feedback. Because a predictable therapeutic result cannot be expected from an incomplete adjustment of the splint's occlusion, the T-Scan is essential for achieving excellence with occlusal corrections performed during OS therapy.

The T-Scan clearly shows to the patient, their pre-operative occlusal problems and their post-operative changes resultant from their receiving optimum care. By showing the T-Scan graphics to the patient, the patient immediately gains a visual understanding of their own occlusal problems through the 2-Dimensional and 3-Dimensional ForceViews. This facilitates the patient's involvement, and raises their appreciation of the clinician's work required to achieve excellence in OS therapy.

OS therapy has also been used to study the physiology of occlusal contacts, and to test the clinical effects of various occlusal designs (Manns, Chan, & Miralles, 1987; Manns, Miralles, Santander, & Valdivia, 1983). Because an OS can be readily modified to test differing non-invasive occlusal contact schemes, they can be worn by the same patient, and evaluated for levels of adaptive comfort. Computerized occlusal analysis can provide verification of the actual occlusion tested, both in clinical patient care, but during research studies, as well, where occlusal problems are being treated. A lack of documentation of the true before and after measured occlusal status has been a significant failing of many published occlusal studies (Dao, Lavigne, Charbonneau, Feine, & Lund, 1994; Pullinger & Seligman, 2000; Truelove, Huggins, Mancl, & Dworkin, 2006; Kidder & Solow, 2014). The T-Scan technology offers a new standard for the validity of occlusal research, because of its time and force measurement and capabilities.

OCCLUSAL ANALYSIS AND THE PHILOSOPHY OF OPTIMAL CARE

Optimal dentistry may be defined as, the education, diagnosis, and treatment that provides a patient with the highest level of comfort, function, and esthetics over the long term, requiring minimal maintenance (Solow, 2011). Codiagnosis, or patient education, is a conversation during which each aspect of the patient's health or disease is shown to, and discussed with the patient. This conversation is the starting point for success, whether the goal is simply to better prevent bacterial problems through improving the patient's oral hygiene technique, or to perform a sophisticated reconstruction because there are many lost and compromised teeth. Patients must understand their oral health status and their occlusal problems, along with the potential solutions available to them, before they can be expected to commit their time, effort, and finances towards undergoing definitive therapy.

A comprehensive examination consists of a preclinical interview, a clinical examination, imaging (radiographs, tomograms, photographs), and an occlusal analysis. The clinician uses this data to create a problems and solutions list. Sharing the exam findings with the patient provides them with the information needed, to make a fully informed decision about what treatment is appropriate for their individual goals. For many patients, participating in this discussion may be the first time that a clinician has taken time with them, to fully evaluate their problems, and include them in the decision-making process. This helps to create a relationship of trust that is based upon professional competency and shared mutual goals, which is in distinct contrast to when a patient passively accepts suggested treatment procedures.

Occlusal Analysis and T-Scan

Many patients have physical signs of excessive force on their teeth that results from the adverse occlusal contact. Tooth wear beyond the patient's chronologic age, perforation of gold crowns, fractured teeth, chipped porcelain, gingival recession, abfractions, bone loss around implants with good oral hygiene, and tooth mobility despite healthy periodontal bone support, are common problems related to ongoing occlusal force overload.

Occlusal analysis is an integral part of the comprehensive examination, that identifies problems, which can be amenable to predictable occlusal treatment. Thorough diagnosis and patient education should always precede the clinician making treatment recommendations and performing corrective procedures. Direct visual observation of the teeth in Centric Relation, Maximum Intercuspation, in mandibular excursions, with mounted diagnostic casts, and T-Scan recordings all have advantages in evaluating the patient's occlusal relationships.

Direct observation of the teeth in static and dynamic (excursive) contact helps the patient to understand why wear facets occur from lateral, protrusive, and crossover contacts. The patient gains an immediate orientation of the importance of occlusion at no cost, while also feeling the effect of their contacts. However, it is difficult for some patients to see small teeth in a hand mirror, and muscle incoordination from occlusal interferences may limit the ability of patients to perform certain excursions. Direct visual observation should be considered a gross evaluation of the occlusal relationships.

Diagnostic casts mounted on a semi-adjustable articulator, with an interocclusal record made when the condyles are physiologically seated, often illustrates occlusal problems that are not detectable with intraoral clinical examination (Figures 1, 2). Direct observation of intercuspated teeth, or ink ribbon marking of the occlusal contacts that occurred in MIP can be inaccurate, because the patient is programmed by their protective neuromuscular response to avoid traumatic occlusal contact on the arc of closure interference closure so that more teeth contact and distribute the force of closure more comfortably (Roth, 1973).

Also, natural teeth can intrude due to the periodontal ligament (PDL) and obscure the actual initial point of contact while adjacent teeth mark. Teeth on stone casts do not intrude and therefore, can accurately identify these interferences. A predictable method to replicate the patient's occlusal relationships on mounted diagnostic stone casts using an anterior deprogrammer with bimanual guidance, has been previously described (Solow, 1999).

The advantages of employing mounted diagnostic casts are):

Figure 1. Mounted diagnostic casts verified in centric relation on a semi-adjustable articulator. The true anterior teeth relationship in the arc of closure is evident. Centric Relation theory postulates that patients typically close in maximum intercuspation to avoid contact on arc of closure interferences, which affects the anterior teeth relationship.

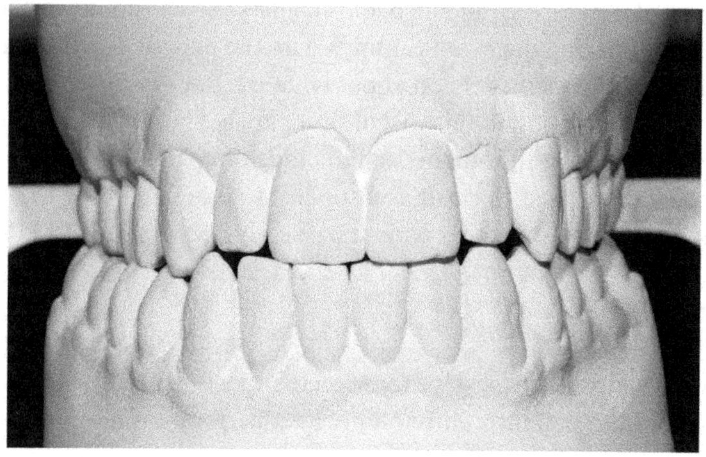

Figure 2. Arc of closure interference clearly shown on tooth #3. The solid stone depict arc of closure interferences accurately when compared to natural teeth, that intrude intraorally upon contact, that allow adjacent teeth to mark.

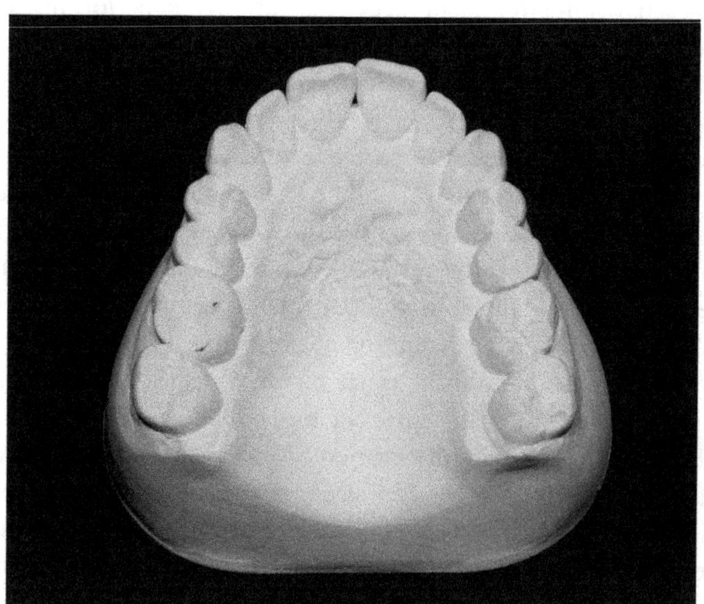

- The clinician can visualize the arc of closure interference.
- The clinician can measure the horizontal and vertical components of the lower arch translation from CR into MIP.
- The casts can be duplicated and then trial equilibrated, and compared to the initial unaltered cast with a wax reduction record, or with the occlusal matrix method, to quantify the actual amount of occlusal correction that would likely be required intraorally.
- During the diagnostic workup, the anterior contact relationships can be evaluated for the presence of proper anterior guidance function.

These objective, precise measurements facilitate predictable treatment planning (Solow, 2005; Solow, 2010; Solow, 2013).

Computerized occlusal analysis (T-Scan 8, Tekscan, Inc., S. Boston, MA, USA) is a high-technology modality that uses a full arch intraoral sensor to record the location, relative force, and the timing of the occlusal contacts. These records are obtained when the patient intercuspates during mandibular closure, or slides in a lateral or protrusive excursive movement. A significant advantage of the T-Scan is that it quickly generates a force movie that can be read frame-by–frame, with 2-Dimensional and 3-Dimensional ForceViews, that shows patients and the clinician where, when, and with how much force, opposing teeth make contact. The net balance of left to right side forces is displayed along with the Center of Force (COF) Icon and trajectory that shows the sum of the left, right, anterior, and posterior force distribution visible during each frame of a recorded occlusal event. Scans can easily be repeated at various stages of a procedure, or at different appointments, to compare, quantify, and document occlusal stability.

The T-Scan system is comprised of a recording handle, which houses an autoclavable sensor support, and a disposable, Mylar-encased 100 um thick sensor that registers occlusal contact at 5-10 um (Figure 3). The handle connects to a computer via a USB port, which transmits the force and timing data into the software for display, playback, and analysis. The system stores all data of each closure and excursion while documenting the occlusal contacts present on an OS, on the natural dentition, on implant-supported restorations, and upon partial or complete dentures.

Figure 3. The T-Scan hand-held recording handle with its U-shaped High Definition recording sensor. The handle attaches to a computer and records occlusal contact relative force and timing data of many mandibular functional movements.

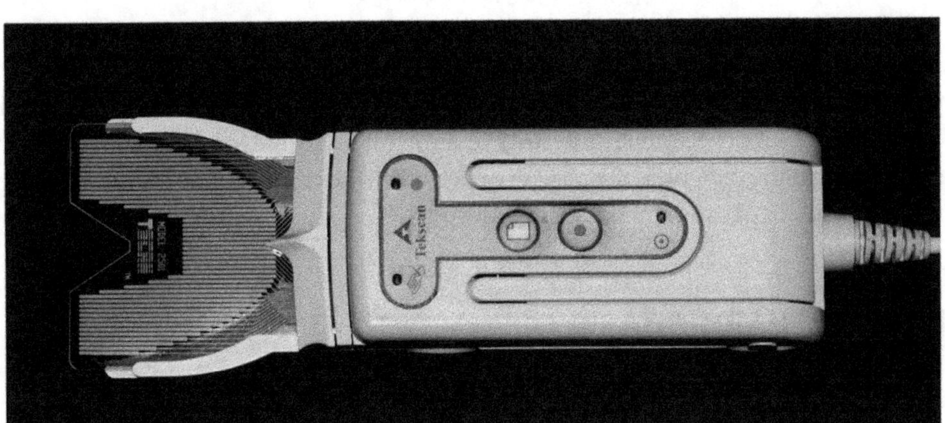

OBJECTIVES OF OCCLUSAL SPLINT THERAPY

After occlusal problems are diagnosed, the clinician and patient may elect to monitor the condition for the progression of signs or symptoms of the teeth, the periodontium, the masticatory muscles, and the Temporomandibular joints (TMJs), that would ultimately warrant some form of definitive treatment. They may also decide that the patient should undergo definitive treatment with orthodontics, occlusal adjustment, or comprehensive occlusal restoration.

Some patients may not be emotionally ready, or financially able to commit to definitive treatment. An OS may be a conservative, affordable, and non-invasive option for these patients. The OS is a removable appliance that covers the occlusal surface of the teeth and gives the clinician control over the relationship of the mandible to the maxilla, for diagnostic and therapeutic purposes (Academy of Prosthodontics, 2005). Nightguards, orthotics, occlusal devices, and bite appliances are synonyms for OS, without indicating the presence of a specific occlusal design.

OS therapy represents an indirect occlusal adjustment of the opposing arch to the OS, performed by manipulating the plastic occlusal surface of the OS. The treatment goals may be protection of teeth and restorations from attrition due to nocturnal bruxism, relief of masticatory muscle pain due to occlusal interferences, decreased tooth mobility from occlusal trauma, or stabilization of tooth position related to adverse forces overloading a reduced periodontium (Clark, 1984a; Lytle, 2001; Boero, 1989). These goals are achieved by shaping the occlusal surface of the OS to optimize the occlusal contacts, and redistribute occlusal force to the opposing dentition.

Importantly, the OS gives the patient the opportunity to preview the possible effects of an occlusal correction made to their teeth, without committing them to definitive treatment. This is an educational process for the patient when they begin to feel comfort and relief of pain, as their teeth, periodontium, and masticatory muscles, are freed from the burden of adverse occlusal force. The clinician cannot substitute descriptive words for this experience. The relief of chronic pain and the appreciation of the details involved in creating excellence with this initial conservative procedure, often prompts patients to ask for definitive treatment. The correction of the occlusion on an existing OS provided the needed educational experience, to drive the patient to want definitive treatment.

All patients should be instructed to bring their OS with them to the comprehensive examination, for evaluation with photographs, inked ribbon, and T-Scan analysis. This gives the clinician the opportunity to explain the deficiencies in the OS, and in some cases perform an occlusal correction so that the patient can understand and experience the improved, physical change.

OS therapy allows the clinician to confirm the tentative diagnosis that was based on the data obtained during the comprehensive examination. If the patient presented with painful masticatory muscles and discomfort of their teeth prior to OS therapy that was completely relieved by the OS therapy, the clinician should have confidence that proceeding to definitive adjustment of the specified, and putative occlusal interferences, will benefit the patient. If the patient experienced no relief, or had an exaggerated emotional response to slight detail changes in the occlusion, definitive occlusal treatment would not be indicated.

THE CLINICAL RESEARCH BASIS FOR OCCLUSAL SPLINT THERAPY

The masticatory system consists of strong, durable structures that are designed to function in a coordinated fashion, while lasting a lifetime. Chronic adverse forces generated by destructive tooth contacts must be absorbed by the teeth and periodontium, but can affect all structures in the system. If these forces are applied with an intensity and duration that exceeds the tolerable limit of these structures, breakdown will ensue. The common effects of physical force overload are: wear, mobility, migration, and fracture of teeth (Dawson, 1989; Ratcliff, Becker, & Quinn, 2001), periodontal destruction (Nunn & Harrel 2001; Harrel & Nunn 2001; Harrel & Nunn, & Hallmon, 2006), muscular fatigue, incoordination, and pain to palpation, and osseous remodeling of the TMJs (Mongini, 1972, 1977, 1980; Israel, Diamond,Saed-Nejad, & Ratcliffe, 1999).

The only predictable protection of teeth from attrition is OS therapy. Although orthodontics, occlusal adjustment, or comprehensive restoration may create an optimal occlusal scheme where posterior teeth are protected by anterior guidance disclusion, the anterior teeth themselves are still susceptible to attrition. Destructive shear forces from bruxism, oral habits, or sleep position are a problem for many patients (Colquitt, 1987). For others, nocturnal OS use may be sufficient to mitigate parafunction, when there is no conscious control of the mandibular position during sleep. Patients that experience progressive tooth discomfort, wear, mobility, or fractures of teeth, despite consistent nocturnal OS use, are more likely exhibiting a daytime occlusal force problem, and 24-hour OS use prior to definitive care, is indicated.

Occlusal Splint Therapy and Masticatory Muscle Problems

OS therapy has been shown to be a consistently effective treatment for masticatory muscle dysfunction that is related to occlusal interferences. Both short-term use (Tsuga, Akagawa, Sakaguchi, & Tsuru, 1989) and long-term use (Sheikoleslam, Holmgren, & Riise, 1986), have been shown to normalize muscle comfort and function. Research has shown that OS therapy reduces pain in the masticatory muscles (Barker, 2004; Clark, 1984b, Okeson, Kemper, & Moody, 1982; Scopel, Costa, & Urias 2005; Ferrario, Sforza, Tartaglia, & Dellavia, 2002), restores the symmetry of their electromyographic (EMG) activity (Humsi, Naeije, Hippe, & Hansson, 1989), reduces the level of EMG activity (Solberg, Clark, & Rugh, 1975; Clark, Beemsterboer, Solberg, & Rugh, 1979), reduces muscular fatigue (Hamada, Kotani, Kawazoe, Yamada, 1982; Kotani, Abekura, & Hamada, 1994), restores muscular coordination (Beard & Clayton, 1980; Crispin, Myers, & Clayton, 1978), restores muscle force (Kurita, Ikeda, & Kurashina, 2000), and restores normal muscle thickness and symmetry (Emshoff & Bertram, 1998).

Achieving a predictable therapeutic result with OS therapy requires the delivery of a defined therapeutic occlusion. Lack of a precise occlusal scheme will alter the occlusal interferences, but does not ensure removal of them, which is inappropriate treatment. There is substantial clinical research to support and define the requirements of an optimal occlusion (Barker, 2004; Wiskott, & Belser, 1995).

The components of an optimal occlusal design are similar for all modalities of treatment that involve the occlusal surfaces of the teeth: OS therapy, occlusal adjustment, comprehensive restoration, orthodontics, and orthognathic surgery. These requirements are (Dawson, 1983):

- Multiple, even, bilateral posterior teeth contact with the condyles physiologically seated.
- Immediate posterior tooth disclusion by the anterior teeth in excursive movements.
- Anterior teeth that function in harmony with the envelope of function, and do not contact heavier than the posterior teeth.

Contacting on an arc of closure interference stimulates an immediate response of the periodontal mechanoreceptors to alter muscle activation (Dawson, 1973; Riise & Sheikholeslam, 1982). One study showed that restored mandibular stability, using an OS with even contacts in CR, avoided the force concentration present on the arc of closure interference, and restored normal muscle contraction levels (Jimenez, 1987). It has also been shown that a lack of posterior tooth contacts places an increased load on the TMJs (Ito, Gibbs, Marguelles-Bonnet, Lupkiewicz, Young, Lundeen, & Mahan, 1986; Spear, 2002).

The removal of artificial occlusal interferences on posterior teeth can normalize muscular activity and symmetry (Clark, Tsukiyama, Baba, & Watanabe, 1999). Posterior tooth contact during mandibular excursions has been shown to stimulate elevator muscle contraction (Williamson & Lundquist 1983; Kerstein & Wright, 1991; Kerstein & Radke, 2012). Another study reported that converting group function lateral excursive contacts into a canine-guided occlusal scheme with a gold casting, reduced elevator muscle EMG activity (Belser & Hannam, 1985). The immediate disclusion of posterior teeth by the anterior teeth within 0.4 seconds of excursive commencement has been shown to relieve hyperactivity of the masseter and temporalis muscles and reduce the symptoms of myofascial pain (Kerstein & wright, 1991, Kerstein, 1993, 1994, 1995, 2010; Kerstein & Radke, 2006, 2012; Kerstein, Chapman, & Klein, 1997; Wang & Yin, 2012).

Occlusal Splint Anterior Guidance: Canine Disclusion vs. Group Function

It is the contact of maxillary and mandibular canines during a lateral excursion that separates the posterior teeth. Group function is the contact of several posterior teeth during a lateral excursion. Because the anterior teeth are smaller than posterior teeth, and are more sensitive to pressure (Coffey, Williams, Turner, Mahan P, Lapointe, & Cornell, 1989), it has been recommended that the during excursions, the anterior teeth should *immediately* and smoothly separate the posterior teeth without, any restriction to the envelope of normal mandibular function (Dawson, 1989).

Canine guidance should be the first choice for lateral excursion contact as the long roots, long inclined crown surface, canine eminence, sensitive innervation, and distance from the TMJ fulcrum of the mandible's Class 3 lever system, allows canine teeth to distribute lateral forces better than posterior teeth. Canine contact during lateral excursion prevents excessive tooth movement of the premolars and molars without inducing deleterious movement of the canine itself (Siebert, 1981). OS anterior guidance contact should place the lateral guidance forces on the teeth with the best periodontal support (Kidder & Solow, 2014). The lateral incisors have small roots and therefore, should typically contact the OS only in the arc of closure absent of direct excursive contact. The canines and central incisors can contact in various patterns during excursive movements where they each take the load separately, sequentially, or simultaneously (Solow, 2013).

Research has shown that clenching solely on anterior teeth, reduced elevator muscle EMG levels are observed compared to when clenching on posterior teeth (Becker, Tarantola, Zambrano, Oquendo. 1999; Manns, Miralles, Valdivia, & Bull, 1989). And clenching on the canine ramp of an OS reduced elevator muscle EMG activity levels, when compared to clenching on an OS in complete MIP contact (Fitins & Sheikholeslam, 1993).

Other studies have shown that OS lateral excursive contact that is placed solely on the canine area, reduced elevator muscle EMG activity levels when compared to a group function OS design (Williamson & Lundquist, 1983; Shupe, Mohamed, Christensen, Finger, & Weinberg, 1984; Manns, Chan, & Miralles, 1987; Manns, Rocabado, Cadenasso, Miralles, & Cumsille, 1993). There was also a study that found no difference in EMG activity levels when OS lateral excursive guiding contacts were solely placed on the canine, or on the first molar. Of note is that canine guidance was recommended by the authors as desirable, due to the canine's better biomechanical position within the arch (Graham & Rugh, 1988; Rugh, Graham, Smith, & Ohrbach, 1989). An alternative anterior guidance design (The Michigan splint) incorporated canine guidance in both lateral and protrusive excursions to simplify adjustment, and to minimize elevator muscle activity (Ramfjord & Ash, 1994).

Congenital absence of the canines in one arch would best be treated by covering that arch with the OS, so that the opposing canines can function optimally against the OS. Congenital absence of both the maxillary and mandibular canines creates a compromised occlusion where the anterior guidance contacts should be placed on the other present anterior teeth that are best able to distribute the lateral guiding force. These teeth are the central incisors or the first premolars. Multiple posterior teeth in a group function should be avoided, due to the high masticatory muscle firing this occlusal design causes (Kerstein & Radke, 2012).

Occlusal Splints and Temporomandibular Joint Problems

OS therapy has a documented positive effect on pain and dysfunction in the TMJs. One study reported that after OS use, relief of pain in the TMJ was noted in 70% of studied patients, but was worsened in 30% (Carraro & Caffesse, 1978). Another study using a Michigan splint design reported that 87% of patients demonstrated improved TMJ pain, 78% demonstrated improved TMJ sounds, and 68% demonstrated improved limitation in movement (Tsuga, Akagawa, Sakaguchi, & Tsuru, 1989). The authors recommended irreversible therapy be employed only after conservative treatment has failed, since a high percentage of patients responded favorably to the OS. An alternative study employing a pivot splint design, where there is only occlusal contact on the molars, reported an 81.2% decrease in TMJ intra-articular pressure (Nitzan, 1994). Lastly, a magnetic resonance imaging study showed that TMJ pain was relieved after three months of maxillary OS use, without the authors reporting any recapture of anteriorly displaced discs (Chen, Boulton, & Gage, 1995).

Occlusal Splint Therapy and the Placebo Effect

The equivocal response of some subjects to various OS occlusal contact schemes have led some researchers to question if there is a placebo effect responsible for the amelioration of Temporomandibular Disorder symptoms (TMD) (Dao, Lavigne, & Charbonneau; Klasser & Greene, 2009). A Placebo is defined as a "procedure with no intrinsic value" (Dorland's Illustrated Medical Dictionary, 1974).

By definition, attributing improvements from OS therapy as being a placebo effect is likely incorrect (Kidder & Solow). OS therapy uses a large, physical device that specifically alters the patient's occlusion, and has been consistently shown to directly affect the highly sensitive, dental-neuromuscular system. Occlusal splints are neither innocuous, nor lack intrinsic value. Instead they are a real prosthesis and a proven treatment. Studies that compare the effect of non-occlusal splints that only cover palatal tissue and not the teeth, with full coverage occlusal splints, consistently show that full coverage splints demonstrate a greater therapeutic effect (Greene & Laskin, 1972; Ekberg, Vallon, & Nilner, 2003; Conti, Santos, Kogawa, de Castro Ferreira Conti, de Araujo Cdos, 2006). Research on non-occluding splints show that they are not innocuous, and can affect the incidence of sleep bruxism episodes (Dube, Rompre, Manzini, Guitard, deGrandmont, & Lavigne, 2004; Harada, Ichiki, Tsukiyama, & Koyano, 2006). Moreover, palatal non-occluding splints were found to suppress masseter muscle activity, such that the authors suggested the lowered muscle activity was possibly related to the palatal splint inducing an altered tongue position (Hasegawa, Okatnoto, Nishigawa, Oki, & Minagi, 2007).

To conclude that the benefit of OS therapy is due to a placebo effect, and is not resultant from the OS occlusal correction, to have any validity, future studies must measure and specify both the preoperative occlusion, and actual test occlusion, on a per subject basis. None of the published studies promoting that the mechanism of OS therapy is a placebo effect, and not a response to the occlusal correction, have done this. Mounted diagnostic casts of the OS, or more conveniently, computerized occlusal analysis scans of the splint's occlusal design, are accurate modalities to verify the occlusion for dental research purposes. Studies that rely on the verbal description of an occlusal scheme, use a non-occlusal splint, or simply assume a therapeutic occlusion is present on the OS because the test splints were adjusted reliably with articulating ink ribbon, do not provide the data needed to verify that a splint's effectiveness was caused solely by a placebo effect.

Occlusal Splint Therapy and Sleep Bruxism

Sleep Bruxism (SB) has been defined as a stereotyped movement disorder, occurring during sleep, that is characterized by tooth grinding or clenching (Lavigne, Khoury, Abe, Yamaguchi, & Raphael, 2008). SB is believed to be a centrally mediated event, but psychological, structural, and peripheral factors, including sleep-disordered breathing, the presence of prolonged excursive occlusal interferences (Kerstein, 1995; Kerstein, Chapman, & Klein, 1997), and some neurochemical mechanisms, may all play a role in its etiology (Bender, 2012).

The pathophysiology of SB may be autonomic self-regulation, whereby airway obstructed breathing leads to sleep microarousals that cause tachycardia. Rhythmic masticatory muscle activity and tooth contact stimulates the trigeminal nerve and induces the trigeminal cardiac reflex that produces bradycardia (Schames, Schames, Schames, & Chagall-Gungur, 2012). SB and clenching may also function to resist airway collapse by reducing negative pressure in the upper airway (Simmons, 2012). One study showed that SB is not related to myofascial TMD symptoms, because the polysomnogram data showed no difference between controls and subjects with myofascial TMD (Raphael, Sirois, Janal, Wigren, Dubrovsky, Nemelivsky, Klausner, Krieger, & Lavigne, 2012). It has been suggested that the reason to treat SB is to limit tooth wear, and not to treat TMD symptoms, such that OS therapy is indicated for patients with SB, to prevent dental damage and manage grinding sounds. But, it is unlikely that OS therapy likely will cure SB (Dao & Lavigne, 1998; Klasser, Greene, & Lavigne, 2010).

OCCLUSAL SPLINT FABRICATION REQUIREMENTS

The OS should be fabricated with a hard material to develop a precise occlusal contact pattern, that fulfills the requirements for an optimal occlusion. Autopolymerized or heat processed methylmethacrylate resin is recommended for strength and durability, as it has been suggested that soft splint materials cannot be accurately adjusted, can increase masticatory muscle EMG activity (Okeson, 1987; Al Quran & Lyons, 1999). The fabrication technique for methylmethacrylate resin OS has been previously described (Lundeen, 1979; Solow, 2011).

Once made, the OS must be stable when seated upon the teeth, and demonstrate no rocking or dislodgement when pressure is applied to one side. Retention is enhanced by covering the buccal surfaces by 2 mm and adjusting the amount of lingual/palatal undercut. The OS should be 1-2 mm thick in the posterior aspect, with a 1-2 mm buccal border for adequate strength (Kidder & Solow, 2014). This will typically create a 2-3 mm splint thickness at the anterior teeth.

The patient's rest position is highly adaptable to this OS thickness. Research shows that each increased vertical dimension generates a new rest position which allows patients to adapt to the vertical dimension change (Carlsson, Ingervall, & Kocak, 1979; Hellsing, 1984). One study illustrated that an increased vertical dimension from 1 mm to 4.42 mm, or 8.15 mm, led to greater muscle relaxation and symptom improvement (Manns, Miralles, Santander, & Valdivia, 1983). Although a thicker splint may have positive clinical effects, it must be thin enough for the patient to comfortably close their lips over the OS (Ramfjord & Ash 1994).

Maxillary and mandibular splints function with the same principles. When evaluating which arch should receive the occlusal splint, it is best to place it on the arch with porcelain restorations, mobile, missing, or crowded teeth, and where there exists uneven incisal and/or occlusal planes.

The OS must be completely comfortable to be consistently worn by the patient. Excessive seating pressure experienced against any tooth, should be adjusted by relieving the intaglio surface. Comfort to the tongue and the lips is ensured by smoothing all surfaces with acrylic resin burs, rubber wheels, and polishing the OS with pumice. The lingual/palatal border should extend 1-2 mm beyond the gingival margin, and taper to a feather edge.

A complete arch coverage design is important for long-term occlusal stability. Segmental arch coverage can intrude the covered teeth and extrude any uncovered teeth, distorting the occlusal plane and creating significant occlusal interferences, when the OS is removed. The general shape of the OS should be flat unless there is a pronounced occlusal plane problem in the opposing arch. Christensen's phenomena, (the separation of posterior teeth as the condyles glide down the articular eminences during protrusion), allows the anterior guidance area of the OS to be relatively flat and still disclude the posterior teeth (Academy of Prosthodontics, 2005). Conversely, a flatter articular eminence inclination requires that the splint's protrusive guidance track be more inclined, to better disclude the posterior teeth.

OCCLUSAL SPLINT DELIVERY AND INK RIBBON OCCLUSAL ADJUSTMENT

Methylmethacrylate acrylic resin distorts during polymerization approximately 5%, correlated to the heat of the setting environment (Danesh, Lippold, Mischke, Varzideh, Reinhart, Dammaschke, & Schafer, 2006). This distortion combined with cast inaccuracy contributes to any OS intraoral misfit. Relining the OS with a thin mix of the same acrylic resin that was used in the fabrication, will ensure stability under loading, while limiting rocking of the splint when seated on the teeth. An effective reline can be accomplished intraorally, or by relining the OS on an accurate stone cast. Once the reline acrylic resin reaches a rubbery consistency, the OS should be repeatedly rotated slightly on and off the teeth on one side of the arch, to develop an internal contour that requires rotation for removal, which improves splint retention and resistance to vertical dislodgement.

Fabrication of the OS on casts mounted with a facebow transfer, and an accurate Centric Relation (CR) record, typically results in a nearly even occlusal contact pattern when the OS is first placed on the teeth. Since most facebow transfers are arbitrary, and do not record the actual mandibular hinge axis, some error in the splint occlusion can occur. If there are sites where the opposing teeth do not contact the OS, acrylic resin can be added to restore contact. Alternatively, adjacent occlusal contacts can be adjusted to reduce the thickness of the OS until all teeth occlude uniformly.

All teeth should mark evenly on the OS coincident with the condyles being physiologically seated. This is predictably done with the patient supine, and the clinician using Dawson Bimanual Guidance to repetitively arc the jaw into CR (Dawson, 1989). The occlusal contacts are then marked with ribbon and modified with laboratory acrylic burs until there appears to be even contact of the opposing teeth against the splint, which is illustrated on the splint by a series of uniformly appearing articulating paper dots. These contacts should be consistently equal when the patient self-closes into the splint, and when the clinician uses Bimanual Guidance to ensure that the condyles are fully seated. Removal of the arc of closure interferences avoids the deflection of the mandible when it enters MIP, and allows the condyles to fully seat into CR at the most anterior-superior aspect of the mandibular fossa, which is coincident with the vector of elevator muscle force (Radu, Marandici, & Hottel, 2004).

To ensure patient comfort in CR, the anterior teeth should not contact heavier than the posterior teeth. A heavier anterior tooth contact can represent an arc of closure interference, and can place excess force on a potentially more sensitive tooth (Johnsen, Krister, Svensson, & Trulsson, 2007). The centric holding cusps (the maxillary palatal and mandibular buccal cusps), are used for posterior tooth contacts. One cusp tip contact per tooth site is desired (Wiskott & Belser, 1995). More contacts per tooth site increase adjustment time but do not necessarily increase mandibular stability. If there is a distortion in the Curve of Wilson resultant from an elongated mandibular lingual cusp, using that cusp as a CR closure contact avoids placing a lateral excursive interference on that cusp, which would occur if the CR contact was located on the shorter buccal cusp.

After proper CR contacts have been established, lateral and protrusive excursions are adjusted so that the posterior tooth contacts remain as small dots, and all excursive guiding contact marks appear as continuous lines (Figure 4). These lines should mark a smooth movement with no interruptions or "hitches" resultant from posterior tooth contact, that can occur as the mandible moves either medio-

Figure 4. A maxillary occlusal splint with 20 um thick ink ribbon marks (Accufilm II, Parkell, Inc. Edgewood, NY. USA). The arc of closure contacts mark as dots, and the lateral and protrusive excursion contacts mark as lines. The size of the dot should be minimal to avoid opposing tooth contact during lateral excursions. The overall shape of the splint is flat.

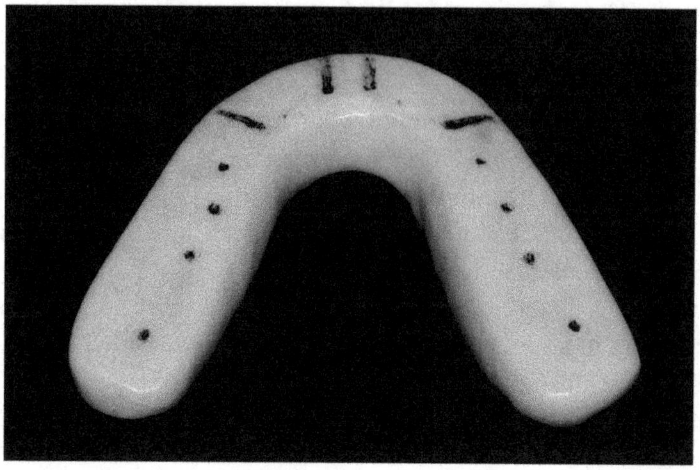

Figure 5. A right lateral excursion showing canine guidance contact with slight separation of the posterior teeth. This guidance design ensures that only vertical force vectors are placed on the posterior teeth, avoiding adverse torquing forces.

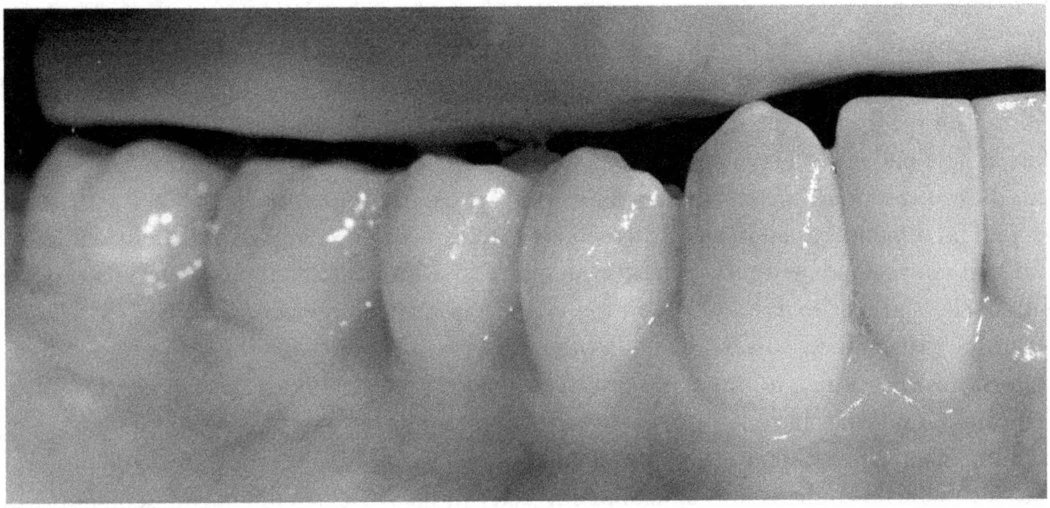

laterally, or lateromedially. Initially, it is common to see small lines extending from the posterior tooth contact dots, indicating contact exists during the lateral excursions. These marks should be removed until all excursive contact is present solely on the anterior teeth, as they can best tolerate the load (Figure 5).

Placing upward and medial pressure at the the gonial angle on the nonworking side of the occlusal splint helps to detect excursive contacts that could occur with intense bruxing (Okeson, 1982). The anterior guidance contact should extend to the full border movement of each excursion. Curving the OS border allows this length of contact without extending the border further horizontally. Crossover contact of the central incisor after a 4-5mm canine mark during lateral excursion creates two short tracks that also minimizes the horizontal dimension of the OS.

Protrusive inclines are adjusted in the same fashion. Continuous line marks indicate that the opposing central incisors contact simultaneously so that force is shared between these teeth. Gaps in the lines would indicate that only one incisor was contacting and absorbing all the excursive force while the other incisor was disengaged from protrusive splint contact.

The protrusive excursion typically shows rapid posterior tooth separation because both right and left condyles glide downward along the inclined articular eminence. During a lateral excursion, only the nonworking side condyle glides down the articular eminence, while the working side condyle rotates. The clinician must therefore, carefully check for posterior tooth excursive contacts during lateral excursive functional movements.

The OS occlusion should also be evaluated with the patient seated upright because the mandible closes in a slightly different arc when it is braced in CR, compared to when the patient is upright. The patient can confirm that all teeth contact evenly, with no anterior teeth contacting harder than the posterior teeth. This adjustment provides freedom in centric to avoid premature anterior tooth contact that can result in fremitus, or tooth discomfort from the postural change.

OCCLUSAL SPLINT REFINEMENT WITH T-SCAN SYSTEM

The same adjustment sequence used during the splint delivery is repeated with a T-Scan computerized occlusal analysis, which assigns force and timing data to each occlusal contact denoted by the marking ribbon. The T-Scan sensor analyzes the occlusal contacts but it does not mark them itself. The thickness of the sensor at 100 um does not interfere with making a correct analysis of the occlusion. The flat OS with the thin, flat recording sensor has virtually the identical arc of closure of the OS alone.

To start, a new patient file is opened, the patient's biological data is entered, and the T-Scan dental arch size is customized to fit the patients arch anatomy. A centric occlusion scan label with Turbo mode (0.003 second incremental scanning) scan speed is selected. The T-Scan sensor is held stable by a plastic support that corresponds with the patient's arch size, that fits outside the OS borders. The sensor is placed intraorally so that the midline 'V' of the support contacts the midline of the OS. The patient is asked to gently close on their posterior teeth, with a caution not to close on the support, and then clench firmly against the OS for one to three seconds. The 1-2 mm facial bulk of the OS creates a horizontal distance from the opposing buccal cusps, so that inadvertent closure on the sensor support is typically not a problem. This facial dimension of the OS should be kept to a minimum for lip comfort, and to ensure that the occlusal contacts are registered correctly in the T-Scan's displayed dental arch outline.

Natural teeth have cusps and fossae that orient the mandible when the patient closes on the sensor. The smooth surface of the sensor and the flat OS do not guide the mandible into an intercuspated position, so it is easy for patients to protrude and register only anterior OS contacts. The clinician should observe the display while using the T-Scan, so that a proper closure on the posterior teeth is being registered for recording. The patient closes several times initially to condition the sensor, and allow the operator to adjust the Sensitivity level to fit the patient's occlusal strength. When the Sensitivity is properly set, the patients occlusal strength range is divided by the T-Scan into 256 differing levels of relative occlusal force.

The T-Scan provides timing data not seen within the ink ribbon marks, and accurately records relative occlusal force with much greater sensitivity than does ink ribbon. An ideal occlusion observed in ink ribbon marks, does not look ideal when measured with the T-Scan. The data from each recorded clench, documents the areas of the OS that requires occlusal refinement. Laboratory carbide burs and rubber wheels are used to adjust the ink ribbon marks that are described by the T-Scan data as being either time-early contacts, force-excessive contacts, or both, until the COF icon sits close to the midline, and the posterior teeth contact with similar force levels.

Mandibular excursions are then adjusted in a similar fashion. The appropriate excursion scan label is chosen, after which the patient is asked to clench on their posterior teeth for one to three seconds, and then move in a lateral or protrusive excursion to the full extent of the border movement. Each excursion type is adjusted completely before the next one is treated. Any visible lateral ink marks leaving a posterior tooth line are removed, and the lateral excursion tracks are smoothed with a rubber wheel. The anterior teeth selected to provide protrusive guidance should contact with equal intensity, to comfortably share the load. The anterior guidance pattern of tooth contact is customized dependent upon the periodontal status and incisal plane.

Posterior teeth have cusps with some roundness, and therefore are not morphologically sharp points. During a lateral movement, as a cusp passes laterally over the OS ink dot marking, slightly different aspects of the cusp tip make contact with the OS, resulting in a prolonged lateral contact time. This can occur despite the dot being small, which implies the presence of only vertical contact. In order to minimize prolonged lateral contact time, it is important for the OS to be fabricated with some inclination of the lateral and protrusive excursion guide tracks, which ensures immediate disclusion of the posterior teeth.

After the T-Scan recordings verify the presence of an optimal occlusion has been created on the OS, the patient should be asked to comment on both the comfort of the OS fit, and of the occlusion. The goal of the OS delivery appointment is for the patient to confirm that the splint fits snugly, creates no discomfort on the teeth, or against the lips, cheeks, or tongue, while both the left and right sides contact evenly during closure, and no anterior teeth contact heavier than do the posterior teeth. Patients cannot be expected to consistently use an OS that seats with pressure on a tooth, rocks on occlusal contact, has a sharp edge, or creates an uneven occlusion.

CLINICAL CASES

The patient presented as an Angle Class I skeletal relationship, with normal incisal overlap and overjet of the anterior teeth (Figure 6). He was concerned about anterior teeth incisal wear and desired protection from nocturnal bruxism. A maxillary OS was fabricated on duplicate diagnostic casts (to preserve the original casts), and was relined intraorally to ensure stability and retention, as a precise therapeutic occlusion cannot be created on an unstable or non-retentive OS. The articular eminence inclination permitted posterior teeth to disclude with a fairly flat anterior guidance exit angle, resulting in a generally flat OS shape (Figure 7).

The maxillary OS was refined with 20 um ink ribbon so that all teeth appeared to contact equally (Accufilm II, Parkell, Inc., Edgewood, NY, USA) on the arc of closure (Figure 4). Anterior guidance was placed on the central incisors and canines. The patient described the occlusion as feeling even and comfortable.

Figure 6. The patient presents as an Angle Class I skeletal relationship with normal incisal overlap and overjet. There are no occlusal plane problems.

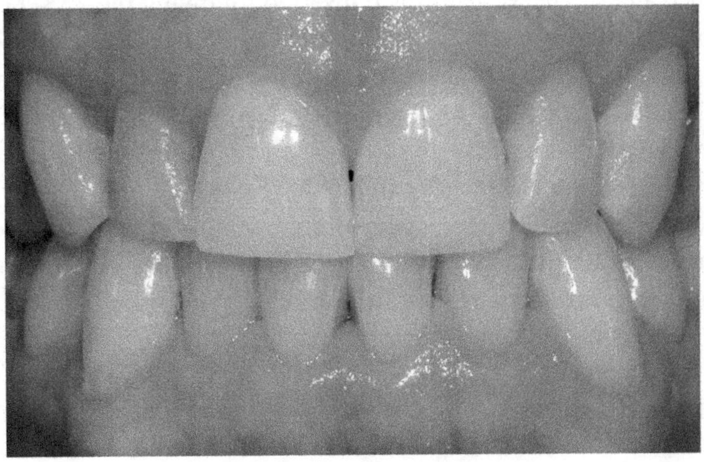

Figure 7. The maxillary occlusal splint has an flat shape. Posterior teeth disclusion in excursions resulted from the articular eminence inclination, and a fairly flat anterior guidance.

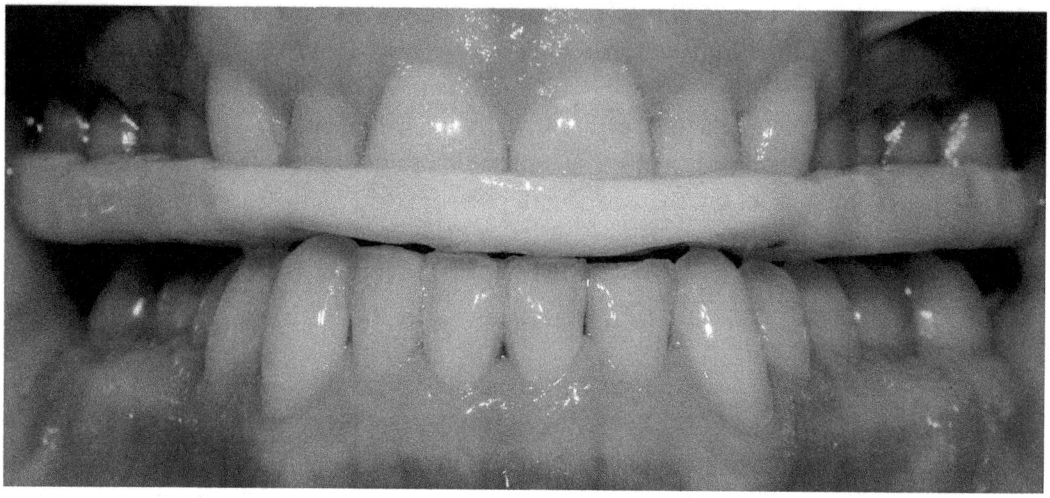

Arc of Closure Evaluation

The T-Scan then recorded the occlusal contact pattern when the patient clenched on their posterior teeth (Figure 8a). Despite the apparent even ink ribbon marks, the T-Scan showed a force distribution that was unbalanced, where tooth #3 received 17.3% of the total force, and tooth #14 received only 0.9%. The occlusal force was also unbalanced on the 2nd premolars, with tooth #4 receiving 5.2% of the total force, and tooth #13 receiving 13.9% of the total force. The anterior teeth were also unbalanced, as tooth #9 received 9.1% of the total force, but tooth #8 received only 2.1% of the total force.

The sites with the heaviest contact were adjusted with laboratory carbide burs after which the T-Scan was reinserted to observe the changes in the occlusal contact force distribution resultant from the initial occlusal adjustments. The occlusal contacts were then marked with the 20 um ink ribbon, the problematic contacts refined once again. The T-Scan was reinserted following the 2nd set of adjustments, as this recording and adjustment sequence method to refine the OS occlusal contacts, was repeated multiple times. By mid-session, the number of contacts increased, the level of individual tooth forces were more equal, but a larger molar tooth #2 at 6.9% total force, received less force than a smaller premolar tooth #4, at 16.0% total force. The anterior teeth were still unbalanced, with tooth #7 receiving 7.5% total force and tooth #10 receiving 2.2% of total force (Figure 8b).

Continued adjustment equalized the number of teeth contacting with similar force levels, and improved the balance of force between the right and left sides, which was confirmed by the COF icon summating in the COF target (Figure 8c). During clenching, the heaviest forces were located on the larger, multiple rooted posterior teeth, and not on the smaller anterior teeth.

Lateral Excursion Evaluation

The right lateral excursive contact was observed solely on the lower right canine against the OS, and verified with ink ribbon marking (Figures 4, and 9). The inclinations of the right canine track and the

Figure 8a. T-Scan ForceView when the patient clenched on the OS, prior to T-Scan guided adjustments. The ForceViews show the point of maximum force level of the B-C clenching plateau. The overall force distribution shifts (COF trajectory pathway) from the right anterior to the left posterior before becoming balanced at the end of closure on the OS (COF icon centered in the target). Teeth pairs #8-9, 3-14, and 4-13, register unbalanced force.

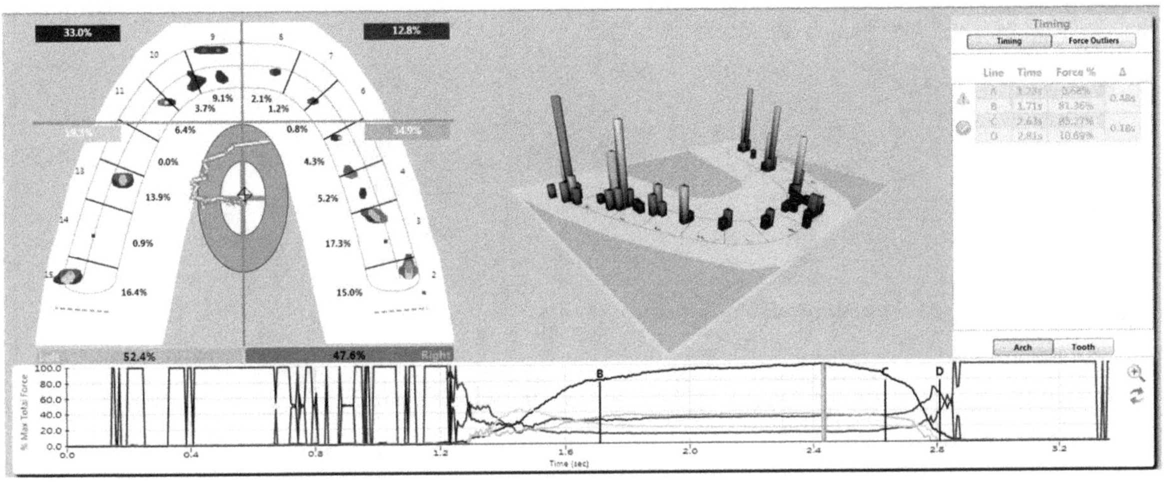

Figure 8b. T-Scan graphs showing closure on the OS at maximum force within the B-C clenching plateau, mid-session during the T-Scan guided adjustments. Note the improved number and level of occlusal contacts with the heaviest forces located on the posterior teeth.

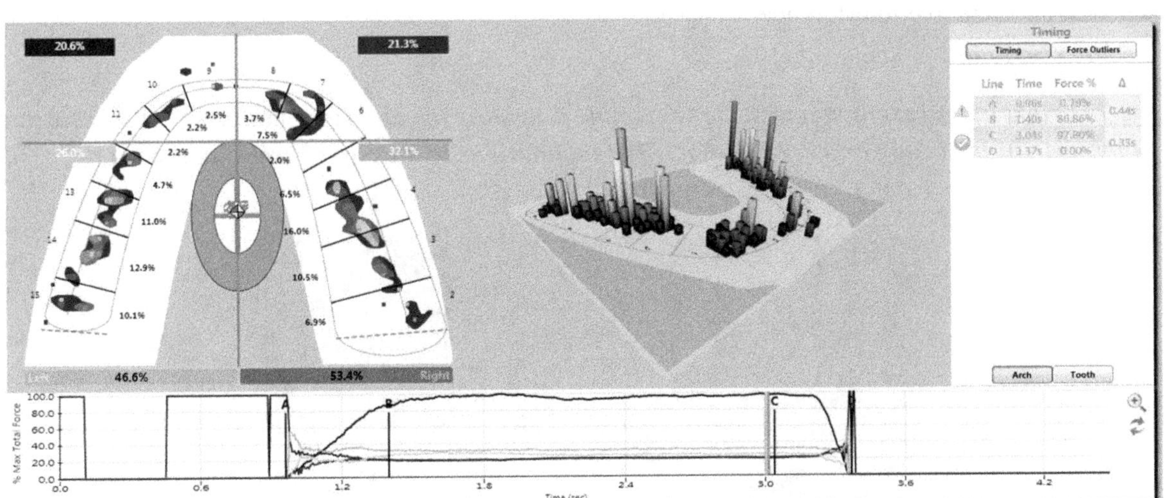

Figure 8c. T-Scan ForceViews showing closure forces present on the OS at the end of the T-Scan guided adjustment session, illustrating the maximum force level of the B-C clenching plateau. There is an optimal occlusion present demonstrating multiple bilateral contacts of similar force levels. The COF icon is in the middle of the target, confirming an optimized right-left and anterior-posterior balance of force.

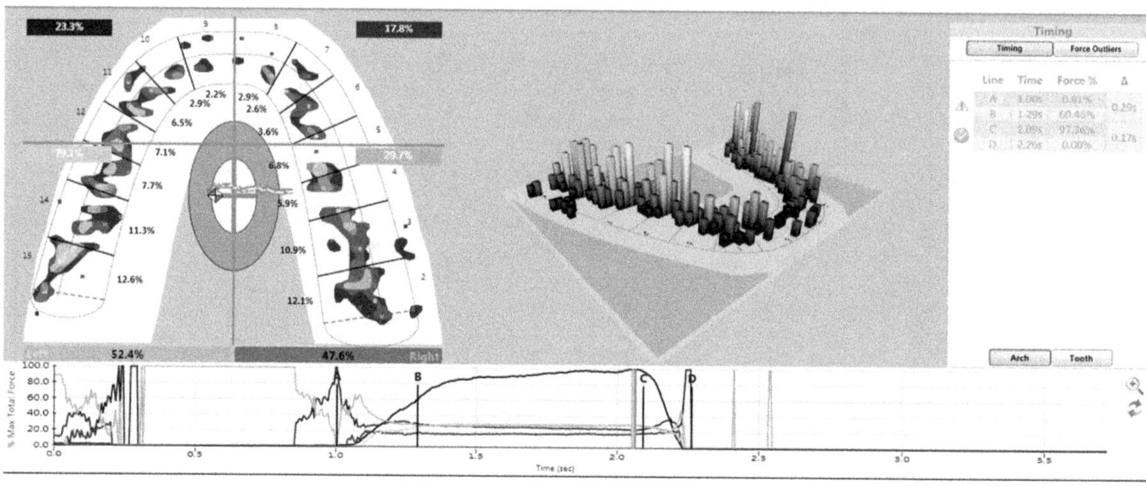

left articular eminence were steep enough to separate all other teeth from contacting the OS. The buccal aspect of the canine track was curved, to minimize the horizontal extent of the OS, and allow canine contact to extend all the way to the end of the excursive movement. The posterior tooth contacts were all dot-shaped ink ribbon markings, which exhibited no lateral ink extensions that would indicate the presence of an excursive interference.

Figure 9. A right lateral excursion with the OS canine providing the anterior guidance that separated all the other teeth from making excursive contact. The inclinations of the canine track and the non-working side articular eminence determine the degree of posterior teeth separation.

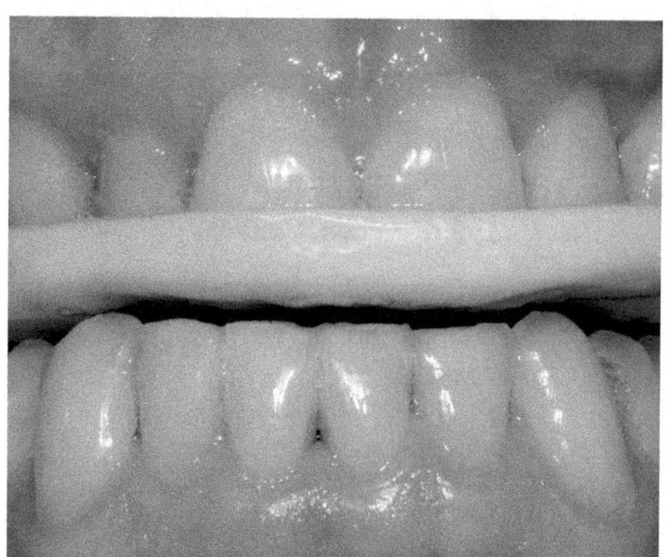

The T-Scan was then inserted intraorally, and the patient was asked to clench on the posterior teeth, and then slide straight right as far as possible (Figures 10a-10c). Within the T-Scan's Force vs. Time Graph (bottom pane of the T-Scan desktop) the black Total Force line rises from 0% force at A, as teeth initially begin to come together and load force onto the OS. Between A and B, more and more contacts engage the OS, until complete intercuspation is reached at B (the A-B time interval determines the Occlusion Time). As the patient clenches and holds the clench on the OS, the Total Force line forms a plateau (between the B-C interval), where the maximum closure force is represented at the 100% moment. At C, the Total Force line then declines as the excursion begins to the right. Throughout the progression of the excursion, the total force percentage drops when the posterior teeth are disengaged, and the anterior guidance begins to separate the posterior teeth, through until there is no force present on the posterior teeth, at all (the C-D time interval determines the Disclusion Time).

The objective of a therapeutic occlusion in lateral excursions is to eliminate any prolonged tooth contact on the posterior teeth. This rapid disengagement of all posterior teeth minimizes masticatory muscle hyperactivity. It has been shown in clinical treatment occlusal adjustment studies that the optimal Disclusion Time is ≤ 0.5 seconds per excursion, which allows for predictable resolution of myofascial pain dysfunction symptoms present in the natural dentition (Kerstein & Wright 1991; Kerstein, 1995; Kerstein, Chapman, & Klein, 1997; Kerstein & Radke, 2012).

It is logical to apply the same excusive timing criteria to OS therapy, since posterior tooth separation from either an OS, or the natural teeth, demonstrates a similar effect on how periodontal mechanoreceptors initiate muscle hyperactivity. However, there are differences between a patient undergoing OS therapy, and having an occlusal adjustment of their natural dentition. Typically, OS therapy is considered a non-invasive and reversible therapy. The alteration of tooth cusp contours is usually not accomplished at this phase of treatment, since the OS itself is adjusted to create an optimal occlusion opposing the existing tooth contours. Additionally, the EMG response from periodontal ligaments covered by a splint

Figure 10a. T-Scan ForceView of the initial right lateral excursion prior to any T-Scan guided adjustments, just after the B-C clenching plateau early in the right excursion. The significant number of, and force levels present on the working side of the OS, indicate a group function is present despite that the ink ribbon marking illustrating what appeared to be clear canine guidance.

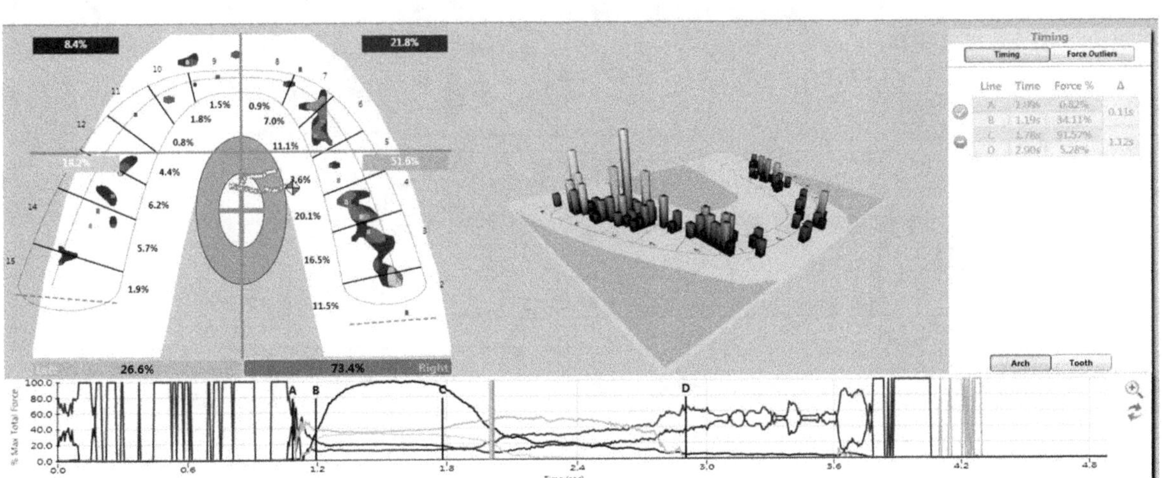

Figure 10b. The T-Scan ForceView mid right excursion, prior to any T-Scan guided adjustments. At 0.537 seconds past point C, there are still multiple posterior teeth making working side contacts, indicating a lack of immediate canine disclusion. Note that the COF trajectory moves right horizontally, towards the teeth involved in the working side group function.

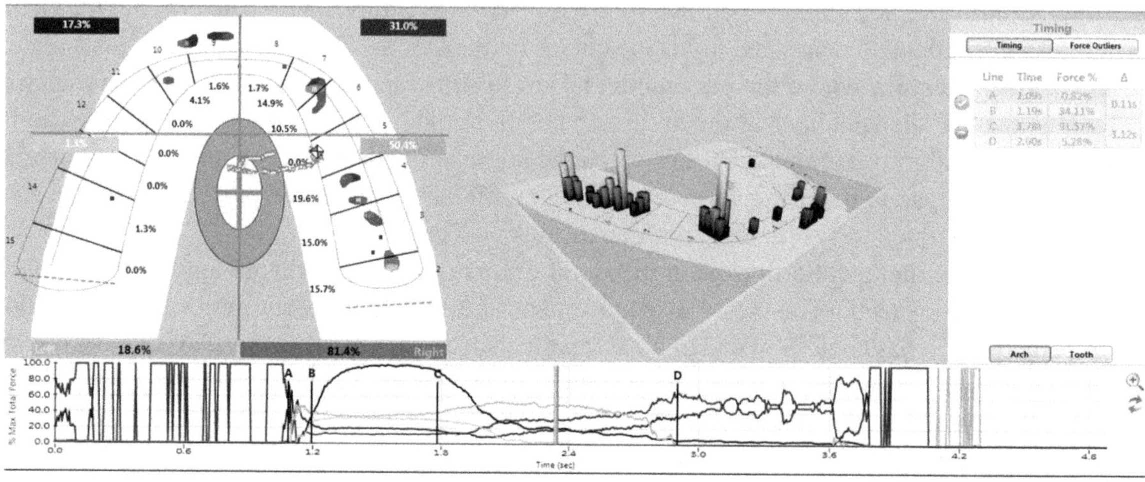

Figure 10c. The T-Scan ForceView at the end of the right lateral excursion, prior to any T-Scan guided adjustments. Note the reduced level of force present in the canine area, compared to the 100% maximum force point located at the B-C plateau. After C, the total force is decreased as masticatory elevator muscle contractions are reduced when the posterior teeth disclude. The low-force level contacts of teeth #s2, 3, 4, and 10, may be artifact resultant from the patient's cheek rubbing against the lateral border of the sensor, which can slightly distort sensor during lateral jaw movements. Here the COF has finally moved forwards to the canine area. The "L-shaped" COF trajectory indicates a group function scheme precedes when the anterior guidance creates the posterior disclusion.

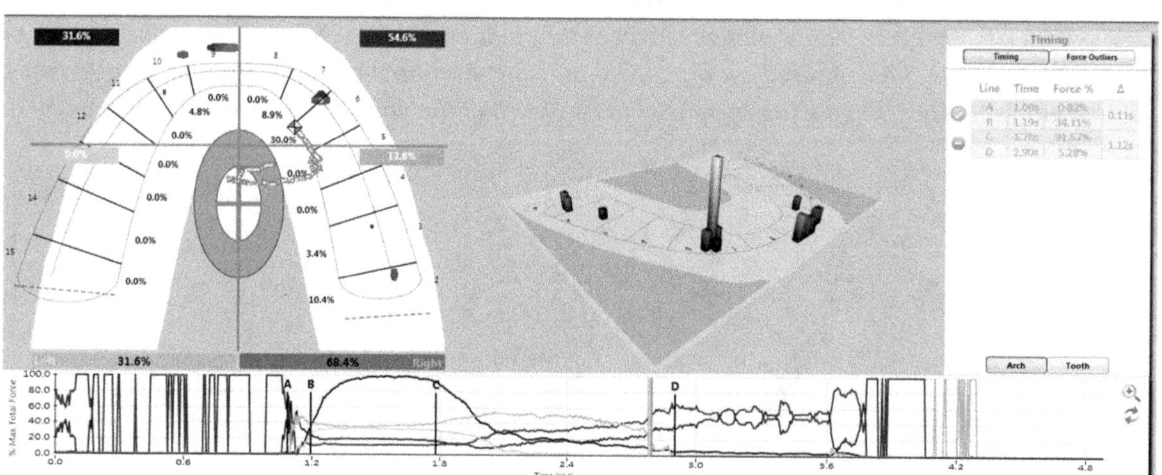

when contacting the opposing tooth, creates far less contraction levels compared to two opposing PDLs simultaneously compressed, without a splint between them.

Dental attrition that results in flattened cuspal contours is considered an indication for OS therapy (Lindfors, Magnusson, & Tegelberg, 2006). If the clinician cannot idealize the opposing cusp morphology, the rounder or flatter cusps may result in longer posterior tooth contact times during lateral excursion, even though the OS posterior tooth contacts appear as pinpoint marks. This occurs when slightly different aspects of the opposing cusp contacts the OS ink dot as the mandible moves excursively, resulting in a longer Disclusion Time than is attainable with occlusal adjustment, or the placement of a comprehensive restoration. Although forming a steeper canine guidance inclination will aid in establishing measurable immediate posterior disclusion and decrease the Disclusion Time within the C-D interval, an excessively steep guidance inclination may conflict with the patient's envelope of function, and create the uncomfortable feeling of being "locked in".

The T-Scan showed that during the right lateral excursion, there existed an initial prolonged Disclusion Time of 1.12 seconds. The posterior teeth contacted on both the working and non-working sides, despite there being OS canine guidance contact and ink ribbon markings that appeared to illustrate ideal right lateral excursive contact dots (Figures 10a and 10b). This prolonged disclusion was due to the flatter morphology of the opposing tooth cusps rubbing against the OS posterior tooth dot-shaped contacts. Low level contact on sites without tooth contact could occur from sensor distortion late in a vigorous lateral excursion, as jaw movement can slightly bend the sensor (Figure10c). The force recorded at the end of this canine guided lateral excursion is less than the maximum force demonstrated during the B-C clenching plateau, because masticatory elevator muscle contraction is decreased when posterior teeth disclude (Becker, Tarantola, Zambrano, Spitzer, & Oquendo, 1999).

If ink ribbon does not show posterior teeth excursive interferences are present on the OS, but the T-Scan does indicate there is prolonged posterior tooth contact present, the treatment options are to increase the inclination of the anterior guidance track by adding acrylic, decrease the size of the involved posterior tooth dots to pinpoints, or recontour and define the opposing contacting cusp tips. Also, further refinement of the arc of closure contacts can deepen the anterior teeth contact depressions in the OS surface relative to the adjacent excursive guidance track. This will increase the inclination of the initial portion of the excursive movement.

This non-ideal OS right lateral excursion was refined with T-Scan guided adjustments that decreased the posterior tooth contact dots to pinpoints, eliminated any acrylic resin contact lateral to the dots, and slightly deepened the CR contacts, so that the right lower canine contacted slightly deeper into the OS. This increased the inclination of the early lateral guidance contact (Figure 11). The opposing dentition was not modified, but the Disclusion Time (C-D interval) was decreased from 1.12 seconds down to 0.40 seconds (Figures 12 a - c). This value surpasses the criteria for natural posterior teeth immediate disclusion of ≤ 0.5 seconds, and represents a near-optimal OS therapeutic occlusion. Note that to achieve this functional improvement, the corrective procedures did not modify the opposing teeth cuspal contours.

The same ink ribbon adjustment sequence was repeated for the left lateral excursion. To demonstrate the variation of anterior teeth contact that provides anterior guidance, the inclination of the left lateral canine guidance track was made slightly shallower than the right, so that only the mandibular left canine contacted for the first 4-5 mm, after which the mandibular right canine also contacted the OS to share the guidance (Figure13). Once the mandibular left canine moved past the border of the OS, the mandibular right canine took over guiding contact, as the mandible moved further left to the full extent of the border

Figure 11. The posterior teeth dots have been decreased in size to pinpoints, and opposing tooth contact lateral to the dots has been eliminated. All CR contacts have been slightly reduced to create a deeper canine indent, and a more inclined early right lateral guidance contact compared to the anterior guidance contours shown in Figure 4.

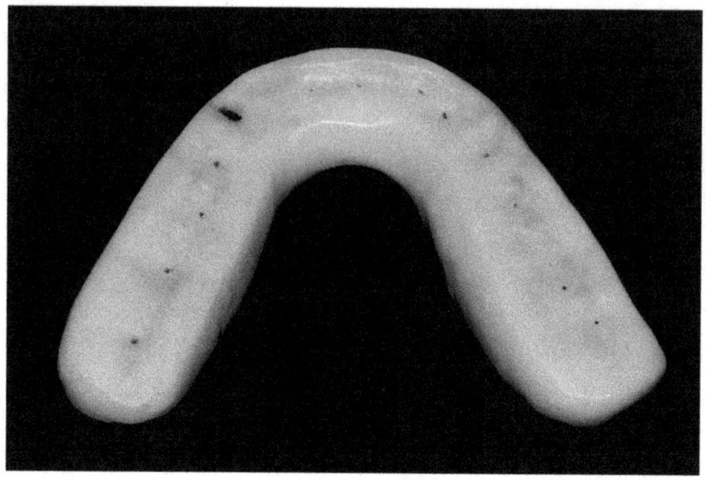

Figure 12a. T-Scan ForceView of the OS right lateral excursion just after the B-C clenching plateau, following T-Scan guided occlusal adjustments. The C-D interval showing the posterior Disclusion Time has been reduced from 1.12 to 0.4 seconds.

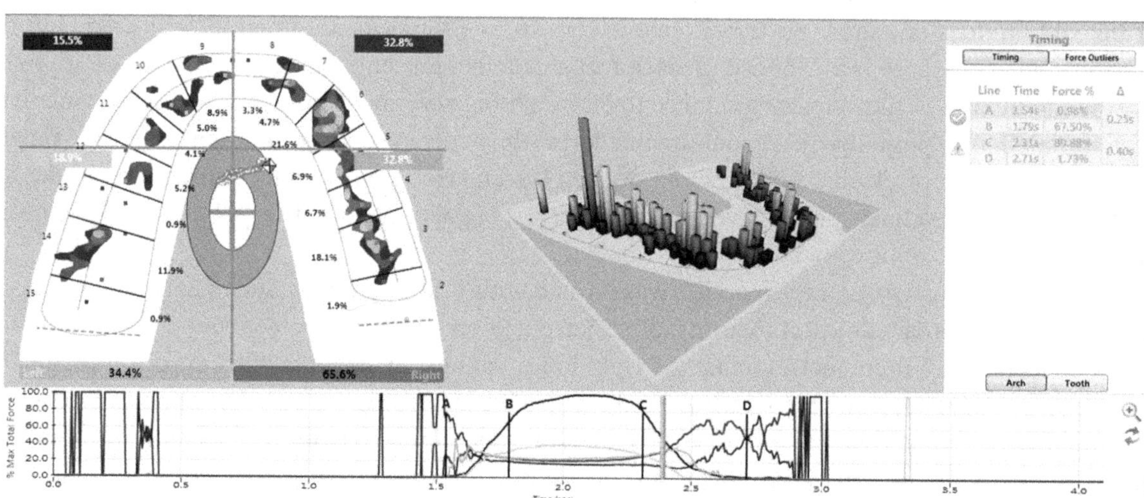

movement. This crossover position contact shared the anterior guidance force between two teeth, while minimizing the OS anterior area width. The excursive tracks can be altered to have either shared, or sequential mandibular canine contact, occurring during the excursive movement.

The T-Scan was then inserted, and the patient was instructed to repeat the same lateral excursive motion to the left side (Figures14a - c).

Figure 12b. T-Scan ForceView of the OS right lateral movement mid-excursion, following T-Scan guided occlusal adjustments. Multiple posterior teeth contact the OS with low level forces. The group function is present 0.2 seconds after the C line, but there is a faster decrease in posterior teeth contact compared to the pre T-Scan guided adjustment condition, shown in Figure 10.

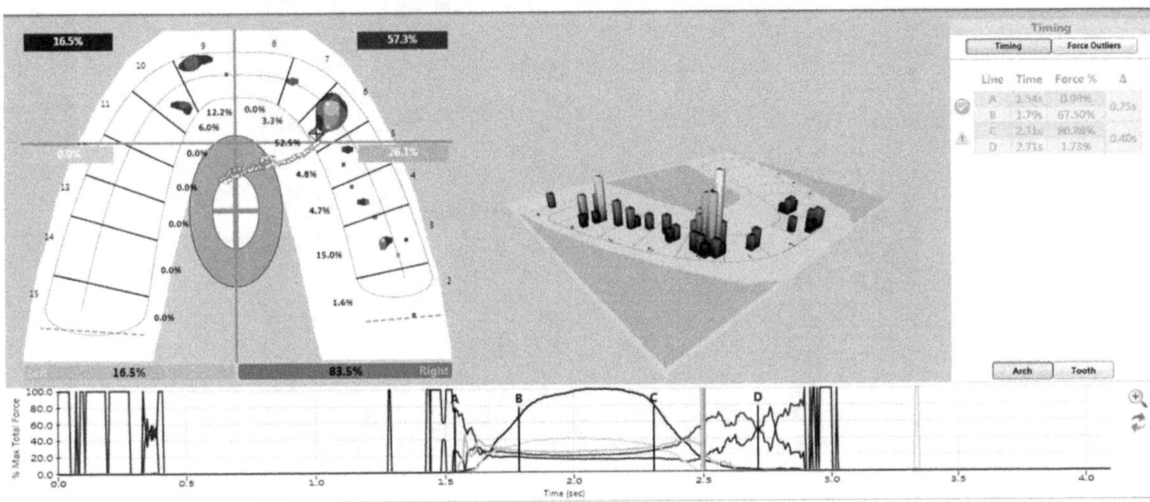

Figure 12c. T-Scan ForceView of the OS at the end of the right lateral excursion, following T-Scan guided adjustments. All excursive contact is solely on the right canine. The pronounced decline in total force that begins at end of the B-C plateau, as the lateral excursion rapidly discludes the posterior teeth.

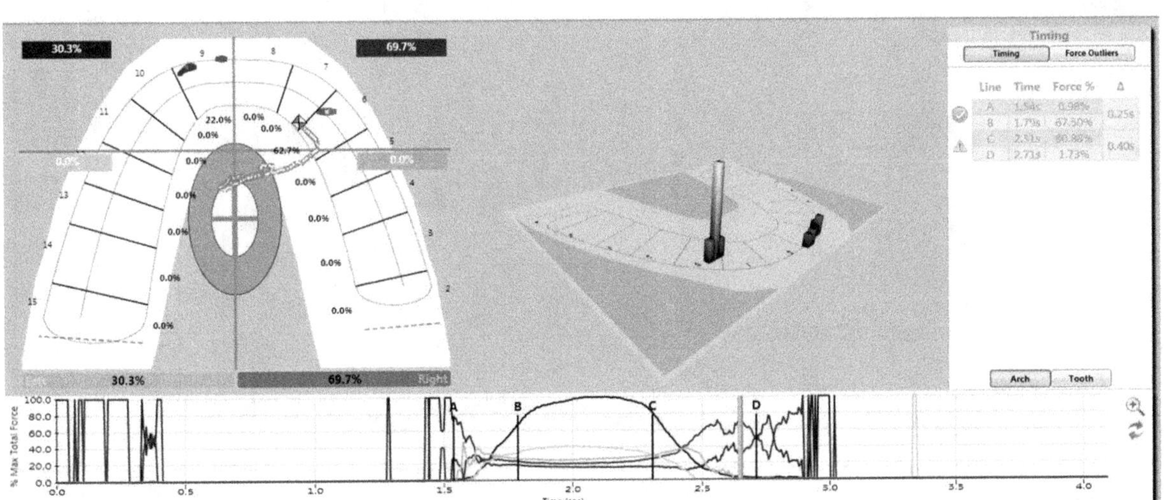

The OS left excursion was refined in the same manner as the right side excursion, by decreasing the posterior ink ribbon dots to pinpoints, eliminating any lateral contact adjacent to the pinpoint, and refining the CR contacts so that the adjacent early lateral guidance track was relatively steepened. The Disclusion Time (C-D interval) was decreased from 1.74 seconds to 0.29 seconds (Figures 15a - c). This decrease was greater than what was achieved on the right side, even thought the left lateral guidance was intentionally shallowed to include the right mandibular canine to share crossover guidance.

Figure 13. The left lateral excursion where, as the left canine nears the end of its contact, the mandibular right canine takes over guidance control on the OS. This contact minimizes the width of the anterior area of the OS, while the curved buccal aspect of the canine track minimizes its horizontal width.

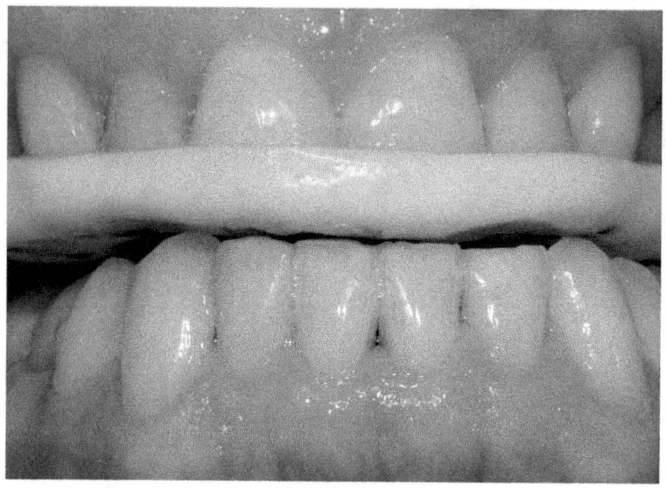

Figure 14a. T-Scan ForceView of the left lateral excursion just after the B-C clenching plateau, prior to any T-Scan guided adjustments. There is significant posterior working contact present on tooth #14, despite that both mandibular canines are in contact with the OS.

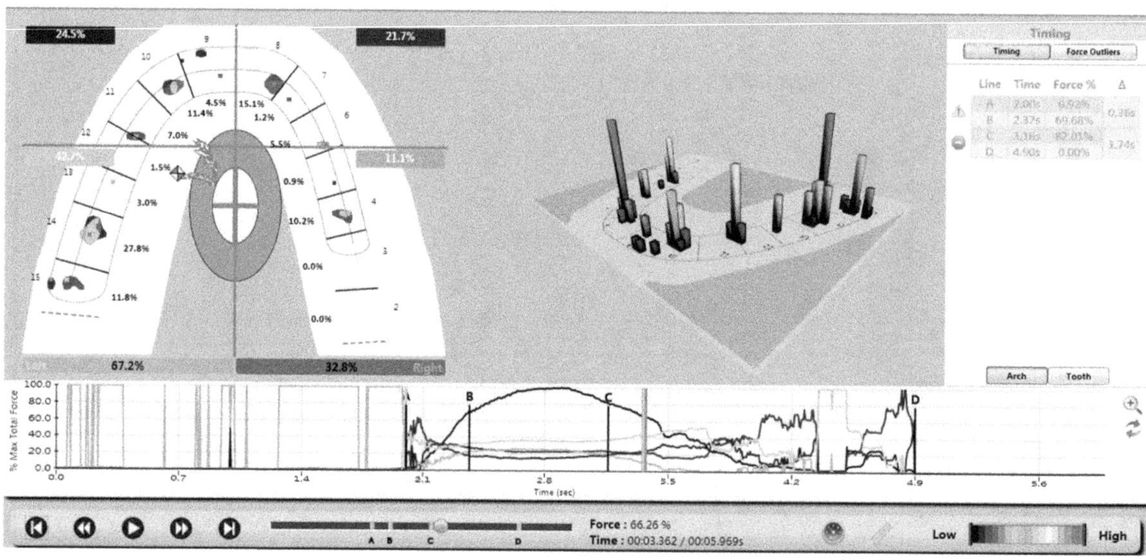

Protrusive Excursion Evaluation

The protrusive excursion contact was placed solely on the central incisors and the patient confirmed a smooth, anteroposterior movement. Ink ribbon marking showed continuous protrusive ink lines on the OS, with no extensions adjacent to the posterior tooth dots (Figures 4 and 16). The T-Scan was then in-

Figure 14b. T-Scan ForceView of the left lateral movement at mid-excursion, prior to T-Scan guided adjustments. At 0.5 seconds past C, there is group function contact of the left posterior teeth visible, as both mandibular canines share the lateral guidance contact.

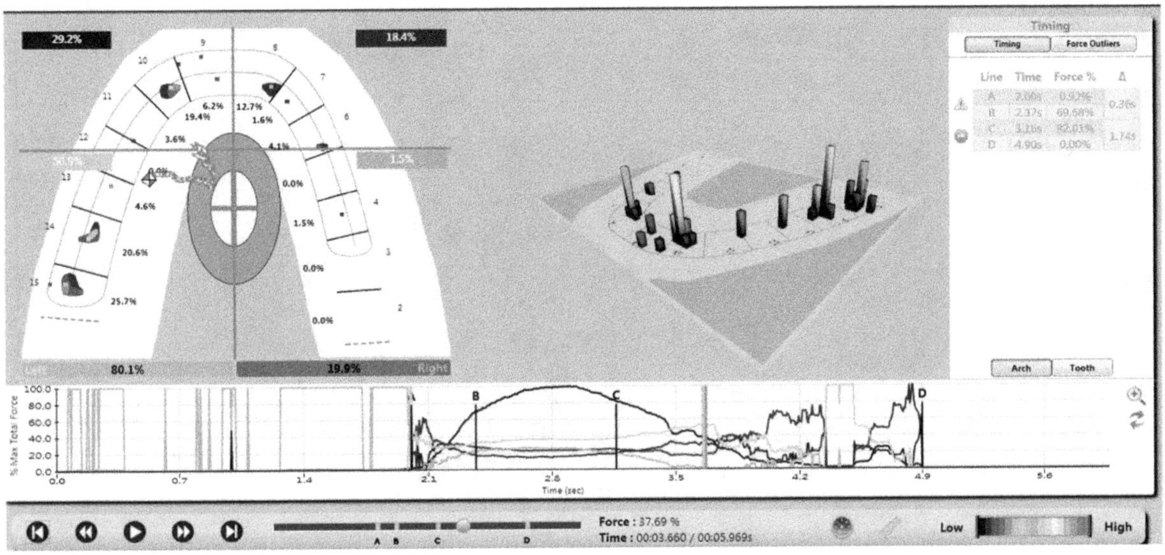

Figure 14c. T-Scan ForceView at the end of the left lateral excursion, prior to any T-Scan guided adjustments. The right mandibular canine is providing the lateral guidance and separating all other teeth from contact with the OS. The low force level contact on tooth #15 is due to distortion of the sensor that can from the cheek rubbing up against and bending the sensor as the patient moves laterally.

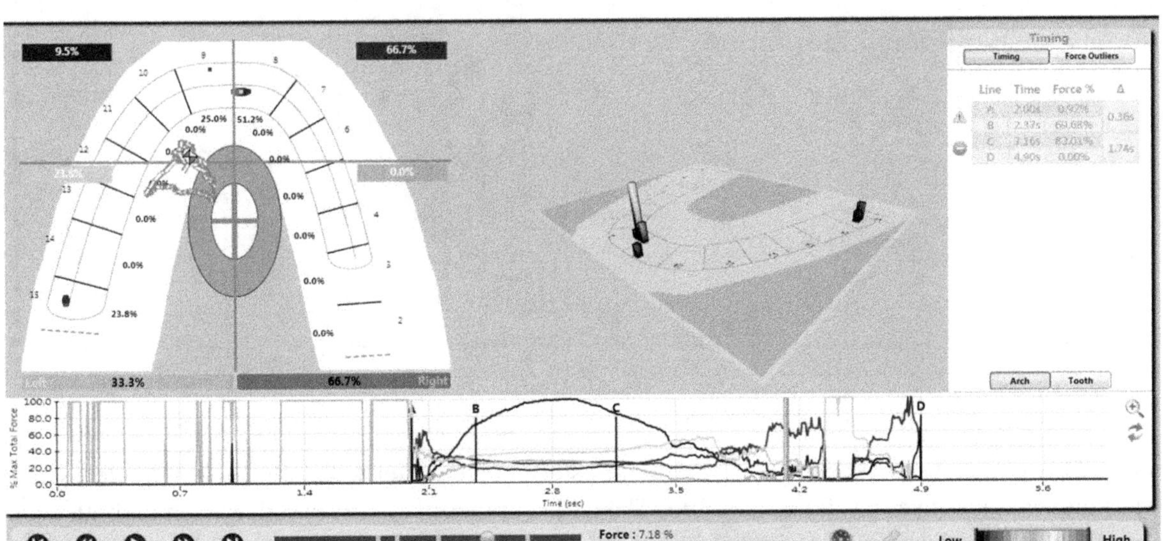

Figure 15a. T-Scan ForceView of the left lateral excursion just after the B-C plateau, following a T-Scan guided adjustment. At 0.1 seconds past the C point, there are posterior teeth contacting the OS early in a group function relationship shared with the left canine.

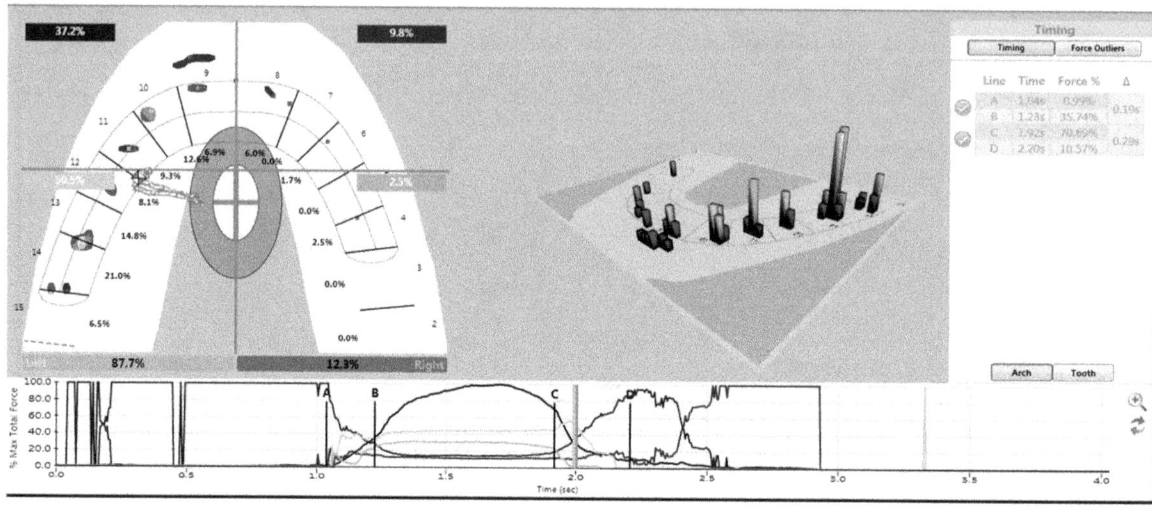

Figure 15b. T-Scan ForceView of the left lateral movement at mid-excursion, after a T-Scan guided adjustment. At 0.2 seconds past the C point, there are no posterior teeth contacting the OS, and two mandibular incisors share the force of the left lateral guidance

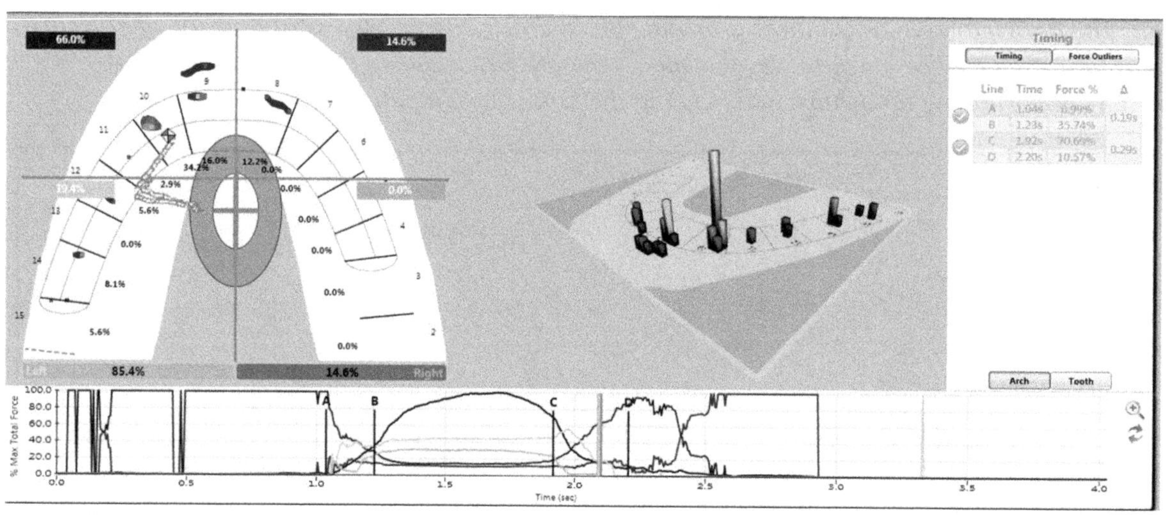

serted and the patient was asked to clench on their posterior teeth, after which the patient made a straight forward movement outward as far as possible. The early contacts were observed as even on both central incisors, but became heavier on tooth #8 at mid-excursion (Figures 17a - c).

The protrusive excursion was adjusted in the same fashion as were the right and left lateral excursions. Acrylic carbide burs and rubber wheels were used to smooth the protrusive tracks, so that the continuous line marks demonstrated equal "ink mark" color intensity (Figures 18a - c). The protrusive

Figure 15c. T-Scan ForceView at the end of the left lateral excursion following a T-Scan guided adjustment. At this point, all excursive force is on the mandibular right canine because the left canine has progressed past the border of the OS. The sequential contact of the mandibular canines creates two short canine guidance tracks and minimizes the buccal dimension of the occlusal splint

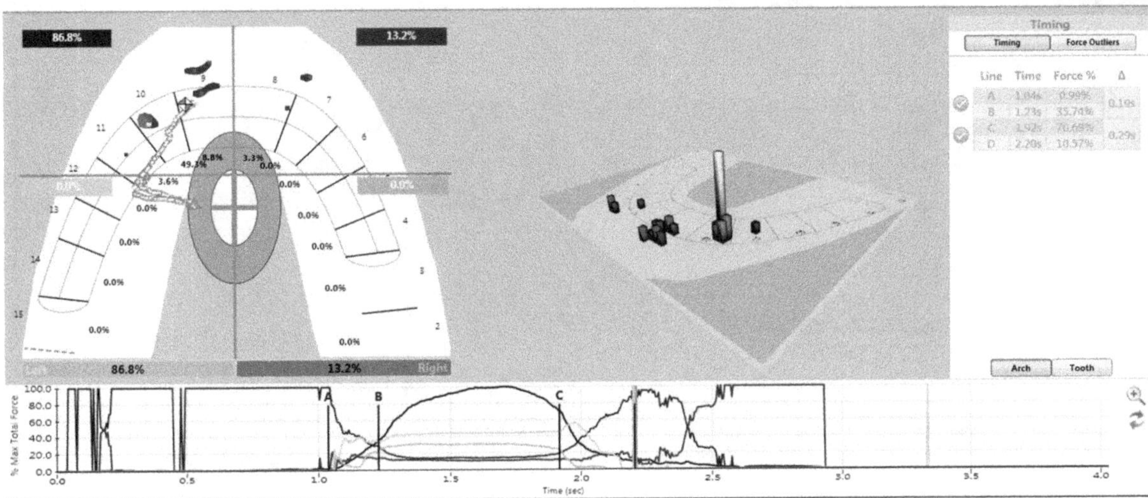

excursion should have even contact distributed on the anterior teeth that can best tolerate the load, for the full extent of the excursion. The grit side of fine sand paper was placed against the OS (the paper backing was placed against the opposing mandibular teeth), and then the patient protruded and retruded while the sandpaper was held against the lower teeth. This motion rubbed the sandpaper forward and backward, planing the OS protrusive contact surfaces of the central incisors, into equalized ink marking contact intensities.

Figure 16. The Protrusive excursion, where the central incisors evenly guide the excursion as all other teeth separate. The inclination of the articular eminence combined with the fairly flat protrusive guidance track, discludes the posterior teeth.

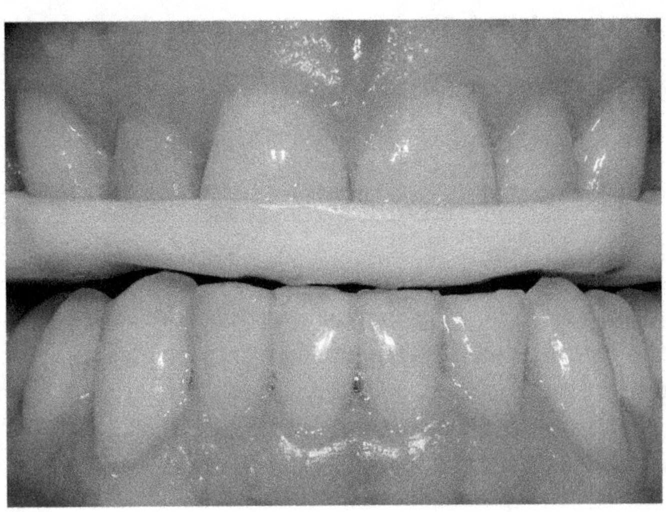

Figure 17a. T-Scan ForceView of the protrusive excursion just after the B-C clenching plateau, prior to any T-Scan guided adjustments. This early portion of the excursion at 0.2 seconds after the C point, shows there is even contact on the central incisors with some right sided posterior tooth contact present.

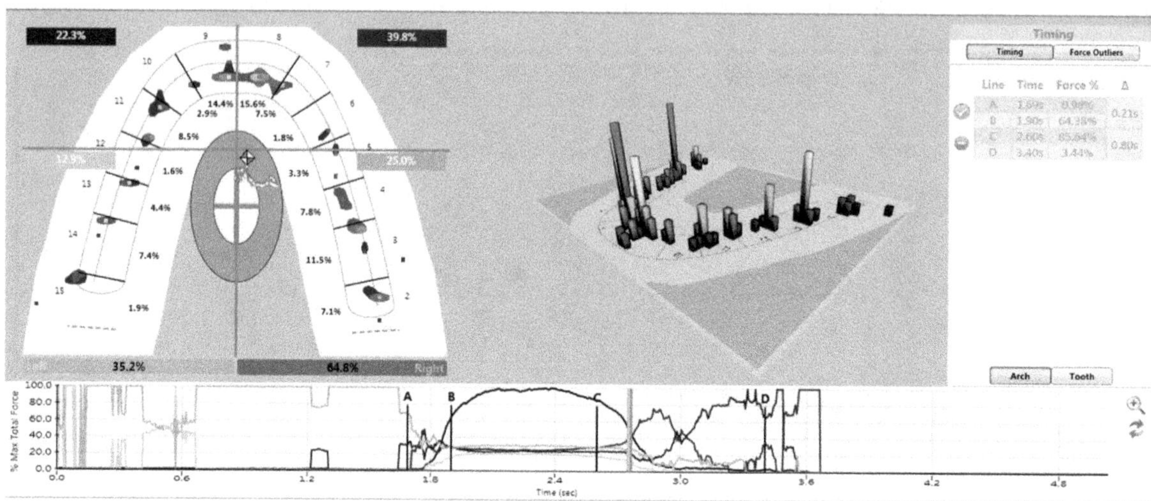

Figure 17b. T-Scan ForceView in the middle of the protrusive excursion, prior to any T-Scan guided adjustments. At 0.5 seconds after the C point, there is virtually no posterior tooth contact present, but the central incisors have unbalanced contacts with tooth #8 demonstrating 46.2% of the total force, compare to tooth #9 demonstrating 36.1% of the total force.

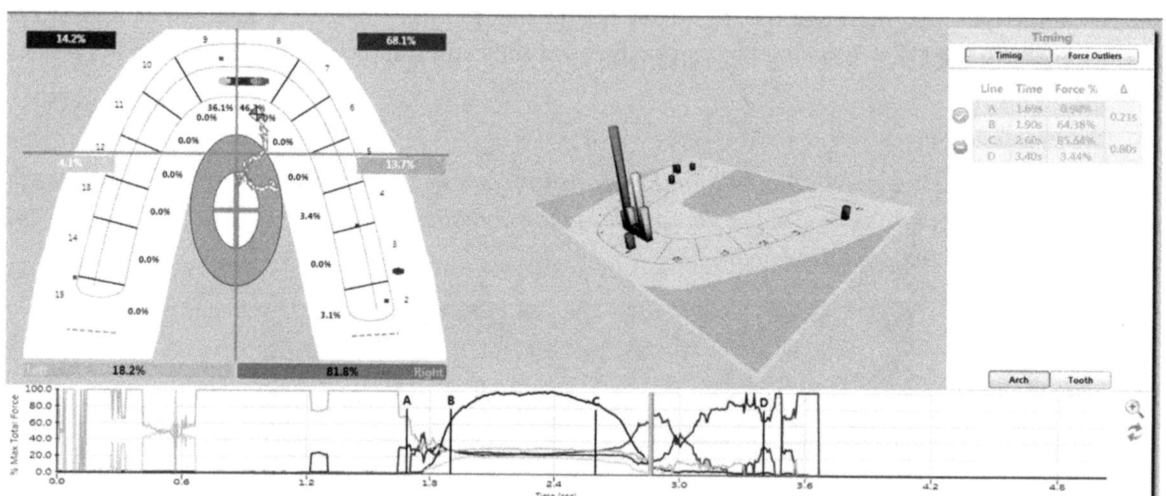

To illustrate a variation of an OS anterior guidance design, the OS was converted into a Michigan splint by grinding away the protrusive contacts on the incisors, and placing all protrusive contact on the on the long rooted canines, while the incisors and canines arc of closure contacts were preserved. Since the protrusive tracks on the canine commence more posteriorly than when the protrusive guidance is present on the central incisor, this design reduces the anterior bulk of the OS for the patient who has a

Figure 17c. T-Scan ForceView at the end of the protrusive excursion, prior to any T-Scan guided adjustments. The protrusive contact remains unbalanced with tooth #9 at 86.9% of the total force, but tooth #8 at 0% of the total force.

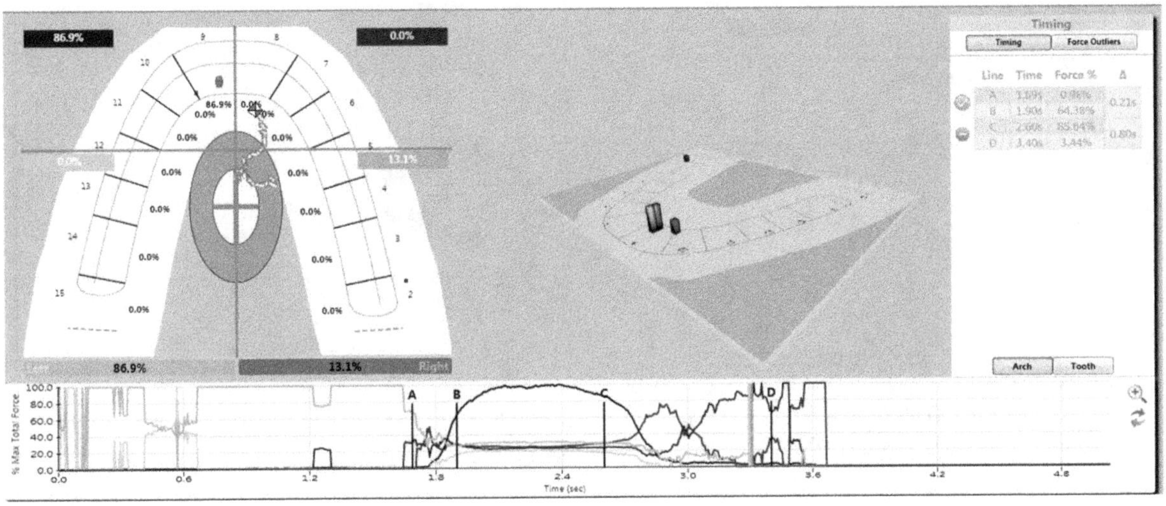

Figure 18a. T-Scan ForceView of the protrusive excursion just after the B-C clenching plateau, following a T-Scan guided adjustment. At 0.2 seconds after the C point, there is virtually no posterior tooth contact present. There is faster posterior tooth disclusion than was seen in Figure 17a.

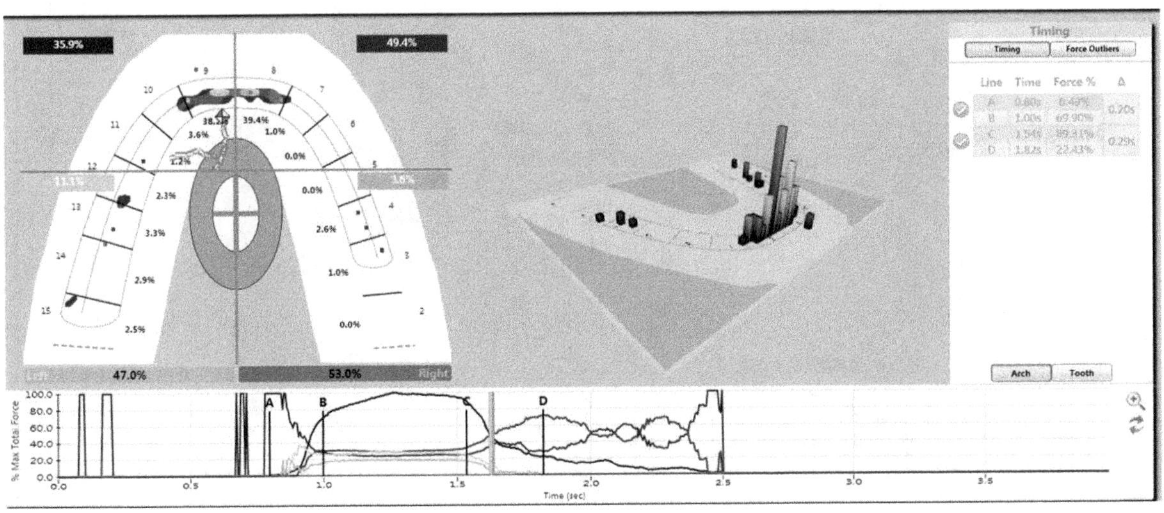

short protrusive range of motion, and provides for a longer excursive track when the patient has a long protrusive range of motion (Figure 19).

The same T-Scan guided adjustment procedure was used to refine the OS after optimal ink ribbon markings were achieved. The change from central incisor protrusive contact to canine protrusive guidance is shown with photographs and T-Scan ForceViews in (Figures 4, 18, 19, and 20a - c).

Figure 18b. T-Scan ForceView in the middle of the protrusive excursion, after a T-Scan guided adjustment. Posterior tooth disclusion is evident with fairly even protrusive guidance forces present on teeth #8 (46.0%) and #9 (41.6%).

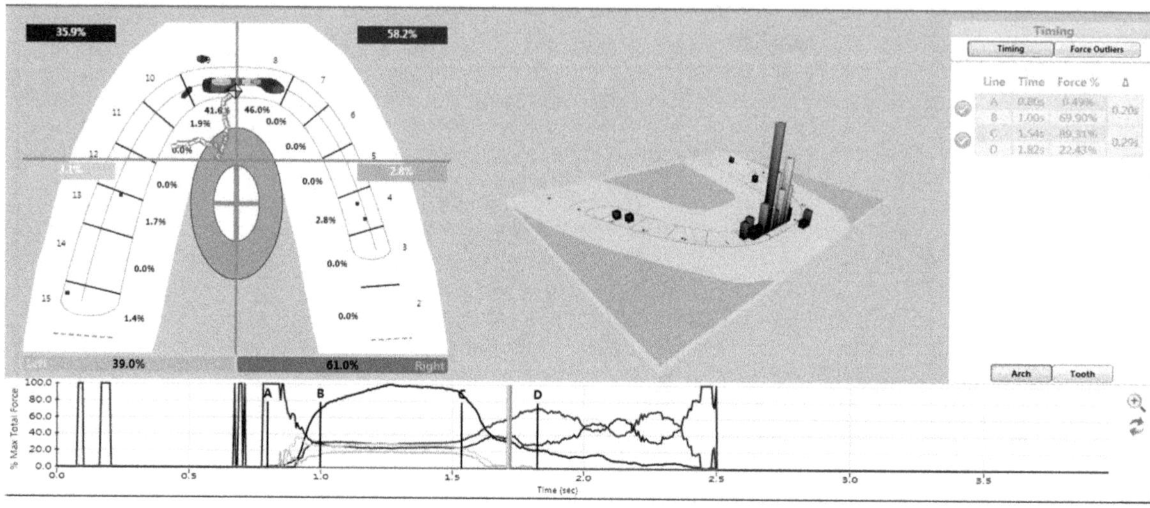

Figure 18c. T-Scan ForceView at the end of the protrusive excursion following a T-Scan guided adjustment. The total force is much more balanced throughout the entire excursion compared to Figure 17c, but ends with tooth #8 at 59.9% of the total force, and tooth #9 at 33.7% of the total force.

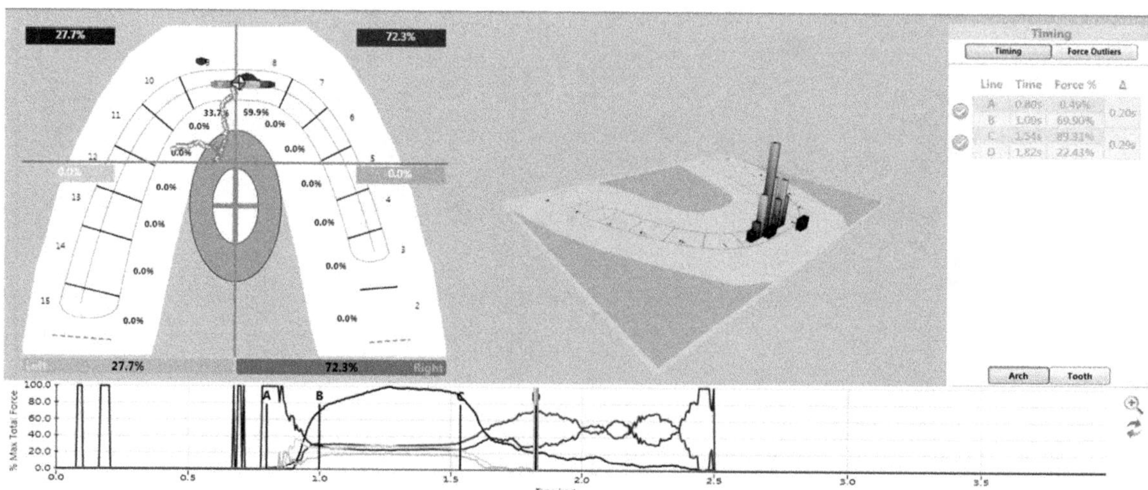

Figure 19. The protrusive anterior guidance has been changed from central incisor contact to canine contact, while the arc of closure contacts on the incisors and canines have been preserved. The canine protrusive track starts more posterior than did the central incisor track. This reduces the OS anterior bulk when the patient has a short protrusive range of motion. When patients have a long protrusive range the longer canine track maintains disclusion of the posterior teeth.

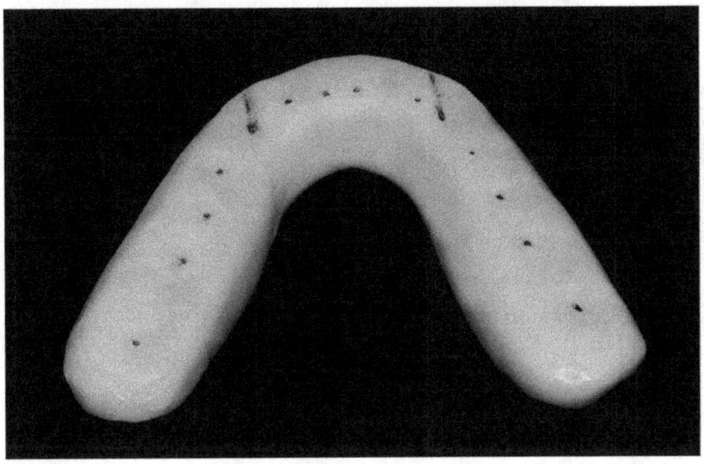

Figure 20a. T-Scan ForceView of the protrusive excursion just after the B-C clenching plateau, following a T-Scan guided adjustment. During the early excursion, there are posterior tooth contacts present, and highly unbalanced anterior quadrants (left anterior = 50.2% of the total force; the right anterior quadrant =24.6% of the total force)

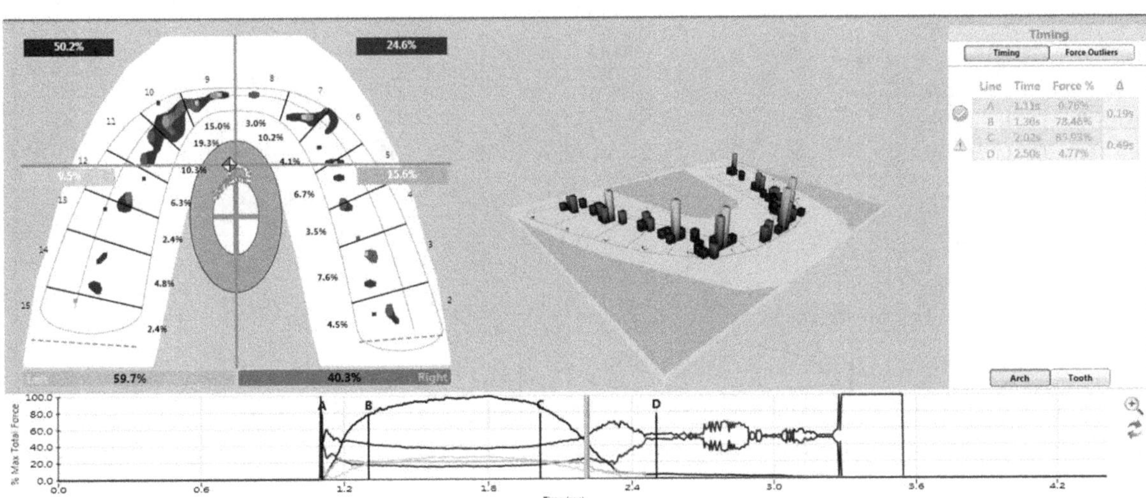

Figure 20b. T-Scan ForceView in the middle of the protrusive excursion, after a T-Scan guided adjustment. At 0.581 seconds past the C point, the lower canine contacts on the occlusal splint are balanced, with tooth #22 = 35.2%, and tooth #27 = 28.0% of the total force. There is minimal posterior tooth contact present

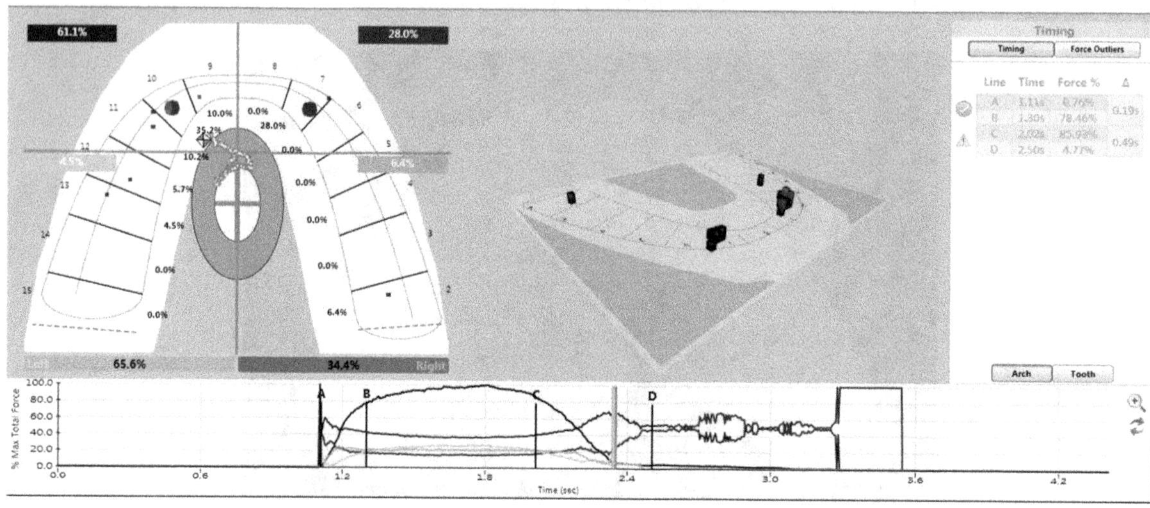

Figure 20c. T-Scan ForceView at the end of the protrusive excursion, after a T-Scan guided adjustment. There are no posterior tooth contacts present, and the canine contact is balanced with #22 = 52.7%, and #27 = 47.3% of total force

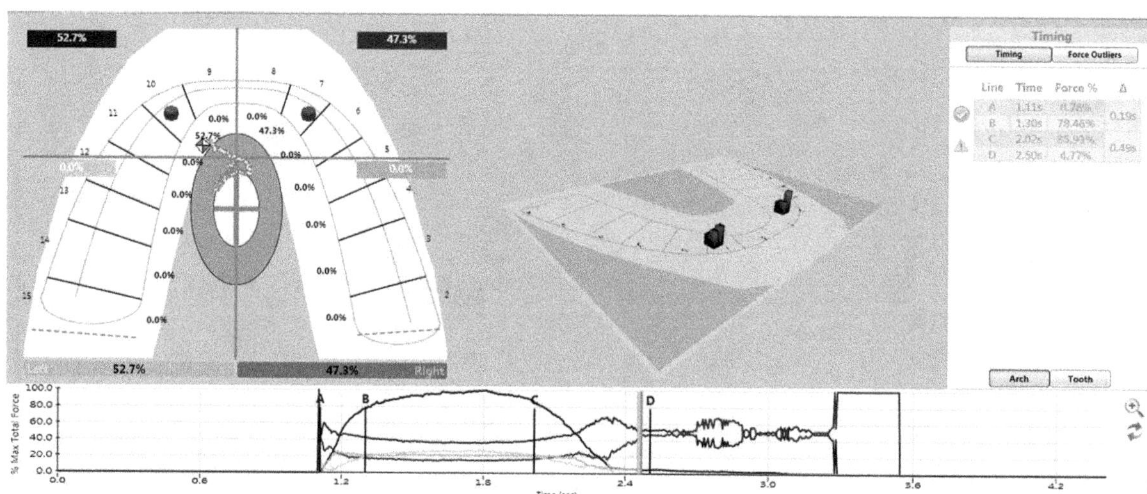

PATIENT RESPONSE TO T-SCAN IN CLINICAL PRACTICE

The T-Scan gives the patient an immediate visual understanding of the diagnosis of occlusal problems by graphically displaying their initial unbalanced force distribution. This is clinically apparent with patients who have had recent restorative procedures, and have not been comfortable after they have undergone multiple occlusal adjustments performed solely with ink ribbon markings.

Patients with an existing OS that has a poor occlusal force distribution, may not have complied with the treatment protocol, and may request that a different type of treatment be rendered. The T-Scan objectively shows these patients where the occlusal contacts are problematic. This co-diagnosis process then begins on a factual basis, with a discussion of the patient's specific problems and their appropriate solutions. Patients often make a strong connection with what they are feeling in their occlusion, and what they clearly see on the computer display. During OS refinement, patients can correlate the sensory changes they are experiencing with the visualized occlusal changes. Involving patients in the details of their care creates an appreciation for what is required of the clinician to achieve excellence in dentistry that is not possible for them to understand when the patient passively receives a procedure.

The T-Scan provides data for both the clinician and the patient. It gives the clinician a scientific basis for assessing occlusal problems, and for determining that the treatment goals have actually been achieved. The T-Scan documents the patient's initial status, and demonstrates when an unbiased, measurable occlusal endpoint of treatment has been achieved. This technology replaces patient feedback from controlling the procedure.

When asked for their occlusal feel input, patients may be unsure of their response, being concerned that their comments may compromise the treatment results. The patient may psychologically question whether the clinician is competent, when they are repetitively asked as to how they "feel". A patient who seeks to control procedures may insist on continual appointments based on their subjective feel or sense. The objectivity of the T-Scan gives the clinician a rational basis for making measured treatment decisions. Patient feedback should be solicited only after all occlusal details have been refined by T-Scan guided adjustments. Both the clinician and patient should be able to observe the change in the quality of occlusion that T-Scan guided treatment achieved, compared to the occlusal end result achieved with ink ribbon marking and patient subjective feel feedback.

POST-OPERATIVE APPOINTMENTS AND MAINTENANCE OF AN OPTIMUM OCCLUSION

Post-operative care should occur 24 hours following OS delivery, if possible. This permits the timely adjustments of any areas that are too tight on teeth, and too sharp on the OS edges that can bother the tongue. Premature contacts on the occlusal surface can also be refined. The delivery of an excellent quality OS that is comfortable to the soft tissues and fulfills all the requirements for an optimal occlusion, tends to minimize the number of post-insertion refinement appointments required. Time invested at the delivery appointment makes it easier for the patient to comply with consistent use of the OS, which remains a bulky foreign object. It is this author's experience that the vast majority of patients can successfully comply with the regimen of OS therapy, when an optimal occlusion and proper fit are both provided.

The post-operative schedule is determined by the patient's structural and symptomatic status. Patients who present with healthy TMJs, little muscle pain, stable teeth, and no problems visible in the associated structures, may need only a single post-insertion appointment. Patients with deteriorating condyles, significant masticatory muscle pain, mobile teeth, and symptoms in the ears or neck, may require a series of refinement appointments.

Teeth in traumatic occlusion respond with increased mobility, as the PDL widens. An OS with optimal occlusion decreases trauma to these teeth, and results in their repositioning within the alveolus. This tooth position change requires that the OS be inspected for minor occlusal changes, which are then adjusted to restore an optimal occlusal contact pattern. OS therapy induces muscle comfort, coordination, and relaxation, as masticatory muscle hyperactivity caused by pre-existing occlusal interferences, is reduced.

Patients often comment that their occlusion feels even and comfortable when wearing the OS, but when it is removed and the patient closes into their natural teeth, the interferences seen on the mounted diagnostic casts are consistently noticeable. This often leads patients to seek out definitive treatment with occlusal adjustment or restoration of their teeth, to match the comfort of their OS.

SOLUTIONS AND RECOMMENDATIONS

Temporomandibular Disorders (TMD) is a non-specific term that refers to pain in the TMJ area or masticatory muscles, limited range of mandibular motion, and the presence of TMJ sounds. Muscle tissue is the most common source of this non-dental orofacial pain (Manfredini, Guarda-Nardini, Winocur, Picotti, Ahlberg, & Lobbezoo, 2012). Acute and chronic myogenous orofacial pain is a commonly reported, significant patient problem. Many myogenous orofacial pains do not follow a natural course of remission, prompting patients to seek medical or dental evaluation.

There is extensive research correlating occlusal problems with pain and dysfunction in the masticatory muscles, and its resolution with occlusal correction. There are also contradictory studies that cannot confirm an occlusal basis for TMD symptomotology. An explanation for this controversy is that studies which show an "absence of evidence" instead of an "evidence of absence", have been unable to form sound conclusions on the relationship between tooth contact time and force aberrations and masticatory muscle problems. In order to scientifically prove that occlusion is not related to myogenous TMD symptoms, both the occlusion prior to treatment, and the altered, therapeutic occlusion must be measured and specified for each subject studied. None of these contrarian studies have provided pre- and post-treatment documentation of the actual occlusal contact time and force status of the occlusion, to plausibly deny a relationship exists between occlusal problems and TMD symptomotology (Kidder & Solow, 2014).

T-Scan documentation is essential for TMD treatment research to have scientific validity. It is a practical device that can be used in any setting, and reports immediate functional occlusal data that specifies the existence of an occlusal problem, while being able to verify the quality of the therapeutic occlusion being tested. A measured change in the occlusal scheme must be quantified before any conclusions can be drawn on the treatment effects resultant from that change.

The T-Scan provides unbiased data and avoids the assumption that an OS is clinically acceptable. This author's experience in 36 years of private practice is that it is rare for a patient to present with an OS that fulfills all the requirements of a therapeutic occlusion. This has been true for OSs fabricated in private practice, and university orofacial pain clinic settings. Scientific studies cannot presume that an OS automatically delivers a therapeutic occlusion, that the occlusion itself is not a test variable, and that without measuring and documenting the occlusal contacts on the OS, the studied OS design cannot be truly optimized.

Clinicians in both daily practice and research settings are the only health care professionals trained to evaluate and treat myogenous orofacial pain that is related to the occlusion. Clinicians are responsible for assessing the structural components of each patient's pain and problem set, and should not make the non-scientific presumption that the occlusion is unrelated to TMD symptoms. No studies have shown an advantage to deleterious forces from occlusal interferences. Although some patients may not have signs or symptoms from an occlusal problem, many patients cannot avoid the effect of traumatic occlusal contact, and would benefit from some form of dental treatment. It is important for restorative clinicians, periodontists, orthodontists, and oral surgeons to have a thorough understanding of how occlusion affects the myogenous orofacial pain and TMD problem set, in order to provide optimal care for their patients.

T-SCAN AND FUTURE DENTAL RESEARCH

Future research should test whether OS therapy yields an equivalent result to the predictable resolution of myogenous orofacial pain that has been seen with precise occlusal adjustment, when diagnosis and treatment are specified by an objective and measured occlusal analysis. Specifically, research should evaluate the effect of OS posterior tooth Disclusion Time on the therapeutic result, and test if the criteria of 0.4 seconds Disclusion Time of natural teeth is appropriate to employ in OS occlusal design. The T-Scan technology provides the real-time data for researchers to know the actual occlusion tested, and the result of the actual treatment provided. This essential data would set a new standard for the validity of OS therapy performed in TMD studies.

Measurement of the timing and force contained within adverse occlusal contacts that commonly cause myogenous orofacial pain, would allow OS therapy research to specify and evaluate differing TMD subject groups. Groups with and without a contact-defined occlusal problem, could be tested for the effects of a measured occlusal change, instead of relying on a non-specific qualifier such as pain, to assess treatment success. The effect of a specific alteration to the occlusal contact time, location, and force with an OS could then be measured, and valid conclusions determined. It is not possible to draw a scientific conclusion on the relationship of occlusion to myogenous orofacial pain when the test group, the control group, and the treatment itself, consist of a spectrum of unknown or problematic occlusions.

Classification of TMD problems centered on masticatory muscle pain, or TMJ disc position, may not be the best approach to organize clinical treatment or research. These structures are seldom directly altered with treatment, rather improvement in comfort and function is related to the indirect effects of physical therapy, pharmacology, and occlusal therapy via an OS, occlusal adjustments, comprehensive restoration, or orthodontics. Reclassifying TMD problems as to a quantified occlusal problem, with subsets defined by muscle pain or TMJ disc position, would facilitate both treatment and research. The dental occlusion and its force on the periodontium can be precisely evaluated and altered. Since the dental occlusion and PDL is an exquisitely sensitive interface, that is highly responsive to adverse forces that affect masticatory muscle, mandibular position, and condyle/TMJ disc integrity, classifying the clinical problem types with measured occlusal parameters is a logical starting point.

A first order of classification may be the extent of present arc of closure interferences, and excursive interferences, which could include the duration of applied force, the intensity of force at individual contacts, and the overall occlusal imbalance between the arch halves. Complete, partial, or the lack of resolution of muscle pain and incoordination from occlusal corrections made with an OS, might be a second level of classification. Combining the information, may give the clinician and researcher the ability to diagnosis the underlying structural occlusion component that is responsible for a complex expression of pain and dysfunction throughout the orofacial system.

An example of classifying TMD problems as previously described is:

- A patient who experienced complete resolution of chronic masticatory muscle pain by OS therapy which was installed with a confirmed (measured) therapeutic occlusion, who without the OS in place demonstrated 30% of their total force was concentrated on an arc of closure interference, and presented with right excursive prolonged posterior Disclusion Time of 1.75 seconds, might be classified as a Myogenous Orofacial Pain of Primary Dental Occlusion Origin.

Another classification might be to connect the physical, structural component of an orofacial pain problem and the patient's psychological or emotional status. The same arc of closure and posterior tooth Disclusion Time problems may affect various patients quite differently. Quantifying the initial occlusal problem may allow clinicians to assess if the problem best treated by structural occlusal correction, or a non-dental approach. Previous research has not developed a classification that correlates a quantified occlusal status combined with a psychological status.

Research on the degree of occlusal refinement needed for therapeutic success in different problem populations could yield data on the probabilities of treatment success with different occlusal correction techniques. For example, if an OS could consistently provide relief from myogenous orofacial pain by the correction of a specified arc of closure interference with a specified level of even and simultaneous occlusal contact, then patients with a similar problem could expect to be treated successfully.

Establishing defined and measured occlusal contact goals for effective treatment with OS therapy would give clinicians and researchers a way to confirm that appropriate treatment was completed. Clinicians would benefit from knowing the level of occlusal accuracy needed for optimal treatment. Specific occlusal contact timing and force distribution criteria could provide guidelines for clinical treatment in orthodontics, restorative dentistry, and occlusal correction for orofacial pain.

CONCLUSION

Occlusal Splint therapy has an important role in comprehensive dental care, as both a diagnostic and therapeutic modality for occlusal problems. An OS provides protection from attrition while assessing the effect of an occlusal correction in a reversible manner. Resolution of myogenous pain with OS therapy can preview the effect of a definitive occlusal correction obtained with equilibration, restoration, or orthodontics. This confirmation of the diagnosis can be essential, before committing to the time, effort, and expense of definitive care. OS therapy gives the patient a physical learning experience on the value of a potential definitive occlusal correction. The OS provides stability in the occlusion so that staged, definitive treatment can be done in the future, without allowing the occlusal function to continually damage the dentition, or perpetuate ongoing pain in the masticatory muscles.

The T-Scan is essential for excellence in OS therapy. It displays accurate, objective data, of the timing and force of tooth contacts during mandibular closure and excursions. This objectivity replaces the reliance on subjective patient feel feedback, or inaccurate ink ribbon markings. The T-Scan can confirm that the OS gives the patient a therapeutic occlusion, instead of a new malocclusion. It can document the nature of the initial occlusal problem, and ensure that all the requirements of a proper OS occlusal design are met. It is the only known way to assess whether the timing of the posterior disclusion by the anterior guidance occurs in an optimal time frame. An important advantage of utilizing the T-Scan in occlusal analysis is that the patient can visualize and understand the problems present within their occlusion, and observe the change on the perfected OS. Patient involvement in their own care is directly related to their appreciation of the clinician's efforts to achieve excellence with the OS therapy.

The T-Scan has important applications to dental research that involves occlusion and TMD symptomotology. The most critical element of performing occlusal therapies with an OS, occlusal adjustment, comprehensive restoration, or orthodontics, is that the therapeutic occlusion delivered to the patient be optimal. Studies that deny a relationship between occlusion and masticatory muscle problems have not documented the force and timing of the occlusal contacts for the initial and test occlusions. These studies lack a scientific basis to conclude that occlusion and masticatory muscle symptoms are unrelated. The T-Scan technology can provide the data that documents occlusal contact timing and force distribution so that future research on TMD patients can compare a documented, precise occlusal correction obtained with OS therapy to the predictable results frequently reported with T-Scan guided occlusal adjustments.

REFERENCES

Academy of Prosthodontics. (2005). The glossary of prosthodontic terms. *The Journal of Prosthetic Dentistry*, *94*, 1–92. PMID:16080238

Al Quran, F. A. M., & Lyons, M. F. (1999). The immediate effect of hard and soft splints on the EMG activity of the masseter and temporalis muscles. *Journal of Oral Rehabilitation*, *26*(7), 559–563. doi:10.1046/j.1365-2842.1999.00421.x PMID:10445474

Barker, D. (2004). Occlusal interferences and temporomandibular dysfunction. *General Dentistry*, *52*, 56–61. PMID:15055673

Beard, C. C., & Clayton, J. A. (1980). Effects of occlusal splint therapy on TMJ dysfunction. *The Journal of Prosthetic Dentistry*, *44*(3), 324–335. doi:10.1016/0022-3913(80)90021-9 PMID:6931225

Becker, I., Tarantola, G., Zambrano, J., Spitzer, S., & Oquendo, D. (1999). Effect of a prefabricated anterior bite stop on electromyographic activity of masticatory muscles. *The Journal of Prosthetic Dentistry*, *82*(1), 22–26. doi:10.1016/S0022-3913(99)70127-7 PMID:10384163

Belser, U. C., & Hannam, A. G. (1985). The influence of altered working-side occlusal guidance on masticatory muscles and related jaw movement. *The Journal of Prosthetic Dentistry*, *53*(3), 406–413. doi:10.1016/0022-3913(85)90523-2 PMID:3857338

Bender, S. (2012). Sleep bruxism: A topical review. *The Journal of the Greater Houston Dental Society*, *83*(5), 10–14.

Boero, R. (1989). The physiology of splint therapy: A literature review. *The Angle Orthodontist*, *59*, 165–180. PMID:2672904

Carlsson, G. E., Ingervall, B., & Kocak, G. (1979). Effect of increasing vertical dimension on the masticatory system in subjects with natural teeth. *The Journal of Prosthetic Dentistry*, *41*(3), 284–289. doi:10.1016/0022-3913(79)90008-8 PMID:283228

Carraro, J. J., & Caffesse, R. G. (1978). Effect of occlusal splints on TMJ symptomatology. *The Journal of Prosthetic Dentistry*, *40*(5), 563–566. doi:10.1016/0022-3913(78)90094-X PMID:281508

Chen, C. W., Boulton, J. L., & Gage, J. P. (1995). Effects of splint therapy in TMJ dysfunction: A study using magnetic resonance imaging. *Australian Dental Journal*, *40*(2), 71–78. doi:10.1111/j.1834-7819.1995.tb03119.x PMID:7786233

Clark, G. T. (1984a). A critical evaluation of orthopedic interocclusal appliance therapy: Design, theory, and overall effectiveness. *The Journal of the American Dental Association*, *108*, 359–364. PMID:6371096

Clark, G. T. (1984b). A critical evaluation of orthopedic interocclusal appliance therapy: Effectiveness for specific symptoms. *The Journal of the American Dental Association*, *108*, 364–368. PMID:6371097

Clark, G. T., Beemsterboer, P. L., Solberg, W. K., & Rugh, J. D. (1979). Nocturnal electromyographic evaluation of myofascial pain dysfunction in patients undergoing occlusal splint therapy. *The Journal of the American Dental Association*, *99*(10), 607–611. PMID:292717

Clark, G. T., Tsukiyama, Y., Baba, K., & Watanabe, T. (1999). Sixty-eight years of occlusal interference studies: What have we learned? *The Journal of Prosthetic Dentistry*, *82*(6), 704–713. doi:10.1016/S0022-3913(99)70012-0 PMID:10588807

Coffey, J. P., Williams, W. N., Turner, G. E., Mahan, P. E., Lapointe, L. L., & Cornell, C. E. (1989). Human bite force discrimination using specific maxillary and mandibular teeth. *Journal of Oral Rehabilitation*, *16*(6), 529–536. doi:10.1111/j.1365-2842.1989.tb01374.x PMID:2600710

Colquitt, T. (1987). The sleep wear syndrome. *The Journal of Prosthetic Dentistry*, *57*(1), 33–41. doi:10.1016/0022-3913(87)90113-2 PMID:3468248

Conti, P. C. R., Santos, C. N., Kogawa, E. M., de Castro Ferreira Conti, A. C., & de Araujo Cdos, R. (2006). The treatment of painful temporomandibular joint clicking with oral splints. *The Journal of the American Dental Association*, *137*(8), 1008–1014. doi:10.14219/jada.archive.2006.0349 PMID:16873326

Crispin, B. J., Myers, G. E., & Clayton, J. A. (1978). Effects of occlusal therapy on pantographic reproducibility of mandibular border movements. *The Journal of Prosthetic Dentistry*, *40*(1), 29–34. doi:10.1016/0022-3913(78)90154-3 PMID:355624

Danesh, G., Lippold, C., Mischke, K. L., Varzideh, B., Reinhart, K. J., Dammaschke, T., & Schafer, E. (2006). Polymerization characteristics of light- and auto-curing resins for individual splints. *Dental Materials*, *22*(5), 426–433. doi:10.1016/j.dental.2005.04.032 PMID:16045980

Dao, T. T. T., Lavigne, G. C., Charbonneau, A., Feine, J. S., & Lund, J. P. (1994). The efficacy of oral splints in the treatment of myofascial pain of the jaw muscles: A controlled clinical trial. *Pain*, *56*(1), 85–94. doi:10.1016/0304-3959(94)90153-8 PMID:8159444

Dao, T. T. T., & Lavigne, G. J. (1998). Oral splints: The crutches for temporomandibular disorders and bruxism? *Critical Reviews in Oral Biology and Medicine*, *9*(3), 345–361. doi:10.1177/10454411980090030701 PMID:9715371

Dawson, P. E. (1973). Temporomandibular joint pain-dysfunction problems can be solved. *The Journal of Prosthetic Dentistry*, *29*(1), 100–112. doi:10.1016/0022-3913(73)90148-0 PMID:4508618

Dawson, P. E. (1983). Determining the determinants of occlusion. *The International Journal of Periodontics & Restorative Dentistry*, *3*, 8–21. PMID:6584415

Dawson, P. E. (1989). *Evaluation, Diagnosis, and Treatment of Occlusal Problems* (pp. 4, 41–46, 282). St. Louis, MO: CV Mosby.

Dorland's Illustrated Medical Dictionary. (1974). Philadelphia, PA: W.B. Saunders Company.

Dube, C., Rompre, P. H., Manzini, C., Guitard, F., de Grandmont, P., & Lavigne, G. J. (2004). Quantitative polygraphic controlled study on efficacy and safety of oral splint devices in toothgrinding subjects. *Journal of Dental Research*, *83*(5), 398–403. doi:10.1177/154405910408300509 PMID:15111632

Ekberg, E. C., Vallon, D., & Nilner, M. (2003). The efficacy of appliance therapy in patients with temporomandibular disorders mainly of myogenous origin. A randomized, controlled, short-term trial. *Journal of Orofacial Pain*, *17*, 133–139. PMID:12836501

Emshoff, R., & Bertram, S. (1998). The short-term effect of stabilization-type splints on local cross-sectional dimensions of muscles of the head and neck. *The Journal of Prosthetic Dentistry*, *80*(4), 457–461. doi:10.1016/S0022-3913(98)70011-3 PMID:9791793

Ferrario, V. F., Sforza, C., Tartaglia, G. M., & Dellavia, C. (2002). Immediate effect of a stabilization splint on masticatory muscle activity in temporomandibular disorder patients. *Journal of Oral Rehabilitation*, *29*(9), 810–815. doi:10.1046/j.1365-2842.2002.00927.x PMID:12366533

Fitins, D., & Sheikholeslam, A. (1993). Effect of canine guidance of maxillary occlusal splint on level of activation of masticatory muscles. *Swedish Dental Journal*, *17*, 235–241. PMID:8134892

Graham, G. S., & Rugh, J. D. (1988). Maxillary splint occlusal guidance patterns and electromyographic activity of the jaw-closing muscles. *The Journal of Prosthetic Dentistry*, *59*(1), 73–77. doi:10.1016/0022-3913(88)90113-8 PMID:3422308

Greene, C. S., & Laskin, D. M. (1972). Splint therapy for the myofascial pain dysfunction (MPD) syndrome: A comparative study. *The Journal of the American Dental Association*, *84*, 624–628. PMID:4500373

Hamada, T., Kotani, H., Kawazoe, Y., & Yamada, S. (1982). Effect of occlusal splints on the electromyographicactivity of masseter and temporalis muscles in bruxism with clinical symptoms. *Journal of Oral Rehabilitation*, *9*, 119–123. doi:10.1111/j.1365-2842.1982.tb00541.x PMID:6951020

Harada, T., Ichiki, R., Tsukiyama, Y., & Koyano, K. (2006). The effect of oral splint devices on sleep bruxism: A 6-week observation with an ambulatory electromyographic recording device. *Journal of Oral Rehabilitation*, *33*(7), 482–488. doi:10.1111/j.1365-2842.2005.01576.x PMID:16774505

Harrel, S. K., & Nunn, M. E. (2001). The effect of occlusal discrepancies on periodontitis. II. Relationship of occlusal treatment to progession of periodontal disease. *Journal of Periodontology*, *72*(4), 495–505. doi:10.1902/jop.2001.72.4.495 PMID:11338302

Harrel, S. K., Nunn, M. E., & Hallmon, W. E. (2006). Is there an association between occlusion and periodontal destruction? *The Journal of the American Dental Association*, *137*(10), 1380–1392. doi:10.14219/jada.archive.2006.0049 PMID:17012716

Hasegawa, K., Okatnoto, M., Nishigawa, G., Oki, K., & Minagi, S. (2007). The design of non-occlusal intraoral appliances on hard palate and their effect on masseter muscle activity during sleep. *The Journal of Cranio-Mandibular Practice*, *25*(1), 8–15. PMID:17304912

Hellsing, G. (1984). Functional adaptation to changes in vertical dimension. *The Journal of Prosthetic Dentistry*, *52*, 867–870. PMID:6595397

Humsi, A. N. K., Naeije, M., Hippe, J. A., & Hansson, T. L. (1989). The immediate effect of a stabilization splint on the muscular symmetry in the masseter and anterior temporal muscles of patients with a craniomandibular disorder. *The Journal of Prosthetic Dentistry*, *62*(3), 339–343. doi:10.1016/0022-3913(89)90346-6 PMID:2810140

Israel, H. A., Diamond, B., Saed-Nejad, F., & Ratcliffe, A. (1999). The relationship between parafunctional masticatory activity and arthroscopically diagnosed temporomandibular joint pathology. *Journal of Oral and Maxillofacial Surgery*, *57*(9), 1034–1039. doi:10.1016/S0278-2391(99)90321-X PMID:10484103

Ito, T., Gibbs, C. H., Marguelles-Bonnet, R., Lupkiewicz, S. M., Young, H. M., Lundeen, H. C., & Mahan, P. E. (1986). Loading on the temporomandibular joints with five occlusal conditions. *The Journal of Prosthetic Dentistry*, *56*(4), 478–484. doi:10.1016/0022-3913(86)90393-8 PMID:3463757

Jimenez, I. (1987). Dental stability and maximal masticatory muscle activity. *Journal of Oral Rehabilitation*, *14*(6), 591–598. doi:10.1111/j.1365-2842.1987.tb00755.x PMID:3481398

Johnsen, S. E., Krister, G., Svensson, K. G., & Trulsson, M. (2007). Forces applied by anterior and posterior teeth and roles of periodontal afferents during hold-and-split tasks in human subjects. *Experimental Brain Research*, *178*(1), 126–134. doi:10.1007/s00221-006-0719-9 PMID:17031682

Kerstein, R. B. (1993). A comparison of traditional occlusal equilibration and immediate complete anterior guidance development. *The Journal of Cranio-Mandibular Practice*, *11*, 126–139. PMID:8495505

Kerstein, R. B. (1994). Disclusion time measurement studies: a comparison of disclusion time between chronic myofascial pain dysfunction patients and nonpatients: a population analysis. *The Journal of Prosthetic Dentistry*, *72*(5), 473–480. doi:10.1016/0022-3913(94)90117-1 PMID:7844746

Kerstein, R. B. (1995). Treatment of myofascial pain dysfunction syndrome with occlusal therapy to reduce lengthy disclusion time- a recall evaluation. *The Journal of Cranio-Mandibular Practice*, *13*, 105–115. PMID:8697496

Kerstein, R. B. (2004). Combining technologies: A computerized occlusal analysis system synchronized with a computerized electromyography system. *The Journal of Cranio-Mandibular Practice*, *22*(2), 96–109. doi:10.1179/crn.2004.013 PMID:15134409

Kerstein, R. B. (2010). Reducing chronic masseter and temporalis muscular hyperactivity with computer-guided occlusal adjustments. *The Compendium of Continuing Education in Dentistry*, *31*, 530–534, 536, 538 passim. PMID:20879206

Kerstein, R. B., Chapman, R., & Klein, M. (1997). A comparison of ICAGD (immediate complete anterior guidance development to mock ICAGD for symptom reductions in chronic myofascial pain dysfunction patients. *The Journal of Cranio-Mandibular Practice*, *15*, 21–37. PMID:9586486

Kerstein, R. B., & Farrell, S. (1990). Treatment of myofascial pain dysfunction syndrome with occlusal equilibration. *The Journal of Prosthetic Dentistry*, *63*(6), 695–700. doi:10.1016/0022-3913(90)90328-A PMID:2102663

Kerstein, R. B., & Radke, J. (2006). The effect of disclusion time reduction on maximal clench muscle activity levels. *The Journal of Cranio-Mandibular Practice*, *24*(3), 156–165. doi:10.1179/crn.2006.026 PMID:16933455

Kerstein, R. B., & Radke, J. (2012). Masseter and temporalis hyperactivity decreased by measured anterior guidance development. *The Journal of Cranio-Mandibular Practice*, *30*, 243–254. PMID:23156965

Kerstein, R. B., & Wright, N. R. (1991). Electromyographic and computer analyses of patients suffering from chronic myofascial pain-dysfunction syndrome: Before and after treatment with immediate complete anterior guidance development. *The Journal of Prosthetic Dentistry*, *66*(5), 677–686. doi:10.1016/0022-3913(91)90453-4 PMID:1805009

Kidder, G. M., & Solow, R. A. (2014). Precision occlusal splints and the diagnosis of occlusal problems in myogenous orofacial pain patients. *General Dentistry*, *62*, 24–31. PMID:24598491

Klasser, G. D., & Greene, C. S. (2009). Oral appliances and the management of temporomandibular disorders. *Oral Surgery, Oral Pathology, Oral Medicine, Oral Radiology. Endodontology*, *107*, 212–223.

Klasser, G. D., Greene, C. S., & Lavigne, G. J. (2010). Oral appliances and the management of sleep bruxism in adults: A century of clinical applications and search for mechanisms. *The International Journal of Prosthodontics*, *23*, 453–462. PMID:20859563

Kotani, H., Abekura, H., & Hamada, T. (1994). Objective evaluation for bite plate therapy in patients with myofascial pain dysfunction syndrome. *Journal of Oral Rehabilitation*, *21*(3), 241–245. doi:10.1111/j.1365-2842.1994.tb01140.x PMID:8057192

Kurita, H., Ikeda, K., & Kurashina, K. (2000). Evaluation of a stabilization splint on occlusal force in patients with masticatory muscle disorders. *Journal of Oral Rehabilitation*, *27*(1), 79–82. doi:10.1046/j.1365-2842.2000.00498.x PMID:10632847

Lavigne, G. J., Khoury, S., Abe, S., Yamaguchi, T., & Raphael, K. (2008). Bruxism physiology and pathology: An overview for clinicians. *Journal of Oral Rehabilitation*, *35*(7), 476–494. doi:10.1111/j.1365-2842.2008.01881.x PMID:18557915

Lindfors, E., Magnusson, T., & Tegelberg, A. (2006). Interocclusal appliances--indications and clinical routines in general dental practice in Sweden. *Swedish Dental Journal*, *30*, 123–134. PMID:17233329

Lundeen, T. F. (1979). Occlusal splint fabrication. *The Journal of Prosthetic Dentistry*, *42*(5), 588–591. doi:10.1016/0022-3913(79)90259-2 PMID:290810

Lytle, J. D. (2001). Occlusal disease revisited: Part II. *The International Journal of Periodontics & Restorative Dentistry*, *21*, 273–279. PMID:11490404

Manfredini, D., Guarda-Nardini, L., Winocur, E., Piccotti, F., Ahlberg, J., & Lobbezoo, F. (2012). Research diagnostic criteria for temporomandibular disorders: A systematic review of axis I epidemiologic findings. *Oral Surgery, Oral Medicine, Oral Pathology, Oral Radiology. Endodontology*, *112*, 453–462.

Manns, A., Chan, C., & Miralles, R. (1987). Influence of group function and, canine guidance on electromyographic activity of elevator muscles. *The Journal of Prosthetic Dentistry*, *57*(4), 494–501. doi:10.1016/0022-3913(87)90024-2 PMID:3471962

Manns, A., Miralles, R., Santander, H., & Valdivia, J. (1983). Influence of the vertical dimension in the treatment of myofascial pain-dysfunction syndrome. *The Journal of Prosthetic Dentistry*, *59*(5), 700–709. doi:10.1016/0022-3913(83)90213-5 PMID:6580439

Manns, A., Miralles, R., Valdivia, J., & Bull, R. (1989). Influence of variation in anteroposterior occlusal contacts on electromyographic activity. *The Journal of Prosthetic Dentistry*, *61*(5), 617–623. doi:10.1016/0022-3913(89)90288-6 PMID:2746532

Manns, A., Rocabado, M., Cadenasso, P., Miralles, R., & Cumsille, M. A. (1993). The immediate effect of the variation of anteroposterior laterotrusive contacts on elevator electromyographic activity. *The Journal of Cranio-Mandibular Practice*, *11*, 184–191.

Mongini, F. (1972). Remodeling of the mandibular condyle in the adult and its relationship to the condition of the dental arches. *Acta Anatomica*, *82*(3), 437–453. doi:10.1159/000143825 PMID:5048605

Mongini, F. (1977). Anatomic and clinical evaluation of the relationship between the temporomandibular joint and occlusion. *The Journal of Prosthetic Dentistry*, *38*(5), 539–551. doi:10.1016/0022-3913(77)90030-0 PMID:269953

Mongini, F. (1980). Condylar remodeling after occlusal therapy. *The Journal of Prosthetic Dentistry*, *43*(5), 568–577. doi:10.1016/0022-3913(80)90333-9 PMID:6928962

Nitzan, D. W. (1994). Intra-articular pressure in the functioning human temporomandibular joint and its alteration by uniform elevation of the occlusal plane. *Journal of Oral and Maxillofacial Surgery*, *52*(7), 671–679. doi:10.1016/0278-2391(94)90476-6 PMID:8006730

Nunn, M. E., & Harrel, S. K.Relationship of Initial Occlusal Discrepancies to Initial Clinical Parameters. (2001). The effect of occlusal discrepancies on periodontitis. I. Relationship of initial occlusal discrepancies to initial clinical parameters. *Journal of Periodontology*, *72*(4), 485–494. doi:10.1902/jop.2001.72.4.485 PMID:11338301

Okeson, J. P. (1987). The effects of hard and soft occlusal splints on nocturnal bruxism. *The Journal of the American Dental Association*, *114*, 788–791. PMID:3475357

Okeson, J. P., Dickson, J. L., & Kemper, J. T. (1982). The influence of assisted mandibular movement on the incidence of nonworking contact. *The Journal of Prosthetic Dentistry*, *4*(2), 174–177. doi:10.1016/0022-3913(82)90108-1 PMID:6955516

Okeson, J. P., Kemper, J. T., & Moody, P. M. (1982). A study of the use of occlusion splints in the treatment of acute and chronic patients with craniomandibular disorders. *The Journal of Prosthetic Dentistry*, *48*(6), 708–712. doi:10.1016/S0022-3913(82)80034-6 PMID:6961210

Pullinger, A. G., & Seligman, D. A. (2000). Quantification and validation of predictive values of occlusal variables in temporomandibular disorders using a multifactorial analysis. *The Journal of Prosthetic Dentistry*, *83*(1), 66–75. doi:10.1016/S0022-3913(00)70090-4 PMID:10633024

Radu, J., Marandici, M., & Hottel, T. L. (2004). The effect of clenching on condylar position: A vector analysis model. *The Journal of Prosthetic Dentistry*, *91*(2), 171–179. doi:10.1016/j.prosdent.2003.10.011 PMID:14970764

Ramfjord, S. P., & Ash, M. M. (1994). Reflections on the Michigan occlusal splint. *Journal of Oral Rehabilitation*, *21*(5), 491–500. doi:10.1111/j.1365-2842.1994.tb01164.x PMID:7996334

Raphael, K. G., Sirois, D. A., Janal, M. N., Wigren, P. E., Dubrovsky, B., & Nemelivsky, L. V. et al. (2012). Sleep bruxism and myofascial temporomandibular disorders: A laboratory-based polysomnographic investigation. *The Journal of the American Dental Association*, *143*(11), 1223–1231. doi:10.14219/jada.archive.2012.0068 PMID:23115152

Ratcliff, S., Becker, I. M., & Quinn, L. (2001). Type and incidence of cracks in posterior teeth. *The Journal of Prosthetic Dentistry*, *86*(2), 168–172. doi:10.1067/mpr.2001.116578 PMID:11514804

Riise, C., & Sheikholeslam, A. (1982). The influence of experimental interfering occlusal contacts on the postural activity of the anterior temporal and masseter muscles in young adults. *Journal of Oral Rehabilitation*, *9*(5), 419–425. doi:10.1111/j.1365-2842.1982.tb01031.x PMID:6957573

Roth, R. H. (1973). Temporomandibular pain-dysfunction and occlusal relationships. *The Angle Orthodontist*, *43*, 136–153. PMID:4511992

Rugh, J. D., Graham, G. S., Smith, J. C., & Ohrbach, R. K. (1989). Effects of canine versus molar occlusal splint guidance on nocturnal bruxism and craniomandibular symptomatology. *Journal of Crandiomandibular Disorders: Facial and Oral Pain*, *3*, 203–210. PMID:2639157

Schames, S. E., Schames, J., Schames, M., & Chagall-Gungur, S. S. (2012). Sleep bruxism, an autonomic, self-regulating response by triggering the trigeminal cardiac reflex. *Journal of the California Dental Association*, *40*(8), 670–676. PMID:22953526

Scopel, V., Costa, G., & Urias, D. (2005). An electromyographic study of masseter and anterior temporalis muscles in extra-articular myogenous TMJ pain patients compared to an asymptomatic normal population. *The Journal of Cranio-Mandibular Practice*, *23*, 194–203. PMID:16128354

Sheikoleslam, A., Holmgren, K., & Riise, C. (1986). A clinical and electromyographic study of the long-term effects of an occlusal splint on the temporal and masseter muscles in patients with functional disorders and nocturnal bruxism. *Journal of Oral Rehabilitation*, *13*(2), 137–145. doi:10.1111/j.1365-2842.1986.tb00646.x PMID:3457133

Shupe, R. J., Mohamed, S. E., Christensen, L. V., Finger, I. M., & Weinberg, R. (1984). Effects of occlusal guidance on jaw muscle activity. *The Journal of Prosthetic Dentistry*, *51*(6), 811–818. doi:10.1016/0022-3913(84)90382-2 PMID:6588202

Siebert, G., & Siebert, G. (1981). Recent results concerning physiological tooth movement and anterior guidance. *Journal of Oral Rehabilitation*, *8*(6), 479–493. doi:10.1111/j.1365-2842.1981.tb00523.x PMID:6947080

Simmons, J. H. (2012). Neurology of sleep and sleep-related breathing disorders and their relationships to sleep bruxism. *Journal of the California Dental Association*, *40*(2), 159–167. PMID:22416635

Solberg, W. K., Clark, J. T., & Rugh, J. D. (1975). Nocturnal electromyographicevaluation of bruxism patients undergoing short-term splint therapy. *Journal of Oral Rehabilitation*, *2*(3), 215–223. doi:10.1111/j.1365-2842.1975.tb00915.x PMID:1056979

Solow, R. A. (1999). The anterior acrylic resin platform and centric relation verification: A clinical report. *The Journal of Prosthetic Dentistry*, *81*(3), 255–257. doi:10.1016/S0022-3913(99)70265-9 PMID:10050110

Solow, R. A. (2005). Equilibration of a progressive anterior open occlusal relationship: A clinical report. *The Journal of Cranio-Mandibular Practice*, *23*, 229–238. PMID:16128358

Solow, R. A. (2010). Diagnosis, equilibration, and restoration of an orthodontic failure. *General Dentistry*, *58*(5), 444–453. PMID:20829170

Solow, R. A. (2011). Occlusal bite splint therapy. In I. M. Becker (Ed.), *Comprehensive occlusal concepts in clinical practice* (pp. 169–214). Hoboken, NJ: Wiley-Blackwell.

Solow, R. A. (2013). Mounted diagnostic casts: The entry into comprehensive care. *General Dentistry*, *61*(5), 12–15. PMID:23928429

Solow, R. A. (2013). Customized anterior guidance for occlusal devices. *The Journal of Prosthetic Dentistry*, *110*(4), 259–263. doi:10.1016/S0022-3913(13)60373-X PMID:24079560

Spear, F. M. (2002). Occlusion in the new millennium: The controversy continues. *Signature (Ramsey, N.J.)*, *7*(2), 18–21.

Truelove, E., Huggins, K. H., Mancl, L., & Dworkin, S. F. (2006). The efficacy of traditional, low-cost and nonsplint therapies for temporomandibular disorder: A randomized controlled trial. *The Journal of the American Dental Association*, *137*(8), 1099–1107. doi:10.14219/jada.archive.2006.0348 PMID:16873325

Tsuga, K., Akagawa, Y., Sakaguchi, R., & Tsuru, H. (1989). A short-term evaluation of the effectiveness of stabilization-type occlusal splint therapy for specific symptoms of temporomandibular joint dysfunction syndrome. *The Journal of Prosthetic Dentistry*, *61*(5), 610–613. doi:10.1016/0022-3913(89)90286-2 PMID:2746530

Wang, C., & Yin, X. (2012). Occlusal risk factors associated with temporomandibular disorders in young adults with normal occlusions. *Oral Surgery, Oral Medicine, Oral Pathology, Oral Radiology, and Endodontics*, *114*(10), 419–423. doi:10.1016/j.oooo.2011.10.039 PMID:22841427

Williamson, E. H., & Lundquist, D. O. (1983). Anterior guidance: Its effect on electromyographic activity of the temporal and masseter muscles. *The Journal of Prosthetic Dentistry*, *49*(6), 816–823. doi:10.1016/0022-3913(83)90356-6 PMID:6576136

Wiskott, H. W. A., & Belser, U. C. (1995). A rationale for simplified occlusal design in restorative dentistry: Historical review and clinical guidelines. *The Journal of Prosthetic Dentistry*, *73*(2), 69–83. doi:10.1016/S0022-3913(05)80159-3 PMID:7722934

ADDITIONAL READING

Alanen, P., & Kirveskari, P. (1990). Disorders in TMJ research. *Journal of Craniomandibular Disorders. Facial and Oral Pain*, *4*, 223–227.

Anderson, G. C., Schulte, J. K., & Goodkind, R. J. (1985). Comparative study of two treatment methods for internal derangement of the temporomandibular joint. *The Journal of Prosthetic Dentistry*, *53*(3), 392–397. doi:10.1016/0022-3913(85)90520-7 PMID:3857335

Becker, I. M. (Ed.). (2012). *Comprehensive occlusal concepts in clinical practice*. Hoboken, NJ: Wiley-Blackwell.

Chen, C. W., Boulton, J. L., & Gage, J. P. (1995). Effect of splint therapy in TMJ dysfunction: A study using magnetic resonance imaging. *Australian Dental Journal*, *40*(2), 71–78. doi:10.1111/j.1834-7819.1995.tb03119.x PMID:7786233

Clark, G. T., Beemsterboer, P. L., Solberg, W. K., & Rugh, J. D. (1979). Nocturnal electromyographic evaluation of myofascial pain dysfunction in patients undergoingsplint therapy. *The Journal of the American Dental Association*, *99*, 607–611. PMID:292717

Crawford, S. D. (1999). Condylar axis position, as determined by the occlusion and measured by the CPI instrument, and signs and symptoms of temporomandibular dysfunction. *The Angle Orthodontist*, *69*, 103–115. PMID:10227550

Dawson, P. E. (1985). Optimum TMJ condyle position in clinical practice. *The International Journal of Periodontics & Restorative Dentistry*, *5*, 10–31. PMID:3862655

Dupont, J. S. Jr, & Brown, C. E. (2006). Occlusal splints from the beginning to the present. *The Journal of Cranio-Mandibular Practice*, *24*(2), 141–145. doi:10.1179/crn.2006.022 PMID:16711277

Kirveskari, P., & Alanen, P. (1991). Scientific evidence of occlusion and craniomandibular disorders. *Journal of Orofacial Pain*, *7*, 235–240. PMID:9116622

Kirveskari, P., Alanen, P., & Jamsa, T. (1989). Association between craniomandibular disorders and occlusal interferences. *The Journal of Prosthetic Dentistry*, *62*(1), 66–69. doi:10.1016/0022-3913(89)90052-8 PMID:2787399

Kirveskari, P., Jamsa, T., & Alanen, P. (1998). Occlusal adjustment and the incidence of demand for temporomandibular disorder treatment. *The Journal of Prosthetic Dentistry*, *79*(4), 433–438. doi:10.1016/S0022-3913(98)70158-1 PMID:9576319

McNeill, C. (1985). The optimum temporomandibular joint condyle position inclinical practice. *The International Journal of Periodontics & Restorative Dentistry*, *5*, 53–77. PMID:3867653

Moses, A. J. (1994). Scientific methodology in temporomandibular disorders: Part I epidemiology. *The Journal of Cranio-Mandibular Practice*, *12*, 114–119. PMID:8055585

Moses, A. J. (1994). Scientific methodology in temporomandibular disorders: Part III diagnostic reasoning. *The Journal of Cranio-Mandibular Practice*, *12*, 259–265. PMID:7828209

Nitzan, D. W. (2001). The process of lubrication impairment and its involvement in temporomandibular joint disc displacement: A theoretical concept. *Journal of Oral and Maxillofacial Surgery*, *59*(1), 36–45. doi:10.1053/joms.2001.19278 PMID:11152188

Nitzan, D. W., & Marmary, Y. (1997). The "anchored disc phenomenon": A proposed etiology for sudden-onset, severe and persistent closed lock of the temporomandibular joint. *Journal of Oral and Maxillofacial Surgery*, *55*(8), 797–802. doi:10.1016/S0278-2391(97)90335-9 PMID:9251606

Poyser, N. J., Porter, R. W., Briggs, P. F., Chana, H. S., & Kelleher, M. G. (2005). The Dahl Concept: Past, present and future. *British Dental Journal*, *198*(11), 669–676. doi:10.1038/sj.bdj.4812371 PMID:15951771

Ramfjord, S. P., & Ash, M. M. Jr. (1981). Significance of occlusion in the etiology and treatment of early, moderate, and advanced periodontitis. *Journal of Periodontology*, *52*(9), 511–516. doi:10.1902/jop.1981.52.9.511 PMID:6793705

Rehany, A., & Stern, N. (1981). The modified Hawley occlusal splint. *The Journal of Prosthetic Dentistry*, *45*(5), 536–541. doi:10.1016/0022-3913(81)90042-1 PMID:6938684

Sheikoleslam, A., & Riise, C. (1983). Influence of experimental interfering occlusal contacts on the activity of the anterior temporal and masseter muscles during submaximal and maximal bite in the intercuspal position. *Journal of Oral Rehabilitation*, *10*(3), 207–214. doi:10.1111/j.1365-2842.1983.tb00114.x PMID:6575162

Tarantola, G. J., Becker, I. M., & Gremillion, H. (1997). The reproducibility of centric relation: A clinical approach. *The Journal of the American Dental Association*, *128*(9), 1245–1251. doi:10.14219/jada.archive.1997.0401 PMID:9297946

Tarantola, G. J., Becker, I. M., Gremillion, H., & Pink, F. (1998). The effectiveness of equilibration in the improvement of signs and symptoms in the stomatognathic system. *The International Journal of Periodontics & Restorative Dentistry*, *18*, 594–603. PMID:10321174

Vallon, D., & Nilner, M. (1997). A longitudinal follow-up of the effect of occlusal adjustment in patients with craniomandibular disorders. *Swedish Dental Journal*, *21*, 85–91. PMID:9291556

Wang, M. Q., He, J. J., Li, G., & Widmalm, S. E. (2008). The effect of physiological nonbalanced occlusion on the thickness of the temporomandibular joint disc: A pilot autopsy study. *The Journal of Prosthetic Dentistry*, *98*(2), 148–152. doi:10.1016/S0022-3913(08)60031-1 PMID:18262016

Wenneberg, B., Nystrom, T., & Carlsson, G. E. (1988). Occlusal equilibration and other stomatognathic treatment in patients with mandibular dysfunction and headache. *The Journal of Prosthetic Dentistry*, *59*(4), 478–483. doi:10.1016/0022-3913(88)90046-7 PMID:3162993

Yamada, K., Hanada, K., Fukui, T., Satou, Y., Ochi, K., Hayashi, T., & Ito, J. (2001). Condylar bony change and self-reported parafunctional habits in prospective orthognathic surgery patients with temporomandibular disorders. *Oral Surgery, Oral Pathology, Oral Medicine, Oral Radiology, and Endodontics*, *92*(3), 265–271. doi:10.1067/moe.2001.117558 PMID:11552142

KEY TERMS AND DEFINITIONS

Canine Guidance: The contact of maxillary and mandibular canines during a lateral excursion, that separates the posterior teeth.

Centric Relation (CR): The braced position of the mandibular condyle/TMJ disc on the most anterior-superior aspect of the articular eminence. This position allows precise, consistent rotation of the mandibular transverse axis, while allowing for relaxation of the lateral pterygoid muscle.

Computerized Occlusal Analysis: The digital record of the timing and relative occlusal force data of tooth contact during mandibular closure and excursions, obtained with the T-Scan 8 Occlusal Analysis System.

Diagnostic Casts: Three dimensional stone casts mounted on a semi-adjustable articulator, that accurately replicates the relationship of the teeth during mandibular closure and excursions.

Group Function: The contact of several posterior teeth during a lateral excursion.

Maximum Intercuspation (MIP): The position where the most teeth contact during mandibular closure.

Occlusal Interference: A tooth contact that concentrates adverse force on a single tooth and prevents other teeth from participating in an optimal occlusal scheme.

Occlusal Splint (OS): A prosthetic appliance that alters the occlusal surface contacts for diagnosis and treatment of occlusion related problems.

This work was previously published in the Handbook of Research on Computerized Occlusal Analysis Technology Applications in Dental Medicine edited by Robert B. Kerstein, DMD, pages 602-648, copyright year 2015 by Medical Information Science Reference (an imprint of IGI Global).

Chapter 10
Occlusal Considerations in the Hypersensitive Dentition

Nick Yiannios, DDS
Private Practice, USA

ABSTRACT

In the literature, Dentinal Hypersensitivity (DH) is considered to arise from exposed dentin and patent dentinal tubules. However, clinical observation of recurrent DH sensitivity indicates it can occur in the presence or absence of exposed dentin. Quantified occlusal contact force and timing parameters have been ignored in studies assessing hypersensitive teeth. This chapter introduces a novel occlusal concept: Frictional Dental Hypersensitivity (FDH). Clinical evidence from combining computerized occlusal analysis and electromyography is presented linking opposing posterior tooth friction and muscular hyperactivity to Dentin Hypersensitivity. This chapter proffers how occlusion, muscular TMD symptoms, and frictional Dentin Hypersensitivity are all related. Lastly, a Pilot Study is presented that used a Visual Numerical Analog scale to quantify Dentin Hypersensitivity resolution observed in symptomatic patients who underwent the Immediate Complete Anterior Guidance Development (ICAGD) coronoplasty. This computer-guided occlusal adjustment eliminated pretreatment FDH symptomatology, further supporting that Dentinal Hypersensitivity has an occlusally-based, frictional etiology.

INTRODUCTION

Dentinal Hypersensitivity (DH) is classically described in the dental literature as a sharp, acute pain of short duration, arising from *open dentinal tubules in vital teeth*, which is diagnosed through a process of exclusion with a thorough dental screening, examination, and history (Porto, Andrade, & Montes, 2009). DH is generally occurs in the cervical regions of teeth, as in the abfractive lesion, or on the occlusal surface where occlusal microtrauma, erosion, abrasion, or attrition, has exposed dentinal tubules.

This chapter will explore how occlusion is frequently linked to the sharp, short duration acute pain, consistent with the clinical diagnosis of Dentinal Hypersensitivity, which can occur *without* exposed dentinal tubules. The included literature will detail how dental occlusion can be one of the primary causative factors in the development of hypersensitive dentitions, resultant from prolonged frictional

DOI: 10.4018/978-1-5225-1903-4.ch010

interactions between opposing teeth in function, and how the same occlusal surface friction can lead to hyperactive muscles, which may over time, cause abfractive events, exposed dentin, and patent dentinal tubules. The new term of Frictional Dental Hypersensitivity (FDH) will be presented, which describes DH of frictional occlusal etiology, *with or without exposed dentin.* The condition known as Traumatic Occlusion (synonymous with occlusal microtrauma and hyperocclusion) will also be defined, compared and contrasted to FDH, as well as to classical DH that involves exposed dentin. The myriad of scientific theories attempting to explain the causation of DH will also be reviewed, along with a discussion of the mechanisms that explain Frictional Dental Hypersensitivity events. A rational protocol for optimum treatment using occlusal adjustment to treat FDH, and the clinical factors that can identify FDH patients whom could benefit from computer-guided occlusal treatment, are detailed, as well.

Proposed Mechanism of Frictional Dental Hypersensitivity

A tooth's pain response from FDH may be indicative of a significant muscular occlusal overload, applied to specific teeth within the functional range of motion. The nociceptive response, which may be inflammatory in origin, and occurs within the pulpal and/or periodontal interface of the overloaded teeth, leads to frequent short duration pain episodes.

It has been documented that excess frictional engagement of the posterior teeth, over time (Disclusion Time > 0.5 seconds) is known to promote hyperactivity of the muscles of mastication (Kerstein & Wright, 1991; Kerstein, 1993; Kerstein & Radke, 2006; Kerstein & Radke, 2012). Hypothetically, if excess muscular hyperactivity could be linked to the nociceptive response that manifested clinically as FDH, then the occlusal adjustment procedure known as Immediate Complete Anterior Guidance Development (ICAGD), could be used to decrease the Disclusion Time to less than 0.5 seconds (Kerstein 1992), and quiesce the hyperactive musculature thereby indirectly eliminating the FDH symptomotology.

ICAGD is a precise and conservative, measurement-driven coronoplasty, which involves a subtractive removal phase and occasionally an additive phase (when orthodontic movements are not an option), to optimize a physiologic change in both occlusal force and timing endpoints. ICAGD has been shown through research and case reports to result in a clinical minimization of periodontal ligament compression time, which indirectly results in the reduction of hyperactive elevator muscle activity down to a more normal functional baseline (Kerstein & Wright, 1991; Kerstein, 1993; Kerstein & Radke, 2006; Kerstein & Radke, 2012).

This chapter will define Dentinal Hypersensitivity (DH), describe theories of its etiology, and discuss the research that points both away from, and towards, a mechanically activated occlusal etiology. It is important to note that the traditional DH concept involves exposed dentinal tubules, while the novel FDH concept does not require or necessarily involve exposed dentinal tubules, FDH *will be implicated as a precursor to the genesis of DH episodes.* Additional chapter content will highlight clinical patient diagnostic procedures, as well as the traditional treatments available for Dentinal Hypersensitivity. Lastly, this chapter will proffer how occlusion, muscular TMD dysfunctional conditions, and frictional DH are all intricately related. A pilot study will be presented that indicates predictable resolution of DH can be achieved following the ICAGD coronoplasty, further supporting the concept of frictionally caused, Dentinal Hypersensitivity (FDH).

BACKGROUND

Section 1: The Definition of and Clinical Characteristics of Dentinal Hypersensitivity

Over the last 150 years, much research has been conducted in an effort to explain why the human dentition may or may not experience episodic bouts of Dentinal Hypersensitivity. Popular theories abound, from the widely accepted Hydrodynamic Theory, to the less accepted Odontoblastic Receptor Theory, to the least accepted Direct Innervation Theory. Correlations between periodontal recession, patent cementoenamel junction (CEJ) interfaces, exposed dentinal tubules, and tooth hypersensitivity are usually well supported, but both professionally applied treatments and over the counter (OTC) medicaments seem to only temporarily lessen DH episodes. It is clear that the dental profession has yet to completely understand the etiology and pathogenesis of this common patient affliction.

In the literature, the term Dentinal Hypersensitivity (DH) has many equivalent meanings, in which most relate the sensitivity episodes to the exposure of dentin and open dentinal tubules that communicate with a vital pulp. This chapter will refer to this classic condition consistently as *Dentinal Hypersensitivity* (DH), despite the many apparent synonyms.

The nomenclature surrounding DH seems confusing, as the literature attempts to organize various conditions under one catchall diagnosis.

Published Dentinal Hypersensitivity (DH) Nomenclature

- Tooth Hypersensitivity/Hypersensitivity/Dental Hypersensitivity.
- Dentinal Hypersensitivity/Cervical Dentinal Hypersensitivity.
- Dentin(e) Sensitivity/Hypersensitivity/Dentin(e) Hypersensitivity.
- Cervical Hypersensitivity/Sensitivity.
- Cemental Hypersensitivity/Sensitivity.
- Root Sensitivity/Hypersensitivity.

Since Blum first documented DH in 1530, most of the literature has reported on clinical trials purporting the efficacy of a given chemical treatment for the malady (Blum, 1530). The theories behind DH causation and treatment are numerous, and to this day, no one etiology, or treatment, is uniformly accepted by Dental Medicine as primary, nor does a single, effective, and permanent treatment exist (Banfield & Addy, 2004; Balaji, Jois, & Kumar, 2012). As such, much remains to be known about DH.

DH may be described as an exaggerated response to non-noxious stimuli (Dababneh, Khouri, & Addy, 1999). The pain is usually a sharp, fleeting, and well-localized pain, which can be distinguished from pulpal pain. Alternatively, Pulpal pain is described as prolonged dull and aching pain that is poorly localized, which persists long after the removal of a stimulus. The distinction between pain of dentinal versus pulpal origin is critical in making a reliable clinical diagnosis. Dentinal Hypersensitivity has been characterized as a short, sharp pain arising from exposed dentin in response to stimuli: typically thermal, evaporative, tactile, osmotic, or chemical, which cannot be ascribed to any other form of dental defect or pathology (Holland, Narhi, Addy, Gangarosa, & Orchardson, 1997).

DH has also been thought to be a form of reversible pulpitis (Bruder & Erickson). In contrast, other researchers argue that due to the short time that symptoms manifest themselves, DH causation is not likely an inflammatory response (West, Lussi, Seong, & Hellwig, 2012). but is considered one of the most painful and chronic of dental conditions (Strassler & Serrio, 2009). The DH condition meets all of the clinical criteria to be classified as a true pain syndrome (Curro, 1990).

Traditionally, it has been advocated that, DH *involves exposed dentin with open dentinal tubule orifices that communicate with a vital pulp* (Pashely, Tay, Haywood, Cooins, & Drisko, 2008). The only time in the literature that DH appears *not to be associated with exposed dentinal tubules*, is with hypersensitivity associated with the vital bleaching of teeth (Swift, 2012). DH that follows vital bleaching is annoying and painful to patients and can appear very similar to that of Dentinal Hypersensitivity. As such, post-operative vital bleaching sensitivity has been thought to involve a similar mechanism to that of non-bleaching Dentinal Hypersensitivity (Swift, 2012).

Reviews on the subject of DH have argued that the term Dentin Sensitivity be considered more appropriate, since there is no evidence that 'hypersensitive' dentin differs clinically in any way from normal dentin, or that a pulpal response is nothing more than a normal reaction to the stimulation of exposed dentin (Dababneh, Houri, & Addy, 1999). However, clinicians recognize that dentin at times, can be extremely sensitive to certain stimuli (Rowe 1985; Tronstad, 1986). Histologically, sensitive dentin presents with two times wider dentinal tubules and a greater number of tubules per area, when compared to dentin without sensitivity (Yoshiyama, Noiri, Ozaki, Uchida, Ishikawa, & Ishida, 1990). This is partly explained by dentin's tubular structure. The intratubular fluid is free to move in response to thermal, osmotic, tactile, or evaporative stimuli (Pashley, 1996). However, clinical experience as well as the literature, have both pointed out that not all exposed dentin is sensitive (Trowbridge, Franks, Korostoff, & Emling, 1980; Rimondini, Baroni, & Carrassi, 1995). Dababneh et. al., in 1999 stated that the clinical usage of the descriptor "DH" as exclusively relating to exposed dentin(e) may not be totally accurate (Dababneh, Khouri, & Addy, 1999). However, the same authors noted that despite these definition discrepancies, the term has been used for decades and is widely accepted by Dental Medicine, to describe a distinct clinical entity.

DH is Diagnosed by Exclusion

A diagnosis of DH is a diagnosis of exclusion, whereby the sensitivity cannot be attributed to any other cause or pathology (Porto, Andrade, & Montes, 2009). Amongst the plethora of dental conditions that can cause DH in the absence of exposed dentin (see Section 9), hyper-occlusion and acute traumatic occlusion are high on the list (Dowell & Addy, 1983; Dawson, 2006). The over-contouring of restorations, as well as typical malocclusions that leave teeth in chronic traumatic occlusion, are both common examples (West, 2006). One might argue that these conditions should be classified as chronic rather than acute because the teeth remain hyper-occluded for long periods of time. Although these often-miniscule occlusal discrepancies are frequently undetected by conventional Dental Medicine diagnostics, and can be relatively innocuous to the patient, DH symptomatology may spontaneously manifest itself when the involved teeth are exposed to the various non-noxious stimuli, over time. Regardless of Dental Medicines acumen at detecting these often microns-thick occlusal contact discrepancies, chronically hyper-occluded teeth are a widespread reality in clinical practice, which can have an enormous impact upon whether a patient experiences hypersensitivity. This chapter focuses primarily on this type of spatial and mechanical occlusal contact aberration that can lead to tooth-borne hypersensitivity symptoms of excessive *frictional* origin, which may or may not involve exposed dentin or open dentinal tubules.

Section 2: Dental Anatomy as It Relates to Dentinal Hypersentivity

The Pulp and Its Possible Inflammatory Response That Can Result in DH

The dental pulp is a connective tissue, akin to other connective tissue structures in the human body. It consists of blood vessels, nerves, interstitial fluid, ground substances, odontoblasts, fibroblasts and other cellular components (Ingle, Bakland, & Baumgartner, 2008). However, unlike most of the other connective tissues of the body, the pulp is encased within a rigid shell made of enamel and dentin. This restrictive environment has little to no room for volumetric expansion, such as occurs during inflammation. Though the pulp consists primarily of sensory fibers, a miniature circulatory system also exists, complete with lymphatics where only 7% of the pulpal volume is vasculature. Due to this tiny vascular component, the blood volume of the pulp is replaced frequently, typically 5 to 14 times every minute (Ingle, Bakland, & Baumgartner, 2008).

Embryologically the pulp, the dentin, and the periodontal tissues, are derived from the ectomesenchyme, while the enamel of the tooth is derived from the separate ectoderm (Ingle, Bakland, & Baumgartner, 2008). Sensory nerve fibers containing the neuropeptide, calcitonin gene-related peptide (CGRP), and substance P (SP), are found throughout the pulp. During tooth crown formation and just before root formation, a subodontoblastic sensory nerve plexus forms in the pulp, with the concomitant appearance of CGRP and SP that is contained within nerve fibers present in the dentinal tubules (Ingle, Bakland, & Baumgartner, 2008). Receptors for these neuropeptides are found surrounding the miniscule pulpal blood vessels, whereby pulpal changes depend upon the type of neuropeptide released.

Due to the encasement of the pulp within its rigid environment, changes in blood flow can have profound effects on pulpal health, ranging from minor ischemia, to necrosis of the pulpal tissue (Ingle, Bakland, & Baumgartner, 2008). The blood flow of the pulp is regulated by sympathetic a-adrenergic vasoconstriction, b-adrenergic vasodilation, the sympathetic cholinergic vasoactive system, and antidromic vasodilation, which is an axon reflex (Ingle, Bakland, & Baumgartner, 2008). These neuropeptides, along with local factors and hormones, influence the smooth muscle tone and therefore the blood flow (Ingle, Bakland, & Baumgartner, 2008).

Vasoconstriction and vasodilation are both possibilities within the pulpal microvasculature. Vasodilators are primarily produced when an inflammatory process initiates, which can compromise the health of pulpal tissues (Ingle, Bakland, & Baumgartner, 2008). If the dentin is covered coronally by enamel and radicularly by cementum, the vitality of the pulp within will usually remain unscathed for a lifetime, unless the apical blood supply is disrupted by excessive orthodontic forces, or severe impact trauma (Ingle, Bakland, & Baumgartner, 2008). The status of the pulpal microcirculation is therefore, a significant factor in maintaining stability and health of the pulp. Lastly, because there is a close relationship of the blood circulation between the periodontal and the pulpal tissues, traumatic inflammation of the periodontal tissues may also extend to the pulp, thereby affecting the pulp's heath (Seltzer & Bender, 1984).

Evidence from animal experiments suggests that pulpal inflammatory reactions may play a role in Dentinal Hypersensitivity (Narhi, Yamamoto, Ngassapa, & Hirvonen, 1994). In contrast, West et. al. in 2012, noted that the status of the pulp when Dentinal Hypersensitivity occurs is not known (West, Lussi, Seong, & Hellwig, 2012). These authors postulated that although the repetitive nature of the symptoms would suggest it, it is *unlikely* there is an acute or chronic inflammatory response taking place within the pulp, due to the short length of time a patient experiences each symptomatic episode.

Dentin and Dentinal Tubules

Dentin is a porous mineralized connective tissue with an organic matrix of collagenous proteins combined with inorganic hydroxyapatite. Dentin is considered to be a vital tissue.

Dentinal tubules are minuscule circular canals found distributed throughout the dentin, which radiate outward from the pulp chamber to the dentinal surface. All tubules possess dentinal fluids, contain a Tomes fiber (a cytoplastic cell process), and an odontoblast that communicates with the pulp. Millions of these tiny tubules permeate the dentin (Figure 1). The tubule density varies from approximately 20,000 tubules/mm^2 (from the CEJ going apically) to approximately 45,000 tubules/mm^2 (from the pulp going coronally) (West, 2006). Dentin and cementum are usually not exposed to the oral environment in ideal health (Reiter, 1980). But when exposure of either occurs, subsequent wearing away of these tissues is possible over time, which can readily lead to exposed dentin, dentinal tubules, and possible DH events.

This variation in dentinal tubule distribution has clinical implications. The closer to the pulp a clinician progresses during operative procedures, the softer the dentin becomes due to the increased area of the fluid-filled dentinal tubules and the decreased amount of calcified matrix (Ingle, Bakland, & Baumgartner, 2008). This tubule wetness increases 20 times when traveling from superficial to deep dentin (Pashley, 1996). Normal human dentin tubules taper from about 3-4 μm at their pulpal end, down to 0.5 μm peripheral diameter, dependent upon the age of the individual (Forsell-Ahleberg, Brannström, & Edwall, 1975). Tubule width is also clinically important, as the *rate of fluid flow* is dependent on the fourth power of the radius of the circular tubules. Doubling tubule diameter therefore results in a 16-fold increase in fluid flow rate.

It must be stressed that the permeability of dentin is not uniform in all areas of the tooth. There is variation, especially on the occlusal surfaces, where only 30% of the tubules are in free communication with the pulp (Pashley, Andringa, Derkson, Derkson, & Kalathoor, 1987). Axial dentin has been shown to be more permeable than occlusal dentin (Richardson, Tao, & Pashley, 1991). Interestingly, sensitive

Figure 1. Scanning electron micrograph of the dentine surface magnified 2000X. (Reprinted with permission from Chu, C.H. (2010). Management of Dentine Hypersensitivity, Dental Bulletin, 15, 3)

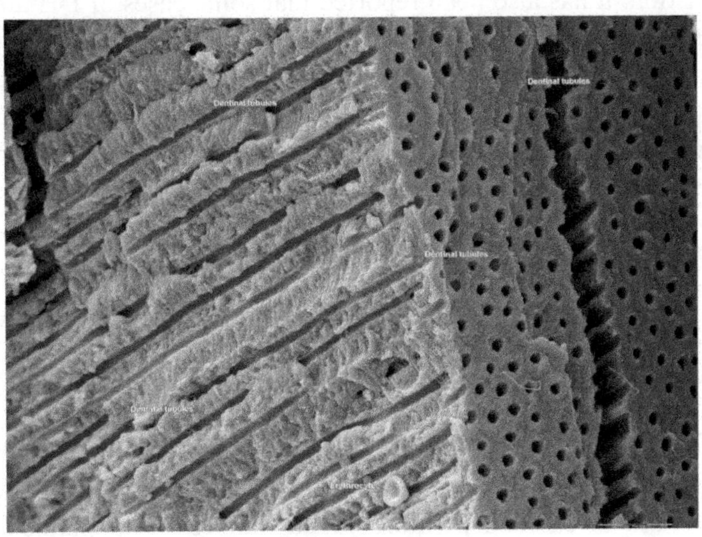

teeth have eight times more (8x), and two times wider (2x), dentinal tubules in the cervical-buccal region than do non-sensitive teeth (West, 2006). In a practical sense, these histological correlations may help explain the frequency of cervical DH symptoms often seen by clinicians in clinical practice.

Dentin permeability can be divided into two broad categories (Pashley, 1996):

- Transdentinal movement of substances through dentinal tubules (such as fluid shifts in response to hydrodynamic stimuli).
- Intradentinal movement of exogenous substances into intertubular dentin (the dentin between the tubules). This occurs during infiltration of hydrophilic adhesive resins into demineralized dentin surfaces after etching, or from the demineralization of intertubular dentin by bacterially derived acids.

Pashley et. al., used radioactive Iodine in the early 1980's, to demonstrate that once dentinal tubules are opened, molecules could readily penetrate through the fluid-filled tubules into the pulp chamber (Pashley, Kehl, Pashley, & Palmer, 1981). This classic study confirmed that if caries, abrasion, abfractions, or fractures, removed either the protective enamel or cementum, dentinal tubules could become exposed allowing a potential communication portal to open between the oral cavity and the pulp. Smaller molecules are more likely to penetrate through the dentinal tubules better than will larger molecules. Although the magnitude of the permeability of the exposed dentin varies with depth, age, time, location, and whether the dentin is sclerotic or infected with bacteria, pulpal irritation can result from hydrodynamic fluid shifts (from thermal, evaporative, chemical and mechanical stimuli), leading to immunologic irritation resultant from bacterial byproducts.

The dentinal fluid may also become contaminated by injurious agents which can permeate to the pulp and cause inflammation (such as from bacterial invasion, and from either endotoxins or exotoxins from caries). Since the size of the tubules (0.5 to 4μm) generally disallows the transport of the larger bacteria themselves, the concentration of these injurious agents in the pulp has been suspected to be responsible for inflammatory events, or abscess creation (Ingle, Bakland & Baumgartner, 2008).

Decreasing pulpal blood flow increases the interstitial fluid concentration of substances that permeate through the dentinal tubule fluids, allowing for higher concentrations of injurious agents to indirectly initiate pulpal inflammation. It has also been reported that some cases of DH are induced from direct exposure of the dentin(e), which may remain sensitive after the tubules are effectively closed. This may be due to pulpal inflammation and consequent sensitization of the intradentinal nerves (Byers & Narhi, 1999; Narhi, Yamamoto, Ngassapa, & Hirvonen, 1994). Sensitization may be described as a heightened or newfound hypersensitivity to noxious, as well as normally innocuous stimulation, following nerve injury (Vera-Portocarrero, Zhang, Ossipov, Xie, Lai, & Porreca, 2006).

Pulpo-Dentinal Innervation

Though the pulp and dentin are two distinct anatomical entities, they both function as a single unit. It is therefore appropriate to discuss the two together when describing shared innervation. The tooth is innervated *almost* exclusively by nociceptive afferents which are the receptors for pain sensations (Lin, Luo, Bai, Xu, & Lu, 2011). Additionally, teeth have unusual neural features, such as dense polymodal nociceptive sensory innervation of the coronal dentin, the pulp, and the vasculature, a sparse autonomic innervation, sensory nerve involvement in dentinal fluid dynamics, neural pulpal blood flow regulation, neural protective reflexes to preserve dental tissues and initiate dental wound healing (Byers & Narhi, 1999). For the most part, sensory afferents are involved in pain mediation (Byers, 1984; Mumford, 1982; Närhi, Jyväsjärvi, Virtanen, Huopaniemi, Ngassapa, & Hirvonen, 1991).

It is known from repeated histological studies that the physical innervation of dentin is limited, with nerve fibers only traversing approximately 1mm into dentin from the pulpo-dentinal interface. Despite this limited innervation, dentin appears to be highly sensitive when there dentinal tubules are patent (Matthews, Andrew, & Wanachantararak, 2000). In mammalian teeth, there is less innervation of root dentin than in crown dentin. The percentage of dentinal tubules towards the crown rgion is more densely innervated than the tubules that are located more apically (Grippo, 1991). At the tip of the pulp horns, a tuft of dense innervation extends 0.5- 1.0 mm into the inner dentin. Gradually there is less dense dentinal innervation as the distance away from the pulp horn increases (Byers & Narhi, 1999), such that nerves are absent in the peripheral dentin (Byers, 1980). Therefore, only the first millimeter or so outwards from the pulpo-dentinal interface possesses significant nervous tissue in the dentinal tubules. The rest of the dentinal tubules up to the dentinoenamel junction is histologically devoid of nervous tissue.

What is less well known, is whether the movement of the fluid within the tubule excites the nerve endings directly, either in the inner ends of the tubules or in the superficial pulp, or whether the odontoblasts play a role in the transduction mechanism (Matthews, Andrew, & Wanachantararak, 2000). The experiments of Brännström suggest that neither odontoblastic processes, nor excitable nerves within dentin are responsible for dentin sensitivity (Brännström, 1966). Brännström's Hydrodynamic Theory is the most accepted working model that is proffered to explain the many symptoms of DH (the Hydrodynamic Theory will be further explained in this chapter's section devoted to the traditional DH theories).

Sensory nerves have a strong impact on the blood circulation of the dental pulp, due to the liberation of vasodilating neuropeptides contained within the main pulp body, as well as in walls of the pulpal blood vessels. Studies indicate that these neuropeptides help with pulpal blood flow (Ingle, Bakland, & Baumgartner, 2008).

Research suggests that unmyelinated C fibers may play a significant role in the perception of dull intradental pain of pulpal inflammatory origin (Närhi, Jyväsjärvi, Virtanen, Huopaniemi, Ngassapa, & Hirvonen, 1991). It seems that intradental C-fibers do not respond to the hydrodynamic stimulation of dentin. They are polymodal, and are activated when external stimuli reach the pulp proper. They primarily mediate the dull pain associated with pulpitis. However, C fibers may have an important modifying effect on dentin(e) sensitivity, because they may release neuropeptides which function in pulpal inflammatory reactions (Närhi, Yamamoto, Ngassapa, & Hirvonen, 1994).

Myelinated A and unmyelinated C nerve fibers are both present in the pulpo-dentinal interface. Most of the A-delta, A-beta and C-fibers have polymodal receptor functions (Byers & Narhi, 1999). Studies indicate that intradental A-type nerve fibers are responsible for the sensitivity of dentin, and are thought to be activated by fluid movements in dentinal tubules (known as the Hydrodynamic Mechanism) (Narhi, Yamamoto, Ngassapa, & Hirvonen, 1994). The swiftest of the group, the intradental A-beta fibers are classified as belonging to the same functional group as A-delta fibers, and both are likely involved with pain sensations induced from the dentin (Narhi, Yamamoto, Ngassapa, & Hirvonen, 1994). It has been postulated that these vibration-sensitive A-beta mechanoreceptors, may cause "pre-pain" warnings of dentinal injury (Dong & Chudler, 1985; Dong & Shiwaku, 1993).

Dong in 1993 found evidence using electro physiologic recording techniques, that some intradentinal receptors in cat canine teeth detect mechanical transients applied to intact enamel (Dong, Shiwaku, Kawakami, & Chudler, 1993). This finding suggested that mammalian pulpo-dentinal innervation might also play an important non-nociceptive role, in detecting tooth contact during mastication and swallowing. Thus, intradentinal receptors not only serve to signal impending tissue damage and harm (nociception), but also may serve to modulate the movements of the entire Stomatognathic system (teeth, masticatory muscles, ligaments, periodontal ligaments Temporomandibular joints and cartilage). The authors determined that some type of fiber exists that communicates with the brainstem, thalamus, and the somatosensory cortex, faster than do the A-delta fibers. These faster sensory fibers have been identified as A-beta fibers (Levy, 2009). Narhi et. al. in 1999 showed using electrophysiological recordings, that intradental A-beta fibers belong to the same functional group as A-delta fibers, and are probably involved with pain sensations induced from dentin (Byers & Narhi, 1999). Later, in 2008, it was demonstrated that the dental pulp is represented in the primary somatosensory cortex, which receives input from intradental A-beta neurons. This work provided a detailed organizational map of the orofacial area, resulting in the addition of the dental pulp to the "sensory homunculus" (Kubo, Shibukawa, Shintani, Suzuki, Ichinohe, & Kaneko, 2008).

Periodontal Ligament and Muscle

Considerations with respect to the muscles of mastication are typically an afterthought in the practice of Dental Medicine. This can be a mistake as relaxed and efficient muscles are the key to a peaceful Stomatognathic system, and predictable restorative dentistry (Dawson, 2006). Williamson, Kerstein, and others using electromyography (EMG), have shown that occlusal interferences of both the centric and excursive variety, can produce muscular hyperactivity (Williamson & Lundquist, 1983; Mahan, Wilkinson, Gibbs, Mauderli, & Brannon, 1983; Kerstein & Wright, 1991; Kerstein & Radke, 2006; Kerstein & Radke, 2012). Kerstein has actually quantified objective occlusal timing parameters that may be used to quiesce hyperactive muscles (Kerstein & Wright, 1991; Kerstein, 1992, Kerstein, 1993, Kerstein, 1995, Kerstein, Chapman, & Klein, 1997; Kerstein & Radke, 2006; Kerstein, 2010, Kerstein & Radke, 2012).

The mechanoreceptors of the periodontal ligament (PDL) as well as intradental A-beta fibers (Kleinfelder & Ludwig, 2002; Levy, 2009) are known to control the loading forces produced by the masticatory muscles. In 1999, it was reported that tactile information from teeth emanates from the low-threshold Ruffini mechanoreceptors in the periodontal ligament and the dento-gingival ligaments, while tooth-related thermal information comes mainly from receptors in the gingival tissues. As such, tooth-related pain can originate in the pulp, dentin, or from the periodontal ligaments (Byers & Narhi, 1999). A 2009 modern scientific review pointed out that the periodontal Ruffini mechanoreceptors are slowly adapting, fire continuously after detecting low frequency vibrations, detect only unilateral force movements, and only perceive the first contact between teeth before shutting down (Levy, 2009). They make the CNS aware that there is an object between the teeth.

Definitions

- **Mechanoreception:** The unconscious sensing or conscious perception of touch, or mechanical displacement arising from stimuli outside the body.
- **Mechanoreceptors:** The sensory end organs which respond to mechanical stimuli such as pressure, vibration, tension and friction.

In contrast to the periodontal Ruffini mechanoreceptors, the A-beta intradental mechanoreceptors are rapidly adapting, fire intermittently after detecting a much wider frequency range of mechanical vibrations, and detect force movements from multiple directions. In addition, these intradental fibers also perceive the texture of the food bolus, and communicate this information to the CNS so that an appropriate efferent muscular response and rhythm results (Levy, 2009). Additionally,Dong's cat studies concluded that the neurophysiologic properties of intradental and periodontal mechanoreceptors are functionally different (Dong & Chudler 1985; Dong & Shiwaku, 1993). After rubbing different grit sandpaper on feline canine teeth, frequency-encoded discharge patterns were found to arise in the trigeminal ganglionic neurons. These discharge patterns were unique to grit size, suggesting that intradental mechanoreceptors are actually able to encode different types of mechanical vibrations (Levy, 2009). Therefore, a combination of intradental and periodontal mechanoreceptor input is theoretically responsible for the perception of the mechanical properties of food brought into the mouth, and for the fine motor control over mastication (Trulsson, Francis, Bowtell, & McGlone, 2010; Levy, 2009).

The influence of directional movement, whether it is axial or orthogonal, depends upon the tooth's position or laterality (Ohmori, Kirimoto, & Ono, 2012). For instance, subjects that lack information from periodontal receptors (such as when anesthetized, or when they present with dental implants), demonstrate a marked disturbance in the control of precisely directed, low occlusal forces, and report the absence of distinct and reliable sensations of where on the tooth a contact is made. These findings strongly suggest that the periodontal and intradental receptors play a significant role in the specification of the level, direction, and point of attack of muscular forces used to hold and manipulate food between teeth (Trulsson, Francis, Bowtell, & McGlone, 2010; Levy, 2009). It is therefore likely that the direction of force application contributes to the reflex response of the human masticatory muscles, with the periodontal mechanoreceptors contributing unilaterally and the intradental A-beta mechanoreceptors contributing omnilaterally.

The complexity of the neural regulation of teeth and adjacent tissues is further demonstrated by the efferent actions that sensory nerve fibers have on blood flow in pulp, periodontal tissues, and within the lip, following stimulation of either the pulp or the lip. This suggests that some afferents branch both inside the tooth, and to the surrounding tissues (Byers & Narhi, 1999).

Levy suggested a paradigm shift in regards to the function of vital teeth (Levy, 2009), where teeth not only act as organs that assist with nourishment for the life of the organism, but that vital teeth should be considered as sensory organs. As such, vital teeth are responsible for orchestrating mechanoreceptive input into the CNS, via both pulpal and periodontal afferent input resultant from the mechanical displacements a tooth undergoes during vibrational, tensile, pressure and frictional changes from the differing consistencies of a given food bolus. All of this feedback assists the masticatory system to successfully manage the task at hand (chewing, swallowing, breathing).

Occlusal force magnitude was described as being affected by the mechanosensory feedback that can restrain muscle activity, and limit structural damage to the teeth, Temporomandibular joints, and the periodontal apparatus. Levy implied that occlusal therapy may actually manipulate mechanosensory neurological streams to the CNS, which can almost instantaneously change jaw muscle activity and oromotor behavior. He stressed that devitalization of teeth supports the contention that less control is afforded the Stomatognathic system without a vital pulp, citing that frequent, uncontrollable forces, that lead often to catastrophic fracture of endodontically treated teeth, as being supportive evidence. Basically, endodontically treated teeth and dental implant-retained prostheses were shown to provide less mechanosensory information than vital teeth. Additionally, occlusal force magnitude (via muscle activity) was implicated as being directly affected by pulpal mechanosensory feedback, as well as by the traditionally accepted, periodontal mechanosensory feedback mechanisms.

Traumatic Occlusion (Also Known as Occlusal Microtrauma, or Hyper-Occlusion)

Traumatic Occlusion can affect the whole tooth, its supporting structures (including the PDL's), and the pulp (Kvinnsland & Heyeraas, 1992). Mechanical forces applied to intact teeth (most frequently through the function of the masticatory muscles), have been shown to activate sensory receptors in the periodontium and the pulp, increase periodontal tissue pressure, and alter blood flow both within the pulp and the periodontium (Kvinnsland & Heyeraas, 1992). Because the forces of occlusal prematurities have been associated with the progression of periodontal disease (Harrel, Nunn, & Hallmon, 2006), reduced periodontal support may decrease the threshold level of periodontal mechanoreceptor function (Takeuchi & Yamamoto, 2008), which can cause changes in occlusal forces (Alkan, Keskiner & Arici, 2006). It is axiomatic that a vicious cycle ensues when the occlusion perpetuates the loss of periodontal support, which over time leads to not only the loss of soft tissue and osseous support, but also to the exposure of the CEJ and cementum, thereby increasing the likelihood of DH occurring (following the traditional theories that rely upon exposed dentin and open dentinal tubules).

Excess frictional engagements of the posterior teeth during excursive movements over time, leads to hyperactivity of the mandibular elevator muscles, namely the masseter, temporalis and medial pterygoid muscles (Dawson 2006; Kerstein & Wright, 1991; Kerstein & Radke, 2006; Kerstein & Radke, 2012). This muscular hyperactivity leads to excess horizontal forces against posterior teeth, increases the compressive load on the TMJ's, and invites excess wear and overload onto the posterior dentition, especially if the patients is a bruxer (Dawson, 2006). Such overload over time, can readily generate excess *frictional* occlusal surface interactions between opposing teeth in function, flexing them during function and inciting tooth sensitivity. A novel term, *Frictional Dental Hypersensitivity* (*FDH*), seems appropriate to describe this occlusally-caused event. It is this authors experience that it is possible to quantify and treat the causation of FDH with digital occlusal analysis, whereas Traumatic Occlusion has been a relatively immeasurable, abstract, and often subjectively treated, occlusal problem.

Section 3: The Prevalence and Potential Etiologies of Dentinal Hypersensitivity

During clinical practice, patients experiencing symptoms of Dentinal Hypersensitivity, often present to their dental practitioner concerned with either an acute or chronic episode of DH. Single or multiple sensitive teeth may be involved, sometimes located in different quadrants. The patient typically describes an inability to eat hot foods, drink cold drinks, comfortably breathe in cold air, or undergo non-invasive dental manipulation that would not ordinarily cause sensitivity. Some patients may even present for dental treatment unaware that they have DH, or assume that the affliction is normal. According to Addy, of those complaining of experiencing DH, only 48% of the patients actually discussed the condition with their dentist, and only half of these individuals sought out the recommended treatment options. As such, it is difficult to arrive at a definitive frequency of appearance. Depending on the study reviewed, the prevalence of DH has been reported to lie between 5% and 57% of the general population (Rees, 2000; Fischer, 1992; Liu et. al., 1998; Taani & Awartani, 2001; Irwin & McCusker, 1996; Clayton et. al., 2002; Al-Sabbagh, et. al., 2004; Rees & Addy; 2002).

Such a wide variation in the epidemiology of DH is difficult to explain, but a selection bias in the recruitment study sample is probable (Splieth & Tachou, 2013). As representative studies involving patients in general dental practice vary greatly between regions and countries, a locale that focuses heavily on preventative care will see DH rates significantly differ from an area where patients seek dental care intermittently, and therefore present with more advanced disease states. An advanced periodontal patient with intermittent bouts of treatment will present with more recession and potential for exposed dentin than a patient who religiously seeks periodontal treatment, whereby the former will be more likely to present with DH. In addition, it has been questioned whether individuals with Dentin Hypersensitivity will seek professional help, especially when dentists themselves are lacking appropriate scientific data to both prevent and treat episodes of hypersensitivity (Splieth & Tachou, 2013).

Potential Dentinal Hypersensitivity Etiologic Processes

Studies indicate that dentinal exposure may result from one or more of the following processes (Chabanski & Gillam, 1997; Ikeda et. al., 1998; Gillam & Orchardson, 2006; Porto, Andrade & Montes, 2009)

- **Poor Oral Hygiene:** Periodontal tissue destruction, loss of supporting bone and root exposure have been directly correlated with low levels of oral hygiene (Mayhew, Jessee, & Martin, 1998). After root exposure occurs, DH often when acids secreted by the plaque biofilm open the dentinal tubules chemically (Wilchgers & Emert, 1997).
- **Lack of or Excessive Tooth Brushing:** Lack of tooth brushing understandably leads to accumulation of dental plaque. Excessive plaque causes gingival inflammation that may lead to migration of the gingiva apically, potentially exposing the cementum, root dentin, or an un-buttressed CEJ (Suge et. al., 2006). Excessive tooth brushing has also been implicated in the appearance of DH where there is exposed dentin (Addy, 2005), perhaps due to the physical removal of the smear layer, which usually occludes the dentinal tubules (Pashley, 1991).
- **Exposure to Non-bacterial Acids in the Diet:** Low pH drinks, drugs, chemical products, and endogenous acids from gastric regurgitation, can lead to chemical dissolution and subsequent opening of dentinal tubules. Typically labeled *erosion*, this process leads to softened enamel in both the cervical and occlusal areas (Eisenburger & Addy, 2002). Acidic insults can lead to greater propensity for DH, and can be associated with abrasion, especially when acidic gastric reflux or acidic dietary consumption is followed immediately by tooth brushing (Wilchgers & Emert, 1997).
- **Periodontal Therapy:** Non-surgical root planning and open flap periodontal surgeries frequently lead to loss of cemental structure and gingival recession. These occurrences lead to a greater propensity for patent dentinal tubules and subsequent episodes of DH (Marini et. al., 2004).
- **Natural Physiologic Causes Leading to Recession and Supraeruption:** Natural aging generally leads to excessive root exposure, and possible DH. Dental extrusion or supraeruption resultant from antagonist tooth loss can also lead to root exposure and DH (Bartold, 2006). Gingival recession should be considered a predisposing factor, rather than a direct cause of DH, as it exposes the root surfaces to the oral environment (Swift, 2005). It was reported that the prevalence, extent, and severity of gingival recession can be correlated with prior orthodontic treatment (Sluzkey & Levin, 2008), as orthodontic movement of teeth outside the labial or lingual plate could lead to dehiscence formation (Joss-Vassalli et. al., 2010; Tugnait & Clerehugh,

2001). Frontolateral bruxism has been also associated with the initiation and/or enhancement of gingival recession (Abbound, Gruner, & Koeck, 2002).

- **Excessive Occlusal Force or Premature Occlusal Contacts:** Occlusal disease in the form of hyper-occlusion, also called chronic *occlusal microtrauma*, has been cited as causative for premature operative, esthetic, or prosthetic failure, including failure of Class V restorations (Ruiz, 2005; Christensen, 1992; Ruiz & Christensen, 2006; Tyas, 1995). In this authors' experience, this hyper-occlusion phenomenon is quite prevalent clinically, and can also lead to symptoms of DH even without dentin and dentinal tubule exposure. DH has been labeled by a number of authors as a symptom of occlusal related disease (Johansson et. al., 2002; Hypersensitivity C.A.B.O.D, 2003; Dawson, 2006; Manshreck, 2009; Splieth & Tachou, 2013). Furthermore, the presence of an active occlusal prematurity has been associated with the progression of periodontal disease (Harrel et. al., 2006; Ruiz & Coleman, 2008).

DH has been deemed more directly related to dentinal exposure through abrasive, erosive, abfractive and periodontal mechanisms (West et. al., 2012), and less typically to occlusal factors, although much recent literature evidence does exist that correlates DH to occlusal contact, abfraction formation and occlusal disease (Mayhew et. al., 1998; Ikeda et. al., 1998; Miller et. al., 2002; Porto et. al.,2009; Grippo et. al., 2012). In addition, some studies directly correlate hyperocclusion to DH (Ikeda eta al. 1987; Ikeda, Nakana & Suzuki, 1998; Coleman, Grippo, & Kinderknecht, 2003). In an extensive study that lasted 17 years, long-term relief of DH was observed in patients who received occlusal equilibration as the primary treatment for their DH condition (Coleman et. al., 2003).

Section 4: Abfraction Formation, Non-Carious Cervical Lesions (NCCLs), and the Concept of Frictional Dental Hypersensitivity

Grippo in 1991, concluded that cervical lesions were the result of flexing of the teeth at the gingival crest, due to heavy bruxing. This flexure resulted in damage to the cervical enamel rods resulting in their loosening, and subsequent flaking away of the tooth structure (Grippo, 1991). This type of occlusally induced, tooth structural damage was termed an "abfraction" (Figure 2).

Figure 2. Cervical abfractions and gingival recession

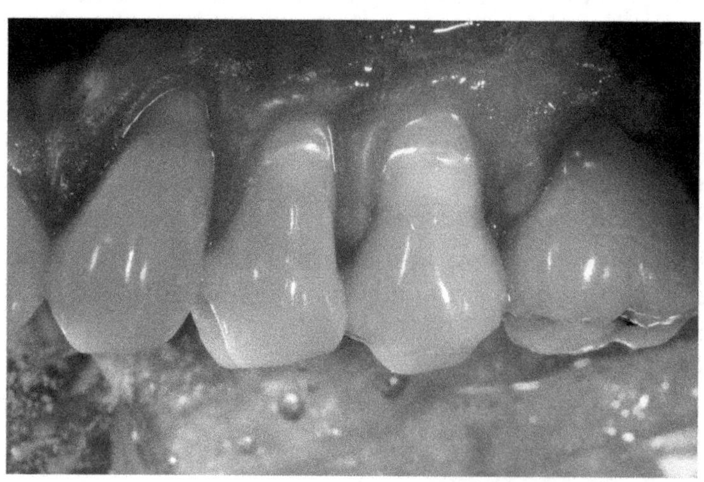

Abfractions have been implicated by some authors to be a predisposing factor of DH (Mayhew, Jessee & Martin, 1998; Ikeda, Nakano, Bando, & Suzuki, 1998; Coleman, Grippo & Kinderknecht, 2000). The association of DH with the distribution and location of abfractive lesions indicates that DH may result from excessive parafunctional or functional occlusal stresses (Coleman, Grippo, & Kinderknecht, 2003). Yoshiyama et. al., found that exposed dentinal tubules resultant from abfraction formation could lead to increasing stimulation of the pulp, and result in DH (Yoshiyama et. al., 1990). Another study reported that working and non-working excursive forces produced 10-20 times greater *flexure* to teeth than did vertical loading forces, such that flexural stresses appeared to play a role in the genesis of both DH and abfractive lesions (Spranger, 1995). Because Abfractions have been definitively implicated in occlusal disturbances (Miller et. al., 2003; Porto et. al., 2009; Grippo, Simring, & Coleman, 2012), occlusion has been deemed one of the many etiological factors of DH (Dowell & Addy, 1983).

The interplay between stress, corrosion, and occlusal surface *friction* seems to be responsible for the formation of non-carious cervical lesions (NCCL's) (Ruiz & Coleman 2008). It has been suggested that when less than five or six teeth have been diagnosed with verified Cervical Dentin Hypersensitivity, the primary etiology is likely *chronic occlusal microtrauma*. In contrast, Coleman & Ruiz found that when there are *greater than* six teeth with Cervical Dentin Hypersensitivity, the primary etiologic factor was more likely *corrosion* due to acidic insult (Ruiz & Coleman 2008).

Figures 3a, 3b, 3c, & 3d illustrate a patient who demonstrated evidence of occlusal frictional trauma, that reported no history of gastric reflux, or excessive intake of acidic foods or beverages. The patient did however, demonstrate an Occlusion Time of 0.51 seconds, a left Disclusion Time of 1.89 seconds, and a right Disclusion Time of 1.65 seconds. It is likely that the cervical abfractions and the cupped-out lesions on the mandibular molar were the result of chronic excessive frictional engagements that induced excessive muscular hyperactivity. Note the extreme wear facets on the buccal cusps of both premolars, which were highly suggestive of excursive muscular hyperactivity and lack of posterior disclusion.

Compared to traumatic occlusion, erosion and DH have been extensively studied. Erosion (caused by extrinsic acids on hard tooth substrate) was considered by Bartlett, to be the most common and important etiological factor in tooth wear (Bartlett 1997). Opponents to the potential occlusal genesis of abfraction formation, argue that many in vitro studies fail to address the cushioning effect of the Periodontal ligament (West, Lussi, Seong, & Hellwig, 2012). Consequently, occlusal trauma alone, cannot satisfactorily

Figure 3a. A first mandibular molar that demonstrated both NCCL, and occlusal wear facets

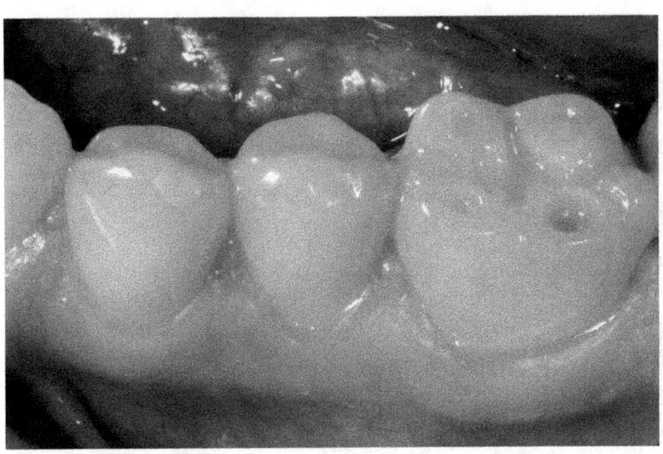

Figure 3b. Mandibular occlusal surfaces of the same patient. The patient described transient generalized symptoms of hypersensitivity throughout the dentition, with exposure of dentin visible solely on both mandibular first molars (one was previously restored)

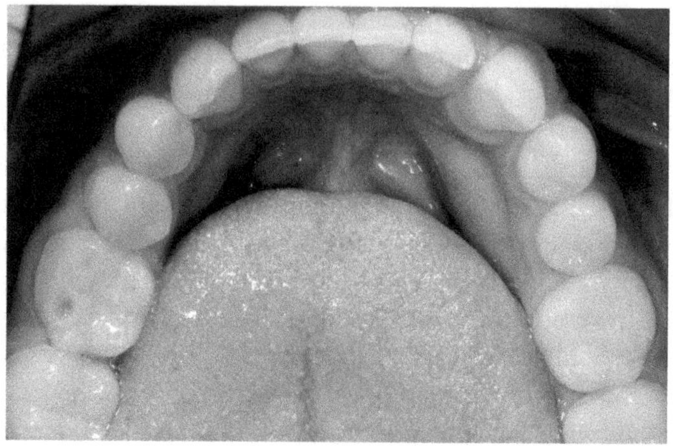

Figure 3c. The same patient's maxillary dentition. Note the lack of exposed dentin and erosive lesions

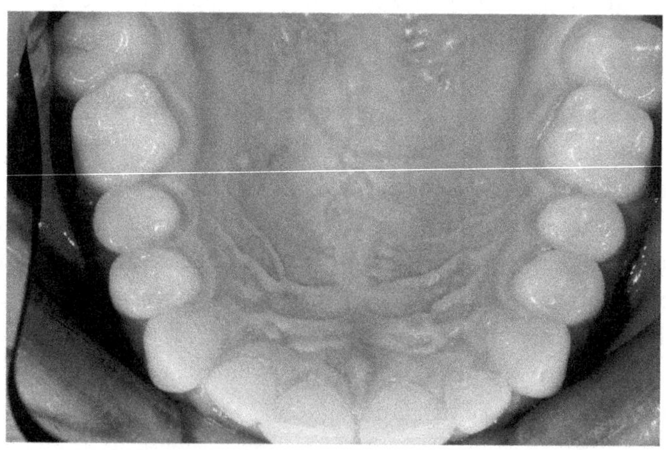

Figure 3d. The same patient's retracted view in MIP

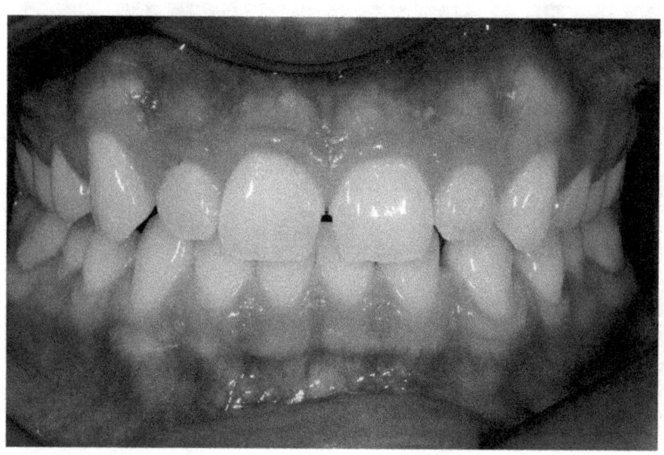

explain the development of NCCL's. The role of occlusal loading in the formation of an NCCL has been considered contributory to a multifactorial event (West, Lussi, Seong, & Hellwig, 2012).

The differing NCCL's appear to result from differing factors:

- **Abfraction:** Occlusion.
- **Erosion:** Acids.
- **Abrasion:** Toothbrushing and toothpaste.
- Combinations of the above.

Attrition from parafunctional bruxism may also play a role in some cases of occlusal Dentinal Hypersensitivity (Bartlett & Smith, 2000; Ekfeldt et. al., 1990). Occlusal surface structure abnormalities have been implicated in the exposure of dentin via attrition, where excess forces may cause abfraction formation and DH (Spranger, 1995).

Arguments against abfractions developing from occlusal forces suggest that many teeth demonstrate the signs of *traumatic occlusion,* but do not develop cervical lesions. Moreover, if abfractions were created exclusively through occlusal overload, both buccal and lingual cervical regions would share in the characteristic notching patterns (West, Lussi, Seong, & Hellwig, 2012). This opinion purports that since most abfractions occur to the buccal of teeth, these lesions are most likely due to excessive and overzealous tooth brushing (West, Lussi, Seong, & Hellwig, 2012). In contrast, a 2003 study found that NCCL's coexist almost systematically with occlusal wear facets (94.5%) and a lack of canine disclusion (77.2%), and that clinical signs of excessive brushing were lacking in a study of 309 abfractive lesions (Miller et. al.,2003).Perhaps, had an untreated patient pool been followed longitudinally, where their occlusions were digitally measured periodically and repeatedly, perhaps traumatic occlusion would have been seen as etiologic to cervical lesion formations over time. A literature search by this author could not produce a single study using T-Scan occlusal analysis that tried to correlate DH to excessive occlusal force, or prolonged occlusal surface friction.

A recent study demonstrated that working side group function increased excursive muscle activity levels more so than did balancing interferences, using Electromyography (BioEMG III, Bioresearch Associates, Milwaukee WI, USA) synchronized in real-time with the T-Scan 8 system (Tekscan Inc, S. Boston, MA USA) (Kerstein & Radke, 2012*)*. This study identified working excursive interferences as being more likely to stimulate muscular hyperactivity than balancing interferences, which is contrary to popular advocated occlusal thought, which implicates balancing contacts as being the most problematic (in regards to inciting muscular hyperactivity) occlusal contacts. This observation helps explain why NCCL's and abfractions primarily appear on the buccal aspects of teeth in patients who present without a crossbite. It is quite plausible that compressive lateroflexion forces would be greatest to the buccal in the working excursion.

Frictional Dentin Hypersensitivity vs. Traumatic Occlusion

Perhaps the answer to occlusion's role in DH appears to be, as of yet, an undocumented etiology. One could argue that a likely etiology is traumatic occlusion or occlusal microtrauma (hyperocclusion) when no exposed dentin exists (West, 2006). Although traumatic occlusion and hyperocclusion might describe similar or even identical conditions, both of these terms do not quantify anything occlusal that is representative of these conditions.

The concept of Frictional Dental Hypersensitivity (FDH) may help explain what most practicing clinicians frequently observe in clinical practice. This DH condition may or may not involve the presence of exposed dentin, and may be objectively diagnosed, with digital occlusal analysis, and readily resolved with the occlusal adjustment procedure known as ICAGD (Kerstein & Wright, 1991; Kerstein, 1992). Rather than simply qualifying the presence of offending occlusal contacts using articulating paper, it is possible with the T-Scan technology, to address the occlusal pathology objectively, by quantifying occlusal contact timing and relative force on teeth that demonstrate DH.

In this author's clinical experience using objective digital data (Tscan/EMG) and opinion, the tooth flexion and lateroflexion resultant from the combination of hyperactive muscles and excessive centric and excursive applied occlusal contact force, often causes DH symptomatology to appear. An increase in intradental A-beta pulpal stimulation, and/or excess periodontal ligament mechanoreceptor stimulation, may be etiologic for DH symptomotology, long before abfractive lesions clinically appear. In addition, such mechanoreceptor stimulations may one day prove to be at least partially etiologic for abfractive lesion formation and the resultant exposed dentin.

Section 5: Widely Accepted Dental Hypersensitivity Theories

1. **Dentinal Receptor Mechanism Theory:** This is an older hypothesis that suggests DH results from direct stimulation of sensory nerve endings in the dentine. However, there is little experimental and microscopic evidence to support this theory, as it seems unlikely that neural cells exist in the sensory portion of the outer dentine (Irvine 1988, Porto et. al., 2009).
2. **Odontoblast Transducer Mechanism:** Proposed by Rapp in 1968, (Rapp et. al., 1968) this theory hypothesized that odontoblasts act as receptor cells, mediating changes in the membrane potential of the odontoblasts through their synaptic junctions with nerves. This could result in a pain sensation within the pulp-dentinal complex. The Odontoblast Transducer Mechanism has little supporting evidence (West, 2008; Porto et. al., 2009).
3. **Hydrodynamic Theory:** To date, the Hydrodynamic Theory is the most widely accepted DH theory (West et. al., 2012, Linsuwanont et. al., 2008). Proposed in 1964, it was theorized that the loss of enamel or cementum in the cervical region leads to the subsequent opening of the dentinal tubules, exposing them to the oral cavity (Brännström & Åström, 1964). External stimuli then induce a rapid outflow of dentinal fluid from within the dentinal tubules. This fluid outflow is believed to indirectly stimulate pulpal nerves by activating mechanoreceptors located at the pulpal-dentinal interface, causing a pain sensation. The means by which the dentinal fluid flow stimulates the nerve impulses is still unknown (Chidchuangchai, Vongsavan, & Matthews, 2007).

The pulpal-dentinal interface mechanoreceptor response to external stimuli are believed to induce rapid myelinated A-delta and A-beta fiber impulse transmission to the cranial pain centers (Ruiz & Coleman, 2008). The flow of dentinal fluid is directly influenced by the linear dimensions between the pulp and the external dentin, the number of open tubules, the tubular diameter, and the configuration of the tubules (Ruiz & Coleman, 2008). One study has shown that larger and more numerous tubules are found in DH teeth, than in normal non-sensitive dentin (Absi et. al., 1987; Swift, 2005). As described previously, a substantial increase in dentinal fluid flow occurs when here exists a combination of larger and greater number of tubules as dentinal tubule diameter increases, which then amplifies an external stimulus response (Swift, 2005).

Based on the Hydrodynamic Theory, Dentinal Hypersensitivity has been considered to be a transient tooth pain. Simply explained, in order to exhibit a response to the external stimuli, the tubules would have to be open at the dentin surface, and patent all the way through to the pulp of a vital tooth. The external stimuli, such as cold air or liquid, could cause a pressure change across the dentin that than activates a nerve response causing a painful sensation. The Hydrodynamic Theory explains thermally induced DH, by suggesting a thermal insult causes a rapid displacement of tubular contents, which then stimulates nerve fibers mechanically at the pulpo-dentinal border (Brännström & Åström, 1964). The thermal expansion or contraction of the fluid within tubules is thought to cause the fluid displacement, such that the rate of temperature change the tooth was subjected to induced a more pronounced response (Matthews, 1977). Therefore, the presence of a high temperature gradient across the dentin surface is needed for this response to manifest (Linsuwanont et. al., 2008).

Pashley postulated that if the hydrodynamic theory was correct, cases of persistent DH were most probably due to one or both of the following events (Pashley et. al., 2008).

- Local pulpal inflammation caused persistent nerve sprouting, or lowering of nerve thresholds.
- Some dentinal tubules remain hyperconductive following individual fluid outflow DH episodes.

The hydrodynamic theory is questioned when the dentinal tubules are not open to the oral environment, but instead are covered by intact enamel and cementum. In clinical situations where bleaching agents are used and cause tooth sensitivity, it is often clinically apparent that exposed dentin is not a prerequisite for this type of DH (Swift, 2005).

However, if the fluid flow is the result of thermal contraction or expansion of the dentin, it should only occur after the hot or cold stimulus actually contacts the anatomical point whereby the dentinal fluid is housed, namely the dentin (Linsuwanont et. al., 2008). However, it has been shown that a patients' thermal sensation precedes the temperature change at the dentinal surface (Linsuwanont et. al., 2007). This precludes the possibility of there being direct thermal stimulation at the pulpo-dentinal border (Trowbridge et. al., 1980; Linsuwanont et. al., 2007).

Questioning the current hypothetical mechanisms of nerve stimulation, thermal expansion or contraction of dentinal fluid, and direct dentin thermal stimulation seems appropriate, as none of these proposed theories adequately explain all clinical DH phenomenona. The alternative mechanistic and inflammatory theories that are presented below, may better explain the rapid DH pain response observed with thermal stimulation, that are noted in both clinical and scientific studies (Pashley, 1990; Linsuwanont et. al., 2008).

Section 6: Alternative Theories Linking Occlusion to Dentinal Hypersensitivity

Alternate mechanisms such as those proposed by Pashley in 1990 (The Stilletto Heel Theory), and Linsuwanont in 2008 (The Strain Deformation Theory), suggest that occlusal overload could lead to sporadic DH symptoms (Linsuwanont et. al., 2008; Pashley, 1990; West et. al., 2012). Over time, such overload has been shown to lead to the abfractive processes with the associated accelerated gingival recession, the micro fractures of the cervical enamel, the exposed dentin, and the patent dentinal tubules (Yoshiyama et. al., 1990). It appears that the patent dentinal tubules are typically what clinicians and researchers focus on as etiologic, while not addressing the occlusal components that may not only begin the process, but also perpetuate the process of DH symptom evolution, with or without the presence of exposed dentinal tubules.

1. **The Neurogenic Inflammatory Theory:** Micro fractures resultant from excess occlusal force, or physiochemical loss of hydroxyapatite crystals, which both affect the cervical regions, may lead to a pulpal neurogenic inflammatory response (Pashley, 1990). It has been postulated that the release of neuropeptides, such as substance P (SP), calcitonin gene-related peptide (CGRP), and neurokinins, may promulgate and intensify Dentin Hypersensitivity.
2. **The Prolonged Disclusion Time, Prolonged Occlusal Surface Friction, Tooth Flexion and Lateroflexion, FDH Theory:** Prolonged PDL compressions resultant from prolonged opposing excursive occlusal surface frictional engagements, have been shown to lead to muscle hyperactivity, whereby the PDL compressions stimulate excessive contractions of the muscles of mastication above their baseline required to move the mandible during function (Kerstein & Wright, 1991;Kerstein 1993; Kerstein & Radke, 2006; Kerstein, 2010; Kerstein & Radke, 2012; Dawson, 2006). The increased contraction levels lead to excessive occlusal and/or parafunctional loads (and consequently excessive frictional, as well as torsional loads) being applied to the dentition (Kerstein 1993). Intricate feedback mechanisms between the PDL, the tooth pulp (perhaps via mechanical stimulation of the intradental A-beta mechanorecptors from tooth deformation), and the Central Nervous System (CNS), lead to a neurogenic inflammatory response due to the torsional flexure within the dental pulp, which may manifest clinically as FDH (Coleman, Grippo, Kinderknecht, 2003, Pashley, 1990). It has been suggested that there is a neurologic influence upon the contraction and relaxation of the muscles of mastication resultant from pulpal stimulation, that likely results from the same tooth torsion and flexion (Sharaw, McGrath, & Dubner, 1982; Coleman, Grippo, & Kinderknecht, 2003).

Mechanosensory Theories

In these theories, external stimuli can cause dentinal fluid movements, and/or induce odontoblastic nerve complex responses, that represent a unique mechanosensory etiology to DH symptoms. In this theory, the odontoblasts are thought to act as sensor cells that elicit the pain of Dentinal Hypersensitivity (Chen et. al., 2003).

1. **The Stiletto Heel Effect:** Physical compression of the occlusal surface is thought to compress the sub-occlusal surface tissues, causing tubule expansion, and hence increased outward fluid flow. A "stiletto heel effect" is where a small surface area contact point will apply great pressure to the occlusal surface of a tooth, flexing the tooth into pain (Pashley, 1990).

A similar, more recent alternative mechanical theory of DH etiology was postulated in 2008.

2. **Strain Deformation Mechanism:** It was shown by using extracted bovine incisors, that a relationship existed between temperature distribution and tooth structure deformation (Linsuwanont et. al., 2008). Thermal stimuli applied to the labial enamel surface resulted in rapid, *almost instantaneous,* development of strain at the pulpal-dentine interface before any temperature change was detected at the DEJ (reducing the plausibility of exposed dentinal tubules as being solely etiologic for DH events). The strain pattern was biphasic; initially the heat produced a contraction of the pulpal surface, followed by an expansion. The reverse was found with cold stimulation. This dentine expansion or contraction suggested that temperature changes at the enamel might exert a physical

force that mechanically induced dentinal fluid flow long before the enamel was able to transmit a temperature change to the DEJ. In short, these researchers found that *mechanically induced deformation of tooth structure may trigger nerve impulses directly*, or may exert mechanically induced fluid flow that triggers nerve activity.

Thermal stimuli have also been hypothesized to cause mechanically induced dentin deformation at the pulpal wall (where most sensory structures are located), which could trigger nerve impulses directly. These theories imply that the physical and structural deformations of teeth directly trigger nerve impulses, and offer a possible alternative DH explanation to the Hydrodynamic Theory for intact teeth with no open dentinal tubules.

Section 7: Occlusion's Role in Muscular Temporomandibular Disorders and Dentinal Hypersensitivity

Modern dentistry typically attempts to control the following three pathologic processes and their effects on the masticatory system:

- Caries.
- Periodontal disease.
- Occlusal disease.

Occlusal disease is undoubtedly, the least understood of the three aforementioned disease processes, possibly due to the minimal exposure that a dental professional experiences during formal education. Continuing education courses offered to practitioners tend to combine an Occlusion curriculum with one on TMD analysis. Given the variability of the different occlusal "camps", it is no wonder why so few engaged in the practice of Dental Medicine, attempt to incorporate occlusal treatments into their everyday practice. This is not an excuse however, since all dentists should be occlusal experts because the functional interactions between opposing arches can wreck havoc with the Stomatognathic system, including causing symptoms of DH (Dawson, 2006). The widespread belief that TMD symptoms are exclusively caused by emotional stress is most likely a fallacy, because the removal of occlusally- related pain, such as is seen with DH, typically alleviates the psychosocial stress of this pain, and other related orofacial pains, including those associated with Temporomandibular disorders (Dawson, 2006).

Occlusal Contact Research and Dentinal Hypersensitivity

In 1987, experimental evidence reported that DH, in the presence of very small premature occlusal contacts (200 μm), and without any present periodontal symptoms, could be treated successfully with occlusal adjustment (Ikeda et. al., 1987). In 1998, the same author observed that light premature occlusal contact (less than 200 μm in height) was able to induce DH symptoms, both objectively using the Tooth Pain Threshold (TPT), and by subjective patient reporting (Ikeda, Nakano, Bando & Suzuki, 1998). These results provided objective data that described the magnitude of a tooth's pain threshold change. Removal of the high occlusal contact was associated with a return to the TPT baseline. The authors concluded that a light premature contact was potentially etiologic for DH, and that occlusal adjustment was the most effective treatment for it (Ikeda, Nakano, Bando & Suzuki, 1998).

Occlusion, Dentinal Hypersensitivity, and Muscular TMD

Parafunctional activities such as bruxism and clenching have been positively correlated with Temporomandibular disorders (Manfredini, et. al.., 2003; Choi, et. al.., 2002; Manschreck, 2009; Molina et. al., 2001; Casanova-Rosado, et. al., 2006; Jerjes, et. al., 2008; Yadav, 2011). DH was reported to be a chronic, often undiagnosed problem that affected many patients with bruxism (Manschreck, 2009). *DH was also one of the most frequently reported symptoms of bruxism* (Yadav, 2011; Jerjes, et. al., 2008; Manschreck, 2009). In a 2007 literature review, Kalamir et. al., reported that only 101 of the 172 papers reviewed, indicated that bruxism correlated to TMD symptoms (Kalamir, Pollard, Vitiello & Bonello 2007). The authors suggested that this variability was primarily due to the lack of a universally accepted definition for both TMD and bruxism, recommending that dental medicine abandon the terms, and replace them with a set of diagnostically appropriate descriptors. Choi et. al., in 2002 concluded in a study of over 27,000 nineteen year-old Korean military servicemen, that bruxism may not be a direct risk factor in TMD, but that the parafunctional clenching habit may be (Choi, Choung, Moon, & Kim, 2002). They found that those men who professed to having a clenching habit were 2.05 times more likely to have limited opening than did the non-habit group. This large study was unusual in that it consisted of males exclusively, whereas most other studies tend to favor a larger percentage of females than males (Choi, Choung, Moon, & Kim, 2002). Lastly, DH has been cited numerous times within the literature, to be a symptom of muscular TMD (Jerjes, et. al., 2008; Emodi-Perlman, et. al., 2008; Melchior, Mazzetto, & Felicio, 2012; Chuang, 2002; De Felicio, et. al., 2006). Manschreck, et. al., in 2009 cited increased DH as a major clinical screening indicator for bruxism, along with muscular facial and mandibular pain, headaches, and earaches (Manschreck, 2009).

Earlier, in 2000, another literature review found that there was little support for the role of occlusion in the management and prevention of signs and symptoms of TMD (DeBoever, Carlsson, & Klineberg, 2000). Manfredini, et. al., reported that bruxism had a stronger relationship with muscular Temporomandibular Disorders than with disk displacement and joint pathologies (Manfredini, Cantini, Romagnoli, & Bosco, 2003). Koh and Robinson concluded in their literature review that occlusal adjustment was not strongly correlated with effective treatment outcomes for TMD (Koh & Robinson, 2004). In a 2012 review article concerning dental occlusion, body posturing and TMD, four authors stated emphatically that occlusion and TMD issues were not related (Manfredini, Castroflorio, Perinetti, & Guarda-Nardini, 2012).

Conversely, high occlusal contacts of only a few microns in size, have been shown to cause TMD dysfunction (Andreson, Schulte, & Aeppli, 1993; Sharma, Rahul, Poduval, Shetty, Gupta, & Rajora 2013). In 1998, Kirveskari reported that numerous controlled clinical trials involving symptomatic subjects had yielded results that would be difficult to explain unless occlusal factors played a causal role in Temporomandibular Disorders. He strongly suggested that research efforts should be intensified to ascertain definitively, occlusion's role in causing muscular TMD symptoms (Kirveskari, 1997).

Ramjford supported the Neuromuscular Theory of DH and that occlusal interferences were a causative factor for TMD symptoms, by noting that regional pain associated with bruxism and myalgia was completely eliminated in subjects after undergoing occlusal equilibration (Bhat, 2010). This theory proposed that the occlusal interferences caused an altered proprioceptive feedback, leading to incoordination and spasm of some of the masticatory muscles (Ash & Ramfjord, 1995). Similarly, Kerstein during the past 25 years, using the T-Scan occlusal analysis technology and the Immediate Complete Anterior Development (ICAGD) coronoplasty protocol (as opposed to using a CR-based equilibration protocol), has presented compelling evidence that occlusion is definitely correlated to muscular TMD symptomotology (Kerstein & Farrel, 1989, Kerstein & Wright, 1991; Kerstein, 1995; Kerstein, Chapman, & Klein, 1997; Kerstein & Radke, 2006; Kerstein, 2010; Kerstein & Radke, 2012). To date, Kerstein's extensive research linking muscular TMD symptomotology to occlusion using digital occlusal analysis and electromyography (EMG) has yet to be replicated or challenged in a peer-reviewed scientific article (personal communication, 2012). In a retrospective study that spanned 17 years, the authors concluded that occlusal equilibration was an appropriate treatment for many cases of DH (Coleman, Grippo, & Kinderknecht, 2000). Finally, in a Canadian survey study, the majority of the dentists and dental hygienists identified *bruxism* and *malocclusion* as triggers for DH, despite neither being regularly identified by researchers, as a major causative DH factor. The authors mailed a questionnaire to 5,000 dentists and 3,000 dental hygienists, where 64% of the dentists and 77% of the hygienists cited bruxism and malocclusion as triggers for DH (Hypersensitivity, C.A.B.O.D., 2003). Other authors challenged the findings, stating that the responding professionals misidentified the etiology of DH, claiming that erosion and exposed tubules caused DH (Strassler & Serio, 2009). Perhaps there existed a condition whereby exposed dentin was not necessarily a prerequisite for DH symptomotology? As such, the surveyed dental health practitioners were likely describing frictionally induced DH (FDH).

Based upon the extensive literature that correlates DH to occlusal factors, muscle hyperactivity, and TMD symptoms, it is this author's contention that that excess frictional interactions that occur between opposing posterior teeth during occlusal function, results in excessive tooth flexure that creates localized FDH events. In the dentate individual, excessive occlusal forces can be generated by hyperactive masticatory muscles, such that decreasing muscular force through the elimination of occlusal interferences, would potentially quiesce FDH events. This chapter has, and will continue to present evidence, that strongly suggests occlusion not only has a significant role in the etiology and management of TMD, but in FDH symptoms, as well.

Section 8: Occlusal Adjustments, Both Old and New

As there seems to be little or no consensus in regards to occlusion's role in the genesis of both DH and TMD (Spranger, 1995; DeBoever, 2000), this widespread disagreement can most likely be attributed to:

- The use of subjectively interpreted occlusal contact marking indicators in the assessment of the occlusion.
- The subjective variable of the quality of the unmeasured occlusal adjustment procedures performed that are typically investigated.

Surprisingly, articulating ribbons have been scarcely studied in the literature. Paper markings are assumed to describe force and time simultaneity, although several researchers have found this assumption, which permeates dental education and daily practice, to be groundless (Rimondini et. al., 1995; Carossa et. al., 2000; Millstein & Maya, 2001; Carey et. al., 2007; Saad et. al., 2008). Studies have shown that paper mark size correlates with forceful contacts only 20 - 38.3% of the time (Qadeer et. al., 2012; Carey et. al., 2007). These recently published studies clearly indicate that the articulating ribbons are a subjective occlusal force detection method, rather than being an objective and accurate force and timing measurement tool. These studies *completely contradict* the ongoing, and widespread belief present throughout many disciplines of Dental Medicine, that articulating paper is a reliable and accurate force descriptor.

Predictable restorative dentistry requires the clinician to (Anderson & Schulte 1993):

- Objectively examine the occlusion.
- Record the occlusion.
- Store the occlusion.
- Transfer the occlusal information.

It is axiomatic that traditional occlusal waxes and articulating ink ribbons do not fulfill the above criterion. Dental professionals should by definition, be occlusal experts, and at the very least have an understanding of the basic TM joint and muscle dynamics that occur within the Stomatognathic system. In order to do so, clinicians must utilize objective, recordable, reproducible, and transferable data. A potential key to understanding that occlusal issues are related to TMD symptoms, would be to remove the subjective components (ribbons, waxes, non-reproducible occlusal adjustment procedures), and replace them with objective metrics (T-Scan 8 digital occlusal analysis) and occlusal adjustment methods that objectively measure physiologic occlusal endpoints, such as is prescribed in the ICAGD coronoplasty (Kerstein, 1992). If one cannot reproducibly measure an event, then it is by definition, an opinion. If one can measure an event reproducibly, then it is a fact.

An important variable that may account for the inability for researchers to consistently correlate occlusal contact patterns to TMD pathogenesis, is the lack of any occlusal measurement employed within existing studies. Alternatively, digital occlusal analysis *does* give the clinician the ability to identify and record the "when" (or timing), and the "how much" (or quantity of relative force) of all the occlusal contacts. The T-Scan software contains a database for patient occlusal data storage and recall, which allows the information to be transferred to other clinicians or researchers. Notably, there are a number of T-Scan-based studies that do definitively correlate occlusal contract patterns to the appearance of TMD symptomotology (Kerstein & Wright, 1991; Kerstein, 1995; Kerstein, Chapman, & Klein, 1997; Kerstein & Radke, 2006; Kerstein & Radke, 2012).

T-Scan 8 technology creates a "movie" of the intercuspation of the opposing teeth, in both centric and eccentric movements, which is recorded in 0.003 second-long increments, while simultaneously providing changing relative force data percentages of every occlusal contact present. This "movie" can be played back, analyzed, and used to identify aberrant frictional and/or mechanical engagements that teeth undergo during functional mandibular movements. As such, dynamic occlusal contact timing sequences and changing contact force percentages are *objectively* and *quantifiably* determined as they occur in real-time, which is in stark contrast to most unmeasured researched approaches that subjectively assess the occlusion with traditional, non-digital occlusal indicators.

A final variable that may account for the inability of investigators to consistently link occlusal issues to TMD symptoms, could lie within the differing mandibular positions advocated by the differing occlusal philosophies, as being "correct". Whole institutions and curriculums have been developed which revolve exclusively around these differing mandibular positional theories:

- **Centric Relation (CR):** The CR position can be determined by a number of methods including Bimanual Manipulation, designed to seat the condyles in the most superior anterior position within the glenoid fossa, with the articular discs interposed.
- **Neuromuscularly Obtained (NM):** This position is determined using TENS (Transcutaneous Electronic Nerve Stimulation), which postures the mandible down and forward from CR and MIP.

Electronically lessened muscular activity levels are employed to locate the mandibular position, instead of relying on anatomic TM Joint structure articulation.

- **The 4/7 Position:** An orthopedically obtained jaw relation that places the condyle/disc assembly out of the glenoid fossa on the slope of the articular eminence, slightly down and forward of Centric Relation and MIP.
- **Maximum Intercuspation (MIP):** Also known as Centric Occlusion (CO), This position is dictated by the teeth themselves, determined when the patient habitually self-closes into complete tooth intercuspation.

MIP has been deemed non-physiologic when dysfunctional symptoms exist, such that the other three mandibular relations have been advocated to employ, to resolve the symptoms resultant from the symptom appearances observed in MIP. This contention has never been scientifically validated. Contrarily to what has been advocated, several Occluso-Muscle Disorder symptom treatment studies exist (since 1991) that all were performed in the MIP position, and have demonstrated rapid and lasting symptom resolution that was obtained from treating specific occlusal force and timing factors in the MIP position (Kerstein & Wright 1991; Kerstein, 1995; Kerstein, Chapman, & Klein, 1997, Kerstein & Radke, 2006; Kerstein & Radke, 2012).

Occlusal Equilibration is an Unmeasured and Subjective Coronoplasty Procedure

In the literature, Occlusal Equilibration is the most frequently quoted and studied of the occlusal adjustment procedures (Jerjes et. al., 2008; Dawson, 2006). One could easily argue that Occlusal Equilibration is not an objectively measured procedure. It is based upon the Subjective Interpretation of articulating paper mark size and color depth, the perceived sound of solid occlusal contact, operator feel, dental assistant involvement, patient subjective occlusal feel, and clench testing, which are combined with the questionable reproducibility of the operator consistently performing Bimanual Manipulation to position the patient into Centric Relation (Kerstein, 2010). The process of traditional Occlusal Equilibration is therefore laden with a highly subjective protocol, whose correctness is based upon positioning the mandible in Centric Relation, and not on precision occlusal contact force and timing measured endpoints (Kerstein, 1993, Kerstein, 2010).

Alternative Occlusal Treatment Protocol: Disclusion Time Reduction with the ICAGD Coronoplasty

A less well known occlusal adjustment procedure termed Immediate Complete Anterior Guidance Development (ICAGD)(Kerstein & Wright, 1991; Kerstein, 1992; Kerstein 1993) is based upon a series of reproducible and precise steps following the objective computerized information gleaned from the T-Scan 8 computerized occlusal analysis technology. This process is objectively undertaken guided by measurement driven, occlusal force and timing data, with studied quantifiable, and physiologic known occlusal endpoints. ICAGD is employed within the MIP position that is self- achieved with patient habitual closure. Data collection and treatment are based upon where patients naturally and optimally function, absent of any iatrogenic mandibular manipulation or repositioning (Kerstein, 1992; Kerstein, 1993).

It has been described that the ICAGD coronoplasty procedure differs greatly from traditional Occlusal Equilibration in that ICAGD involves precise measurement of force and timing relating to *excursive* movements made from maximum intercuspation (MIP), rather than from Centric Relation (CR) (Kerstein, 1993).

ICAGD also differs greatly from the neuromuscular approach, in that the patient is treated in their MIP position and not from a TENS-determined mandibular relation. Muscular relaxation is obtained from within the patient's own physiology (as determined by pre and post treatment simultaneously recorded, electromyography data), and not from external electrical stimuli pulsing the muscle into a transient relaxed state (Kerstein, 1993; Kerstein, 2004; Kerstein & Radke, 2012).

Importantly, ICAGD does not rely upon preoperative models and the unknowns involved when transferring adjustments from articulated models to the mouth. The recorded pretreatment T-Scan data guides the coronoplasty that is performed in the mouth, where corrections can be immediately checked for occlusal parameter measured endpoint precision, thereby eliminating all of the subjectivity that unmeasured occlusal adjustments are fraught with.

The ICAGD procedure revolves around the measurement of the Disclusion Time (DT) (Kerstein & Wright, 1991). The DT measures *the amount of time* required for the posterior teeth to completely *frictionally* disengage during a mandibular excursion (Kerstein, 1993). This timing measurement is recordable only with the T-Scan system. These prolonged posterior tooth frictionally engaged time-durations are recorded and quantified with the T-Scan 8 sensor interposed, as the patient self-closes into MIP,

Table 1. Differences between traditional CR occlusal equilibration vs. ICAGD

	Equilibration	ICAGD
Armamentarium	ribbon/Shim stock	ribbon/T-Scan 8
Articulator	required	N/A
Diagnostic Casts	required	N/A
Pretreatment appliance use advisable (Splint)	yes	N/A
Goal	guided CR closure	timed immediate posterior disclusion
Initial adjustment step	centric relation (guided closure)	excursive movements from an unguided closure
Closure position	CR-CO coincident (guided closure)	CO anterior to CR and often to pre-treatment MIP (unguided)
Importance of lateral Interferences	potentially damaging forces placed on teeth	prolonged compression time of PDLs incites excess muscle activity
Importance of timing of The Anterior Guidance	not measured	measured, and must be immediate, & quantifiable ($\leq$0.41 seconds per excursion)
Changes in quantity of molar contact	increased	decreased
Specific quantifiable Occlusal endpoints	no	yes
Measurably reproducible	no	yes
Effect on masticatory Muscles	variable effects reported	decreased hyperactive masseter and temporalis muscles, statistically
Periodontal Ligament Influence	not considered a significant factor; it is most important to locate CR	Most important structural entity treated with ICAGD coronoplasty

holds their teeth in MIP for approximately 2 seconds, and then commences a lateral excursive movement as the mandibular teeth rub across the maxillary teeth, so that all excursive frictional interactions are recorded. From this protocol, both the Occlusion Time (the measured time duration from first contact made in closure to the initial moment of static and complete intercuspation; optimal OT ≤0.2 seconds) (Kerstein & Grundset, 2001), and the Disclusion Time (the measured time duration for posterior teeth to completely frictionally disengage during an excursion, until only anterior teeth exclusively control the remainder of the excursion; optimal ≤ 0.4 seconds), can be digitally quantified.

Kerstein has repeatedly demonstrated that prolonged Disclusion Time is intricately related to myogenous pain and symptoms (this author has repeatedly observed DH frequently accompanies myogenous symptoms since implementing ICAGD in 2008). Additionally, Kerstein has also repeatedly shown that when the ICAGD adjustment procedure is performed properly, requiring the utilization of the T-Scan technology to achieve precise, measured physiologic occlusal endpoints, the myogenous symptoms can be readily resolved and remain absent across passing time (Kerstein 1993; Kerstein, 1995). In a published 9-year recall study of 102 patients who had undergone ICAGD, statistically significant reductions in muscular TMD symptomotology for the subject group, were lasting from between 2-9 years post treatment (Kerstein, 1995).

Immediate Complete Anterior Guidance Development (ICAGD) is the coronoplasty procedure that clinically accomplishes the desired *Disclusion Time Reduction* (DTR). The T-Scan system aids the operator in both the isolation of, and the precise corrective reduction of, the prolonged excursive tooth-to-tooth occlusal surface frictional interactions. In clinical cases where there exists a lack of anterior tooth coupling, the posterior frictional durations cannot be properly shortened without damaging the involved posterior teeth from excessive coronoplasty. Here it becomes necessary to alter the anterior open contacts with additive restorative procedures, to couple the non-contacting anterior teeth, or alternatively employ orthodontic tooth movement to couple the non-contacting teeth. These restorative additions assist in creating an anterior guidance contact arrangement that will disengage the posterior teeth in ≤ 0.5 seconds per excursion (Kerstein, 1992). It should be noted that the bonded additions alone, will not routinely disclude the posterior teeth in the desired ≤0.5 second-long timeframe. To achieve that level of precision post treatment, the bonded additions must be followed directly with the clinician performing the ICAGD coronoplasty.

Although articulating ribbon is used to mark the teeth during ICAGD, the operator does not subjectively interpret its appearance, but instead only proceeds with adjustments after cross-matching the paper ink marks present on the frictionally involved teeth, with the recorded digital force and timing data. This greatly reduces a clinician's propensity to adjust false "high" and "low" force contacts present in both the centric and eccentric movements. Repeated articulating ribbon markings that are cross-referenced with follow-up T Scan data, are then targeted by the clinician by employing miniscule occlusal adjustments, to objectively and predictably accomplish a favorable post treatment Disclusion Time Reduction (Kerstein, 2010). Typically the excursions are adjusted *initially* (right, left, and protrusive) to reduce the DT ≤ 0.5 per excursion, after which the Occlusion Time is adjusted as needed to accomplish an OT of ≤0.2 seconds. Usually the OT automatically falls beneath this 0.2 second threshold, when the excursive occlusal adjustments have been properly refined to measure ≤ 0.5 seconds.

The excursive Disclusion Time (DT) has been shown to be extremely important in both elevating (when prolonged) and controlling (when properly shortened to ≤ 0.5seconds per excursion) levels of elevator muscle activity (Kerstein &Wright, 1991; Kerstein & Radke, 2006; Kerstein, 2010; Kerstein & Radke,

2012). In this author's experience, this prolonged excusive timing can also be consistently correlated with active DH symptoms. Excess frictional engagements seem to not only cause muscular hyperactivity, but also increase a tooth's lateral flexion. This flexion results from muscle overload, induced by prolonged PDL compressions that occurs simultaneously with the prolonged excursive frictional occlusal surface engagements (Kerstein, 1992; Kerstein, 2010, Kerstein & Radke, 2012).

Tooth flexion and deformation *over time*, contributes to the fracture of enamel crystals in the cervical region of teeth, as well as in the exposure of coronal and root surface dentin (Osborne-Smith, Burke, & Wilson, 1999), such that these abfracted lesions have been linked to DH symptoms (Mayhew, Jessee, & Martin, 1998, Ikeda, Nakano, Bando, & Suzuki, 1998). This excess lateroflexion is likely also *etiologic for FDH symptomatology* that appears clinically prior to any dentin exposure observed in the progression of the abfractive disease process.

Section 9: The Diagnosis and Traditional Clinical Management of Dental Hypersensitivity

Diagnosing Dental Hypersensitivity

DH is typically a diagnosis of exclusion, forcing a practitioner to eliminate other potential etiologies that present with similar symptomatology (Hypersensitivity C.A.B.O.D. 2003; van Loveren, 2013). Clinicians therefore, must *exclude* any alternative causes of the short and sharp dentinal pain, so as to make a correct DH diagnosis.

Alternate Conditions That Mimic Dentin Hypersensitivity

- Chipped, cracked or fractured teeth causing exposed dentin.
- Failing restorations.
- Post-operative vital bleaching sensitivity.
- Poorly placed dentin pins.
- Irreversible and reversible pulpal responses, to either caries and/or restorative treatment.
- Inappropriate application of various medicaments during cavity preparation.
- Cracked tooth syndrome, often in heavily restored teeth.
- Acute occlusal hyper-function of teeth.
- Palatogingival groove and other enamel invaginations.
- Ditching of restorative margins and surface wear on composites.
- Incorrect placement of dentine adhesives leading to nanoleakage.
- Caries.
- Metallic restorations placed without proper insulation.
- Congenitally open cementum-enamel junction.
- Hypoplastic enamel.
- Certain periodontal conditions that result in tissue loss and recession.
- Atypical facial Odontolgia.
- Transient post-operative restorative sensitivity.

Usually the reported history of DH alone may be clinically confounding (Davies, Gray, Linden, & James, 2001; Porto, Andrade, & Montes, 2009). As noted earlier, vital tooth bleaching may cause a reversible pulpitis (Byers, 1985; Swift, 2005). It is therefore necessary to ask the patient if they are actively bleaching their teeth during their DH reported oral history.

DH Clinical Diagnostic Testing

Traditionally, dentists have used an exploratory probe, or jets of air from a triple syringe sprayed onto the exposed root surface, to provoke a DH response from the patient (Gillam & Orchardson, 2006). Because unregulated air blasts have resulted in obtaining inconsistent results when clinicians attempt to assess DH, Coleman published a novel "Air Indexing" method, that could determine individual patient DH threshold responsiveness (Coleman & Kinderknecht, 2000). Regulated "puffs" of room temperature air, directed at the root from a distance of 0.5 cm, sprayed at a 45^0 angle to the long axis of the tooth, for 0.5 to 1 second long duration, can predictably grade a tooth's DH response. Prior sprayed air studies were far more subjectively accomplished, as unregulated amounts of air was sprayed in prolonged and variable blasts, which dehydrated dentin and caused an inconsistent, iatrogenically induced DH response. A detailed explanation of using the Air Indexing technique in the diagnosis of Cervical Dentinal Hypersensitivity, can be found in Chapter 9.

Although somewhat inconsistent, tactile stimulus using a probe has been considered one of the easiest and fastest methods available to diagnose suspected DH (Gillam & Orchardson, 2006). Of all the tested stimuli, cold has been reported to be the most problematic DH stimulus, and is routinely employed in clinical trials as the test stimulus. Cold water (more so than warm water) has been shown to elicit a very consistent DH response (Brännström, 1966: Kleinberg, Kaufman, & Confessore; 1990: Addy, 2000, Walters, 2005).

The severity of DH pain experienced in response to a known stimulus has been diagnostically quantified by several subjective pain assessment methods (Holland, Narhi, Addy, Gangarosa, & Orchardson 1997; Gillam & Orcardson, 2006):

- A Verbal Descriptive Scale (VDS) described by the subject as slight, moderate, or intense.
- A Behavior Rating Scale (BRS).
- A Visual Analogue Scale (VAS).
- A Numerical Scale (NS).

Of these, the Visual Analogue Scale (VAS) has been deemed a more reliable pain assessment method for clinical settings, when compared to the Verbal Rating Scale (Banos, Boshch, Canellas, Bassols, Ortega, & Bigorra, 1989). However, a separate study found that the Visual Analogue Scale and the Verbal Descriptive Scale were uncertain, subjective measurements of TMD pain, while the Numerical Scale was found to be the most objective pain reporting determination (Le Resche, Burgess, & Dworkin, 1988).

Traditional Treatments for Dentinal Hypersensitivity in Teeth With Exposed Dentin and Patent Dentinal Tubules

The majority of DH cases are thought to result from gingival recession and tooth erosion (Strassler, Drisko, & Alexander, 2008). What appears to be absent from the proposed pathogenesis however, is the possibility that excessively long frictional occlusal contacts may be potentially contributory to the observed recession and erosion. Regardless of the theoretical etiology, the two principal traditionally advocated treatment options are to desensitize the nerve (making it less responsive to stimulation), or to occlude the dentinal tubules (preventing fluid flow) (Marvin 2008).

- **Desensitize the Nerve:** This is accomplished by ionic diffusion, which increases the concentration of potassium ions that can act on pulpal nerve sensorial activity (Ling & Gillam, 1996; Porto, Andrade, & Montes, 2009). Typically, over the counter (OTC) medicaments and desensitizing toothpastes are applied to the tooth surface to create the needed ionic diffusion.
- **Occlusive Therapy that Seals Over the Open Dentinal Tubules:** This approach prevents fluid flow in and out of the involved teeth (Pashley 1986; Porto, Andrade, & Montes, 2009). Fluoride, oxalate, and chloride-containing agents are applied during professional desensitizing treatments.

Paine et. al., found that home use mouthwashes and dentifrices containing fluoride, potassium nitrate, and strontium acetate, helped reduce DH and prevent caries (Paine, Slots, & Rich, 1998). In contrast however, other authors report that despite the widespread use of fluoride dentifrices, no significant decrease in DH had been reported with fluoride applications (Gillam & Orchardson, 2006). Mild cases of DH seemed to respond (at least palliatively) to the above-listed traditional treatments when there exists exposed dentin.

It is this author's experience and clinical observation that in cases of FDH with or without exposed dentin, employing the ICAGD coronoplasty to accomplish a Disclusion Time Reduction (DTR), often improves DH symptomotology, even when traditional treatments are ineffective. This predictably occurs when the T-Scan confirms that the OT ≥ 0.2 seconds, and the DT is ≥ 0.5 seconds, and companion EMG data confirms the presence of masticatory muscle excursive hyperactivity. These clinical findings, when combined with the Results of an FDH Pilot Study (described below), support the premise that excessively long occlusal surface frictional engagements are etiologic for DH, and that the ICAGD coronoplasty is a viable and predictable treatment option for DH symptoms.

Diagnostic Criteria for Utilizing ICAGD in the Treatment of Dentin Hypersensitivity

The following criteria can aid the clinician in determining if ICAGD may be applied in the treatment of DH:

- Chronic history of DH symptomotology.
- Positive response to cold water swish (transient sharp pain).
- FDH/DTR Scaling questionnaire (below) suggestive of DH and accompanying Occlusal Muscle Disorder (OMD).
- Non-responsiveness to previous traditional DH treatments, with or without exposed dentin.

- Disclusion Time (DT) recordings illustrating a DT that is $\geq$0.5 seconds, and the DH sensitive teeth are exhibiting some of the prolonged excursive contacts.
- Occlusion Time (OT) recordings illustrating an OT that is $\geq$0.2 seconds (measured from the time-moment of first tooth contact until the patient achieves static intercuspation).

Section 10: The Use of Computer-Guided Occlusal Analysis and Therapy in the Treatment of Frictional Dental Hypersensitivity

This portion of the chapter will describe a Pilot Study in which frictional occlusal factors are central to the symptom appearances observed in FDH patients. This study illustrates that treating the occlusion with precisely timed *computer-guided* occlusal adjustments that are non-subjective, can resolve DH symptomotology predictably. This study is, as of yet unpublished, such that this chapter will be the first reporting of this author's' T-Scan-guided DH treatment findings.

The Specific Aims of this study were to try to correlate FDH improvements in DH sensitive patients using the ICAGD coronoplasty as the sole treatment for the DH condition. Occlusal and muscular improvements from the ICAGD treatment, were monitored with the T-Scan 8/BioEMG III synchronization module (Tekscan, Inc. S. Boston, MA; Bioresearch Assoc., Milwaukee, WI, USA)

Genesis of the FDH Study

In an ongoing practice of General Dentistry, the author noticed that when performing the ICAGD coronoplasty to accomplish DTR on Occluso-muscle Disorder patients, that often the initial adjustments accomplished with high speed burs and water and air irrigation, would result in the patient experiencing *short, sharp painful moments consistent with DH.* As these initial adjustments were followed in the same patient visit by other T-Scan guided excursive friction corrections, *the DH symptoms would abate often by mid-treatment,* despite the clinician using the same high speed burs, with similar air and water irrigation, regardless of whether or not there existed pre treatment exposed dentin. As the ICAGD procedure progressed, many patients reported that they no longer felt uncomfortable with the air and water spray touching their teeth, which was in stark contrast to what they had reported a few minutes prior.

At subsequent recall appointments, many of these same patients would not only present with a significant improvement in their muscular TMD symptomotology, but also *a profoundly decreased incidence of DH symptomotology*. Many patients did not even consciously realize that they had DH symptoms until the symptoms were relieved following undergoing the DTR treatment. Other patients reported being able to drink cold beverages, consume ice cream, and even enjoy a popsicle, which were foods they had not been able to comfortably consume prior to undergoing the DTR treatment. Such repeated clinical observations made over a 2-year period prompted this author to undertake a pilot study, to assess Disclusion Time Reduction's effect on chronic DH symptomotology.

Material and Method

Thirty-two patients with ongoing DH symptoms were asked to participate in the study that was conducted in a private practice setting. This study was conducted over a 6-month period of observation that included male and female patients, ranging in age between 16 to 75 years.

The subject inclusion criteria were:

- A history of ongoing DH symptoms (positive transient sharp and painful cold water swish)
- Class I occlusal classification with anterior coupling or near coupling
- A lack of caries, immediate restorative, or periodontal needs
- No history of locking TMJ's
- The ability to open > 30mm vertically
- Piper Classifications 1, 2, 3a, 3b, 4a (Droter, 2005), as diagnosed with Joint Vibration Analysis (JVA, Bioresearch Assoc., Milwaukee, WI, USA – see Chapter 6) in combination with clinical TM joint findings limited to solely popping or clicking
- History of Occluso-muscular Disorder chronic symptomotology

The subject exclusion criteria were:

- A Class II or III malocclusion with poor anterior tooth coupling or anterior open bite
- Large open canine contact
- A deep overbite
- Patients with a history of open-flap periodontal surgery
- Confirmed or suspected carious, endodontically involved, or periodontally compromised teeth
- Piper Classification 4b, 5a or 5b, diagnosed with Joint Vibration Analysis and clinical data interpretation (these Piper classifications represent typically unstable and adapting Temporomandibular joints)
- Inability to open >30mm
- Significant deviation upon opening and concurrent facial asymmetry
- Prior history of TM Joint surgery

Potential participants that met the inclusion criteria were informed of the known complications of DTR and ICAGD (Kerstein, 2002; Kerstein, 2010) before undergoing any occlusal treatment, after which they signed a Consent Form. They were given the opportunity to query the dental practitioner about ICAGD, and also had the opportunity to reject participation within the study for any reason.

FDH/DTR Scaling Questionnaire: A Hybrid Visual Analog Scale and Numerical Scale (VAS/NS) Used to Assess Patient Subjective Perceptions about Dentinal Hypersensitivity and Masticatory Muscle Hyperactivity

To measure a patient's rapid and transient DH response to ice cold water and latent masticatory muscle hyperactivity symptomotology, a combination Tooth Sensitivity Pain Scale (with an integrated hybrid Visual Analog Scale (VAS) and Numerical Scale (NS)) and a Muscular Hyperactivity questionnaire was created by the author (see Appendix). The FDH study included subjects who completed a non-treatment day diagnostic scale, a pre-operative treatment day scale, and a post-operative treatment result scale, that together assessed the patients hypersensitivity and masticatory muscle resolution to the ICAGD/DTR treatment.

The pre-treatment questionnaire was given with a *5 second long cold ice water swish test* helped to identify patients that might benefit from the ICAGD/DTR treatment, while this same questionnaire and ice water swish post-operatively, served as a follow-up re-evaluation tool.

The first section (A) of the questionnaire used a hybrid visual analog scale (VAS)/numerical scale (NS) to determine the patient's subjective assessment of their DH, based upon an intraoral cold ice water swish. The initial diagnostic cold water swish was followed by a 2nd five second long ice water swish that occurred minutes prior to commencing ICAGD/DTR on the day that the treatment was to be rendered. This repeated cold water swish confirmed the previous DH response, as each patient acted as his or her own control. A third cold water swish and questionnaire was given post treatment on the day of treatment, to re-assess the patient's condition after undergoing the ICAGD/DTR treatment, and when possible, in the authors private practice setting, weeks or months later.

The second section, (B), of the questionnaire identified the presence of signs and symptoms of occlusally related disease, including masticatory muscle hyperactivity. The third section (C) served to identify dental concerns such as endodontic and intracapsular disease states that would be less likely to be respond to computer-aided occlusal adjustment treatment. Individuals that presented with DH and numerous "yes" responses to the (B) section, with few to no responses in the (C) section, underwent additional evaluation consisting of a Joint Vibration Analysis, muscle palpation, a range of motion assessment, and T-Scan 8/BioEMG III recordings of their Occlusion and Disclusion Times, to confirm their applicability for the study.

Joint Vibration Analysis (JVA)

Joint Vibration Analysis (JVA, Bioresearch Associates, Milwaukee, WI, USA) is a TM joint screening tool that assesses of the health of the cartilaginous Temporomandibular Joint discs *while in function* (see Chapter 6). JVA records vibrations within the TM joints, which are displayed in proprietary software for analysis (Figure 4). Vibration-less readings generally coincide with healthy intracapsular cartilage. Vibration-laden readings indicate with less healthy TMJ cartilage. This data can be correlated with known stages of TM joint damage (gleaned from actual TM surgical correlations), and with Pipers' classification of the TM joints (Ishigaki, Bessette, & Maruyama 1994; Droter 2005). The recorded vibration values are cross-referenced to a flowchart that aids the clinician in diagnosing various TM joint conditions.

JVA has been shown to be an effective method of determining whether cartilage damage exists in the TM Joints, before the commencement of any clinical treatment (Mazzeto, Hotta, & Mazzetto, 2009). The importance of the JVA screening is that it helps to determine the likelihood that the subjects occlusion will predictably maintain an occlusal alteration, due to a digitally verified set of stable and adapted temporomandibular joints. If both TMJ's are identified as having little to no internal structural damage, the discs are likely stable and adapted such that the clinician will most probably have predictable success with the ICAGD procedure. If the discs are unstable and non-adapted, or structural damage has evolved beyond solely soft tissue displacement type (based upon JVA interpretation), altering the occlusion could be potentially problematic. Here the TMJ's are likely to remodel, with resultant changes of the hinge axis during the disc's structural adaptation, which can alter the mandibular closure and excursive paths over time, also altering the occlusion in the process. An example of a JVA recording is presented in Figure 5.

Muscle Palpation

Intraoral palpation of the lower head of the lateral pterygoid muscle has been included in study protocols and examinations of the masticatory system, as has the extra oral palpation of the anterior belly of the temporalis, and the superficial belly of the masseter muscles (Jerjes, Upile, Abbas, Kafas, Vourvachis,

Figure 4. The JVA headset is placed over the bilateral Temporomandibular joints (TMJ's), to detect vibrational energies emanating from both TMJ capsules.

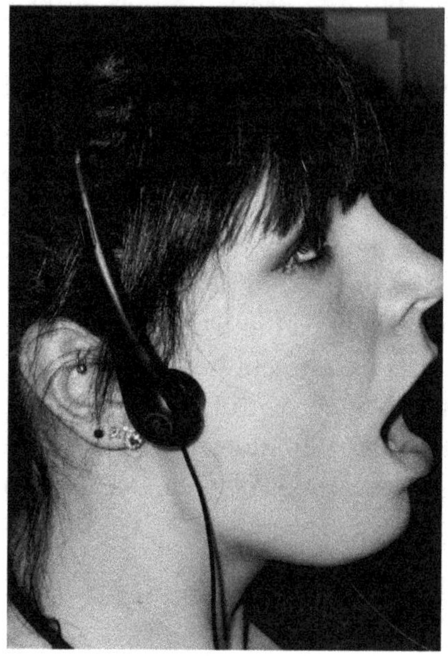

Figure 5. Sample pre-operative JVA Recording where the top of the sine wave (labeled C in green for closed) signifies complete intercuspation, and the bottom of the sine wave (labeled O in green for open) signifies maximum opening. This closure was repeated six times while an average of the waveform energy was computed within the JVA software. This trace indicated that the right TM joint appeared within normal limits, while the left TM joint vibrations indicated ligament laxity, or partial disc displacement with reduction. This patient could be included within the pilot study, as there were no significant internal derangements

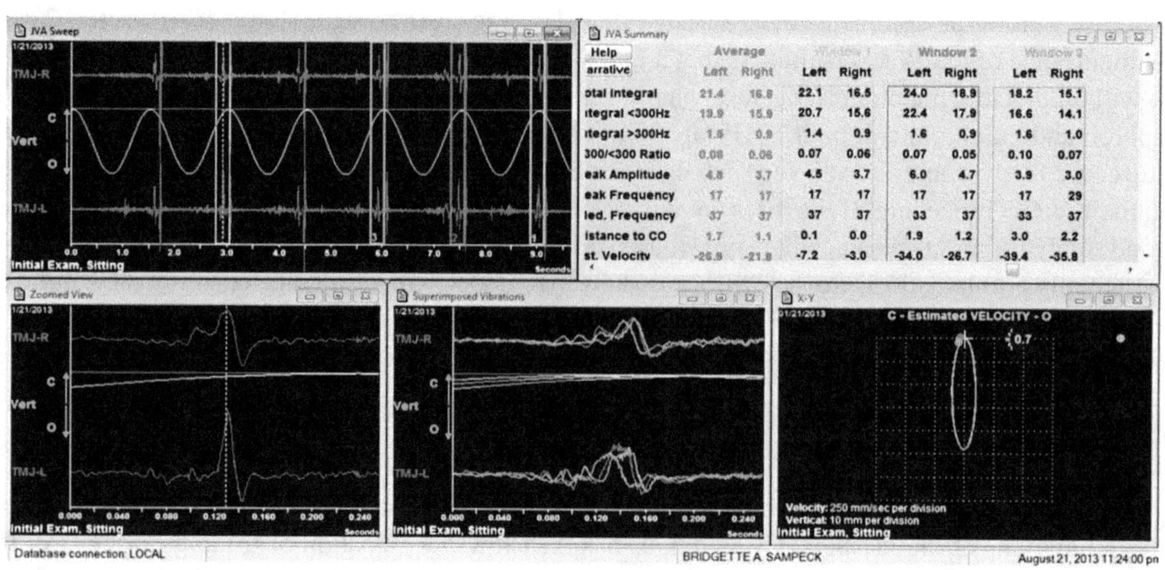

& Hopper, 2008; Tarantola, Becker, Gremiilion, & Pink, 1998). Palpation is by far the most common method of assessing myofascial pain sensitivity (Ekberg & Nilner, 2006; Tarantola, Becker, Gremiilion & Pink, 1998). Therefore within the study protocol, elevator and accessory muscles of mastication (including the neck muscles) were palpated. A positive tenderness response although subjective, was considered highly suggestive of a muscular disorder (Figures 6, 7, and 8).

Range of Motion (ROM)

Manual measurements of each patient's vertical range of motion were obtained. Values > 30mm allowed for inclusion in the study, with values > 40mm considered optimal. Any detected deviation upon opening was not considered problematic unless the deviation remained present through to full opening. A full opening deviation is highly consistent with an intracapsular disorder that is not likely to resolve predictably with ICAGD/DTR therapy (Kerstein, 1995).

The T-Scan 8/BioEMG III Evaluation

The T-Scan 8/BioEMG III (Figure 9) was used to measure the occlusal contact pattern and (at a minimum) the bilateral masseter and anterior temporalis muscle activity response to those occlusal contacts. On occasion when treating muscular TMD, the accessory muscles of mastication were also studied using EMG. The accessory muscles included the bilateral sternocleidomastoid, digastric, and the trapezius muscles. For an FDH pre treatment analysis, it has been this author's experience that only the masseter (MM) and temporalis (TA) muscles are necessary to analyze.

The T-Scan/EMG combination system was then employed diagnostically, to confirm the presence of excursive muscular hyperactivity (Kerstein, 2004, Kerstein, 2010; Kerstein & Radke, 2012). Hyperactive excursive EMG data combined with near normal JVA interpretation, muscle tenderness during palpation, a > 30 mm range of motion, and a FDH/DTR Scaling Questionnaire suggestive of FDH with or without exposed dentin confirmed the need for implementing ICAGD/DTR treatment. Patients who met these specific criteria were included in the Pilot Study, and ultimately underwent the ICAGD coronoplasty.

Figure 6. Clinical extraoral palpation of the right and left anterior temporalis muscles

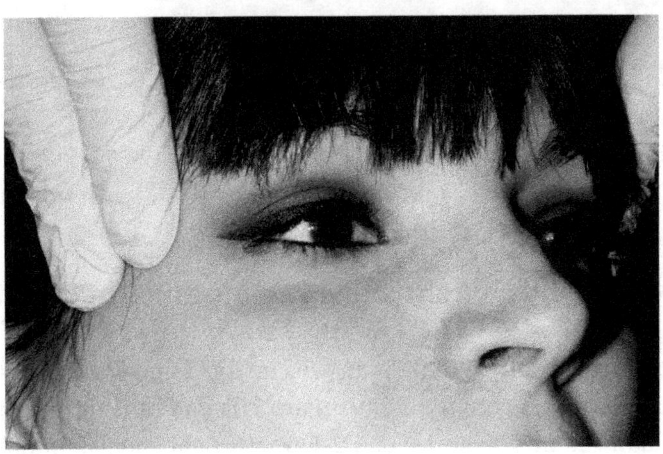

Figure 7. Palpation of the superficial right masseter muscle

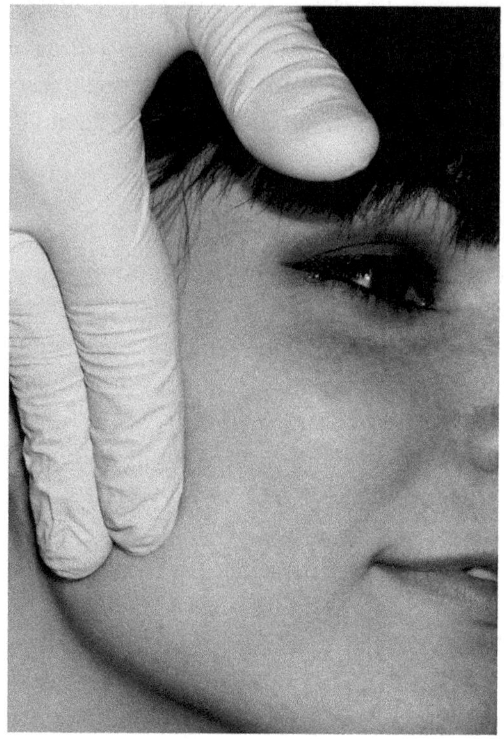

Figure 8. Intraoral palpation of the left inferior belly of the lateral pterygoid muscle. Tenderness is common in patients with masticatory muscle hyperactivity, and often resolves following ICAGD/DTR treatment

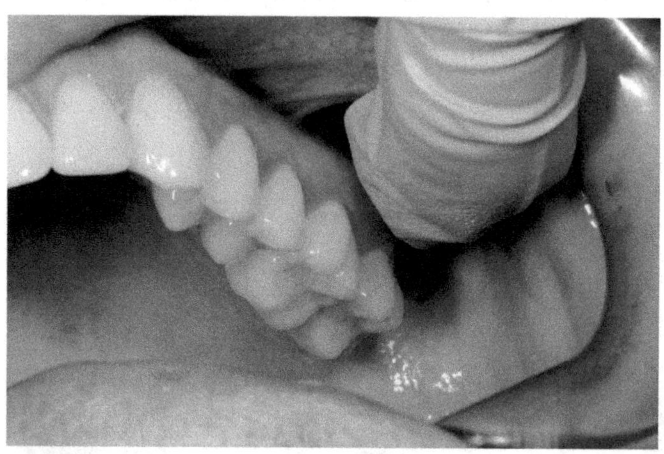

T-Scan 8/Electromyography Synchronization Module Interpretation

Figures 10 a and b illustrates an example of T-Scan Disclusion Time data (Figure 10a and b; left pane) synchronized with BioEMG muscle activity data (Figure 10a and b; right pane) from the same patient illustrated in the JVA data of Figure 5. The T-Scan 2-Dimensional and 3-Dimensional ForceViews (up-

Figure 9. The BioEMG III system can study the superficial bellies of up to 4 bilateral muscle pairs. The anterior temporalis and masseter muscles are routinely studied, whereas only two of three accessory muscle groups can be studied, dependent upon the patients' symptomotology

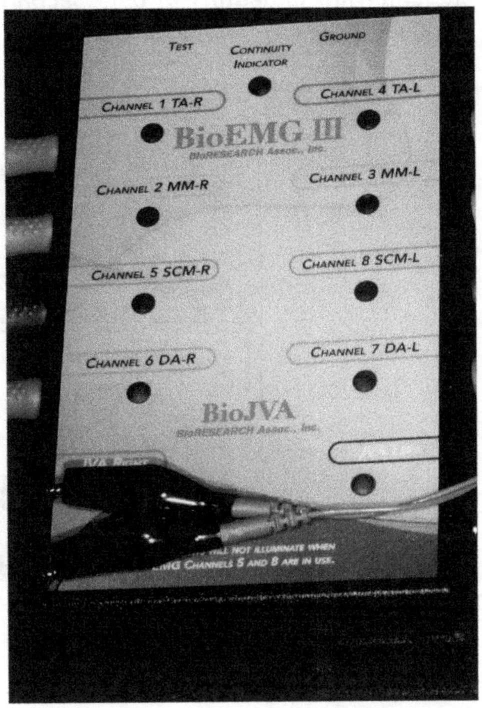

per T-Scan pane) and the temporalis and masseter EMG horizontal bar graph (lower EMG pane), both illustrate a particular recorded instant. Whereas the T-Scan Force vs. Time graph (lower T-Scan pane) and the upper EMG waveform pane illustrates the entire recorded event from initial closure into MIP, through to the commencement and execution of a right excursion. During the initial closure, the patient required 0.44 seconds to reach MIP (A-B), after making the initial tooth contact at A (T-Scan Timing pane). The T-Scan software indicated that the OT is not healthy, being twice as long as physiologic (OT $\leq$ 0.2 seconds). The patient then clenched their teeth firmly together for approximately 1.0 seconds (from line B up to line C in both data sets), before making a right excursion that began at the C line. The excursion evolved for 0.34 seconds (DT = 0.34 seconds), after which only the anterior teeth contact, and no posterior teeth remained in contact (at the D line). In the T-Scan Force vs. Time graph after C (bottom T-Scan pane), the Total force generated decreased (the black line dropped) when the patient disengaged their teeth to move into the excursion. Note that the left temporalis muscle is hyperactive after the C line (EMG upper pane) which is an unusual occurrence, as the non-working temporalis muscle routinely will shut down at line C when the mandible commences an excursion to the opposite side of the head. If this patient demonstrated short left excursive Disclusion Time ($\leq$ 0.5 seconds), then only the prolonged Occlusion Time would be treated to lessen any FDH responsive teeth.

Figure 10a. The T-Scan/EMG desktop at MIP (0.119 seconds after activation of the recording) of the patient described in Figure 5, just before a subsequent right excursive movement was made. The occlusal force and timing data (left pane) sits side-by-side with the synchronized EMG data (right pane). The Occlusion Time is prolonged, and somewhat unhealthy at 0.44 seconds duration. However, the right Disclusion Time is 0.34 seconds long, which is well under the 0.5 second-long physiologic, healthy limit

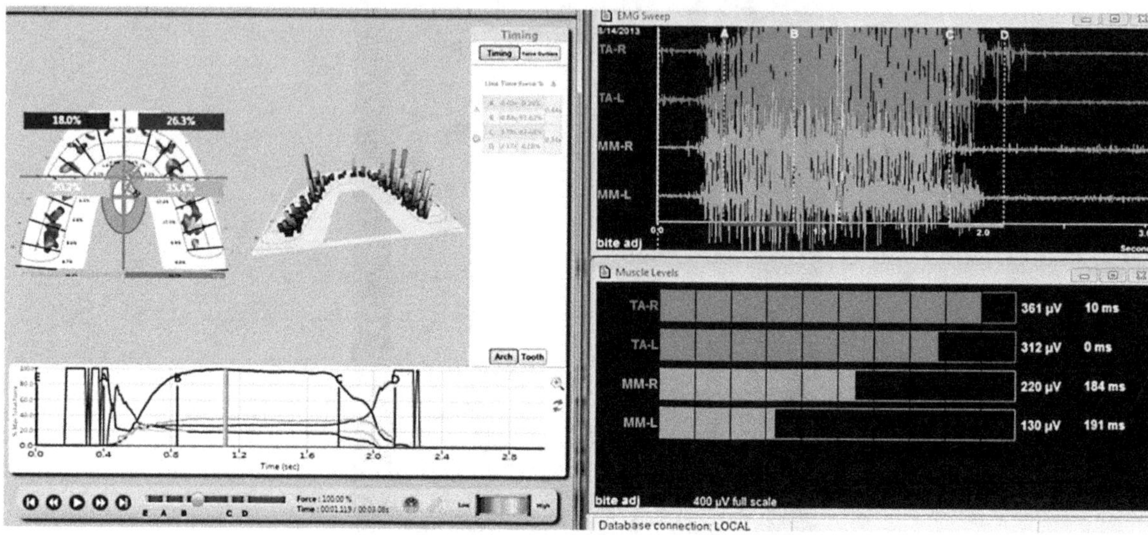

Figure 10b. The same data as in Figure 10a, with labeling to expedite interpretation of both the occlusal function and the muscular response to the occlusal function

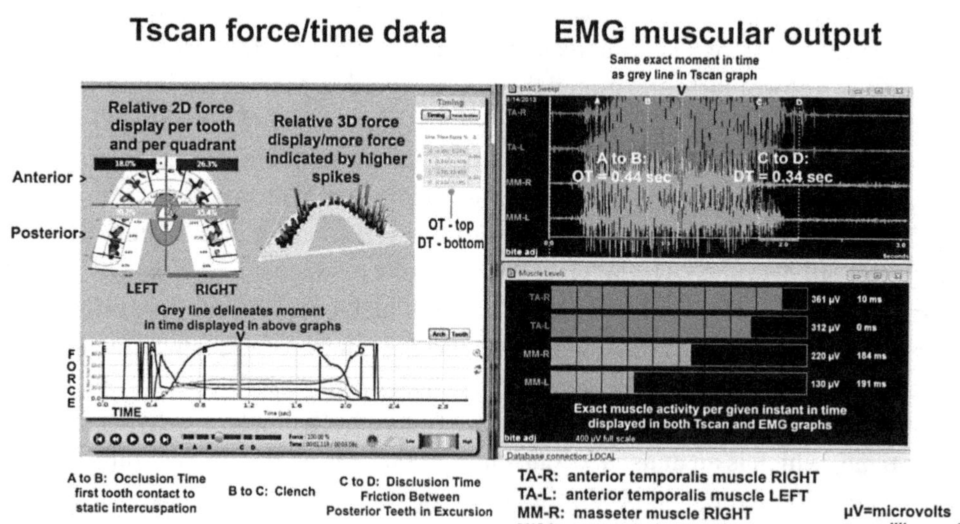

Interpretation of the EMG Portion of T-Scan/EMG Data

The surface electrodes applied to the skin over the bulk muscle detect microvoltage discharge made by the muscle during contractions. Resting muscles report lower microvolt readings than do working muscles, but there is always a muscle tonus present and micro-electrical discharge evident even in the resting state. In general, when the T-Scan/EMG data illustrates readings of less than 8-10 μv present in the elevator muscles (the anterior temporalis and the masseter), the elevators are considered as resting, while less than 2-4 μv is considered resting for the accessory muscles (the anterior digastric, sternocleidomastoid, and trapezius muscles). Microvolt readings that are greater than these resting values would signify that the involved muscle is hyperactive, even in the resting state (resting state assumes that the patients muscles of mastication are in a clinical baseline and in an non-contracted state).

When the BioEMG is utilized alone (without the T-Scan 8 synchronization), it will likely report slightly lower muscle activity values than when the BioEMG is synchronized with the T-Scan. The synchronized version functions slightly differently than when the EMG operates alone because the EMG Time cursor, when synchronized with the T-scan, is narrowed to approximate the *time-width* of a single T-Scan movie frame. A wider time-width provides more of an average of the muscle activity levels present, whereas a narrower time-width will more closely report sudden increases and decreases present within the recorded EMG data. Thus, with a narrower time-width, the peaks will appear higher and the valleys will appear lower. There is an Option in the EMG synchronization, which allows the clinician to analyze the EMG portion of a T-Scan/EMG recording, as if it were recorded separately [Go to *Options*, and select *Switch Display Mode* (personal communication with Mr. John Radke of Bioresearch Associates, Milwaukee WI, USA).

Performing the ICAGD Coronoplasty

The ICAGD technique is described in detail, in Chapter 7

The necessary armamentarium for ICAGD is:

- **Subtractive Phase:** Universally performed in an incremental fashion, which is directed with new and repeated T-Scan/EMG recorded data every few minutes to verify the progress and correctness of the coronoplasty:
    - T-Scan 8/BioEMG III.
    - Coarse round diamond bur for initial coronoplasty.
    - Fine round diamond and rubber cups for final polishing.
    - Accufilm II articulating ribbon (Parkell, Inc. Farmingdale, NY, USA).
- **Additive Phase:** (Figure 11) Performed *when* canine or anterior contact does not exist, or is worn away such that conservative subtractive measures alone cannot reduce the DT values below 0.5 seconds:
- T-Scan 8/BioEMG III.
- Accufilm articulating ribbon.
- Composite bonding system that combines good esthetics with physical load resistance when used to re-tip incisal edges of canines and/or anterior teeth (used to restore the lost, or absent canine guidance).

Figure 11. Beginning of application of composite to a left maxillary canine to facilitate a shorter (faster) Disclusion Time for this patient. Incisal-facial-lingual composite is bonded to place, if the Disclusion Time is not below 0.5 seconds after the subtractive phase of ICAGD has been properly completed

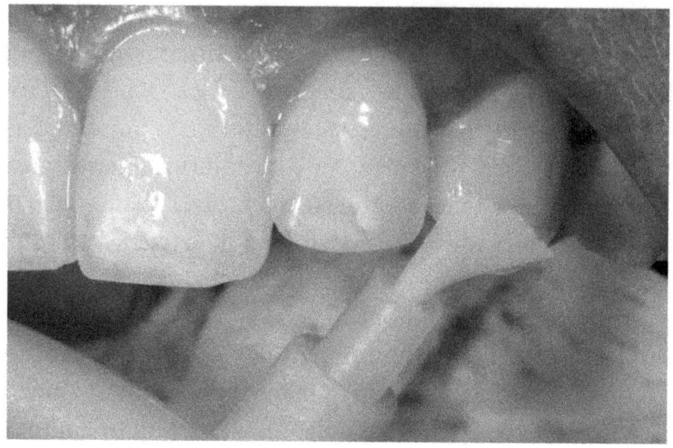

CASE REPORT

T-Scan 8/EMG Diagnostic Recordings of an Occluso-Muscle Disorder Patient Who Demonstrates FDH

In the below FDH case report of a pilot study patient, for brevity only the right excursive functional data is presented, although both the right and left excursions were treated. The figures and captions will sequentially describe the case details.

Data Acquisition Phase

- **Chief Complaint:** "My cheek muscles are usually very sore, especially by the end of the day. I can't chew gum or eat crunchy foods. I think I clench and grind my teeth at night, too. Two of my old dentists each made me a bite splint, and those did not help at all. Sometimes, I think wearing them even made me worse… I also have a hard time drinking and eating cold things like ice cream and it drives me crazy! I miss not being able to drink iced tea and eat ice cream more than you know!"
- **Medical History:** Non-contributory
- **Dental History:** History of orthodontic treatment 15 years prior. No periodontal treatments experienced, or pathology present. No restorative needs. Three composite fillings and one porcelain crown were present in good repair.
- **Questionnaire & Cold Water Swish:** The patient reported on the Tooth Sensitivity Pain Scale (the 1st section of FDH/DTR Scaling Questionnaire), a 6 out of 10 DH response to the ice cold water swish. The patient described the DH as being a sharp, generalized and transient pain. The same DH response was noted at both the diagnostic appointment and the pre-operative appointment. These findings indicated the likelihood of occlusally activated FDH.
- **JVA Findings:** (Figure 13)

Figure 12. Facial retracted pre-operative view of patient in MIP

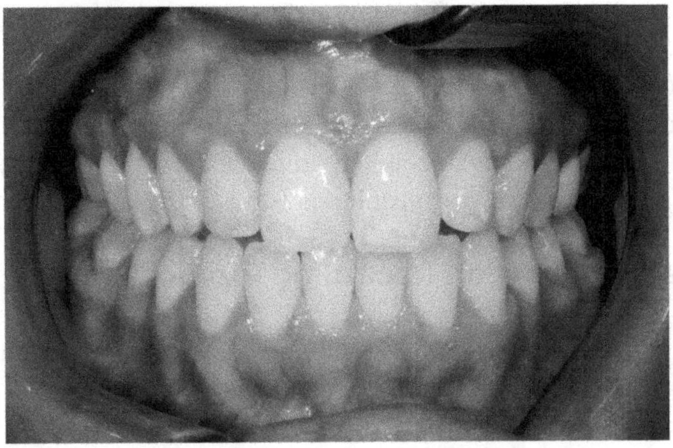

- **Right TMJ:** Piper 4a indicative of chronic adapted disc displacement with reduction (DDR)
- **Left TMJ:** Piper 4a indicative of chronic adapted disc displacement with reduction (DDR)

Notes: The abnormal vibrations in both TM Joints occurred at full opening, bilaterally.

Muscle Palpation Findings -
Left Anterior Temporalis: tender
Right Anterior Temporalis: tender
Left Masseter: tender
Right Masseter: normal

Figure 13. Pre-operative JVA data suggestive of bilateral chronic adapted disc displacement with reduction (DDR)

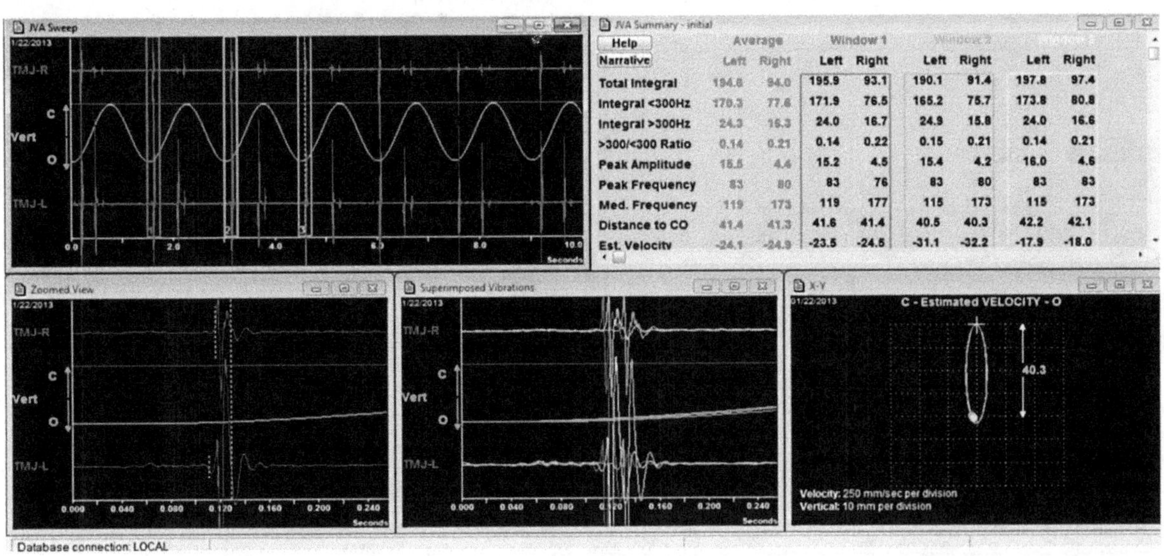

Left Inferior Belly Lateral Pterygoid: tender
Right Inferior Belly Lateral Pterygoid: tender
Vertical ROM - 40 mm with no deviation
Preliminary evaluation of the anterior teeth -
The patient presented with slight incisal edge wear visible on all four canine teeth. The maxillary canines were more worn than their mandibular counterpart teeth, but no exposed dentin was visible on any tooth. 1-2 mm of facial recession was apparent on teeth #'s 5 and 30.

Right Excursive Data Acquisition Recording Protocol

The patient was trained to perform proper right excursive movements commenced from MIP prior to capturing any definitive T-Scan/EMG data. The patient was then instructed to self occlude into MIP and clench their teeth together for 1-2 seconds, before commencing an unguided right excursive movement that continued until the posterior teeth were completely separated, and only anterior teeth were in contact (Figures 14, 15, 16, 17 & 18). The resultant data generated was assessed for proper A/B/C/D line placement to study the Occlusion Time (A-B timing), the Disclusion Time (C-D timing), and the presence of excursive muscular hyperactivity (within the EMG data between C-D).

It should be noted that in a physiologic, efficient, and ideal right excursive movement, the right anterior temporalis should do most of the work, while the left anterior temporalis and both masseter muscles should relax shortly after C, and stay relaxed throughout the remainder of the excursive movement.

Right Excursive Data Analysis

The OT in this patient is relatively fast and healthy at 0.2 seconds, and the relative force percentages are fairly well distributed between quadrants. However, the DT = 0.95 seconds, such that this patient was experiencing tension in the left masseter muscle (MM-L), and the right and left temple muscles (TA-R & TA-L).

Figure 14. Right excursion at MIP, 1.389 seconds into the recording

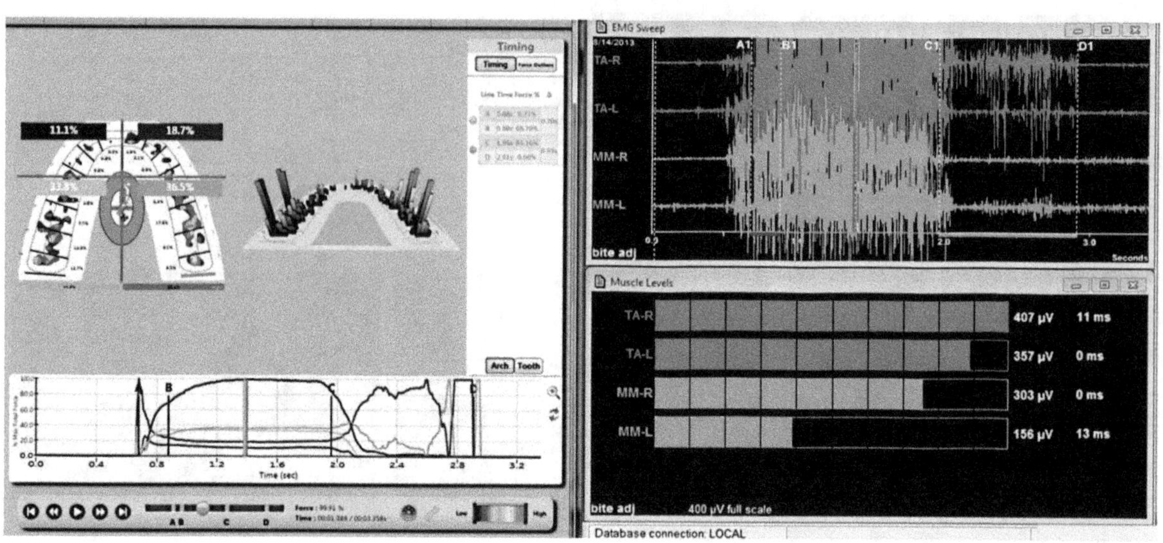

Figure 15. Right excursion, just past the C line at 2.019 seconds

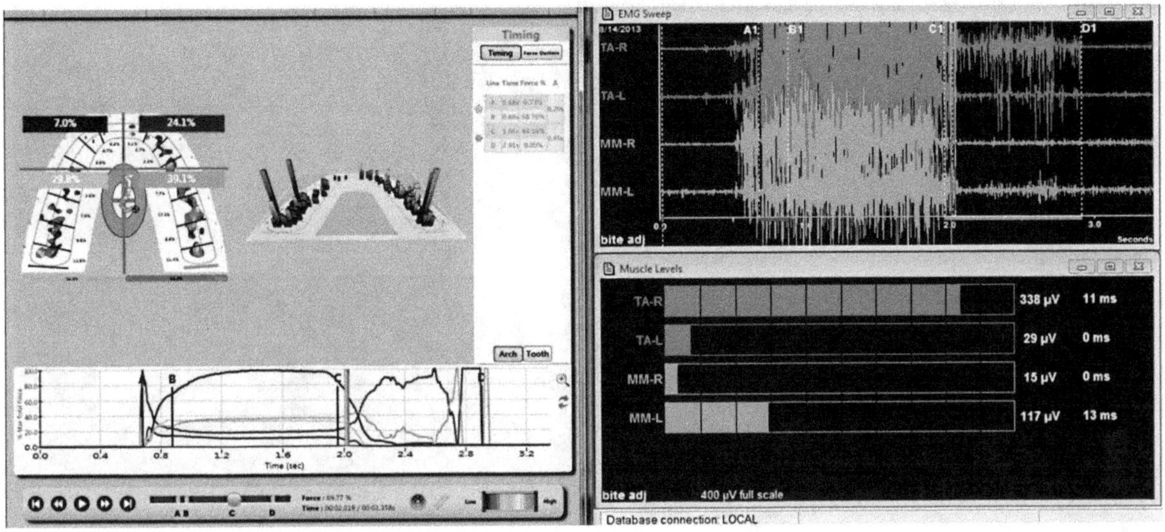

As the patient leaves MIP and begins the right excursion, notice the 2 relative occlusal force spikes present on the left side of the T-Scan 3-Dimensional Force View signifying excessive friction is present in the left posterior quadrant, which has heightened the left masseter muscle activity levels (MM-L). The right anterior temporalis (TA-R) is working (as it should be) during the right excursion. But the left temporalis should be resting below 8μv, but is elevated at 29μv. Note that the left masseter is very hyperactive at 117μv, and both the TA-L and MM-L are also hyperactive after C. Both of these muscles should be resting during in the right excursion.

This MM-L and TA-L hyperactivity is due to excessive friction occurring at this point *in time* into the excursion. This excessive hyperactivity is what causes excessive torsional flexing of the involved posterior teeth, resulting in FDH symptoms.

Slightly later, excess force still remains on the right posterior teeth, but the friction on the left molars has decreased considerably. Due to the left side decrease in friction, the left masseter has calmed considerably, as has the left temporalis. This relaxed state is short lived however, as the excessive friction reappears in less than 0.3 seconds more, as the patient moves further to the right (Figure 17).

At 2.408 seconds, notice that 83% of the force lies solely in the right anterior quadrant, which is a positive occurrence. There remains however, 17% of the force present on the working side posterior teeth, which results in a large increase in left temporalis electrical output (note the increase to 81 μv in the TA-L, up from 11μv only 0.1 second before. The left masseter also increases its output slightly (23μv). This 17% force present in the right posterior quadrant has resulted in a huge increase in muscular hyperactivity, and excessive torsional flexure of the involved teeth.

0.5 second later into the right excursion nearing its end, the left temporalis should be resting near the 8uv range, but instead, it is 4 times higher resting at 30 μv, despite that no posterior working or balancing frictional engagements are present. The left masseter is twice as active as it should be, demonstrating at 21 μv rather than the resting in the 8-10 μv range. This hyperactivity overwhelms the capability of aerobic metabolism to produce enough ATP (Adenosine Tri Phosphate), which leads to excess lactic acid accumulation and subsequent muscular ischemia, with the resultant manifestation of muscular TMD symptoms.

Figure 16. Right excursion further past the C line at 2.089 seconds

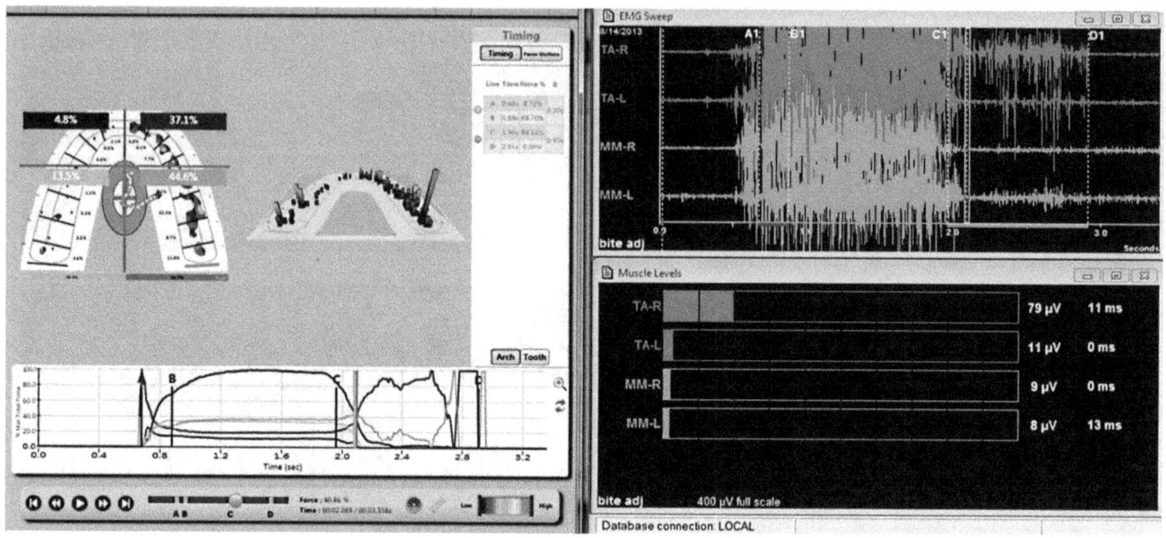

Figure 17. Right excursion further past C line at 2.408 seconds

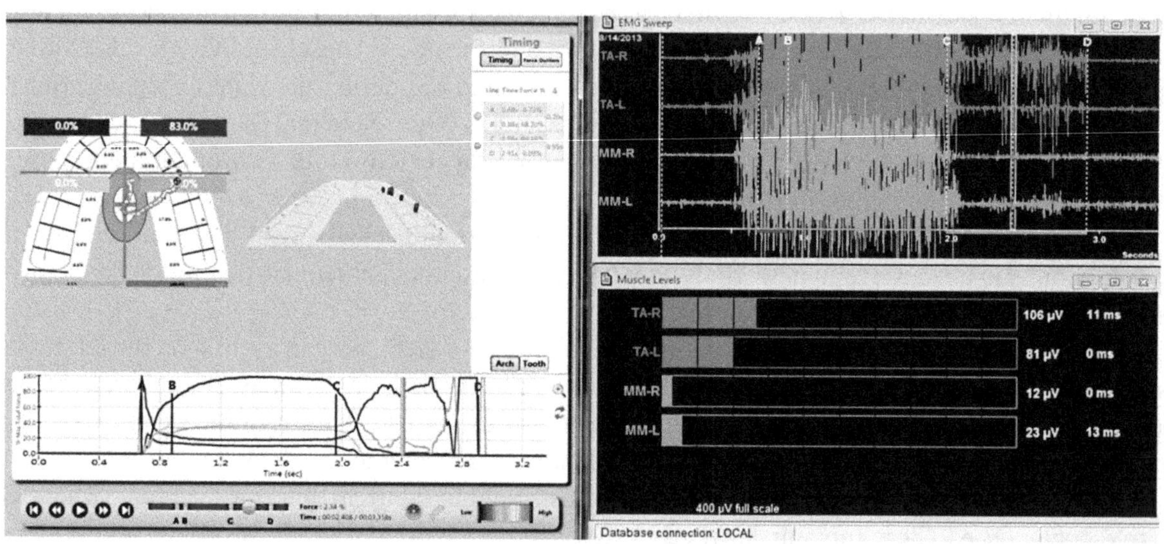

Diagnosis

Occluso-muscle Disorder (OMD)
Frictional Dental Hypersensitivity (FDH)

ICAGD/DTR Treatment Begins With the Subtractive Phase

After thoroughly drying the teeth, the patient is asked to close into MIP and repeat the unguided excursive movements with articulating paper held between the teeth. Then, the cross-referencing of the ink

Figure 18. Right excursion, just before D line at 2.9 seconds

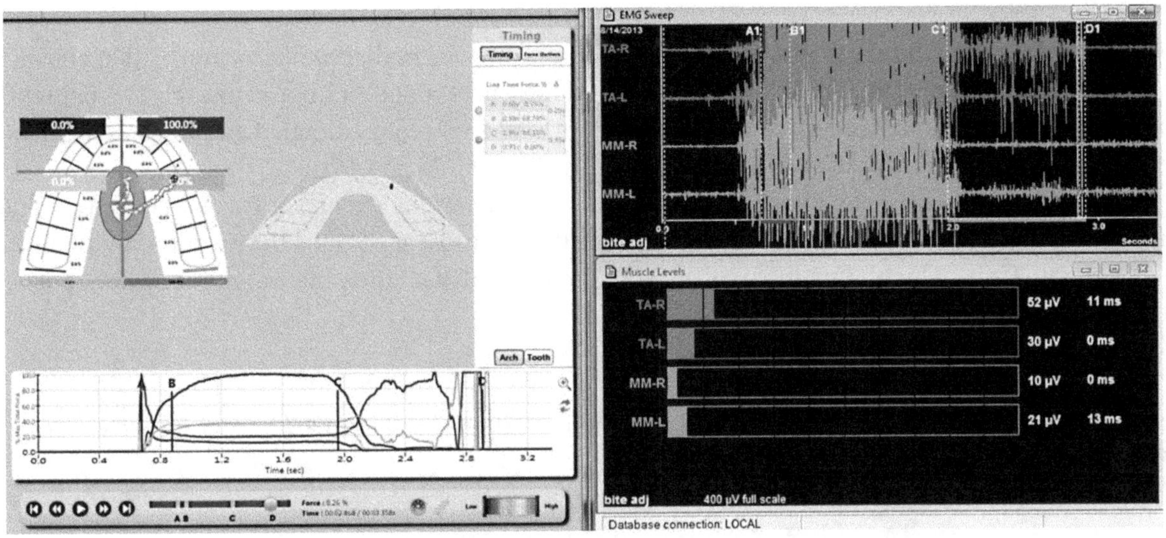

marks with the computer data, locates the problematic frictional contacts introrally. Next, the removal of any T-Scan defined hyperoccluded excursive contacts present in the excursive movements were then treated. The clinician can apply the BULL rule (Buccal Upper; Lingual Lower) for class I occlusions that present without posterior crossbite. Removal of the working and non-working frictional marks on the buccal inclines of the maxillary molars and premolars, and lingual inclines of the mandibular molars was accomplished, *leaving the MIP contacts intact and untouched.*

Every few minutes, T-Scan/EMG excursive recordings were remade, followed by articulating ribbon marking and occlusal adjustments to incorrect contacts, to check the procedure's progress, until the Disclusion Time was shorter and faster than pre treatment, and Center of Force icon (COF) was moving more anteriorly. A more anterior COF is desirable because it signifies decreased posterior tooth force concentration. When the initial excursion had been properly discluded, the same process was accomplished to the opposite excursive movement, again cross-referencing the articulating ribbon marks with the T-Scan/EMG data, deferring to computerized data to guide which ink marks were problematic. Repeating the occlusal data acquisition and ribbon marking was performed until the DT was shorter and faster ($\leq$ 0.5 seconds in the 2nd excursion). If a short enough DT was not attained, the additive phase should be commenced by bonding appropriate canine(s) until a DT $<$ 0.5 seconds is accomplished on both right and left excursive movements. Commence bonding of the incisal-lingual or the incisal-facial-lingual to the canines as needed, to facilitate a DT of $\leq$ 0.5 seconds.

It is important to use common sense when removing posterior frictional interferences. One may not necessarily acquire a DT $\leq$ 0.5 seconds with only subtractive removal of a given right or left excursion. Properly performed, the subtractive phase will increase the muscular efficiency of the maxillomandibular movements due to decreased PDL compression, but as needed, the additive phase may be implemented subsequently, by bonding the anterior teeth (usually the canines) to decrease the DT even further.

The Additive Phase

In this case, the patient received direct bonded IFL composites on both maxillary canines that enhanced the posterior disclusion (as conservative subtractive measures alone did not bring the DT below 0.5 seconds). The mandibular canines, though slightly worn, did not require bonded additions as the maxillary bondings alone facilitated a DT of ≤ 0.5 seconds (Figure 19a and 19b).

Only after adjusting the right and left excursions (and *rechecking* excursive DT's if composite additions were implemented), should the operator finish the adjustment of the MIP position, by dialing in the Occlusion Time, which often requires minimal improvements. Often the excursive corrections will optimize the MIP closure timing to be ≤ 0.2 seconds.

Figure 19a. The addition of composite to the incisal, facial and lingual surfaces of the maxillary left canine to effect a swifter Disclusion Time (DT)

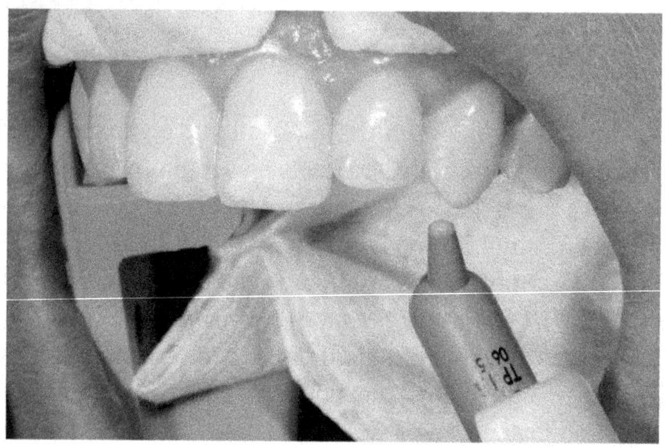

Figure 19b. Post operative MIP view of composite additions to both maxillary canines after the additive phase. The photograph was taken prior to final contour and polishing, to exaggerate the canine composite addition

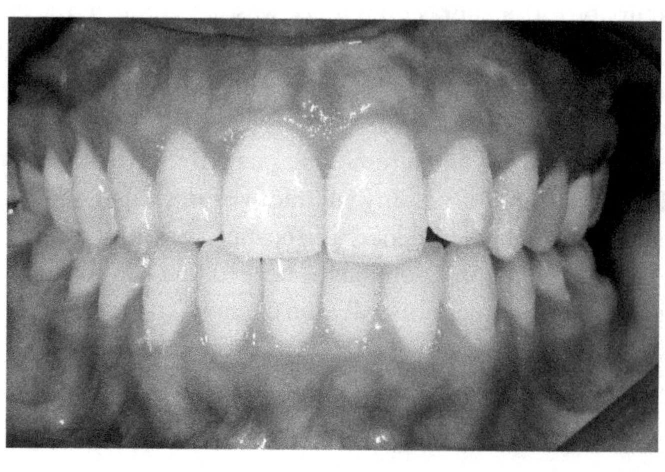

This patient did not require any significant MIP refinement, as her right and left excursive adjustments automatically centered a slightly anterior COF icon position. This anterior movement is a positive result of ICAGD, and one of the many differences that this occlusal adjustment process possesses over the traditional CR operator-guided equilibration. Decreased posterior frictional engagement leads to decreased molar occlusal contact, that leads to decreased PDL compressions, which leads to decreased muscular hyperactivity and decreased tooth torsional flexing. It should be noted that the light posterior contacts that remain in central fossa, marginal ridges, and cusp tips, will suffice over time to maintain a stable post-ICAGD occlusal adjustment treatment.

The ICAGD occlusal adjustment was completed by polishing any rough areas with appropriate diamonds, cups and pastes, after which the post-operative excursive data was recorded, bilaterally (Figures 20-23 show only the right excursive post op data).

Day of Treatment Post-Operative ICAGD/DTR Right Excursive T-Scan/EMG Data

In the timing pane of the T-Scan data, notice the OT = 0.17 seconds, and the DT = 0.35 seconds. These are both well within healthy tolerances. When comparing the pre-operative MIP data (Figure 14) to the post-operative MIP, the TA-R decreased from 407µv pre-operatively, to 280µv post-operatively. The TA-L decreased from 357µv pre-operatively to 260 µv post-operatively. The MM-R decreased from 303 µv pre-operatively to 156 µv post-operatively, and the MM-L decreased from 156 µv pre-operatively to 137 µv post-operatively. The patient's muscular output at MIP decreased in all four measured muscles resultant from the ICAGD/DTR corrections.

Less than 0.01 second after the patient left MIP, note that the TA-R is firing as it should be, and that the TA-L has almost reached the resting state (13µv, close to the 8-10 µv resting range). The MM-R and MM-L are just slightly hyperactive at this point in the excursion.

Figure 20. Post ICAGD/DTR right excursion at MIP, 1.149 seconds

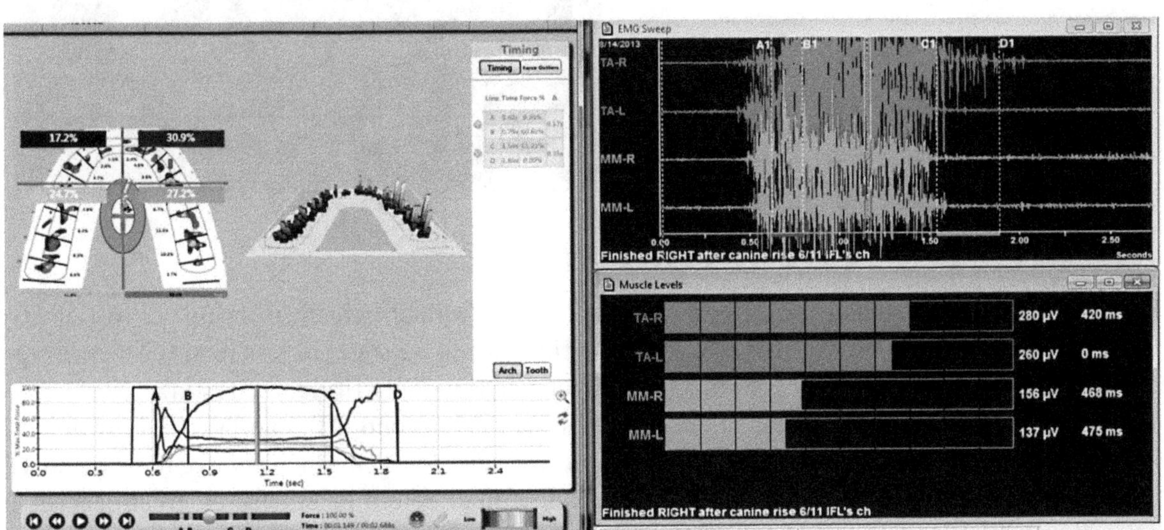

Figure 21. Post ICAGD/DTR right excursion, just past the C line at 1.589 seconds

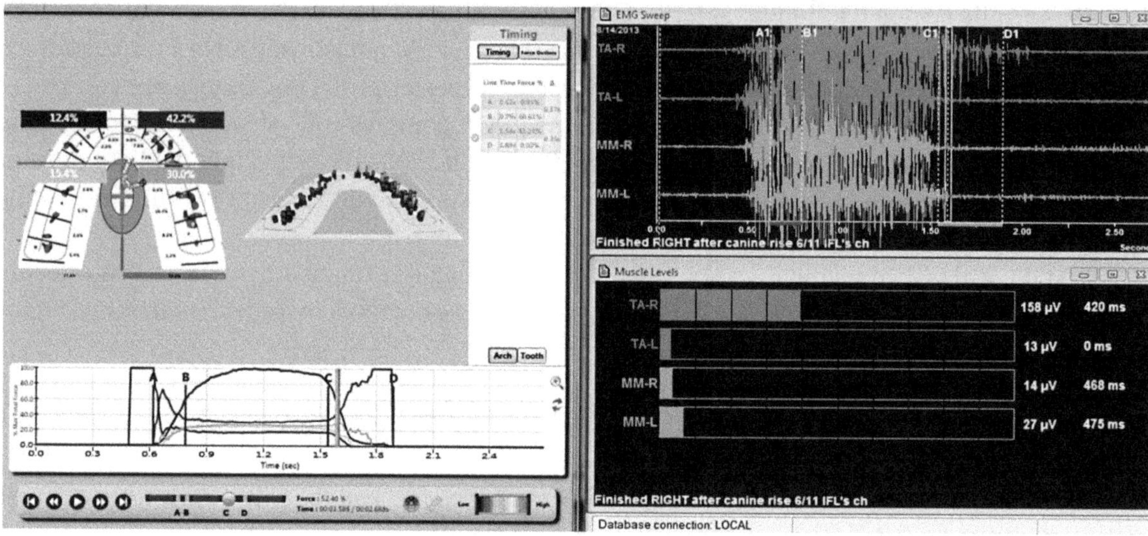

Figure 22. Post ICAGD/DTR right excursion 0.05 seconds past C line, at 1.639 seconds

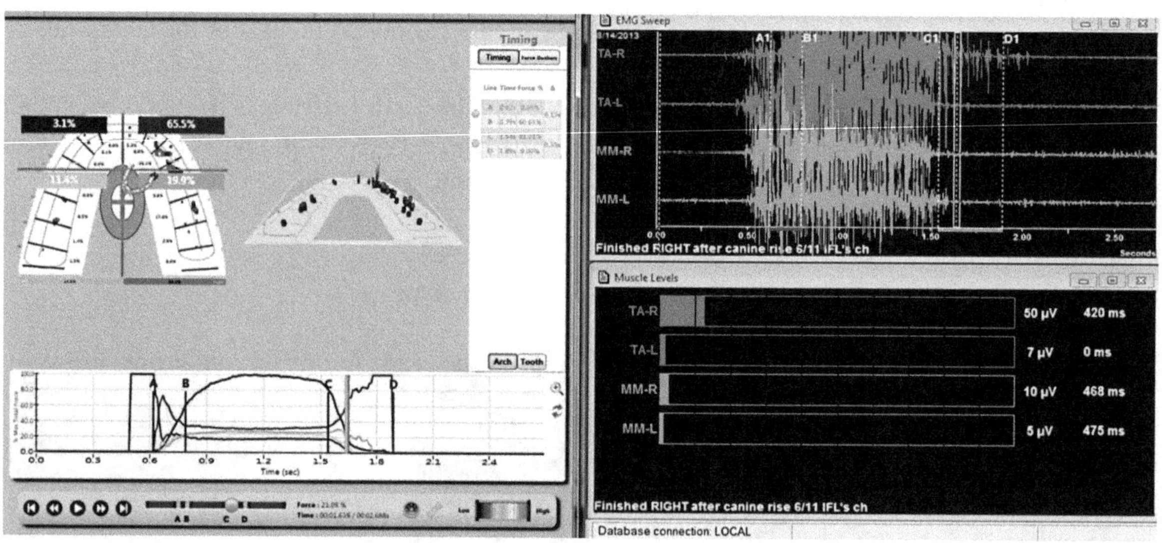

0.05 seconds later (than in Figure 21), notice that the TA-R is much quieter (working very efficiently), and that the TA-L, MM-L, and MM-R are all approaching a resting state. In less than 0.2 seconds past the C line (~1.57 seconds), the muscles that should not be excessively firing, are resting.

Here the excursion is nearly finished, just short of the 0.35 second DT time. Notice how quiet the muscles are, including the TA-R, which is primarily responsible for the right excursive movement. This patients "masticatory machine" is now far more efficient than before ICAGD/DTR treatment, as the muscles are no longer excursively hyperactive.

Figure 23. Post ICAGD/DTR right excursion, just before the D line at 1.879 seconds

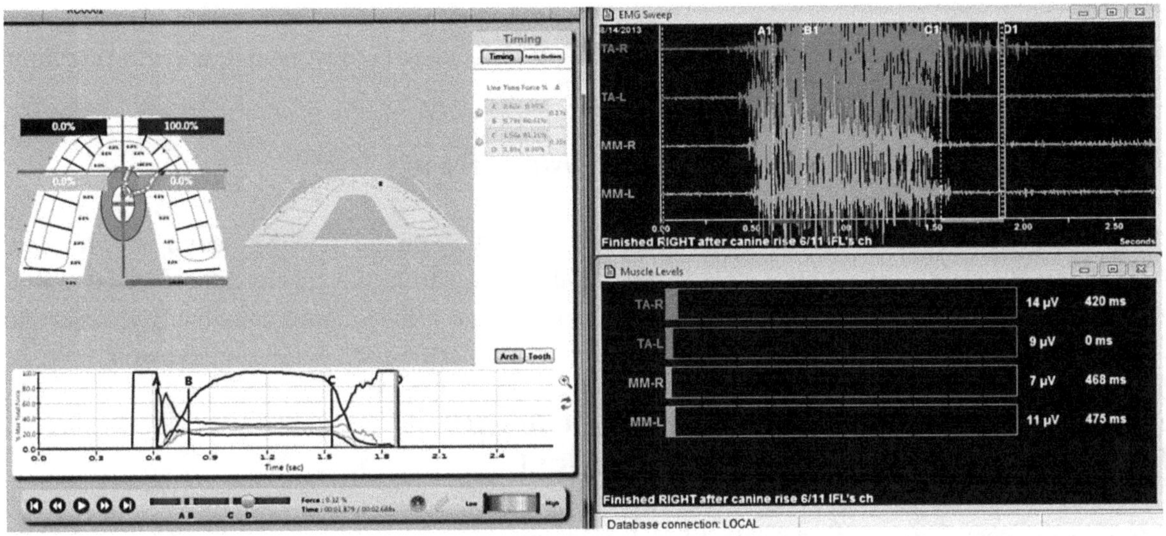

More efficient muscles demand less ATP. Aerobic metabolism will now be sufficient for the patient to produce enough energy to fuel the more efficient muscles. Hence, the anaerobic glycolytic pathways will no longer be needed to create supplemental ATP for these muscles, and the resultant decrease of the now, unnecessary glycolytic lactic acid byproducts, will result in these muscles becoming less ischemic. Over time, the patient will metabolize the excess lactic acid, and in the coming weeks feel dramatic muscular hyperactivity symptomatology relief. In addition, these consequences will not only lead to more relaxed muscles, but to decreased and more balanced forces throughout the occlusal design, with reduced tooth torsional flexing such that the patient will experience fewer FDH episodes.

Protrusive Consideration

Protrusive excursions are typically less necessary to treat (Kerstein & Wright, 1991; Kerstein, Chapman & Klein, 1997; Kerstein & Radke, 2012) unless there is substantial anterior overjet, a reverse smile line, significant anterior wear is present, or mesioversion and/or tipping of posterior teeth are present. If any of these conditions exist, the clinician should ensure the protrusive DT $\leq$0.5 seconds. The above case did not require protrusive measurement, as none of the above listed conditions were present.

CR Consideration

At no point in this case study, or any other treated patient in the pilot study, was the Centric Relation (CR) position or the CR pathway interferences verified, nor were either considered as part of the treatment protocol.

Occlusal Splint Consideration

At no point in this case study, or any other treated patient included within the pilot study, were occlusal splints utilized, either pre-operatively or post-operatively.

Treatment Times

All patients were treated in a single 30 - 60 minute ICAGD occlusal adjustment session to accomplish T-Scan 8/EMG III-guided DTR therapy.

Post-Treatment Questionnaire and Cold Water Swish Test

At 6-week recall, the patient reported experiencing a 1 out of 10 on the VAS/NS scaling portion of the questionnaire, after swishing ice water. This was notably down from the reported 6 out of 10 that was reported pre-operatively. The patient's post-operative treatment-related comments involved descriptors such as "...unbelievably relaxed", "...cold drinks are no problem", and "...no more tension".

Subject Group Response Results to the ICAGD/ DTR Treatment of the Cold Water Swish Test

Thirty-two subjects who presented with FDH symptoms, participated in the Cold Water Swish Test twice before, and once after undergoing ICAGD. Their collective data is presented in Figure 24, which shows the Means and Standard Deviations, and Medians for each group listed. Because the subjects reported ordinal number subjective responses, it was necessary to use a non-parametric statistic like the one-sided Wilcoxon Signed Rank for Paired Difference test. Non-parametric statistics assume the data are less precise (which they typically are when the data is subjective), and are less likely to lead to a type 1 statistical error, which is the finding of a significant difference when none exists. All of the cold water swish test data values are subjective, therefore, using a non-parametric statistic assumes there is less precision in the patient "estimates" of their pain levels (Figure 24).

In addition to reporting the Medians (the central tendency of the subject group), it was also valid to calculate means of the Cold Water Swish Test reported subjective ordinal number responses for comparison group to group, because the arbitrary "zero" for each patient is presumably the same before and after treatment. The Standard Deviation is descriptive of the variability of the group's response estimates, as well as their ability to describe the responses. The reason to employ the "paired" Wilcoxon Signed Rank Difference test, was because each patient's reported values were being compared to the same patient's reported values before and after treatment.

Within this group of thirty-two treated patients, no negative results were reported (no treated patient reported a worsened Cold Water Swish Test result after ICAGD). The postoperative responses showed definitive statistically significant differences from the pretreatment and control responses ($p < 0.005$) (Figure 24).

Figures 25a and 25b graphically illustrate the change in response distribution seen from pretreatment to post ICAGD treatment. The pretreatment cold water pain response ranged from 0 - 9, with many patients reporting a pretreatment range from 4 - 8 (Figure 25a). The post ICAGD cold water pain response data ranged only from 0 - 3, with most patients reporting zero cold water swish test pain (Figure 25b).

Discussion

As this is the first ICAGD/FDH treatment study ever performed, its findings cannot confirm or contradict other similar studies. However, the results of this pilot study do corroborate the findings of other authors

Figure 24. Preoperative, Control, and Postoperative ICAGD, Cold Water Swish Test response data of 32 subjects with FDH symptoms. The Means and Standard Deviations, and Medians for each group illustrate a statistically significant change resulted from the ICAGD treatment (p <.005).

Wilcoxon Signed Rank for Paired Difference

(0 = no pain to 10 = extreme pain)		C	P	C-P		
Patient	**Pre op Cold Water Swish Response**	**Control Cold Water Swish Response**	**Post-op Cold Water Swish Response**	**Difference**	**Rank of Difference**	**Negative difference**
01	8	8	2	6	25	
02	2	2	1	1	4	
03	3	4	3	1	4	
04	2	2	0	2	9	
05	4	4	2	2	9	
06	8	8	0	8	30	
07	8	8	2	6	25	
08	5	5	2	3	13	
09	3	3	2	1	4	
10	4	4	0	4	18.5	
11	8	8	2	6	25	
12	3	3	0	3	13	
13	4	4	0	4	18.5	
14	7	7	0	7	28.5	
15	2	2	1	1	4	
16	7	7	0	7	28.5	
17	4	4	1	3	13	
18	7	7	2	5	22	
19	3	3	0	3	13	
20	4	3	2	1	4	
21	9	9	0	9	31	
22	2	2	0	2	9	
23	1	1	0	1	4	
24	4	4	0	4	18.5	
25	2	0	0	0	0	
26	4	4	0	4	18.5	
27	4	4	1	3	13	
28	7	7	1	6	25	
29	8	8	2	6	25	
30	5	5	1	4	18.5	
31	5	5	1	4	18.5	
32	2	2	1	1	4	
Median	*4*	*4*	*1*			
Mean	*4.65625*	*4.59375*	*0.90625*		*T-positive*	*T-Negative*
SD	*2.322531642*	*2.421135098*	*0.92838309*	*sum*	*496*	*0*
With n = 32 and with alpha = 0.005 for a one-tailed test, the critical value of T negative < 160						

(previously cited in this chapter), who have concluded that occlusal function plays an etiologic role in the DH condition. Specifically, this study illustrated that occlusal surface friction promoted episodes of DH that were readily resolved with a specific occlusal therapy (ICAGD) aimed at treating the prolonged frictional durations. All thirty-two studied patients did respond post-operatively with statistically significant lessened DH sensitivity responses. What was not specifically and objectively followed in this pilot study, was whether the studied patients possessed areas of recession, abfraction, or exposed dentin. However, the author does recall that numerous test subjects presented without any exposed dentin while experiencing frequent episodes of cold sensitivity.

Figure 25a. Pre ICAGD treatment Cold Water Swish Test pain level distribution

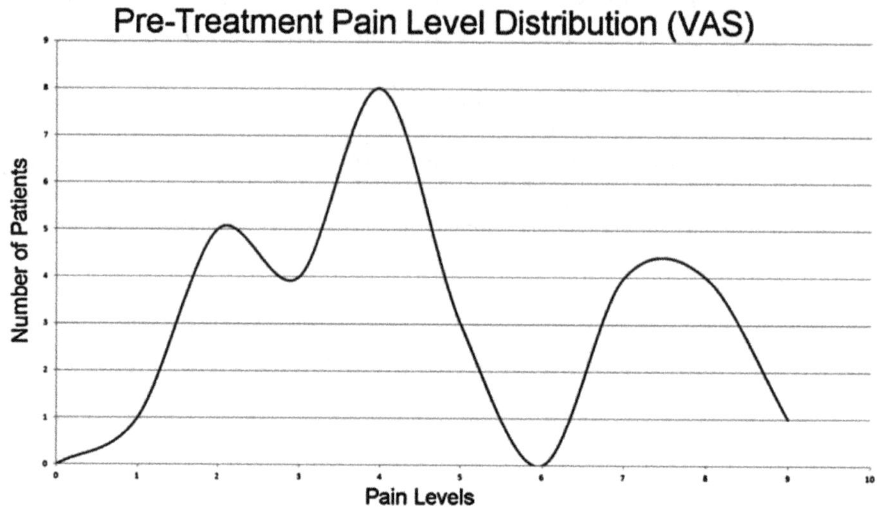

Figure 25b. Post ICAGD treatment Cold Water Swish Test pain level distribution

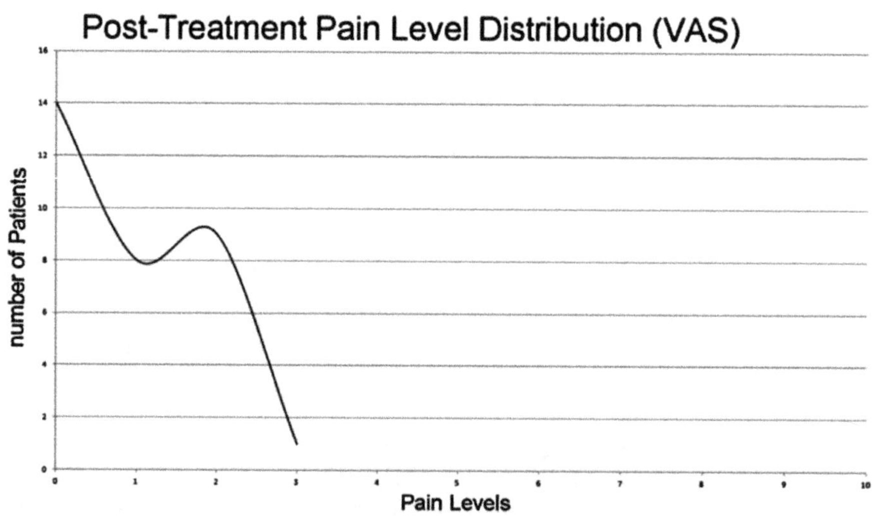

The findings of the Pilot Study are in agreement with previously performed occlusal treatment research that attempted to resolve Dental Hypersensitivity (Coleman et. al., 2003), despite that the two studies employed two differing DH detection methods, and two differing occlusal adjustment techniques. This study used a cold (ice) water swish to detect a DH sensitivity response, whereas Coleman used the Air Indexing method. Both methods satisfied the classic DH definition for why teeth can be hypersensitive; fluid flow was induced resultant from a cold water application to teeth, or the air desiccation of the fluid-filled dentinal tubules caused the resultant fluid flow. As such, it would seem that both techniques were practical methods of assessing a tooth's hypersensitive response.

The occlusal adjustment technique employed in this pilot study differed from Coleman's method (habitual closure contacts and excursive movement friction were treated using the T-Scan 8, versus using a Centric Relation-based, unmeasured, and non-quantified equilibration that was performed solely with articulating ribbon). The results with ICAGD performed in MIP obtained similar symptom resolution as did the CR based occlusal equilibration. With similar DH sensitivity improvements obtained in both studies, it would seem logical that the chosen occlusal position was not a factor in the symptom resolution. Instead, the rendered occlusal treatment in both studies addressed the excessive force issue present on the involved teeth that was repetitively over time, cyclically applied to these teeth by the muscles of mastication.

The key factor in DH evolution appears to be that excess occlusal surface friction leads to excessive Periodontal Ligament compression (PDL), which directly increases muscle contractions that increase the lateroflexion of tooth structure. Frictional Dental Hypersensitivity would therefore likely result from strain and deformation. The physical and thermal insults on teeth cause an instantaneous physical deformation of the dentin, which then triggers nerve impulses bio-mechanically, even without patent dentinal tubules. It is possible that this bio-mechanical trigger involves the activation of the intrapulpal and omnidirectional A-beta myelinated nerve fibers, given the rapid FDH resolution that was clinically observed within the studied population shortly after ICAGD was performed.

It is also probable over time that repeated torsional and frictional insults will lead to exposed dentin through abfractive events and occlusal surface wear faceting. A worsening factor to the wear and abfractive processes that would occur simultaneously during the frictional tooth torsional deformation, is that excess muscular forces result and overload the teeth when the PDL mechanoreceptors are compressed for prolonged periods. This is the mechanism by which PDL compressions hyperfunction the masticatory musculature (Kerstein & Radke, 2012).

What was not statistically analyzed in this Pilot Study, was the subjective questioning of the subjects as to the appearance and resolution of dysfunctional muscular symptoms consistent with masticatory muscle hyperactivity. All thirty-two patients returned for their recall Cold Water Swish assessments after having enough time to experience changes in both tooth sensitivity and muscular symptomotology. Most subjects reported that their muscular hyperactivity symptomotology had typically abated after the friction had been removed from their teeth. These oral reports coincide with the symptomatic results observed in the ICAGD studies performed by Kerstein since 1991.

During this author's ICAGD treatment performed on a pool of muscularly dysfunctional patients, using the force and timing data provided by the T-Scan 8 with the simultaneous muscular activity level data provided by the BioEMG, it became apparent that hyperactive masticatory musculature is not only linked to dysfunctional muscle symptomotology, but to DH symptomotology, as well. The observation that hypersensitive teeth became non-sensitive minutes into the ICAGD procedure, which also induced a concomitant relaxation of the masticatory musculature, strongly suggests that DH is probably not solely due to an inflammatory response to external stimuli. It is more likely that a strain deformation mechanism is at least partially responsible for DH symptomotology, in addition to neuropeptides causing a rapid change in pulpal vascularity. This strain deformation mechanism would help to explain the almost instantaneous hypersensitivity changes that were observed within the study patient pool.

It has been shown that reducing occlusal surface friction reduces masticatory muscle hyperactivity via decreased Periodontal Ligament compressions (Kerstein & Wright, 1991; Kerstein & Radke, 2012). Decreased muscle hyperactivity leads to lessened lateroflexion of the teeth, because the masticatory apparatus loads the teeth with less muscle force when there is rapid excursive movement separation of the posterior teeth. Less lateroflexion of the teeth leads to less tooth strain and deformation. Fewer PDL compressions lead to less frequent physical compression of both the periodontal and pulpal vasculature, leading to a decreased nociceptive response to stimuli that can trigger DH events. It also seems plausible that excessive muscular activity, occlusal surface friction, and tooth lateroflexion together over time, would lead to abfractive formation, exposed dentin, and open dentinal tubules, which are the very signs that researchers traditionally look towards as explanations for DH events.

This pilot study's finding that all thirty-two subjects reported a significant decrease in their dentinal hypersensitivity response after undergoing the objective, computer-guided ICAGD procedure, strongly indicates that FDH does exist, and the of presence FDH symptoms indicates that sensitive teeth are likely under excessive excursive frictional forces. Additionally, the study data suggests that computer-guided occlusal intervention is a highly efficacious treatment for the FDH condition. Perhaps then, through computer-guided occlusal intervention performed prophylactically, clinicians could likely stave off the appearance of this precursor condition, by addressing the prolonged occlusal surface excursive friction that leads to the appearance of Frictional Dental Hypersensitivity (FDH).

SOLUTIONS AND RECOMMENDATIONS

Dental Medicine should give serious consideration to the little known alternate occlusal adjustment protocol known as ICAGD. This method depends upon the precise quantification of friction, timing, and relative force gathered pre treatment using the T-Scan 8 technology. It is possible that Dental Medicine may not have previously noticed FDH as a condition, since the quantifiable ICAGD protocol using digital occlusal analysis is less frequently employed than is traditional Occlusal Equilibration.

Dental Medicine also should impartially compare the protocols between ICAGD and Occlusal Equilibration, with the realization that the latter is dependent upon iatrogenic manipulation, while the former is virtually independent of iatrogenic influences. The entire process is performed with the patient self-articulating into their habitual closure position, and with the patients performing their very own natural mandibular movements. Alternatively, Equilibration relies upon the questionable transference of the occlusal contacts to articulated casts with inherent transfer inaccuracies (incorrect maxillomandibular relationship, impression distortions, lack of periodontal ligaments present on study casts, articulator mounting errors, stone contraction setting errors, and subjectively reducing the models to simulate this subtle change to the actual patient). ICAGD on the other hand, requires no impressions, no CR manipulation, and no articulators. Instead, the patient's own dentition is measured intraorally, allowing for a precise analysis of the interactions that the teeth, the muscles, the central nervous system (CNS), the TMJ's, and the PDL's share. As this chapter has highlighted, occlusal instabilities and muscular hyperactivity may result from only microns of excessive frictional tooth contacts.

Qualification alone is insufficient to accomplish a measurable and consistently predictable change; only when *quantification* is added into the equation, may predictable outcomes result in the patient possessing stable and adapted TM joints. Occlusion = WHERE (articulating ribbon) + WHEN (T-Scan 8) + HOW MUCH (T-Scan 8). Only when these three influences are taken into consideration together, may a practitioner truly and predictably manipulate the occlusions' influence upon the Stomatognathic system.

This author's observations regarding ICAGD affecting DH resolution have been predictable and quantifiable. Simply stated, Dental Medicine now has at its disposal a modality in the T-Scan, whereby occlusal contact relative force and time durations can be precisely measured. This is in contrast to the past when only the qualification of occlusal contacts was possible using articulating ribbons, waxes and other non-digital occlusal indicators. This digital technology elucidates the previously untreatable parameters of timing, force, and friction, and when combined with the BioEMG technology, provides solid evidence that muscular hyperactivity, once controlled, prevents susceptible teeth from experiencing bouts of FDH.

Based upon the literature, little consideration is given to DH being a symptom of TMD. Perhaps the "minor affliction" of Dentin Hypersensitivity is truly a sign or symptom of changes occurring in the Stomatognathic system. Maybe the term "Dentin Sensitivity" is generally factual, in that transient DH events are part of what nature designed dentin to do for the human organism. Perhaps the sensory organs that are the teeth, may secondarily act as "stop meters" for the Stomatognathic system, relaying nociceptive, tactile, thermal, and proprioceptive information back to the CNS, assisting the organ in its own preservation, and the preservation of the entire Stomatognathic system. It is conceivable that DH might *warn* the central nervous system that a spatial imbalance exists, by detecting in its earliest stages, long before an abfraction results in exposed dentin and open dentinal tubules and that excess torsional forces are present within the occlusal scheme.

In 2009, Levy described "teeth as sensory organs", and made several salient statements that lend credibility to Disclusion Time Reduction and its positive influence on frictional DH (Levy, 2009). He stated that patients with canine and incisive guidance had fewer contacting teeth during excursions, and had less mechanosensory information to integrate than would patients presenting with group function and non-working side interferences. As the number of interfering tooth contacts present during excursive movements increases, the CNS is compelled to orchestrate more midcourse corrections to accomplish the oromotor movement, resulting in additional muscular hyperactivity.

It has been shown in monkeys that slowly adapting periodontal mechanoreceptors are more numerous around the anterior teeth than around posterior teeth (Byers & Dong, 1989). Levy subsequently postulated that the tactile thresholds for anterior teeth are lower than those of posterior teeth. This author's routine usage of surface electromyography (EMG) in the practice of occlusal therapy supports the contention that patients routinely and predictably demonstrate a diminished ability to generate high elevator muscular forces when only anterior teeth contact. An example of this has been observed in more traditional TMD treatment approaches that utilize anterior deprogramming splints, where only anterior teeth contact and the posterior teeth are completely left out of contact.

That being said, if excessive posterior occlusal interferences (and subsequent hyperactive masticatory muscle activity) are definitively linked to hypersensitive teeth, it is axiomatic that the ICAGD coronoplasty may prove far more effective than Centric Relation Occlusal Equilibration in the treatment of FDH for 2 main reasons:

- Centric Relation Occlusal Equilibration increases the quantity of molar contact, directly increasing the mechanosensory output, which potentially increases muscular hyperactivity by the mechanisms repeatedly illustrated throughout this chapter. In contrast, the ICAGD occlusal adjustment predictably results in decreased quantity of molar contact, predictably and routinely decreasing muscular output.
- Centric Relation Occlusal Equilibration does not possess objective, quantifiable endpoints.
- The ICAGD method does possesses objective endpoints that are quantifiable and reproducible, while establishing statistically significant reductions in hyperactive muscle activity levels.

Should muscular hyperactivity consistently lead to FDH events, it makes sense that where indicated, Dental Medicine should turn to the ICAGD method to definitively address hypersensitive teeth.

FUTURE RESEARCH DIRECTIONS

Research on Dentinal Hypersensitivity has traditionally focused on patent dentinal tubules, and how best to eliminate any communication with a vital pulp, by applying surface treatments to the open tubules. Pulpal communication is what researchers have been typically concerned with, while not necessarily studying the causative occlusal component, which may not only begin the process of DH, but likely also perpetuate the process over time.

Future research therefore, should be undertaken to definitively link occlusal surface friction's role to the etiology and treatment of DH, as well as to completely understand the pathophysiology behind the FDH process. Should occlusal factors prove to be a primary etiology of Frictional Dental Hypersensitivity, then traditional treatments for Dentinal Hypersensitivity would only temporarily mask the symptoms, without lessening the ongoing occlusal disease that promotes repetitive FDH symptomatic episodes.

More research should be conducted to firmly understand the physiologic reasons why measured occlusal adjustments diminish Dentinal Hypersensitivity and Frictional Dental Hypersensitivity. Carefully conducted studies that incorporate a standardized, measurable method of diagnosing Dentinal Hypersensitivity, such as the Air Indexing method, could track the identification of recessed periodontal tissue heights and abfractive lesions. This type of study would further elucidate the role occlusion plays in root surface structural breakdown, and in Dentinal Hypersensitivity symptomotology.

A study could be designed using the T-Scan/BioEMG synchronization technologies, to assess the potential viability of a muscular overload/FDH/DH etiology. This analysis could confirm that excess occlusal force leads to wear and abfractive sequelae, making it possible for clinicians to better predict and prevent muscular overload to the system, and thereby limit abfractive and wear occurrences from initiating FDH episodes.

Ideally, a comprehensive longitudinal study should be undertaken, that attempts to correlate prolonged occlusal surface friction with both Cold Water Swish Test sensitive teeth with or without exposed dentin and abfractions, and the muscular hyperactivity symptoms often exhibited in FDH sensitive patients.

Another interesting study could attempt to correlate vital bleaching sensitivity with FDH, as it also seems plausible that hyperactive masticatory muscles and the FDH that results, might decrease the bleached teeth's' tolerance to the bleaching agent's concentrated chemical and osmotic insult. A study of this type could include a control group that would first undergo ICAGD prior to vital bleaching, that would be compared to a bleaching population that had no pre-bleaching occlusal adjustment, where neither population was given desensitizing medicaments to sequester any post-operative bleaching sensitivity. If the group with prior ICAGD treatment experienced a profound reduction in post bleaching sensitivity, it would further indicate that FDH could be a plausible forbearer to other types of DH events.

CONCLUSION

Pain is referred to as the fifth vital sign, and is an important reason for which patients seek health care (McCafeery & Parson, 1999). Dental Hypersensitivity has been labeled a true pain syndrome that crosses all cultures and continents (Curro, 1990). As such, it behooves modern Dental Medicine to investigate all treatments that may sequester this clinical problem. A 2009 literature review stated that the predisposing factors associated with DH must be controlled or eliminated, by educating the patient regarding the excessive intake of acidic foods, provide guidance on proper tooth brushing techniques, and by performing an analysis of the occlusion (Porto, Andrade, & Montes, 2009).

This chapter described the potential etiologies and treatment of hypersensitive teeth, while discussing the research that points towards a mechanically activated, occlusal etiology. A Pilot Study that employed objectively controlled occlusal adjustments, that led to a marked consistent decrease in the appearance of Dental Hypersensitivity within the treated patient population, was also described. The objective occlusal data supplied by the T-Scan 8 technology, to direct a measured coronoplasty that reduced frictional durations during excursive movements, also reduced or eliminated the hypersensitive episodes present in the studied subjects. The addition of surface Electromyography used in combination with the T-Scan, leaves little room for error in obtaining an ideal muscular response resultant from a properly performed and precisely measured occlusal adjustment procedure. In addition, a new term, Frictional Dental Hypersensitivity was introduced, that describes the DH phenomenon that can occur without exposed dentin or open dentinal tubules. Lastly, a paradigm shift was presented that suggests Dental Medicine consider accepting that occlusal factors are central to both TMD muscular conditions, and Frictional Dentinal Hypersensitivity symptomatology.

Over the last 150 years, much research has been conducted in an effort to explain why the human dentition may or may not experience episodic bouts of Dentinal Hypersensitivity. Conventional theories abound, from the widely accepted Hydrodynamic Theory, to the less accepted Odontoblastic Receptor Theory, to the least accepted Direct Innervation Theory. Correlations between periodontal recession, patent CEJ interfaces, exposed dentinal tubules, and bouts of hypersensitivity, are usually well supported, but these correlations may be incomplete. Alternatively, many authors clearly consider hypersensitivity to be a direct result of an occlusal problem. This chapter supports the contention that occlusion plays a significant role in the evolution of DH symptoms, and that the early identification of Frictional Dental Hypersensitivity may herald the onset of more frequent Dentinal Hypersensitivity events, over time.

REFERENCES

Abboud, M., Grüner, M., & Koeck, B. (2002). Anterior Crowding–Just an Esthetic Problem? *Journal of Orofacial Orthopedics. Fortschritte der Kieferorthopadie*, *63*(4), 264–273. doi:10.1007/s00056-002-0033-5 PMID:12198742

Absi, E. G., Addy, M., & Adams, D. (1987). Dentine hypersensitivity. *Journal of Clinical Periodontology*, *14*(5), 280–284. doi:10.1111/j.1600-051X.1987.tb01533.x PMID:3475295

Addy, M. (2002). Dentine hypersensitivity: New perspectives on an old problem. *International Dental Journal*, *52*(Suppl 1), 367–375. doi:10.1002/j.1875-595X.2002.tb00936.x

Addy, M. (2005). Tooth brushing, tooth wear and dentine hypersensitivity—are they associated? *International Dental Journal*, *55*(Suppl 4), 261–267. PMID:16167604

Addy, M., Mostafa, P., & Newcombe, R. G. (1987). Dentine hypersensitivity: The distribution of recession, sensitivity and plaque. *Journal of Dentistry*, *15*(6), 242–248. doi:10.1016/0300-5712(87)90045-5 PMID:3480906

Al-Sabbagh, M., Andreana, S., & Ciancio, S. G. (2004). Dentinal hypersensitivity: Review of aetiology, differential diagnosis, prevalence, and mechanism. *Journal of the International Academy of Periodontology*, *6*(1), 8. PMID:14964489

Alkan, A., Keskiner, I., Arici, S., & Sato, S. (2006). The effect of periodontitis on biting abilities. *Journal of Periodontology*, *77*(8), 1442–1445. doi:10.1902/jop.2006.060025 PMID:16881814

Anderson, G. C., Schulte, J. K., & Aeppli, D. M. (1993). Reliability of the evaluation of occlusal contacts in the intercuspal position. *The Journal of Prosthetic Dentistry*, *70*(4), 320–323. doi:10.1016/0022-3913(93)90215-A PMID:8229882

Ash, M. M., & Ramfjord, S. P. (1995). *Occlusion*. Philadelphia, PA: W.B. Saunders Co.

Balaji, V. C., Jois, H. S., & Kumar, M. P. (2012). Approaching Dentin Hypersensitivity. *Ranchi University Journal of Dental Surgery*, *1*(2), 1.

Banfield, N., & Addy, M. (2004). Dentine hypersensitivity: Development and evaluation of a model in situ to study tubule patency. *Journal of Clinical Periodontology*, *31*(5), 325–335. doi:10.1111/j.1600-051X.2004.00488.x PMID:15086613

Banos, J. E., Bosch, F., Canellas, M., Bassols, A., Ortega, F., & Bigorra, J. (1989). Acceptability of visual analogue scales in the clinical setting: A comparison with verbal rating scales in postoperative pain. *Methods and Findings in Experimental and Clinical Pharmacology*, *11*(2), 123. PMID:2709918

Bartlett, D., & Smith, B.G. (2000). Definition, classification and clinical assessment of attrition, erosion, and abrasion of enamel and dentine. *Tooth Wear and Sensitivity*, 87-92.

Bartlett, D. W. (1997). The causes of dental erosion. *Oral Diseases*, *3*(4), 209–211. doi:10.1111/j.1601-0825.1997.tb00042.x PMID:9643213

Bartold, P. M. (2006). Dentinal hypersensitivity: A review. *Australian Dental Journal*, *51*(3), 212–218. doi:10.1111/j.1834-7819.2006.tb00431.x PMID:17037886

Bhat, S. (2010). Etiology of temporomandibular disorders: The journey so far. *International Dentistry South Africa*, *12*, 4.

Blum, M. (1530). *Artzney buch wider Allerbi.* Krancheyton und Gebrechen der Tzeen.

Brännström, M. (1966). Sensitivity of dentine. *Oral Surgery, Oral Medicine, and Oral Pathology*, *21*(4), 517–526. doi:10.1016/0030-4220(66)90411-7 PMID:5218158

Brännström, M., & Åström, A. (1964). A study on the mechanism of pain elicited from the dentin. *Journal of Dental Research*, *43*(4), 619–625. doi:10.1177/00220345640430041601 PMID:14183350

Bruder, G.A., & Erickson, T.E. (n.d.). *Color Atlas of Endodontics*. Philadelphia, PA: Elsevier Science.

Byers, M. R. (1980). Development of sensory innervation in dentin. *The Journal of Comparative Neurology*, *191*(3), 413–427. doi:10.1002/cne.901910307 PMID:7410601

Byers, M. R. (1984). Dental sensory receptors. *International Review of Neurobiology*, *25*, 39–94. doi:10.1016/S0074-7742(08)60677-7 PMID:6206015

Byers, M. R. (1985). Sensory innervation of periodontal ligament of rat molars consists of unencapsulated Ruffini-like mechanoreceptors and free nerve endings. *The Journal of Comparative Neurology, 231*(4), 500–518. doi:10.1002/cne.902310408 PMID:3968252

Byers, M. R., & Dong, W. K. (1989). Comparison of trigeminal receptor location and structure in the periodontal ligament of different types of teeth from the rat, cat, and monkey. *The Journal of Comparative Neurology, 279*(1), 117–127. doi:10.1002/cne.902790110 PMID:2492311

Byers, M. R., & Narhi, M. V. O. (1999). Dental injury models: Experimental tools for understanding neuroinflammatory interactions and polymodal nociceptor functions. *Critical Reviews in Oral Biology and Medicine, 10*(1), 4–39. doi:10.1177/10454411990100010101 PMID:10759425

Camps, J., & Pashley, D. (2003). In vivo sensitivity of human root dentin to air blast and scratching. *Journal of Periodontology, 74*(11), 1589–1594. doi:10.1902/jop.2003.74.11.1589 PMID:14682655

Carey, J. P., Craig, M., Kerstein, R. B., & Radke, J. (2007). Determining a relationship between applied occlusal load and articulating paper mark area. *The Open Dentistry Journal, 1*(1), 1–7. doi:10.2174/1874210600701010001 PMID:19088874

Carossa, S., Lojacono, A., Schierano, G., & Pera, P. (2000). Evaluation of occlusal contacts in the dental laboratory: Influence of strip thickness and operator experience. *The International Journal of Prosthodontics, 13*(3), 201. PMID:11203632

Casanova-Rosado, J. F., Medina-Solís, C. E., Vallejos-Sánchez, A. A., Casanova-Rosado, A. J., Hernández-Prado, B., & Ávila-Burgos, L. (2006). Prevalence and associated factors for Temporomandibular disorders in a group of Mexican adolescents and youth adults. *Clinical Oral Investigations, 10*(1), 42–49. doi:10.1007/s00784-005-0021-4 PMID:16311741

Chabanski, M. B., & Gillam, D. G. (1997). Aetiology, prevalence and clinical features of cervical dentine sensitivity. *Journal of Oral Rehabilitation, 24*(1), 15–19. doi:10.1046/j.1365-2842.1997.00471.x PMID:9049914

Chen, S., Rio, C., Ji, R. R., Dikkes, P., Coggeshall, R. E., Woolf, C. J., & Corfas, G. (2003). Disruption of ErbB receptor signaling in adult non-myelinating Schwann cells causes progressive sensory loss. *Nature Neuroscience, 6*(11), 1186–1193. doi:10.1038/nn1139 PMID:14555954

Chidchuangchai, W., Vongsavan, N., & Matthews, B. (2007). Sensory transduction mechanisms responsible for pain caused by cold stimulation of dentine in man. *Archives of Oral Biology, 52*(2), 154–160. doi:10.1016/j.archoralbio.2006.09.009 PMID:17109813

Choi, Y. S., Choung, P. H., Moon, H. S., & Kim, S. G. (2002). Temporomandibular disorders in 19-year-old Korean men. *Journal of Oral and Maxillofacial Surgery, 60*(7), 797–803. doi:10.1053/joms.2002.33249 PMID:12089696

Christensen, G. J. (1992). A look at state-of-the-art tooth-colored inlays and onlays. *The Journal of the American Dental Association, 123*(9), 66–67. PMID:1517520

Chu, C. H. (2010). Management of dentine hypersensitivity. *Dental Bulletin, 15*, 3.

Chuang, S. Y. (2002). Incidence of temporomandibular disorders (TMDs) in senior dental students in Taiwan. *Journal of Oral Rehabilitation*, *29*(12), 1206–1211. doi:10.1046/j.1365-2842.2002.00968.x PMID:12472858

Clayton, D. R., McCarthy, D., & Gillam, D. G. (2002). A study of the prevalence and distribution of dentine sensitivity in a population of 17–58-year-old serving personnel on an RAF base in the Midlands. *Journal of Oral Rehabilitation*, *29*(1), 14–23. doi:10.1046/j.1365-2842.2002.00805.x PMID:11844027

Coleman, T. A., Grippo, J. O., & Kinderknecht, K. E. (2000). Cervical dentin hypersensitivity. Part II: Associations with abfractive lesions. *Quintessence International*, *31*(7), 466. PMID:11203968

Coleman, T. A., Grippo, J. O., & Kinderknecht, K. E. (2003). Cervical l Dentin Hypersensitivity. Part III: Resolution following occlusal equilibration. *Quintessence International*, *34*, 427–434. PMID:12859087

Coleman, T. A., & Kinderknecht, K. E. (2000). Cervical dentin hypersensitivity. Part I: The air indexing method. *Quintessence International*, *31*(7), 461. PMID:11203967

Curro, F. A. (1990). Tooth hypersensitivity in the spectrum of pain. *Dental Clinics of North America*, *34*(3), 429. PMID:2197119

Dababneh, R. H., Khouri, A. T., & Addy, M. (1999). dentine hypersensitivity: Dentine hypersensitivity - an enigma? A review of terminology, mechanisms, aetiology and management. *British Dental Journal*, *187*(11), 606–611. PMID:16163281

Davies, S. J., Gray, R. J. M., Linden, G. J., & James, J. A. (2001). Occlusal: Occlusal considerations in periodontics. *British Dental Journal*, *191*(11), 597–604. PMID:11770945

Dawson, P. E. (2006). *Functional Occlusion: from TMJ to Smile Design* (1st ed., pp. 14, 18, 23, 26, 42, 146, 394). Philadelphia, PA: Elsevier Health Sciences.

De Boever, J. A., Carlsson, G. E., & Klineberg, I. J. (2000). Need for occlusal therapy and prosthodontic treatment in the management of temporomandibular disorders. *Journal of Oral Rehabilitation*, *27*(8), 647–659. doi:10.1046/j.1365-2842.2000.00623.x PMID:10931259

de Felício, C. M., Mazzetto, M. O., de Silva, M. A., Bataglion, C., & Hotta, T. H. (2006). A preliminary protocol for multi-professional centers for the determination of signs and symptoms of temporomandibular disorders. *The Journal of Cranio-Mandibular Practice*, *24*(4), 258–264. doi:10.1179/crn.2006.041 PMID:17086855

Dong, W. K., Chudler, E. H., & Martin, R. F. (1985). Physiological properties of intradental mechanoreceptors. *Brain Research*, *334*(2), 389–395. doi:10.1016/0006-8993(85)90239-2 PMID:3873270

Dong, W. K., Shiwaku, T., Kawakami, Y., & Chudler, E. H. (1993). Static and dynamic responses of periodontal ligament mechanoreceptors and intradental mechanoreceptors. *Journal of Neurophysiology*, *69*(5), 1567–1582. PMID:8389830

Dowell, P., & Addy, M. (1983). Dentine hypersensitivity-A review. *Journal of Clinical Periodontology*, *10*(4), 341–350. doi:10.1111/j.1600-051X.1983.tb01283.x PMID:6309917

Droter, J. R. (2005). An orthopaedic approach to the diagnosis and treatment of disorders of the temporomandibular joint. *Dentistry Today*, *24*(11), 82–84. PMID:16358802

Eisenburger, M., & Addy, M. (2002). Erosion and attrition of human enamel in vitro part I: Interaction effects. *Journal of Dentistry*, *30*(7), 341–347. doi:10.1016/S0300-5712(02)00048-9 PMID:12554116

Ekberg, E., & Nilner, M. (2006). Treatment outcome of short-and long-term appliance therapy in patients with TMD of myogenous origin and tension-type headache. *Journal of Oral Rehabilitation*, *33*(10), 713–721. doi:10.1111/j.1365-2842.2006.01659.x PMID:16938099

Ekfeldt, A., Hugoson, A., Bergendal, T., & Helkimo, M. (1990). An individual tooth wear index and an analysis of factors correlated to incisal and occlusal wear in an adult Swedish population. *Acta Odontologica*, *48*(5), 343–349. doi:10.3109/00016359009033627 PMID:2251924

Emodi-Perlman, A., Yoffe, T., Rosenberg, N., Eli, I., Alter, Z., & Winocur, E. (2008). Prevalence of Psychologic-, Dental, and Temporomandibular Signs and Symptoms Among Chronic Eating Disorders Patients: A Comparative Control Study. *Journal of Orofacial Pain*, *22*(3), 201–208. PMID:18780533

Fischer, C., Fischer, R. G., & Wennberg, A. (1992). Prevalence and distribution of cervical dentine hypersensitivity in a population in Rio de Janeiro, Brazil. *Journal of Dentistry*, *20*(5), 272–276. doi:10.1016/0300-5712(92)90043-C PMID:1452864

Forssell-Ahlberg, K., Brannström, M., & Edwall, L. (1975). The diameter and number of dentinal tubules in rat, cat, dog and monkey: A comparative scanning electron microscopic study. *Acta Odontologica*, *33*(5), 243–250. doi:10.3109/00016357509004629 PMID:823791

Garberoglio, R., & Brännström, M. (1976). Scanning electron microscopic investigation of human dentinal tubules. *Archives of Oral Biology*, *21*(6), 355–362. doi:10.1016/S0003-9969(76)80003-9 PMID:1066114

Gillam, D. G., Bulman, J. S., Eijkman, M. A. J., & Newman, H. N. (2002). Dentists' perceptions of dentine hypersensitivity and knowledge of its treatment. *Journal of Oral Rehabilitation*, *29*(3), 219–225. doi:10.1046/j.1365-2842.2002.00812.x PMID:11896837

Gillam, D.G., & Orchardson, R. (2006). Advances in the treatment of root dentine sensitivity: mechanisms and treatment principles. *Endodontic Topics, 13*(10), 13-33.

Grippo, J. O. (1991). Abfractions: A new classification of hard tissue lesions of teeth. *Journal of Esthetic and Restorative Dentistry*, *3*(1), 14–19. doi:10.1111/j.1708-8240.1991.tb00799.x PMID:1873064

Grippo, J. O., Simring, M., & Coleman, T. A. (2012). Abfraction, Abrasion, Biocorrosion, and the Enigma of Noncarious Cervical Lesions: A 20-Year Perspective. *Journal of Esthetic and Restorative Dentistry*, *24*(1), 10–23. doi:10.1111/j.1708-8240.2011.00487.x PMID:22296690

Harrel, S. K., Nunn, M. E., & Hallmon, W. W. (2006). Is there an association between occlusion and periodontal destruction?: Yes- occlusal forces can contribute to periodontal destruction. *The Journal of the American Dental Association*, *137*(10), 1380–1392. doi:10.14219/jada.archive.2006.0049 PMID:17012716

Holland, G. R., Narhi, M. N., Addy, M., Gangarosa, L., & Orchardson, R. (1997). Guidelines for the design and conduct of clinical trials on dentine hypersensitivity. *Journal of Clinical Periodontology*, *24*(11), 808–813. doi:10.1111/j.1600-051X.1997.tb01194.x PMID:9402502

Hollstein, W. (1933). Untersuchungen uber das "dickenunter scherdingsvermogen" bei naturlichen zahnen und insbesondere bei festsitzendem und herausnehmbarem abgestutzten ersatz. *Dtch Mschr Zahnheik, 51*, 385.

Hypersensitivity, C. A. B. O. D. (2003). Consensus-based recommendations for the diagnosis and management of dentin hypersensitivity. *Journal (Canadian Dental Association), 69*(4), 221–226. PMID:12662460

Ikeda, T., Nakano, M., Bando, E., & Suzuki, A. (1998). The effect of light, premature occlusal contact on tooth pain threshold in humans. *Journal of Oral Rehabilitation, 25*(8), 589–595. doi:10.1046/j.1365-2842.1998.00295.x PMID:9781861

Ikeda, T., Nakano, M., Bando, E., & Suzuki, A. (1998). The effect of light premature occlusal contact on tooth pain and threshold in humans. *Journal of Oral Rehabilitation, 25*(8), 589–595. doi:10.1046/j.1365-2842.1998.00295.x PMID:9781861

Ikeda, T., Yasumura, H., Yokoyama, M., Mima, S., Yamamoto, I., Kubo, Y., & Bando, E. (1987). A report of hypersensitive teeth induced by abnormal occlusal contacts. *Nippon Hotetsu Shika Gakkai Zasshi, 31*(1), 36–42. doi:10.2186/jjps.31.36 PMID:3506681

Ingle, J. I., Bakland, L. K., & Baumgartner, C. (2008). *Ingle's Endodontics* (6th ed.). Lewiston, PA: PMPH-USA.

Irvine, J. H. (1988). Root surface sensitivity: A review of aetiology and management. *Journal of the New Zealand Society of Periodontology, 66*, 15. PMID:3078601

Irwin, C. R., & McCusker, P. (1996). Prevalence of dentine hypersensitivity in a general dental population. *Journal of the Irish Dental Association, 43*(1), 7–9. PMID:9584750

Ishigaki, S., Bessette, R. W., & Maruyama, T. (1994). Diagnostic accuracy of TMJ vibration analysis for internal derangement and/or degenerative joint disease. *The Journal of Cranio-Mandibular Practice, 12*(4), 241. PMID:7828206

Jacobsen, P. L., & Bruce, G. (2001). Clinical l Dentin Hypersensitivity: Understanding the causes and prescribing a treatment. *The Journal of Contemporary Dental Practice, 2*(1), 1. PMID:12167939

Jerjes, W., Upile, T., Abbas, S., Kafas, P., Vourvachis, M., Rob, J., & Hopper, C. (2008). Muscle disorders and dentition-related aspects in temporomandibular disorders: Controversies in the most commonly used treatment modalities. *International Archives of Medicine, 1*(1), 23. doi:10.1186/1755-7682-1-23 PMID:18973654

Johansson, A., Unell, L., Carlsson, G. E., Söderfeldt, B., & Halling, A. (2002). Gender difference in symptoms related to temporomandibular disorders in a population of 50-year-old subjects. *Journal of Orofacial Pain, 17*(1), 29–35. PMID:12756928

Joss-Vassalli, I., Grebenstein, C., Topouzelis, N., Sculean, A., & Katsaros, C. (2010). Orthodontic therapy and gingival recession: A systematic review. *Orthodontics & Craniofacial Research, 13*(3), 127–141. doi:10.1111/j.1601-6343.2010.01491.x PMID:20618715

Kalamir, A., Pollard, H., Vitiello, A. L., & Bonello, R. (2007). TMD and the problem of bruxism; a review. *Journal of Bodywork and Movement Therapies, 11*(3), 183–193. doi:10.1016/j.jbmt.2006.11.006

Kerstein, R. B. (1992). Disocclusion time-reduction therapy with immediate complete anterior guidance development to treat chronic myofascial pain-dysfunction syndrome. *Quintessence International*, *23*(11), 735–747. PMID:1305288

Kerstein, R. B. (1993). A comparison of traditional occlusal equilibration and immediate complete anterior guidance development. *The Journal of Cranio-Mandibular Practice*, *11*(2), 126. PMID:8495505

Kerstein, R. B. (1995). Treatment of myofascial pain dysfunction syndrome with occlusal therapy to reduce lengthy disclusion time-a recall evaluation. *The Journal of Cranio-Mandibular Practice*, *13*(2), 105–115. PMID:8697496

Kerstein, R. B. (2004). Combining Technologies: A computerized occlusal analysis system synchronized with a computerized electromyography System. *The Journal of Cranio-Mandibular Practice*, *22*(2), 96–109. doi:10.1179/crn.2004.013 PMID:15134409

Kerstein, R. B. (2010). Reducing chronic masseter and temporalis muscular hyperactivity with computer-guided occlusal adjustments. *The Compendium of Continuing Education in Dentistry*, *31*(7), 530–543. PMID:20879206

Kerstein, R. B., Chapman, R., & Klein, M. (1997). A comparison of ICAGD (immediate complete anterior guidance development) to mock ICAGD for symptom reductions in chronic myofascial pain dysfunction patients. *The Journal of Cranio-Mandibular Practice*, *15*(1), 21–37. PMID:9586486

Kerstein, R. B., & Farrel, S. (1990). Treatment of myofascial pain dysfunction syndrome with occlusal equilibration. *The Journal of Prosthetic Dentistry*, *63*(6), 695–700. doi:10.1016/0022-3913(90)90328-A PMID:2102663

Kerstein, R. B., & Grundset, K. (2001). Obtaining measurable bilateral simultaneous occlusal contacts with computer-analyzed and guided occlusal adjustments. *Quintessence International*, *32*(1), 7–18.

Kerstein, R. B., & Radke, J. (2006). The effect of Disclusion Time Reduction on maximal clench muscle activity level. *The Journal of Cranio-Mandibular Practice*, *24*(3), 156–165. doi:10.1179/crn.2006.026 PMID:16933455

Kerstein, R. B., & Radke, J. (2012). Masseter and temporalis excursive hyperactivity decreased by measured anterior guidance development. *The Journal of Cranio-Mandibular Practice*, *30*(4), 243–254. PMID:23156965

Kerstein, R. B., & Wright, N. (1991). An electromyographic and computer analysis of patients suffering from chronic myofascial pain dysfunction syndrome; pre and post - treatment with immediate complete anterior guidance development. *The Journal of Prosthetic Dentistry*, *66*(5), 677–686. doi:10.1016/0022-3913(91)90453-4 PMID:1805009

Kim, H. Y., Chung, G., Jo, H. J., Kim, Y. S., Bae, Y. C., Jung, S. J., & Oh, S. B. (2011). Characterization of dental nociceptive neurons. *Journal of Dental Research*, *90*(6), 771–776. doi:10.1177/0022034511399906 PMID:21364091

Kirveskari, P. (1997). The role of occlusal adjustment in the management of Temporomandibular disorders. *Oral Surgery, Oral Medicine, Oral Pathology, Oral Radiology, and Endodontology*, *83*(1), 87–90. doi:10.1016/S1079-2104(97)90097-4 PMID:9007930

Kleinberg, I., Kaufman, H. W., & Confessore, F. (1990). Methods of measuring tooth hypersensitivity. *Dental Clinics of North America*, *34*(3), 515. PMID:2197125

Kleinfelder, J. W., & Ludwig, K. (2002). Maximal bite force in patients with reduced periodontal tissue support with and without splinting. *Journal of Periodontology*, *73*(10), 1184–1187. doi:10.1902/jop.2002.73.10.1184 PMID:12416777

Koh, H., & Robinson, P. G. (2004). Occlusal adjustment for treating and preventing Temporomandibular joint disorders. *Journal of Oral Rehabilitation*, *31*(4), 287–292. doi:10.1046/j.1365-2842.2003.01257.x PMID:15089931

Kubo, K., Shibukawa, Y., Shintani, M., Suzuki, T., Ichinohe, T., & Kaneko, Y. (2008). Cortical representation area of human dental pulp. *Journal of Dental Research*, *87*(4), 358–362. doi:10.1177/154405910808700409 PMID:18362319

Kurthy, R. (2009). *Solving Teeth Whitening Sensitivity*. Retrieved from www.evolvedental.com

Kvinnsland, I., & Heyeraas, K. J. (1992). Effect of traumatic occlusion on CGRP and SP immunoreactive nerve fibre morphology in rat molar pulp and periodontium. *Histochemistry*, *97*(2), 111–120. doi:10.1007/BF00267300 PMID:1373126

Le Resche, L., Burgess, J., & Dworkin, S. F. (1988). Reliability of visual analog and verbal descriptor scales for" objective" measurement of temporomandibular disorder pain. *Journal of Dental Research*, *67*(1), 33–36. doi:10.1177/00220345880670010601 PMID:11039041

Levy, J. H. (2009). Teeth as Sensory Organs. *Vistas. Aegis Publications*, *2*(3), 14–19.

Lilja, J., Nordenvall, K. J., & Bränström, M. (1982). Dentin sensitivity, odontoblasts and nerves under desiccated or infected experimental cavities. A clinical, light microscopic and ultrastructural investigation. *Swedish Dental Journal*, *6*(3), 93. PMID:6955990

Lin, M., Luo, Z. Y., Bai, B. F., Xu, F., & Lu, T. J. (2011). Fluid mechanics in dentinal microtubules provides mechanistic insights into the difference between hot and cold dental pain. *PLoS ONE*, *6*(3), e18068. doi:10.1371/journal.pone.0018068 PMID:21448459

Ling, T. Y., & Gillam, D. G. (1996). The effectiveness of desensitizing agents for the treatment of cervical dentine sensitivity (CDS)--a review. *The Journal of the Western Society of Periodontology/Periodontal Abstracts*, *44*(1), 5. PMID:9477862

Linsuwanont, P., Palamara, J. E. A., & Messer, H. H. (2007). An investigation of thermal stimulation in intact teeth. *Archives of Oral Biology*, *52*(3), 218–227. doi:10.1016/j.archoralbio.2006.10.009 PMID:17109811

Linsuwanont, P., Versluis, A., Palamara, J. E., & Messer, H. H. (2008). Thermal stimulation causes tooth deformation: A possible alternative to the hydrodynamic theory? *Archives of Oral Biology*, *53*(3), 261–272. doi:10.1016/j.archoralbio.2007.10.006 PMID:18037388

Litonjua, L. A., Andreana, S., Bush, P. J., Tobias, T. S., & Cohen, R. E. (2003). Noncarious cervical lesions and abfractions: A re-evaluation. *The Journal of the American Dental Association*, *134*(7), 845–850. doi:10.14219/jada.archive.2003.0282 PMID:12892441

Liu, H. C., Lan, W. H., & Hsieh, C. C. (1998). Prevalence and distribution of cervical dentin hypersensitivity in a population in Taipei, Taiwan. *Journal of Endodontics*, *24*(1), 45–47. doi:10.1016/S0099-2399(98)80213-6 PMID:9487867

Lussi, A., Seong, J., & Hellwig, E. (2012). Dentin hypersensitivity: Pain mechanisms and aetiology of exposed cervical dentin. *Clinical Oral Investigations*, 1–11.

Mahan, P. E., Wilkinson, T. M., Gibbs, C. H., Mauderli, A., & Brannon, L. S. (1983). Superior and inferior bellies of the lateral pterygoid muscle EMG activity at basic jaw positions. *The Journal of Prosthetic Dentistry*, *50*(5), 710–718. doi:10.1016/0022-3913(83)90214-7 PMID:6580440

Manfredini, D., Cantini, E., Romagnoli, M., & Bosco, M. (2003). Prevalence of bruxism in patients with different research diagnostic criteria for Temporomandibular disorders (RDC/TMD) diagnoses. *The Journal of Cranio-Mandibular Practice*, *21*(4), 279. PMID:14620701

Manfredini, D., Castroflorio, T., Perinetti, G., & Guarda-Nardini, L. (2012). Dental occlusion, body posture and Temporomandibular disorders: Where we are now and where we are heading. *Journal of Oral Rehabilitation*, *39*(6), 463–471. doi:10.1111/j.1365-2842.2012.02291.x PMID:22435603

Manschreck, T. C. (2009). Compulsive bruxism: How to protect your patients' teeth. *Current Psychiatry*, *8*(3), 24.

Markowitz, K., & Kim, S. (1992). The role of selected cations in the desensitization of intradental nerves. *Proceedings of the Finnish Dental Society. Suomen Hammaslaakariseuran Toimituksia*, *88*, 39. PMID:1508896

Marvin, K. (2008). Bright, white, and sensitive: An overview of tooth whitening and Dentin Hypersensitivity. *Dentistry Today*, *27*, 80–81. PMID:18505029

Matthews, B. (1977). Responses of intradental nerves to electrical and thermal stimulation of teeth in dogs. *The Journal of Physiology*, *264*(3), 641–664. PMID:557544

Matthews, B., Andrew, D., & Wanachantararak, S. (2000). *Biology of the dental pulp with special reference to its vasculature and innervation. In Tooth Wear and Sensitivity* (pp. 39–51). London, UK: Martin Dunitz.

Mayhew, R. B., Jessee, S. A., & Martin, R. E. (1998). Association of occlusal, periodontal, and dietary factors with the presence of non-carious cervical dental lesions. *American Journal of Dentistry*, *11*(1), 29. PMID:9823083

Mazzeto, M. O., Hotta, T. H., & Mazzetto, R. G. (2009). Analysis of TMJ vibration sounds before and after use of two types of occlusal splints. *Brazilian Dental Journal*, *20*(4), 325–330. doi:10.1590/S0103-64402009000400011 PMID:20069257

Melchior, M. D. O., Mazzetto, M. O., & Felício, C. M. D. (2012). Temporomandibular disorders and parafunctional oral habits: An anamnestic study. *Dental Press Journal of Orthodontics*, *17*(2), 83–89. doi:10.1590/S2176-94512012000200016

Miller, N., Penaud, J., Ambrosini, P., Bisson-Boutelliez, C., & Briançon, S. (2003). Analysis of etiologic factors and periodontal conditions involved with 309 abfractions. *Journal of Clinical Periodontology*, *30*(9), 828–832. doi:10.1034/j.1600-051X.2003.00378.x PMID:12956659

Millstein, P., & Maya, A. (2001). An evaluation of occlusal contact marking indicators. A descriptive quantitative method. *The Journal of the American Dental Association*, *132*(9), 1280–1286. doi:10.14219/jada.archive.2001.0373 PMID:11665355

Molina, O. F., Dos Santos, J., Mazzetto, M., Nelson, S., Nowlin, T., & Mainieri, É. T. (2001). Oral jaw behaviors in TMD and bruxism: A comparison study by severity of bruxism. *The Journal of Cranio-Mandibular Practice*, *19*(2), 114–122. PMID:11842862

Mumford, J. M. (1982). *Orofacial pain: etiology, diagnosis and treatment*. Edinburgh, UK: Livingstone.

Närhi, M., Jyväsjärvi, E., Virtanen, A., Huopaniemi, T., Ngassapa, D., & Hirvonen, T. (1991). Role of intradental A-and C-type nerve fibres in dental pain mechanisms. *Proceedings of the Finnish Dental Society. Suomen Hammaslaakariseuran Toimituksia*, *88*, 507–516. PMID:1508908

Närhi, M., Yamamoto, H., Ngassapa, D., & Hirvonen, T. (1994). The neurophysiological basis and the role of inflammatory reactions in dentine hypersensitivity. *Archives of Oral Biology*, *39*, 523–530. doi:10.1016/0003-9969(94)90184-8 PMID:7702462

Ohmori, H., Kirimoto, H., & Ono, T. (2012). Comparison of the physiological properties of human periodontal-masseteric reflex evoked by incisor and canine stimulation. *Frontiers in Physics*, *3*, 233. PMID:22754541

Orchardson, R., & Gillam, D. G. (2000). The efficacy of potassium salts as agents for treating dentin hypersensitivity. *Journal of Orofacial Pain, 149*(1), 9-19.

Osborne-Smith, K. L., Burke, F. J. T., & Wilson, N. H. F. (1999). The aetiology of the non-carious cervical lesion. *International Dental Journal*, *49*(3), 139–143. doi:10.1002/j.1875-595X.1999.tb00898.x PMID:10858746

Paine, M. L., Slots, J., & Rich, S. K. (1998). Fluoride use in periodontal therapy: A review of the literature. *The Journal of the American Dental Association*, *129*(10), 69–77. doi:10.14219/jada.archive.1998.0023 PMID:9448348

Pashley, D. H. (1986). Dentin permeability, dentin sensitivity, and treatment through tubule occlusion. *Journal of Endodontics*, *129*(10), 465–474. doi:10.1016/S0099-2399(86)80201-1 PMID:3465852

Pashley, D. H. (1990). Mechanisms of dentin sensitivity. *Dental Clinics of North America*, *34*(3), 449–473. PMID:2197121

Pashley, D. H. (1991). Smear layer: Overview of structure and function. *Proceedings of the Finnish Dental Society. Suomen Hammaslaakariseuran Toimituksia*, *88*, 215–224. PMID:1508877

Pashley, D. H. (1996). Dynamics of the pulpo-dentin complex. *Critical Reviews in Oral Biology and Medicine*, *7*(2), 104–133. doi:10.1177/10454411960070020101 PMID:8875027

Pashley, D. H., Andringa, H. J., Derkson, G. D., Derkson, M. E., & Kalathoor, S. R. (1987). Regional variability in the permeability of human dentine. *Archives of Oral Biology*, *327*(7), 519–523. doi:10.1016/S0003-9969(87)80014-6 PMID:3479091

Pashley, D. H., Kehl, T., Pashley, E., & Palmer, P. (1981). Comparison of in vitro and in vivo dog dentin permeability. *Journal of Dental Research*, *60*(3), 763–768. doi:10.1177/00220345810600031801 PMID:6937512

Porto, I. C., Andrade, A. K., & Montes, M. A. (2009). Diagnosis and treatment of dentinal hypersensitivity. *Journal of Oral Science*, *51*(3), 323–332. doi:10.2334/josnusd.51.323 PMID:19776498

Qadeer, S., Kerstein, R., Kim, R. J. Y., Huh, J. B., & Shin, S. W. (2012). Relationship between articulation paper mark size and percentage of force measured with computerized occlusal analysis. *The Journal of Advanced Prosthodontics*, *4*(1), 7–12. doi:10.4047/jap.2012.4.1.7 PMID:22439094

Rapp, R., Avery, J. K., & Strachan, D. S. (1968). *Possible role of the acetylcholinesterase in neural conduction within the dental pulp* (pp. 309–311). Birmingham, AL: University of Alabama Press.

Rees, J. S. (2000). The prevalence of dentine hypersensitivity in general dental practice in the UK. *Journal of Clinical Periodontology*, *27*(11), 860–865. doi:10.1034/j.1600-051x.2000.027011860.x PMID:11073330

Rees, J. S., & Addy, M. (2002). A cross-sectional study of dentine hypersensitivity. *Journal of Clinical Periodontology*, *29*(11), 997–1003. doi:10.1034/j.1600-051X.2002.291104.x PMID:12472992

Reiter, D. (1980). Concepts of dental occlusion. *American Journal of Otolaryngology*, *1*(3), 245–255. doi:10.1016/S0196-0709(80)80096-2 PMID:7004222

Richardson, D., Tao, L., & Pashley, D. H. (1991). Dentin permeability: Effects of crown preparation. *The International Journal of Prosthodontics*, *4*(3), 219–225. PMID:1810312

Rimondini, L., Baroni, C., & Carrassi, A. (1995). Ultrastructure of hypersensitive and non-sensitive dentine. *Journal of Clinical Periodontology*, *22*(12), 899–902. doi:10.1111/j.1600-051X.1995.tb01792.x PMID:8613556

Rowe, N. H. (1985). *Hypersensitive dentin: origin and management*. Ann Arbor, MI: University of Michigan.

Ruiz, J. L., & Coleman, T. A. (2008). CE 2 Occlusal Disease Management System: The Diagnosis Process. *Compendium-Newton*, *29*(3), 148. PMID:18468301

Saad, M. N., Weiner, G., Ehrenberg, D., & Weiner, S. (2008). Effects of load and indicator type upon occlusal contact markings. *Journal of Biomedical Materials Research. Part B, Applied Biomaterials*, *85*(1), 18–22. doi:10.1002/jbm.b.30910 PMID:17618516

Seligman, D.A., & Pullinger, A.G. (1991). The role of functional occlusal relationships in temporomandibular disorders: A review. *Journal of Craniomandibular Disorders: Facial & Oral Pain*, *5*(4), 265.

Seltzer, S., & Bender, I. B. (1984). *The Dental Pulp: Biologic Considerations in Dental Procedures*. Baltimore, MD: Lippincott Williams & Wilkins.

Sharav, Y., McGrath, P. A., & Dubner, R. (1982). Masseter inhibitory periods and sensations evoked by electrical tooth pulp stimulation in patients with oral-facial pain and mandibular dysfunction. *Archives of Oral Biology*, *27*(4), 305–310. doi:10.1016/0003-9969(82)90159-5 PMID:6953948

Sharma, A., Rahul, G. R., Poduval, S. T., Shetty, K., Gupta, B., & Rajora, V. (2013). History of materials used for recording static and dynamic occlusal contact marks: A literature review. *Journal of Clinical and Experimental Dentistry*, *5*(1), 48–53. doi:10.4317/jced.50680 PMID:24455051

Slutzkey, S., & Levin, L. (2008). Gingival recession in young adults: Occurrence, severity, and relationship to past orthodontic treatment and oral piercing. *American Journal of Orthodontics and Dentofacial Orthopedics*, *134*(5), 652–656. doi:10.1016/j.ajodo.2007.02.054 PMID:18984397

Splieth, C. H., & Tachou, A. (2013). Epidemiology of dentin hypersensitivity. *Clinical Oral Investigations*, 1–6. PMID:23224064

Spranger, H. (1995). Investigation into the genesis of angular lesions at the cervical region of teeth. *Quintessence International*, *26*(2), 149–154. PMID:7568726

Strassler, H. E., Drisko, C. L., & Alexander, D. C. (2008). *Dentin hypersensitivity: its inter-relationship to gingival recession and acid erosion*. Newtown, PA: Aegis Publications.

Strassler, H. E., & Serio, F. G. (2009). *Dentinal hypersensitivity: etiology, diagnosis and management. In Academy of Dental Therapeutics and Stomatology* (pp. 2–7). Aegis.

Suge, T., Kawasaki, A., Ishikawa, K., Matsuo, T., & Ebisu, S. (2006). Effects of plaque control on the patency of dentinal tubules: An in vivo study in beagle dogs. *Journal of Periodontology*, *77*(3), 454–459. doi:10.1902/jop.2006.050159 PMID:16512760

Swift, E. J. Jr. (2005). Tooth sensitivity and whitening. *The Compendium of Continuing Education in Dentistry*, *26*(9Suppl 3), 4–10. PMID:17042087

Taani, D. Q., & Awartani, F. (2001). Prevalence and distribution of dentin hypersensitivity and plaque in a dental hospital population. *Quintessence International*, *32*(5), 372–376. PMID:11444069

Tabbara, N. (2009). Temporomandibular disorders (TMDs): A note from the field. *Journal of the Lebanese Dental Association*, *46*, 37–41.

Takeuchi, N., & Yamamoto, T. (2008). Correlation between periodontal status and biting force in patients with chronic periodontitis during the maintenance phase of therapy. *Journal of Clinical Periodontology*, *35*(3), 215–220. doi:10.1111/j.1600-051X.2007.01186.x PMID:18190555

Tarantola, G., Becker, I. M., Gremiilion, H., & Pink, F. (1998). The Effectiveness of Equilibration in the Improvement of Signs and Symptoms in the Stomatognathic System. *International Journal of Periodontal and Restorative Dentistry*, *18*(6), 595–603. PMID:10321174

Tillis, T. S., & Keating, J. S. (2005). Dentin hypersensitivity. In E. M. Wilkins (Ed.), *Clinical Practice of the Dental Hygienist* (9th ed.). Baltimore, MD: Lippincott, Williams & Wilkins.

Trowbridge, H. O., Franks, M., Korostoff, E., & Emling, R. (1980). Sensory response to thermal stimulation in human teeth. *Journal of Endodontics*, *6*(1), 405–412. doi:10.1016/S0099-2399(80)80216-0 PMID:6935330

Trulsson, M., Francis, S. T., Bowtell, R., & McGlone, F. (2010). Brain activations in response to vibrotactile tooth stimulation: A psychophysical and MRI study. *Journal of Neurophysiology*, *104*(4), 2257–2265. doi:10.1152/jn.00565.2010 PMID:20668275

Trulsson, M., & Johansson, R. S. (1996). Encoding of tooth loads by human periodontal afferents and their role in jaw motor control. *Progress in Neurobiology*, *49*(3), 267–284. doi:10.1016/S0301-0082(96)00016-0 PMID:8878305

Tugnait, A., & Clerehugh, V. (2001). Gingival recession—its significance and management. *Journal of Dentistry*, *29*(6), 381–394. doi:10.1016/S0300-5712(01)00035-5 PMID:11520586

Türker, K. S. (2002). Reflex control of human jaw muscles. *Critical Reviews in Oral Biology and Medicine*, *13*(1), 85–104. doi:10.1177/154411130201300109 PMID:12097240

Tyas, M. J. (1995). The Class V lesion - Aetiology and restoration. *Australian Dental Journal*, *40*(3), 167–170. doi:10.1111/j.1834-7819.1995.tb05631.x PMID:7661762

van Loveren, C. (2013). Exposed cervical dentin and Dentin Hypersensitivity summary of the discussion and recommendations. *Clinical Oral Investigations*, *17*(S1Suppl 1), 73–76. doi:10.1007/s00784-012-0902-2 PMID:23224117

Vera-Portocarrero, L. P., Zhang, E. T., Ossipov, M. H., Xie, J. Y., King, T., Lai, J., & Porreca, F. (2006). Descending facilitation from the rostral ventromedial medulla maintains nerve injury-induced central sensitization. *Neuroscience*, *140*(4), 1311–1320. doi:10.1016/j.neuroscience.2006.03.016 PMID:16650614

Walters, P. A. (2005). Dentinal hypersensitivity: A review. *The Journal of Contemporary Dental Practice*, *6*(2), 107–117. PMID:15915210

West, N.X. (2006). Dentine hypersensitivity. *Monographs in Oral Science: Dental Erosion, from Diagnosis to Therapy, 20*, 173-189.

West, N. X. (2008). Dentine hypersensitivity: Preventive and therapeutic approaches to treatment. *Periodontology*, *48*(1), 31–41. doi:10.1111/j.1600-0757.2008.00262.x PMID:18715354

Williamson, E. H., & Lundquist, D. O. (1983). Anterior guidance: Its effect on electromyographic activity of the temporal and masseter muscles. *The Journal of Prosthetic Dentistry*, *49*(6), 816–823. doi:10.1016/0022-3913(83)90356-6 PMID:6576136

Yadav, S. (2011). A Study on Prevalence of Dental Attrition and its Relation to Factors of Age, Gender and to the Signs of TMJ Dysfunction. *The Journal of Indian Prosthodontic Society*, *11*(2), 98–105. doi:10.1007/s13191-011-0076-7 PMID:22654349

Yoshiyama, M., Noiri, Y., Ozaki, K., Uchida, A., Ishikawa, Y., & Ishida, H. (1990). Transmission electron microscopic characterization of hypersensitive human radicular dentin. *Journal of Dental Research*, *69*(6), 1293–1297. doi:10.1177/00220345900690061401 PMID:2355124

ADDITIONAL READING

Absi, E. G., Addy, M., & Adams, D. (1992). Dentine hypersensitivity–the effect of toothbrushing and dietary compounds on dentine in vitro: An SEM study. *Journal of Oral Rehabilitation*, *19*(2), 101–110. doi:10.1111/j.1365-2842.1992.tb01086.x PMID:1517870

Al-Sabbagh, M., Andreana, S., & Ciancio, S. G. (2004). Dentinal hypersensitivity: Review of aetiology, differential diagnosis, prevalence, and mechanism. *Journal of the International Academy of Periodontology*, *6*(1), 8. PMID:14964489

Bakke, M. (1993). Mandibular elevator muscles: Physiology, action, and effect of dental occlusion. *European Journal of Oral Sciences*, *101*(5), 314–331. doi:10.1111/j.1600-0722.1993.tb01127.x PMID:8248735

Bergamini, M., Pierleoni, F., Gizdulich, A., & Bergamini, C. (2008). Dental occlusion and body posture: A surface EMG study. *The Journal of Cranio-Mandibular Practice*, *26*(1), 25–32. PMID:18290522

Ferrario, V. F., Serrao, G., Dellavia, C., Caruso, E., & Sforza, C. (2002). Relationship between the number of occlusal contacts and masticatory muscle activity in healthy young adults. *The Journal of Cranio-Mandibular Practice*, *20*(2), 91–98. PMID:12002835

Glaros, A. G., Forbes, M., Shanker, J., & Glass, E. G. (2000). Effect of parafunctional clenching on temporomandibular disorder pain and proprioceptive awareness. *The Journal of Cranio-Mandibular Practice*, *18*(3), 198–204. PMID:11202838

Khan, A., & Hargreaves, K. M. (2010). *Animal models of orofacial pain. Analgesia* (pp. 93–104). New York City: Humana Press.

Kimoto, K., Fushima, K., Tamaki, K., Toyoda, M., Sato, S., & Uchimura, N. (2000). Asymmetry of masticatory muscle activity during the closing phase of mastication. *The Journal of Cranio-Mandibular Practice*, *18*(4), 257–263. PMID:11202845

Mahan, P. E., Wilkinson, T. M., Gibbs, C. H., Mauderli, A., & Brannon, L. S. (1983). Superior and inferior bellies of the lateral pterygoid muscle EMG activity at basic jaw positions. *The Journal of Prosthetic Dentistry*, *50*(5), 710–718. doi:10.1016/0022-3913(83)90214-7 PMID:6580440

Nguyen, C., Ranjitkar, S., Kaidonis, J. A., & Townsend, G. C. (2008). A qualitative assessment of non-carious cervical lesions in extracted human teeth. *Australian Dental Journal*, *53*(1), 46–51. doi:10.1111/j.1834-7819.2007.00009.x PMID:18304241

Piancino, M. G., Bracco, P., Vallelonga, T., Merlo, A., & Farina, D. (2008). Effect of bolus hardness on the chewing pattern and activation of masticatory muscles in subjects with normal dental occlusion. *Journal of Electromyography and Kinesiology*, *18*(6), 931–937. doi:10.1016/j.jelekin.2007.05.006 PMID:17616401

Raphael, K. G., & Ciccone, D. S. (2008). *Psychological aspects of chronic orofacial pain. Orofacial Pain and Headache* (pp. 57–74). Edinburgh: Elsevier. doi:10.1016/B978-0-7234-3412-2.10004-5

Rees, J. S. (2006). The biomechanics of abfraction. *Proceedings of the Institution of Mechanical Engineers. Part H, Journal of Engineering in Medicine*, *220*(1), 69–80. doi:10.1243/095441105X69141 PMID:16459447

Robertson, L. T., Levy, J. H., Petrisor, D., Lilly, D. J., & Dong, W. K. (2003). Vibration perception thresholds of human maxillary and mandibular central incisors. *Archives of Oral Biology*, *48*(4), 309–316. doi:10.1016/S0003-9969(03)00006-2 PMID:12663076

Wright, E. F. (2008). Pulpalgia contributing to temporomandibular disorder-like pain; a literature review and case report. *The Journal of the American Dental Association*, *139*(4), 436–440. doi:10.14219/jada.archive.2008.0186 PMID:18385027

Zuñiga, C., Miralles, R., Mena, B., Montt, R., Moran, D., Santander, H., & Moya, H. (1995). Influence of variation in jaw posture on sternocleidomastoid and trapezius electromyographic activity. *The Journal of Cranio-Mandibular Practice*, *13*(3), 157–162. PMID:8949854

KEY TERMS AND DEFINITIONS

Dentinal Hypersensitivity: A sharp, acute pain of short duration arising from *open dentinal tubules* in response to a normally innocuous stimulus, which is diagnosed through a process of exclusion with a thorough dental screening, examination, and history.

Disclusion Time: A measurable T-Scan occlusal parameter that computes the elapsed time required for teeth to leave static intercuspation until all posterior teeth bilaterally completely disengage, and only the anterior teeth remain in contact.

Frictional Dental Hypersensitivity (FDH): A nociceptive response to tooth torsion and flexion induced from excessive occlusal surface frictional engagements of posterior teeth during mandibular excursions. FDH presents as a sharp, acute, transient pain that mimics, and may precede Dentinal Hypersensitivity. FDH, unlike Dentinal Hypersensitivity, does not always involve exposed dentin and patent dentinal tubules.

Lactic Acid: A water-soluble byproduct of anaerobic glucose metabolism produced during muscle contraction. Excess levels of lactic acid can lead to myalgic symptoms in muscular TMD patients.

Mechanoreception: An unconscious sensing, or a conscious perception of touch or mechanical displacement, arising from stimuli outside of the body.

Mechanoreceptors: Sensory nerve end organs which respond to mechanical stimuli, such as pressure, vibration, tension and *friction.*

Sensitization: A heightened or newfound hypersensitivity to noxious stimuli, or normal innocuous stimulation following nerve injury.

Tooth Flexion: A deviation or bend of a tooth that is restricted to the root portion of a tooth.

This work was previously published in the Handbook of Research on Computerized Occlusal Analysis Technology Applications in Dental Medicine edited by Robert B. Kerstein, DMD, pages 358-428, copyright year 2015 by Medical Information Science Reference (an imprint of IGI Global).

APPENDIX

A) Tooth Sensitivity Pain Scale (TSPS)

Patient:	Pre-op
Date:	Post-op

Rate your pain on a scale from 0 to 10:

0 – no pain whatsoever
1 – I almost never feel it
3 – I'm aware of it several times a week
5 – Pain that just barely needs store bought medication
7 – I really should see my dentist
9 – I must have stronger medication and need to see my dentist today!
10 – The worst possible pain!

Please describe your tooth sensitivity pain to a 5 second ice water swish:

No Pain										Very Painful
0	1	2	3	4	5	6	7	8	9	10

B) Occlusion/Bite Related Questions (PLEASE CIRCLE THE NUMBER IF YES)

Do you:

1 – Drink cold drinks through a straw to prevent a painful response in your teeth?
2 – Experience that your tooth sensitivity pain dissipates rapidly?
3 – Have trouble eating crunchy or chewy foods?
4 – Have trouble drinking a cold drink or eating ice cream?
5 – Experience pain in your teeth when breathing in cold air, that dissipates when you close your mouth and breathe through your nose?
6 – Experience a transient sensitivity pain in several of your teeth, or over a general area?
7 – Feel that your jaw and cheek muscles are often tight?
8 – Notice that chewing gum or chewy foods makes your jaw tired?
9 – Clench or grind your teeth?
10 – Notice that you consciously keep your lower teeth from touching your upper teeth because your teeth hurt slightly if not?
11 – Find yourself sticking your tongue between your front teeth sometimes?

C) Less Related to Occlusion Questions (PLEASE CIRCLE THE NUMBER IF YES)

Do you:

12 – Feel that your tooth sensitivity pain lingers long after the hot or cold stimulus is gone?
13 – Experience lingering pain after separating your teeth between crunchy foods?
14 – Feel that cold makes the pain in your tooth or teeth feel better?
15 – Experience pain in your tooth or teeth that wakes you up at night?
16 – Notice that you consciously keep your lower teeth from touching your upper teeth because your teeth hurt unbearably, if not apart?
17 – Find that you must put something between your front teeth or the pain is unbearable?
18 – Think that you know exactly the one tooth that is causing your pain?
19 – Feel that you cannot open your jaw as far as you used to?
20 – Feel that hot drinks are intolerable and lead to a very painful response?

Chapter 11
Segmentation and Feature Extraction of Panoramic Dental X-Ray Images

Pedro H. M. Lira
National Laboratory for Scientific Computing, Brazil

Gilson A. Giraldi
National Laboratory for Scientific Computing, Brazil

Luiz A. P. Neves
Federal University of Parana, Brazil

ABSTRACT

Automating the process of analysis of Panoramic X-Ray images is important to help dentist procedures and diagnosis. Tooth segmentation from the radiographic images and feature extraction are essential steps. The authors propose a segmentation approach based on mathematical morphology, quadtree decomposition for mask generation, thresholding, and snake models. The feature extraction stage is steered by a shape model based on Principal Component Analysis (PCA). First, the authors take the quadtree decomposition of a low-pass version of the original image and select the smallest blocks to generate a mask. Then, the original image is processed by Otsu's thresholding. The result is improved by morphological operators and the quadtree mask is applied to address overlapping, a common problem in X-ray images. The obtained regions are searched and the larger ones are selected to find tooth candidates. The boundary of the obtained regions are extracted and aligned with the shape model in order to recognize the target tooth (molar). The selected curve is used in a search method to initialize a snake technique. Finally, morphometric data extraction is performed to obtain tooth measurements for dentist diagnosis. Experiments show the advantages of the proposed method to extract teeth from X-Ray images and discuss its drawbacks.

DOI: 10.4018/978-1-5225-1903-4.ch011

1. INTRODUCTION

In the last decades, medical imaging techniques have been applied to scan human body for clinical purposes (diagnoses and surgical planning) and medical science studies like anatomy and physiology. The area incorporates imaging technology based on radiography (projection or fluoroscopy), nuclear medicine, endoscopy, microscopy (for human pathological investigations), tomography, magnetic resonance imaging, among others (Suetens, 2002). From the viewpoint of computer science, each one of these modalities needs specific algorithms and mathematical methods for automating the process of image analysis (Suri, 2005).

The Panoramic X-Ray images are obtained through projection radiography devices and are very popular as a first tool for diagnosis in odontological protocols (Figure 1). The panoramic X-ray is a cheap and very useful tool for dentist diagnosis. It has a low level of radiation, is comfortable and very quickly for the patient to have taken. The panoramic X-ray shows the dentist a patient's nasal area, sinuses, jaw joints, teeth and surrounding bone. It can reveal cysts, tumors, bone irregularities, among other problems. So, automating the process of analysis of such images is an important application. However, it is a difficult task due to the structures overlapping and texture patterns commonly observed in such images.

Tooth segmentation from dental X-ray films is an essential step for automating diagnosis as well asforensic procedures like postmortem identification (Said et al., 2006). For these applications, the segmentation step must be followed by features extraction. Approaches in image segmentation can be roughly classified in: (a) Contour Based methods, like snakes and active shape models (Suri, 2005); (b) Region based techniques (Zhou & Abdel-Mottaleb, 2005); (c) Optimization approaches (Fukunaga, 1990) ;(d) Clustering methods, like k-means, Fuzzy C-means, Hierarchical clustering (Jain et al., 1999) and (e) Thresholding methods (Sezgin & Sankur, 2004).

Snake models are 2D deformable models that can integrate image data, an initial estimated, prior shape information (active shape model) in a single extraction process (Black & Yuille, 1993). Region-based methods attempt to group regions following some homogeneity criterion. Optimization approaches rely on an objective function, that combines the input image and constraints, and some optimization process for separating foreground from the background in an image. Clustering methods (in general) apply statistics and machine learning to partition N pixels into K clusters ($K<N$). Thresholding techniques compute a global threshold to distinguish objects from their background. They are low computational cost and effective tools to segment objects in a scene. Also, it is simple to implement these techniques in a computer language (Kanungo at al., 1994).

There are few researches dedicated to the specific problem of dental radiograph image segmentation. Projection histograms, thresholding, mathematical morphology, contrast enhancement are common techniques applied in this area (Jain & Chen, 2004; Zhou & Abdel-Mottaleb, 2005; Nomir & Abdel-Mottaleb, 2005). Recently, it was proposed a work that also applies zonal masks in the Fourier domain to address overlapping (Lira et al., 2009), which is a very common problem in panoramic X-ray images, as we can see in Figure 1.

In this paper, we focus on segmentation, recognition and feature extraction in panoramic X-ray images, like the one picture on Figure 1. The segmentation stage is based on quadtree decomposition and mathematical morphology for mask generation, thresholding and snake models. Quadtree image representation is very useful for image procession because it allows to recursively simplifies the image field. For instance, in (Dua et al., 2010) we find a methodology that performs edge detection only in the leaves and their parents which have 1×1 and 2×2 block sizes. In our case, firstly, we take the quadtree

Figure 1. A typical panoramic x-ray image

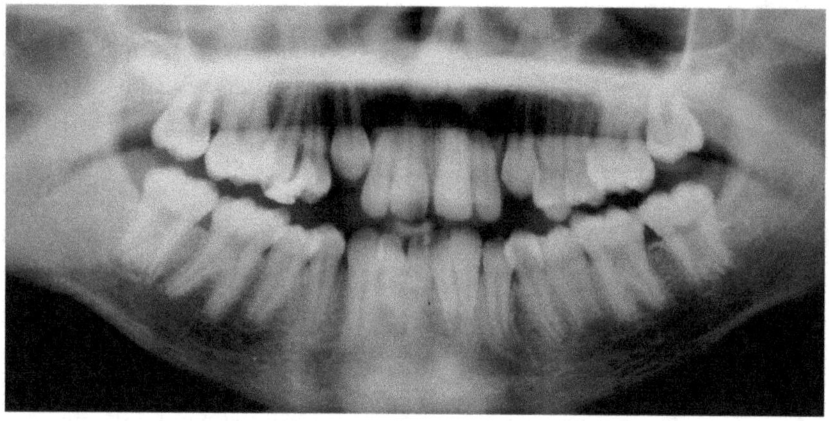

decomposition of a low-pass version of the original image and select the smallest blocks which shall lie nearby object boundaries. These blocks are used to generate a mask for a further search instead of directly applying edge detection filters, like in (Dua et al., 2010).

Then, the original image is processed by Otsu's thresholding. The result is improved by morphological operators in order to fill holes and discard artifacts and processed by the mask obtained in the previous step. We perform a XOR operation between the mask and the binary image to address overlapping, a common problem in X-ray images.

Among the obtained regions the largest ones are selected to find out the tooth candidates. The boundary of those regions are extracted, through a simple 2D marching-cubes like technique. The result is aligned with a shape model (mean shape) that is generated through a database of manually segmented teeth provided by the Odontological Department of Federal University of Rio de Janeiro, Brazil.

Next, we perform the boundary analysis, in the model parameter space, to select the teeth among the aligned curves. Next, using the mean shape, it is performed a search around these curves to find the best site to initialize a snake for improving the result. In the last stage of the pipeline it is performed some measurements for dentist diagnosis. In the experimental results we discuss the efficiency of the proposed pipeline for tooth segmentation and feature extraction and compare it with the work presented in (Lira et al., 2009).

2. DATABASE SAMPLES

The database was provided by the Odontological Department of Federal University of Rio de Janeiro, Brazil. It contains a set of 30 panoramic X-ray images, taken for radiological examinations in usual dentistry protocols. Each image was digitized with 300 dpi resolution, in gray level scale of 8 bits and looks like the one pictured on Figure 1. The dentist team selects in each image a window with containing the tooth of interest (in this case, the molar), which generates the database pictured in Figure 2.

It is interesting to perform some comments about these images and the tests that oriented the steps of the method to be described next. Figure 3(a) shows a sample of the database and Figures 3(b)-(c) picture the zero-crossing images for some values of the gaussian parameter (we use the laplacian of gaussian

Figure 2. Some samples of the image database used in the tests

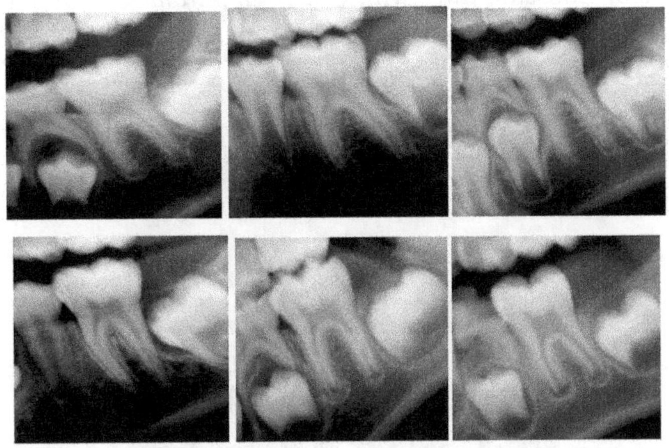

filter). The observed result reflects the textured nature of these images and we observe that we almost lost the shape of the structure of interest.

Figure 3(d) shows another example using median filter and Canny edge detector. The results is better than the laplacian one, but we need a non-trivial pos-processing stage to discard unwanted edges and to reconstruct the pre-molar, probably using a watershed operator. On the other hand, Otsu's technique gives a more valuable result, as we can observe in Figure 3(e). However, it cannot deal with overlapping. So, we decided to get a rough segmentation through Otsu's method and, in a further step, to improve this result with another technique, in this case, the quadtree decomposition. The section 3 describes the pipeline in details.

3. PROPOSED METHOD

Our proposed method is divided into four main steps: (a) Shape Model Generation; (b) Image Pre-processing; (c) Boundary Extraction and Analysis; (d) Morphometrics Data Extraction. Figure 4 shows the main stages of the proposed methodology.

Each tooth has a characteristic shape in the Panoramic X-ray image. Therefore, we can train a shape model in order to incorporate the prior knowledge about the target shape (the molar). The shape model will be used in the tooth identification (recognition) and snake model initialization (Figure 4).

3.1. Shape Model Generation

We consider an object to be described by points, referred to as landmark points. These points may represent the boundary of the object or some structures of interest in the images of a database.

In general, the landmark points are (manually) determined in a set of s training images. From these collections of landmark points, a point distribution model (Jain, 1989) is constructed as follows. The landmark points are stacked in shape vectors:

Figure 3. (a) Original image; (b) Laplace of Gaussian filter with Gaussian parameter σ=0.3 and edge threshold 0.7; (c) Laplace of Gaussian filter with Gaussian parameter σ=0.3 and edge threshold 0.9; (d) Result of median filter with window size 5×5 and Canny edge detector with edge threshold 0.15; and (e) Binarization obtained with Otsu's thresholding

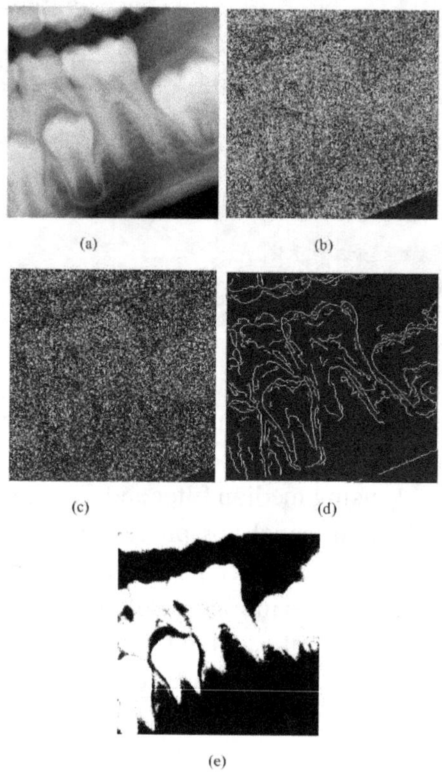

$$x^i = \left(x_1^i, y_1^i, x_2^i, y_2^i, \ldots, x_n^i, y_n^i\right),\ i = 1, 2, \ldots, s, \tag{1}$$

where $\left(x_j^i, y_j^i\right)$ refers to the landmark *j* for the image *i*.

Principal component analysis (PCA), or KL-Transform (Jain, 1989), is applied to the shape vectors by computing the mean shape:

$$\overline{x} = \frac{1}{s}\sum_{i=1}^{s} x^i, \tag{2}$$

the covariance matrix:

$$S = \frac{1}{s-1}\sum_{i=1}^{s}\left(x^i - \overline{x}\right)\left(x^i - \overline{x}\right)^T, \tag{3}$$

Figure 4. Pipeline of the proposed method

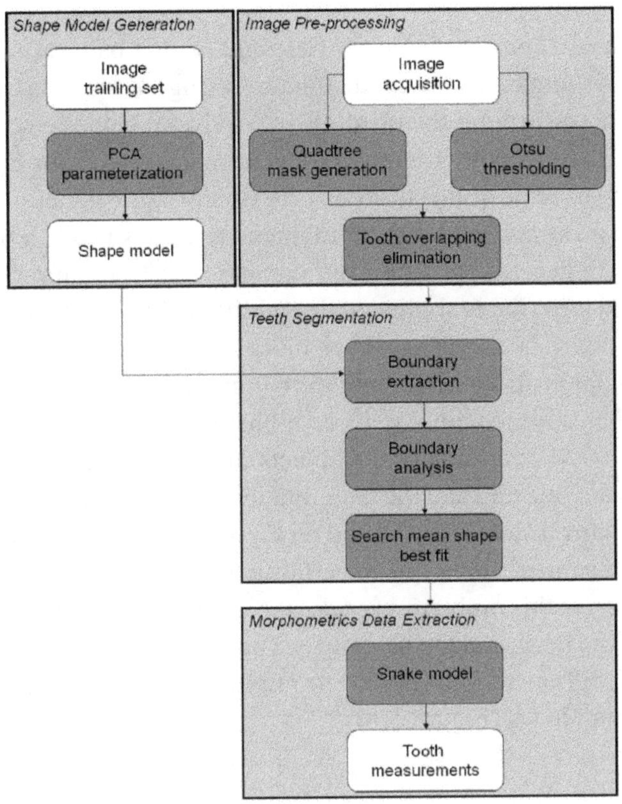

and the eigenvectors of the covariance matrix:

$$\{\varphi_1, \varphi_2, \ldots, \varphi_{2n}\}, \tag{4}$$

The eigenvectors corresponding to the largest t eigenvalues λ_i are retained in a matrix Φ. A shape can now be approximated by:

$$x = \overline{x} + \Phi \cdot b, \tag{5}$$

where b is a vector of t elements containing the model parameters, computed by:

$$b = \Phi^T \left(x - \overline{x}\right), \tag{6}$$

In this work we use a set of manually segmented images to generate the shape model. Their teeth boundaries are aligned with a selected one among these images. This alignment is implemented by a feature extraction discussed later, in section 3.3.

3.2. Image Pre-Processing

Panoramic X-ray images have a complex intensity field and texture patterns, as we can see on Figure 1. So, the user selects a window containing the tooth of interest (Figure 5(a)) and a low-pass filter is applied to smooth the image before performing the quadtree subdivision. Quadtree decomposition is a known image analysis technique that works by dividing a square image into four equal-sized square blocks, and then testing each block to see if it meets some criterion of homogeneity. In our case, we compute the difference between the maximum and minimum intensity values inside a block and compare it with a pre-defined threshold T (in general, T=12 for our database). If (min–max)>T, it is subdivided again into four blocks, and the test criterion is applied to those blocks. This process is repeated iteratively until each block meets the criterion. The result may have blocks of several different sizes. The smallest ones (around 4×4 pixeis, in this application) shall lie in the boundaries of the objects, as we can see in Figure 5(b). We have observed that this technique is more robust than traditional edge detection methods to reveal the information about the boundary of the objects in X-ray images.

So, the smallest blocks are selected and the resulting image is processed by morphological operators (erosion and flood fill) to generate a mask, pictured on Figure 5(c). Besides the quadtree, we process the original image by the Otsu's thresholding process (Otsu, 1979). We observe overlapping between the teeth in Figure 5(d). To address this problem, we take the mask obtained from the quadtree and perform a XOR operation between the mask and Otsu's image. The result, shown in Figure 6(a), is processed by a binary erosion and flood fill operation in order to improve the result obtained by quadtree mask by suppressing small islands and holes (Figure 6(b)).

Figure 5. Image pre-processing: (a) Original Image; (b) Quadtree blocks selection; (c) Mask generation; (d) Otsu's image

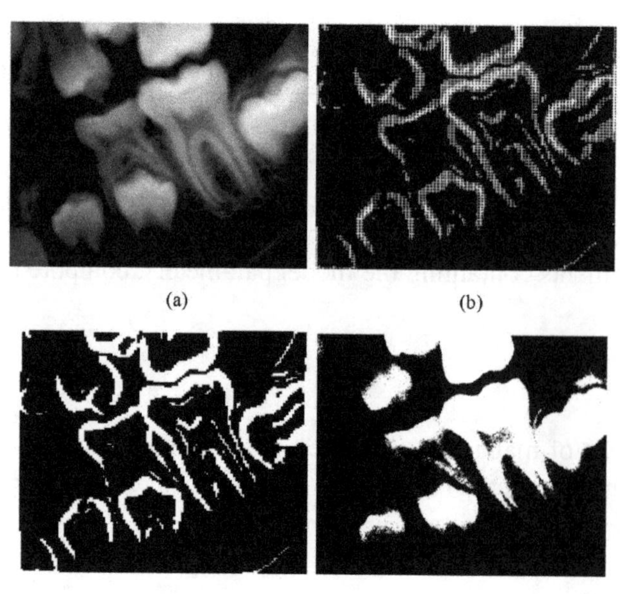

Figure 6. Tooth overlapping elimination: (a) Result of XOR operation and (b) Result of XOR plus morphological operations

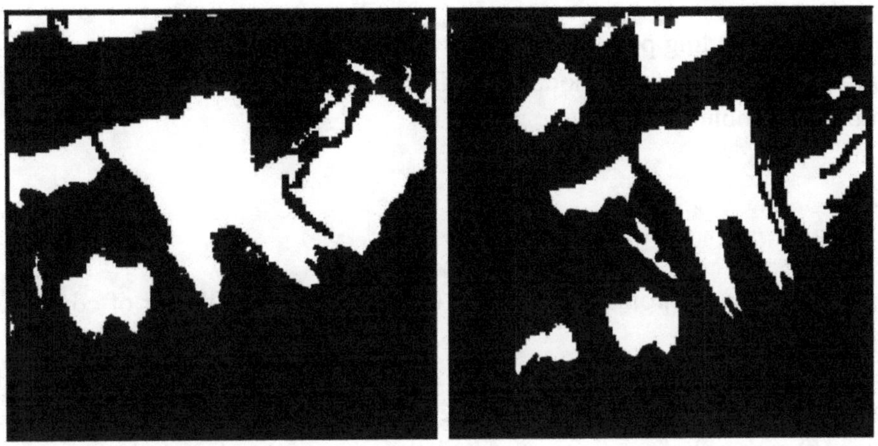

(a) (b)

Among the obtained regions the smaller ones are discarded by using a simple area threshold. Besides, regions that touch the image boundary are also discarded because we know that they do not represent the target. At the end of this process, we find out the tooth candidates.

3.3. Boundary Extraction and Analysis

The boundary of the regions that were segmented on the image pre-processing step (section 3.2) are extracted, through a simple 2D marching-cubes like technique. The obtained curves are tuned to guarantee that they have the same number N of points of the mean shape $\bar{x}$, given by expression (2). Then, we perform the correspondence between each curve and that mean shape. So, a feature vector is computed for each point according to the following expression (Ip & Shen, 1998):

$F_i = [f_{i1}, f_{i2}, \ldots, f_{iM}]$, $i=1,2,\ldots,N$,

$$f_{ij} = \begin{vmatrix} x_{i-j} & x_i & x_{i+j} \\ y_{i-j} & y_i & y_{i+j} \\ 1 & 1 & 1 \end{vmatrix},$$

where $M = \lfloor (N-1)/2 \rfloor$.

Then, at the end of this computation for both curves, we find two feature vectors, $\Phi^k = [F_1 F_2 \ldots F_N]$, with k=1,2, by concatenating the feature vectors of the curve 1, the model, and the curve 2. In Ip and Shen (1998), the correspondence between the two curves is obtained through an optimized algorithm that searches for the cyclic permutation π of points of curve 2 that solves the problem:

$$\min_{\pi}\left\|\pi\left(\Phi^{2}\right)-\Phi^{1}\right\|. \tag{7}$$

The N pairs of corresponding points in both curves are used to seek for the best affine transformation that aligns the input curve to the model one. The target transformation A is obtained solving the following optimization problem:

$$\min_{A}\left\|Y-AX\right\|. \tag{8}$$

where Y is the vector of control points in the input curve and X is the vector of corresponding control points in the model one.

Then, we perform the boundary analysis step in order to select the teeth among the aligned curves. This is performed in the model parameter space. We compute the parameter vector b_i for each curve, by solving expression (6) with $x=x_i$, for i=1,2,... and rank the curves according to the 2-norm of the obtained vector parameters. The ones which 2-norm fall in the interval [0, 500] are considered to be teeth. That range was experimentally obtained by using the training images.

Once the tooth is identified (Figure 7), we need to reconstruct its boundary which was corrupted by the quadtree mask and the morphological erosion operation. We align the mean shape $\overline{x}$, generated in the section 3.1, to the recognized object. However, only translation and rotation are used in this time. Next, the mean shape's main axes is computed by PCA to perform a search along of it. In this search we translate the mean shape along the main axes direction in order to seek for a curve that maximizes the image energy as follows:

$$\max_{\lambda}\sum_{i}\nabla I\left(\hat{x}^{i}+\lambda r\right).$$

where $\hat{x}$ is the aligned mean shape, r is the main axes direction and the real parameter λ defines the search range (usually, $-20\leq\lambda\leq20$). The obtained curve is used to initialize a simple snake technique to get the desired result. This process is described in the section 3.4.

Figure 7. Tooth recognition: (a) Tooth identification; (b) The mean shape alignment; (c) The mean shape best fit

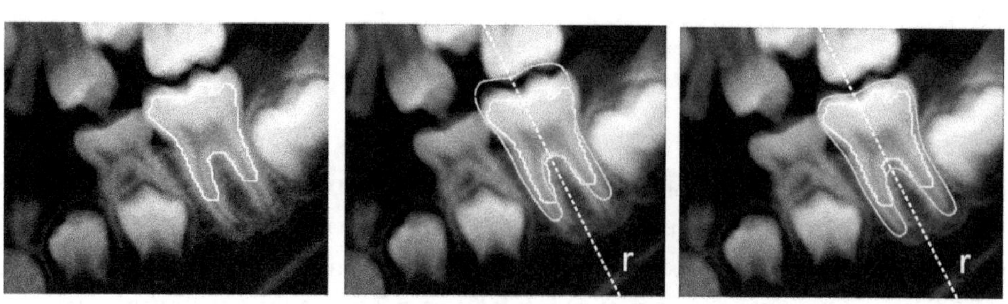

(a) (b) (c)

3.4. Morphometrics Data Extraction

We apply a discrete snake model (Giraldi et al., 2003), which is defined as a set of N points (snaxels) whose positions:

$$\{x^i = (x_i, y_i),\ i=0,\ldots,N-1\}, \tag{10}$$

are connected in series to form a closed contour.

It is convenient to define a rigidity force to minimize the local curvature and normal force, given respectively, by:

$$\beta_i = \alpha\left(x^i - \frac{1}{2}\left(x^{i-1} + x^{i+1}\right)\right), \tag{11}$$

$$F_i = k\vec{n}_i, \tag{12}$$

where n_i defines the normal force in the point (x_i, y_i) and k,α are force scale parameters. The external force is defined in function of the image data:

$$f_i = w\nabla \|\nabla I\|^2, \tag{13}$$

The evolution equation for the snake model is finally given by:

$$x^i_{(t+\Delta t)} = x^i_t + \Delta t\left(\beta^t_i + f^t_i + F^t_i\right), \tag{14}$$

In this stage, when the snake stops moving we re-compute the matching between the snake and the mean shape and re-initialize the snake model with the matching result. In this way, the snake evolution keeps a compromise between the extracted boundary and the tooth shape. The stopping criterion can be an upper bound for the number of iterations or small displacement of the snake in an iteration; that is:

$$\max_i \left\| x^i_{(t+\Delta t)} - x^i_t \right\| < \varepsilon. \tag{15}$$

Finally, the feature extraction in panoramic X-ray images is performed. Along of the main axes we determine two measures: crown-body (CB) and root (R) lengths. The former is obtained through the distance from the deepest pit to the furcation. The latter is the distance from the furcation to the root apex. Finally, we compute the ratio CB/R as shown in Figure 8. These measurements are the morphometrics data of this research.

Figure 8. (a) The scheme for crown-body (CB) and root (R) measurements; (b) Experimental result of an image

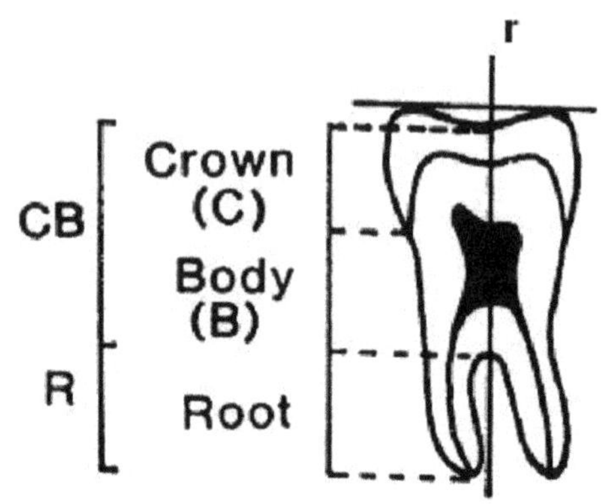

(a)

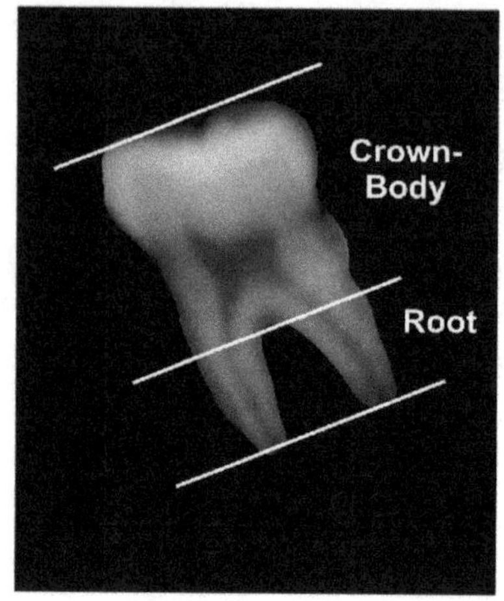

(b)

4. EXPERIMENTAL RESULTS

Figure 9 shows a typical image that we have used in our experiments. The setting of parameters was done through experimentation. The best results for the snake model was obtained with $\alpha=100$ (for any i), $w=6.0$ and $k=2.5$, $\Delta t=0.3$ and the number of iterations of the snake scheme of section 3.4 was 120. The quadtree threshold is $T=12.0$ and the area threshold, used to discard artifacts, is $(1/20)A_{TOTAL}$, where A_{TOTAL} is the area of the whole image.

Figure 9(b) shows the Otsu's thresholding result. The selected blocks of the quadtree and the generated mask are pictured on Figure 9(c) and 9(d), respectively.

The XOR between the quadtree mask and the Otsu's result is shown on Figure 9(e). We observe that the overlapping was properly addressed in this case. However, we must select the tooth among the curves presented on Figure 9(f). It is performed through the matching between each obtained curve and the mean shape of expression (2), taken as the reference curve. Then, we compute the parameter vectors b_i and take the ones which 2-norm fall in the range [0, 550] to recognize the teeth (Section 3.3). The search, based on expression (9), is performed with the result of the recognition process shown in Figure 10, obtaining the results shown in Figures 10(a) and 10(b).

The snake model is initialized with the result of the search process shown in Figure 10(c). Following section 3.4, each time the snake stops moving the matching between the snake and the mean shape is computed, according to the method of section 3.3. The result (transformed mean shape) is used to re-initialize the snake model. Figures 10(d)-(e) show the final snake iteration and segmentation result, respectively. Figure 11 shows another results obtained with the proposed methodology. The result is suitable for dentist analysis although some details were lost nearby the deepest pit and the root apex due to low contrast in the tooth boundaries

Figure 9. Experimental results: (a) Original image; (b) Otsu's image; (c) Quadtree boundary; (d) Quadtree mask; (e) Quadtree segmentation; (f) Image boundaries

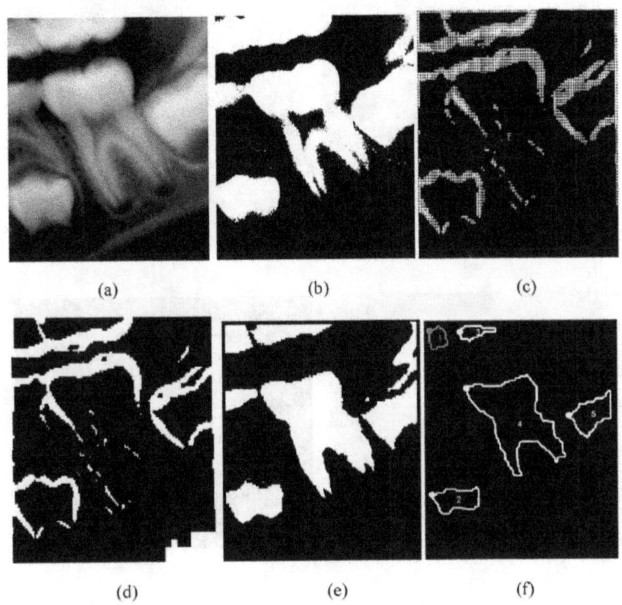

Figure 10. Snake based segmentation: (a) Recongnized Boundary; (b) The mean shape aligned; (c) The mean shape best fit; (d) Snake iteration result; (e) Snake segmentation result

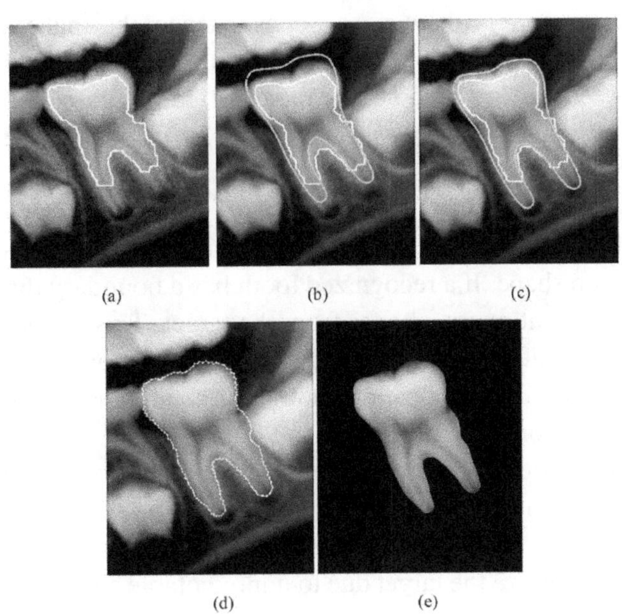

Figure 11. (a) Tooth recognition; (b) Mean shape pose; (c) Snake output; (d) Final result

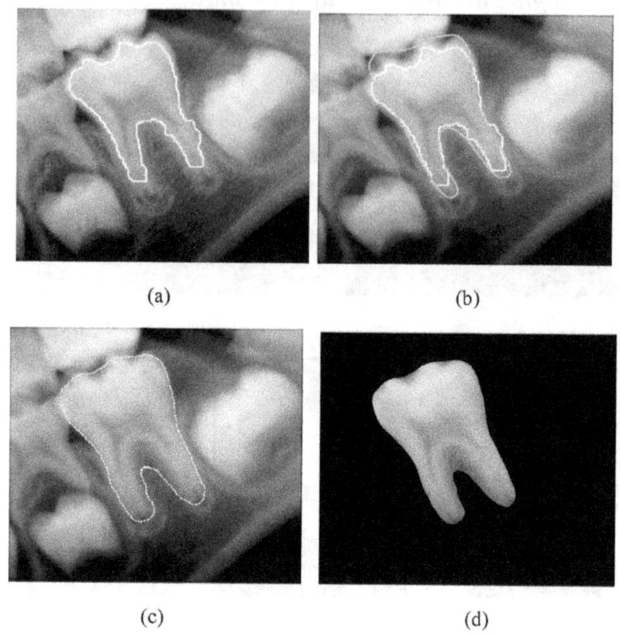

Besides the overlapping, in such images, the outer scale corresponding to the separation between the objects is (in general) finer than the inner scale of the objects of interest. The corresponding problem falls into a category known as *two-scale problems*. As a consequence, the snake model may evolve toward another object nearby the target, as we can observe in Figure 12. Also, we must add to this problem the non-trivial patterns of the intensity field nearby the teeth. In this case, both the snake initialization, based on the search for the best mean shape position (Figure 12(c)) and the snake evolution result (Figure 12(d)) may be corrupted by this problem generating an undesirable result that incorporates regions out of the target, as we can see in Figures 12(d) and 12(e).

Besides, the snake initialization process is also very sensitive to the standard deviation of the training curves respect to the mean shape. If a recognized tooth has a boundary that deviates too much from the mean shape than the initialization may be far from the target. This happens because the process of searching for a curve that solves the problem (9) involves only translation of the mean shape. Fortunately, in a set of 30 training images a visual inspection shows that the method achieves the desired result in 22, which indicates that it is a promising methodology.

Another point is the recognition process based on the parameter vector b_i (expression (6)). Up to now, we are supposing that there is only one tooth of interest in the selected region (molar) and we are applying the corresponding shape model. If there are more than one tooth with similar shapes in the image this process may fail to recognize the target due to unpredictable shape variances generated through the image acquisition process.

The main drawback of our methodology is the overlapping between the teeth. Figure 13 shows this point: we observe that the quadtree mask was not able to separate the segments. In Lira et al. (2009) it is proposed a Zonal Mask in the Fourier domain, a band-pass filter, for addressing the overlapping. This proposal is able to solve this problem for Figure 13(a). However, we have observed that it may harms the image (Figure 13(c)). Further developments and studies are necessary in order to address this problem.

Figure 12. (a) Performed recognition; (b) Initial mean shape position; (c) Result obtained through the search for the best mean shape position (equation (9)); (d)-(e) Final segmentation shows lost of details and incorporation of regions nearby the tooth

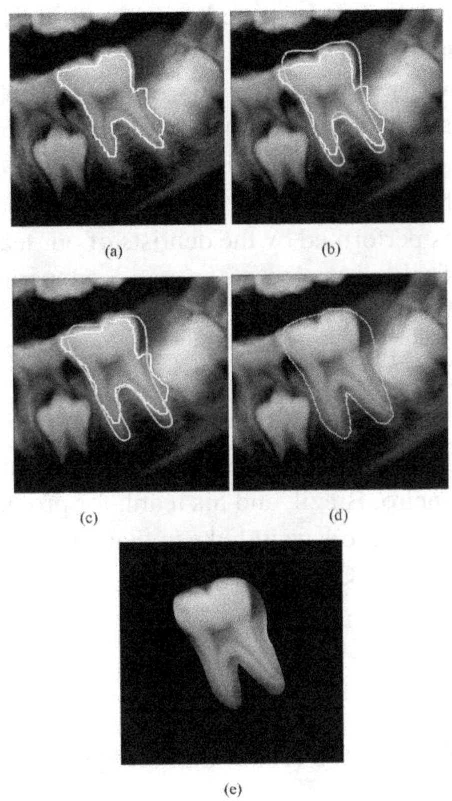

Figure 13. Overlapping problem: (a) Original image; (b) Quadtree segmentation; (c) Zonal mask segmentation

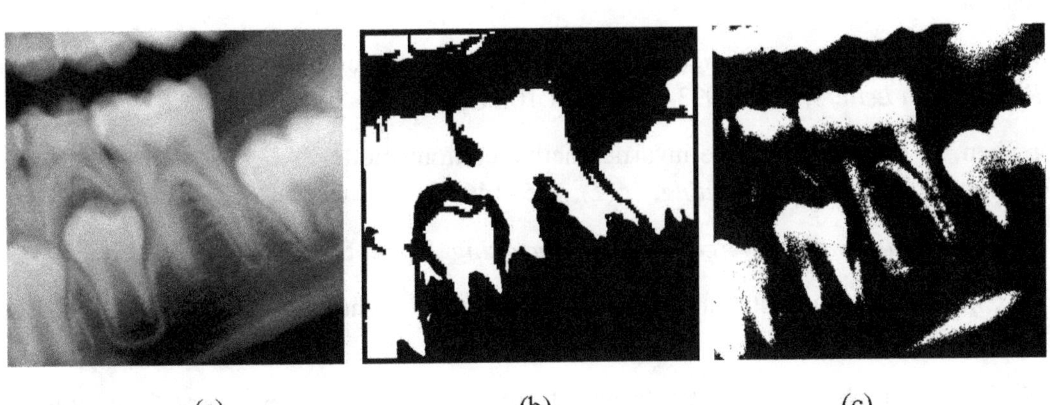

5. CONCLUSION AND FUTURE WORK

In this paper we present a method for automatic segmentation and feature extraction for dental X-ray images. The proposed method has been implemented using traditional image processing techniques, a discrete shape model and shape analysis (PCA).

The experimental results show that it is a promising technique, but needs improvements. In future works, texture analysis techniques and a better solution to address the tooth overlapping have to be studied for inclusion in the proposed method. Besides, adaptive techniques based on wavelets or pyramid models must be considered to improve the robustness against parameter choice. The obtained results will be compared with manual evaluations performed by the dentists of our team. So, some statistics are going to be generated in order to quantify the precision of the proposed method.

ACKNOWLEDGMENT

The authors would like to thank Prof. Dr. Marcelo de Castro Costa, of the Odontological Department of Federal University of Rio de Janeiro, Brazil, and his team, for providing the database image and for valuable discussions. In addition, the authors would like to thank the financial support provided by PCI-LNCC, CAPES (grant 094/2007), and INCT-MACC.

REFERENCES

Black, A., & Yuille, A. (Eds.). (1993). *Active vision*. Cambridge, MA: MIT Press.

Dua, S., Kandiraju, N., & Chowriappa, P. (2010). Region quad-tree decomposition based edge detection for medical images. *Open Med Inform Journal*, *4*, 50–57.

Fukunaga, K. (1990). *Introduction to statistical patterns recognition* (Vol. 18). New York, NY: Academic Press.

Giraldi, G., Strauss, E., & Oliveira, A. (2003). Dual-T-Snakes model for medical imaging segmentation. *Pattern Recognition Letters*, *24*(7), 993–1003. doi:10.1016/S0167-8655(02)00223-4

Ip, H., & Shen, D. (1998). An affine-invariant active contour model (AI-snake) for model-based segmentation. *Image and Vision Computing*, *16*(2), 135–146. doi:10.1016/S0262-8856(97)00051-6

Jain, A. (1989). *Fundamentals of digital image processing*. Upper Saddle River, NJ: Prentice-Hall.

Jain, A., & Chen, H. (2004). Matching of dental x-ray images for human identification. *Pattern Recognition Letters*, *37*(7), 1519–1532.

Jain, A. K., Murty, M. N., & Flynn, P. J. (1999). Data clustering: A review. *ACM Computing Surveys*, *31*(3), 264–323. doi:10.1145/331499.331504

Kanungo, T., Dom, B., Niblack, W., & Steele, D. (1994). A fast algorithm for mdl-based multi-band image segmentation. In *Proceedings of the IEEE Conference on Computer Vision and Pattern Recognition* (pp. 609-616).

Lira, P. H. M., Giraldi, G. A., & Neves, L. A. P. (2009). An automatic morphometrics data extraction method in dental x-ray image. In *Proceedings of the International Conference on Biodental Enginnering*, Porto, Portugal (pp. 77-82).

Nomir, O., & Abdel-Mottaleb, M. (2005). A system for human identification from x-ray dental radiographs. *Pattern Recognition Letters*, *38*(8), 1295–1305.

Otsu, N. (1979). A threshold selection method from gray-level histograms. *IEEE Transactions on Systems, Man, and Cybernetics*, *9*(1), 62–66. doi:10.1109/TSMC.1979.4310076

Said, E., Nassar, D., Fahmy, G., & Ammar, H. (2006). Teeth segmentation in digitized dental x-ray films using mathematical morphology. *IEEE Transactions on Information Forensics and Security*, *1*(2), 178–189. doi:10.1109/TIFS.2006.873606

Sezgin, M., & Sankur, B. (2004). Survey on image thresholding techniques and quantitative performance evaluation. *Journal of Electronic Imaging*, *13*(1), 146–165. doi:10.1117/1.1631315

Suetens, P. (2002). *Fundamentals of medical imaging*. Cambridge, UK: Cambridge University Press.

Suri, J., Wilson, D., & Laxminarayan, S. (2005). *Handbook of biomedical image analysis*. New York, NY: Springer.

Zhou, J., & Abdel-Mottaleb, M. (2005). A content-based system for human identification based on bitewing dental X-ray images. *Pattern Recognition Letters*, *38*(11), 2132–2142.

This work was previously published in Nature-Inspired Computing Design, Development, and Applications edited by Leandro Nunes de Castro, pages 306-320, copyright year 2012 by Medical Information Science Reference (an imprint of IGI Global).

Section 3

Education, Literacy, and Health Services

Chapter 12
Using Online Social Networks for Increasing Health Literacy on Oral Health

Ziauddin Ahmed
Bangladesh Institute of Health Sciences, Bangladesh

Karishma Sharmin Haque
Bangladesh Institute of Health Sciences, Bangladesh

Suptendra Nath Sarbadhikari
Bangladesh Institute of Health Sciences, Bangladesh

Khurshida Khanom
Bangladesh Institute of Health Sciences, Bangladesh

Karimon Nesha
University of Dhaka, India

Kazi Rumana Ahmed
Bangladesh Institute of Health Sciences, Bangladesh

ABSTRACT

A descriptive study was conducted among the members of Oral Health group on a social media network (Facebook) through the Internet. The objective of this study was to explore online interactions on oral health among the Internet users. The study was divided into two parts. First part included content analysis of Oral Health group interactions during the period of July 2011 to April 2012 and second part included online survey findings. All the postings and their discussions in "Oral Health" group were collected and analyzed by using both qualitative and quantitative methods. Total 427 group members were included, 65.84% members were recruited by administrator (admin) and 34.16% by other members of Oral Health group. Among the group members 110 (23%) members were actively participating in group interactions. A total 384 interactive messages were exchanged between the members on 194 discrete topics were discussed (in average 2 messages exchanged per topic). The flow of group interactions mostly occurred between dental professional to dental professional 78%, followed by general to general 3%, dental professional to general 9%, general to dental professional 10%. Opinion of survey respondents about the oral health group online interactions were found as appreciative (52%), "modern technology of learning is useful"(34%), "improves clinical knowledge of professionals"(26%), "improves oral hygiene knowledge and practice"(22%), and "helps to solve oral health problems"(38%). Online oral health group appears to be an effective platform for sharing information, experiences and advice on oral health among the Internet users.

DOI: 10.4018/978-1-5225-1903-4.ch012

INTRODUCTION

An internet-based discussion group was formed by dental and public health professionals. Its purpose was to facilitate discussion and exchange of ideas and information on oral health between dental professionals and others to assess its usefulness as an educational tool, platform for discussion and medium for exchange of ideas on oral health. Oral health is fundamental to general health and well-being. In general, poor oral health has a negative impact on quality of life, influencing eating abilities, personal confidence, mental health, social interaction, personal relationships, general health and well-being and enjoyment in life. Proper dental hygiene can prevent gum disease or digestive disorders and results give a bright healthy smile. On the other hand, neglected oral health can increase the risk of serious health conditions, such as heart disease and diabetes. In other words, a healthy mouth helps create a healthy body, so taking care of teeth and gums is a must. Adequate knowledge about oral health is considered to be an essential prerequisite for health-related behavior (Ashley, 1996). Also, studies have shown that there is an association between increased knowledge and better oral health (Hamilton, 1991; WoodGrove, 1987). It has been demonstrated that health education intervention can effectively change knowledge and practice regarding oral health.

Today, millions of people use the internet on a regular basis. So, naturally, much of this activity has been focused on health. Online health tools have the potential to help people manage their health and health care, but little is known about the use of different kinds of eHealth tools across the population (Baur & Kanaan, 2006; Lorenceet et al, 2006). In 2003, an estimated 12.5 million online health-related searches were conducted globally each day. However, aggregate figures do not tell us about what people are actually doing when they interact with online health-related content and tools.

By sharing knowledge on oral hygiene, one can help improve the overall oral health of a community. In this era of globalization, the internet is the best option for dissemination of knowledge on oral health so that a large number of people can benefit from it. The rapid growth of social networking that has been observed over the last two to three years is indicative of its entry into mainstream culture and its integration into the daily lives of many people. Hence, this study on online interaction on oral health is a step forward towards smooth and quick dissemination of knowledge on oral health.

METHODOLOGY

This was a descriptive study including a retrospective review of qualitative and quantitative data obtained from the posts on the discussion forum along with a survey involving the participants. All the posts and related discussions between 1stJuly 2011 and30thApril 2012 in "Oral Health" Facebook group wall were collected manually and the interactions were studied and analyzed by using both qualitative and quantitative methods. Further an online anonymous survey was conducted (using SurveyMonkey) using a semi-structured questionnaire regarding oral health among the group members during March, 2012. The web link of Survey monkey questionnaire form was posted to Facebook oral health group wall and members were requested to respond. For Quantitative method, data were analyzed with SPSS version-15. The textual interactions in the group were subjected to content analysis. The flows of interactions were categorized as between general people to general people, general people to dental professionals, dental professionals to dental professionals, dental professionals to general people. Ethical approval was obtained from the Institute Review Board of Bangladesh Institute of Health Sciences (BIHS). The participants were administered informed consent for voluntary participation, maintaining confidentiality and allowing them to withdraw themselves at any stage of the study. After cleaning and checking for missing variables, data were coded, compiled and analyzed. Some data were further processed to extract the themes from the online interaction in the Facebook oral health group. The findings obtained are presented in Figure 1: Direction of flow of discussions, Topic of discussions, Media preferred for postings, Respondents' opinion about oral health group.

RESULTS

The findings obtained are presented in the following section:

- Direction of flow of discussions;
- Topic of discussions;
- Media preferred for postings;
- Respondents' opinion about oral health group.

Results are discussed in two parts. First part includes content analysis of oral health group and second part includes survey findings.

Figure 1. Conceptual framework

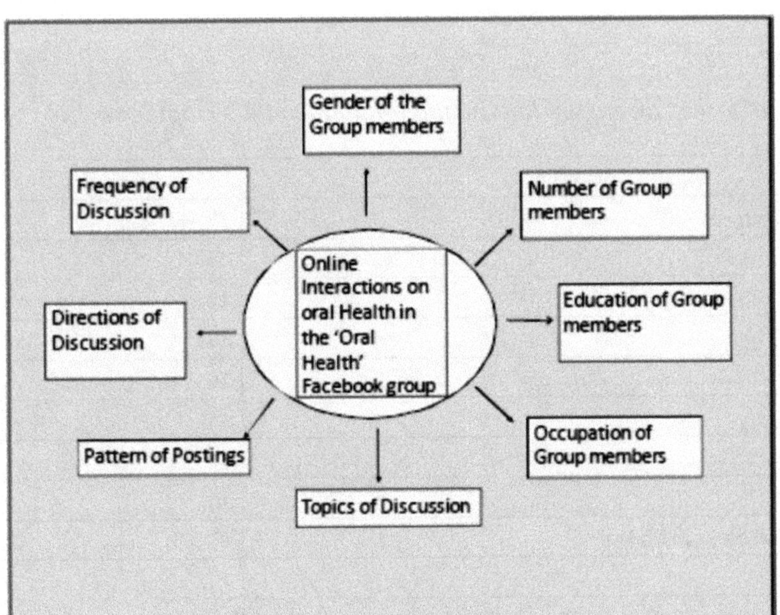

Note: Web address of Facebook Oral Health group:
(http://www.facebook.com /home.php?sk=group_190478537654194&ap=1)

Content Analysis of Oral Health Group Interactions

As of April, 2012, there were 427 members within the oral health group. 281(65.84%) members were recruited by Administrators (admin) and 146 (34.16%) members by other members. Among them 3 person were administrators (admin) and rest were members. A total 384 messages were exchanged within 194 separate discussions (postings) (1.9 message per discussion, range = 0-32). Among 427 group members 110 members were actively participating in group interaction by sending, sharing and liking the messages.

The various topics discussed in the group are shown in Table 1. After coding, the discussion topics fell under 11 major categories, of which 19% topics were found on oral and dental case management, 15% found on oral health tips, 19% topics were on modern technologies in dentistry and 10% on Fluoride in dentistry. The subject of dental care seeking and surgical procedure was discussed 16 times each thorough separated posting.

Different initial posting patterns were classified into five categories. A majority of the posting were in the form of text (32%) followed by video (23%), Web addresses (20%), questions (16%) and pictures (20%).

Interactions had multi-directional flows. Dental professional to dental professional occurred most often(78%). The proportions of the other categories of interactions were general to general (3%), dental professional to general (9%), and general to dental professional (10%).

Survey Results

A total of 50 individuals from the 'Oral health' group responded to the survey. Though, males comprised of a larger fraction of the group, the survey had a higher proportion of female respondents (58%). Mean age of survey respondents was 26.28± 8.074 years.

Table 1. Frequency of topics discussed among the group members (topics n=194)

Topic of Discussion	Frequency	%
Oral and dental case management	37	19
Oral health tips	28	15
Modern technologies in dentistry	18	9
Fluoride in dentistry	19	10
Dental care seeking	16	8
Dental information seeking	15	8
Surgical procedure	16	8
Teaching and learning	10	5
Source of free online dental books and videos	9	5
Dental restorative materials	10	5
Others (Basic anatomy, New course and training Prospect of dentistry)	16	8
Total	194	100

Survey respondents' point of view about the oral health group online interactions were coded as appreciative (52%), modern technology of learning is useful (34%), improves clinical knowledge of professionals (26%), improves oral hygiene knowledge and practice (22%), helps to solve oral health problems (38%), reduces treatment cost (4%) and removes misconception (4%)(Table 2).

DISCUSSIONS

Although, there has been considerable research on the impact of the internet on medical care in general, its impact on dentistry has been less intensively examined. A recent survey in an English Strategic Health Authority concluded that only 45% of practices had access to the internet (Johnet et al., 2003). No such study on dentistry and the internet has been conducted in Bangladesh. This study of online interaction in oral health was conducted in order to understand the key areas covered in this discussion as well as to identify major features and user interactions with the content for potential use in educating and updating the group members. The results of our study demonstrated that the group members of oral health discussion forum on Facebook received the support and information they seek when looking at the online discussion forum.

The present study found a higher proportion of patient– dentist discussions on an internet dental health information forum than previously reported by Chestnut and Reynolds (2006). This difference may be due to the fact that the present data were collected in 2012, six years after Chestnut and Reynolds' study. In addition, while several studies (Ahmad, 2006; McMullan, 2006) found health professionals' reservations toward conversation with patients particularly due to time constraints, participants in the present study reported not having such concerns. The differences in the above findings may be explained by a high number of specialists in the present study, who were more willing to discuss dental health issues with their patients. As opposed to the hectic pace of work in public clinics, the work of dental specialists is often done in private clinics, where the schedule is more relaxed and there is usually a higher awareness of the importance of provider– patient communication. In recent years, there have been quite a few studies dealing with web-based health communications (Atkinson, 2009; Dale, 2010; Sarbadhikari, 2011) where multi-disciplinary interactions have led to new knowledge generation and clarification of common disbeliefs and myths.

Table 2. Survey respondents' opinion about the usefulness of the Oral Health Facebook group

Respondents Opinions about Oral Health Group Interactions	Number	Percentage
Appreciative	26	52
Modern technology of learning is useful	17	34
Improves clinical knowledge of professionals	13	26
Improves oral hygiene knowledge and practice	11	22
Helps to solve oral health problems	19	38
Reduces treatment cost and removes misconception	2	4
Improves professional relationship	2	4
No opinion	2	4

*Multiple opinions

Further studies are needed to establish the following findings such as* Specialists in dentistry were more willing to discuss dental health information with their patients on the internet; *Dentists with high professional self-efficacy had a positive attitude toward patients who wished to discuss dental health information with them.

The dental community should seek to enhance the professional self-efficacy of its members in order to enable them to adequately deal with their patients' needs. This may be done both in dental schools and through continuing professional education. The interpretation and coding of the forum posts, although done following models and framework proposed in previous literature, was conducted by only one researcher and as such may have introduced some subjective bias.

CONCLUSION

The aim of this study was to explore different aspects of online interactions on oral health among internet users both dental professionals and general population. The expert comments and guidance provided there was appreciated by all the participants. The flow of interactions occurred in multiple directions: general people to general people, general people to dental professionals, dental professionals to dental professionals and dental professionals to general people. In most of the cases, the information receivers expressed their gratitude towards the information providers. Survey respondents had positive attitude towards online interaction for knowledge improvement related to oral health. In this study, dental professionals were found to be more interested in sharing their knowledge, views and experience. Online oral health group appears to be an effective platform sharing information, experiences and advice on oral health among the internet users. Findings of this study imply that computer-assisted, interactive social networking and information technology could be important tools and should be evaluated more closely for its potential to improve oral health care.

REFERENCES

Ahmad, F., Hudak, P. L., Bercovitz, K., Hollenberg, E., & Levinson, W. (2006). Are physicians ready for patients with Internet based health information? *Journal of Medical Internet Research, 8*(3), e22. Retrieved January 10, 2012, from http://www.ncbi.nlm.nih.gov/pmc/articles/PMC2018833/

Ashley, F. P. (1996). Role of dental health education on preventive dentistry in prevention of dental disease. In J. J. Murray (Ed.), *Oxford University Press*.

Atkinson, N. L., Saperstein, S. L., & Pleis, J. (2009). Using the internet for health-related activities: Findings from a national probability sample. *Journal of Medical Internet Research, 11*(1). doi:10.2196/jmir.1035 PMID:19275980

Baur, C., & Kanaan, S. B. (2006). *Expanding the reach and impact of consumer e health tools.* Rockville, MD: Office of Disease Prevention and Health Promotion, US Department of Health and Human Services. Retrieved from http://www.health.gov/communication/ehealth/ehealthTools/

Chestnutt, I. G., & Reynolds, K. (2006). Perceptions of how the Internet has impacted on dentistry. *British Dental Journal, 200*(3), 161–165. doi:10.1038/sj.bdj.4813195 PMID:16474364

Dale, J. (2010). *Linking food, oral health and social interaction: Developing a multi-disciplinary approach to oral health promotion*. Health Sciences Research Institute.

Hamilton, M. E. C. W. (1991). Oral health knowledge and habits of senior elementary school students. *Journal of Public Health Dentistry*, *51*(4), 212–219. doi:10.1111/j.1752-7325.1991.tb02217.x PMID:1941772

John, J. H., Thomas, D., & Richards, D. (2003). Questionnaire survey on the use of computerisation in dental practices across the Thames Valley Region. *British Dental Journal*, *195*(10), 585–590. doi:10.1038/sj.bdj.4810734 PMID:14631436

Lorence, D. P., Park, H., & Fox, S. (2006). Assessing health consumerism on the Web: A demographic profile of information seeking behaviors. *Journal of Medical Systems*, *30*(4), 251–258. doi:10.1007/s10916-005-9004-x PMID:16978004

McMullan, M. (2006). Patients using the Internet to obtain health information: How this affects the patient health professional relationship. *Patient Education and Counseling*, *63*(1-2), 24–28. doi:10.1016/j.pec.2005.10.006 PMID:16406474

Sarbadhikari, S. N. (2011). Unlearning and relearning in online health education. In R. Biswas & C. M. Martin (Eds.), *User-driven healthcare and narrative medicine* (pp. 294–309). Hershey, PA: IGI Global.

WoodGrove, J. C. G., & Gylbier, S. (1987). Understanding dental attendance behavior. *Community Dental Health*, *4*, 215–221. PMID:3477305

This work was previously published in the International Journal of User-Driven Healthcare (IJUDH), 3(2); edited by Ashok Kumar Biswas, pages 51-58, copyright year 2013 by IGI Publishing (an imprint of IGI Global).

Chapter 13
An Evaluation of Oral and Dental Health Services in Turkey and in the Member States of the EU in Terms of Economy

Abdülkadir Işık
Namık Kemal University, Turkey

Özge Selvi Yavuz
Namık Kemal University, Turkey

Seda Suat
Sevgi Dental Clinic, Turkey

Gamze Yıldız Şeren
Namık Kemal University, Turkey

Berkay Habiboğlu
Thrace Development Agency, Turkey

ABSTRACT

Dental health expenditures are a big part of general health expenditures. In Turkey, oral health services are provided by both private practitioners and government sections. In 2012, approximately 7 million fillings were made by government clinics. According to Turkish Dental Association data, in the same year, the number of fillings that Turkish citizens needed was 247 million. Even if the entire budget of the Health Ministry of Turkey were spent for these fillings, it is impossible to handle this demand. In 2012, in the European Union with 24 member countries, dental health spending was close to 74 billion Euro. Because of this financial burden, Turkey and the other countries are trying to find cost-effective methods to minimize dental health spending. This chapter emphasizes dental health conditions of both Turkey and European Union, firstly, and then successful and cost-effective strategies are discussed.

INTRODUCTION

Every year thousands of Turkish Liras (TL) are spent for dental health. In this study, we will discuss how to use the resources more effectively. We will be explaining the dental health services in the EU and in Turkey and will mention the projects applied to reduce the economic effects of dental health services before the conclusion part.

DOI: 10.4018/978-1-5225-1903-4.ch013

COST ITEMS IN ORAL AND DENTAL HEALTH SERVICES

Calculating properly the cost of a service plays a role not only in the control and audit of the costs, but also in the efficient allocation of resources. Various cost centers appear in health care units and this issue prevents to calculate the costs exactly. Therefore, the classification method started to be used in determining the cost of health care. Generally costs are divided into three groups as follows: direct costs, indirect costs and immaterial costs (Elliott& Payne 2008):

- **Immaterial Costs:** Immaterial costs are the most difficult ones to express monetarily. Costs of pain due to tooth decay take part in immaterial costs.
- **Indirect Costs:** Indirect costs occur because of the loss of work force of the patient or of the person who takes care of the patient.
- **Direct Costs:** Direct costs are the costs related to the medical care services and can be calculated at market prices. Direct costs are divided into two groups, direct medical costs and direct non-medical costs. This separation can be made in oral and dental health services as follows: Direct dental costs and direct non-dental costs.
    - **Direct Non-Dental Costs:** These costs include foods, drinks, transportations and accommodations.
    - **Direct Dental Costs:** Direct dental costs are divided into three groups:
- **Fixed Costs:** The building where the service is provided, building-related expenses and service investments are included in this group. Dental units, all equipment, instruments and systems are included in this group.
- **Semi Fixed Costs:** Personal expenses are included in this group.
- **Variable Costs:** Drugs and consumables used for treatment are included in this group.

ORAL AND DENTAL HEALTH PROFILE OF TURKEY

In Turkey, oral and dental health problems are among the most important health problems. Oral diseases affect 96% of the individuals and the losses suffered by the country's economy is quite large.

According to Turkish Dental Association's report published in 2011, there are 24.203 dentists working actively. Turkish population was 74.724.269 in 2011. So in 2011 there were 3087 patients per dentist. The distribution of the dentists actively employed is, 60% of them work in private clinics, 29% of them work for the Ministry of Health, 10% of them work at faculties, and 1% for other institutions (Table 1).

We can see the current situation below in terms of the number of treatments provided and the number of treatments needed. But considering the number of treatments needed in our country, these numbers seem very low (Figure 1).

In February 2010, the first results of "Health for your mouth" project were published. 3040 persons from 7 different regions and from 9 different age groups participated in this project, which was ongoing for four years. The results of the project are:

1. 1 of every 3 people in Turkey do not have the habit of brushing their teeth.
2. In a year a person has less than one toothbrush.

Table 1. The number of treatments provided by dentists working for the Ministry of Health in 2010

Name of Treatment	Number
Filling	4.739.103
Root canal operation	752.206
Detertraj	4.954.240
Tooth extraction	6.369.715
Removable denture	944.276
Fixed partial denture	3.043.235

Table 2. The number of treatments in 2010

Name of Treatment	Number
Filling	247.000.000
Tooth extraction	35.000.000
Root canal operation	8.700.000
Detertraj	39.500.000

Figure 1. The distribution of dentists who are actively employed

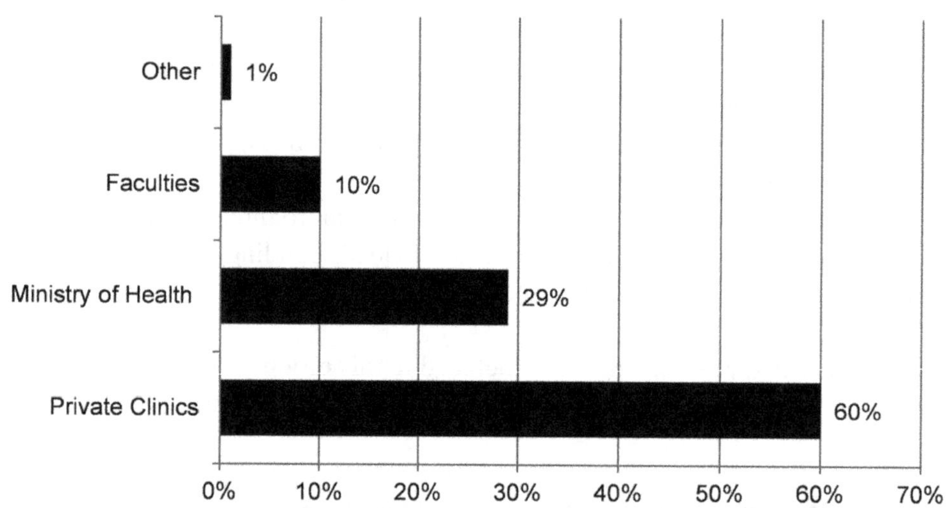

Figure 2. Number of treatments needed in Turkey in 2010

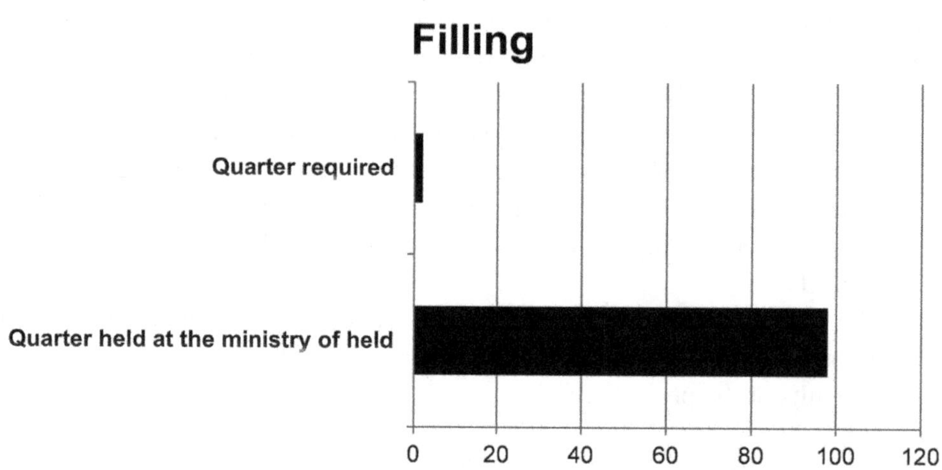

   a. Annual consumption of toothpaste is 440 grams, it is 870 grams in France, 703 grams in Germany.
3. Frequency of going to the dentist is 0.9 per a year, it's 5 times a year in the European Union countries
4. While the tooth decay ratio is 35% for 0-4 age group, it's 90% for 10-15 age group.
   a. Evaluating the results of the project, it's obvious that in oral and dental health services, our country is far more behind than the developed countries.

ORAL AND DENTAL HEALTH PROFILES OF EU MEMBER COUNTRIES

Distribution of Oral Diseases in EU Member Countries

In the last 30 years, the percentage of young adults and children who have tooth decays highly reduced. Simultaneously the percentage of individuals who lost their teeth reduced too. These developments are the result of better life conditions, changed nutrition habits, augmented usage of fluoride and fluorinated toothpaste and the emergence of new oral hygiene techniques.

However, the averages based on population may hide the disequilibrium in oral health. The researches show that even if the childhood tooth decays dropped, there's a disequilibrium among some minority-ethnic groups and some social classes (Watt & Sheiham 1999, Locker 2000, Sabbah 2007). In the east of Europe, tooth decay is a serious problem for lots of groups that are socio-economically behind all of the member countries (Figure 2 and Table 1). For example, in Spain, the number of tooth decays of young adults who are the members of lower socio-economic classes are twice more than the ones who are the members of upper socio-economic classes (Spanish Dental Association 2010).

The researches show that especially the tooth decay ratios of children coming from lower socio-economic classes are much more than the ones coming from other classes and they generally are not treated (Droz 20006). A research done in Denmark showed that the oral and dental health disequilibrium is obvious between the families migrated to Denmark and the ones living in Denmark for more than one generation.

When we look at Table 1 and Figure 2, we see that during the last 30 years, the tooth decay prevalence of 12 years old groups dropped obviously. In the Eastern European countries, the drop is less obvious.

Europe's Situation in Periodontal Health

Even if there are lots of research about Europe's periodontal situation, gathering trustful information is still a serious problem. Advanced periodontitis impacts 5-20% of the adult population worldwide and is the main cause of teeth losses (Petersen 2005, Philstrom 2005, Jin 2011). In Europe, more than 50% of the population are suffering from periodontitis and 10% of the population from advanced periodontitis (König, 2011). Here appears the misleading part: When the older population has more tooth in mouth, the number of teeth having periodontal problems increases. Also, when the population consists of individuals who lose their teeth in early ages, periodontal diseases appear rarely since there's no tooth.

Europe's Situation in Oral Cancers

Oral cancer is globally the 8th most common cancer type (Johnson, 2011). In 2008, there was 132.000 head and neck cancer. 62.800 of them ended with the death (Ferlay, 2010).

Table 3. The comparison of daft scores of 12 years old group in 1980's and in 2000's. (WHO, 2012b)

Country	80s' DMFT Scores	2000s' DMFT Scores
Austria	3.8 (1984)	1.04 (2002)
Cyprus	2.2 (1990)	0.65 (2003-2004)
Denmark	5 (1980)	0.7 (2008)
France	4.2 (1987)	1.23 (2006)
Germany	3.8 (1989)	0.7 (2005)
Ireland	2.6 (1984)	1.4 (2001)
Italy	4.9 (1986)	1.1 (2004-2005)
Lithuania	4.5 (1983)	3.7 (2005)
Poland	4.4 (1985)	3.2 (2003)
Romania	3.1 (1986)	2.8 (2000)
Spain	4.2 (1984)	1.3 (2005)
England	3.1 (1983)	0.7 (2008-2009)

Figure 3. The comparison of dmft scores of 12 years old group in 1980S and in 2000S (who 2012B)

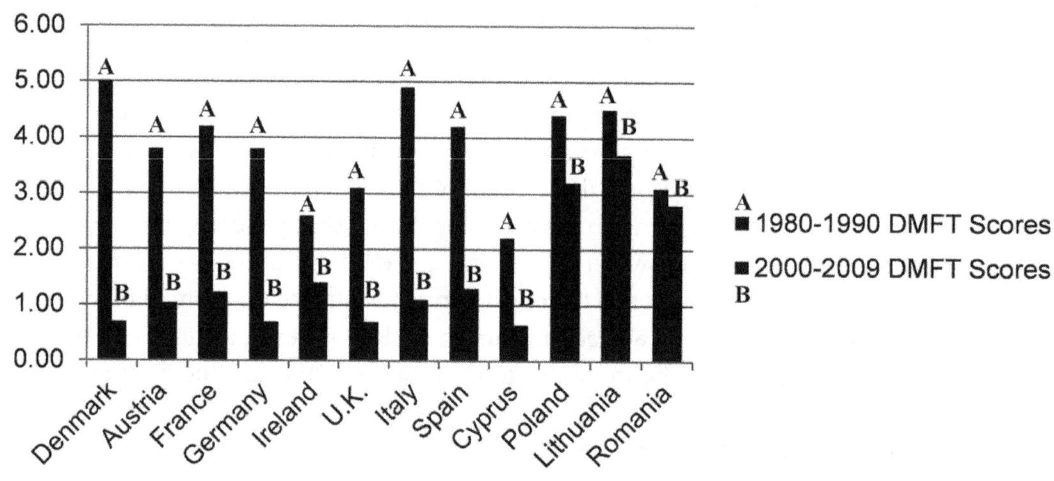

There's a strong relation between oral cancer incidence and socio-economic situation. The most disadvantaged, poorest groups face with highest cancer ratios (Menvielle 2005, Conway 2007, Conway 2008, Warnakulasuriye 2009).

Oral cancer incidences are differences among the EU countries, this is because of the regional differences in being exposed to risk factors. The highest incidence speed in 100.000 persons belongs to Spain with 6,7 and to Hungary with 9,4 (Figure 3)

Figure 4 shows the mortality in Europe. While Slovakia, ABD and Hungary have the highest mortality, Cyprus and Iceland have the lowest (IARC 2012c). In many countries of Europe and Asia, mortality due to oral cavity cancers declined seriously (Garavello 2010).

Figure 4. Lid and oral cavity cancer incidence speed of EU member countries among 100.000 persons (IARC 2012b, GLOBOCAN 2008)

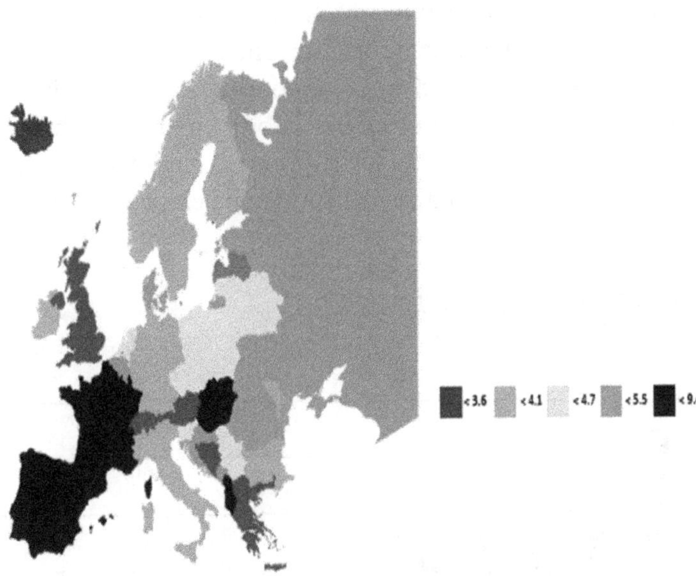

Figure 5. Lid and oral cavity cancer mortality speed of EU member countries among 100.000 persons (IARC 2012b, GLOBOCAN 2008)

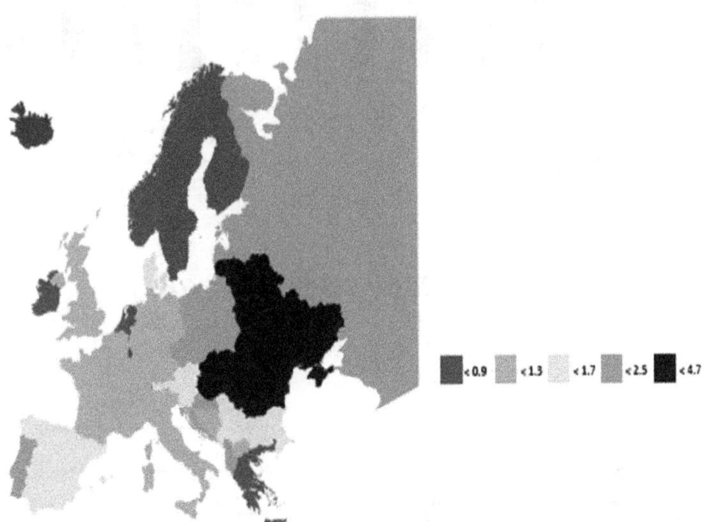

Survival rates change obviously upon geographical regions for oral cavity and oropharynx cancers. The survival rates of rich people are higher like in the other cancer types (Edwards & Jones, 1999). Researches in this area shows that five-year survival rate in Eastern Europe countries is 23% while it's 51% in North Europe countries (Zigon, 2011).

The Cost of Oral Diseases in Europe

In EU member countries, the general health expenditures including dentistry are directly related to the country's welfare which is measured by gross national income.

Expenditures made for oral diseases exceed the expenditures caused by other diseases, even in high-income countries. It's interesting to spend lots of money in order to treat tooth decays and the complications caused by them instead of taking into account preventive applications especially when thinking of cost-effectiveness (Pitts, 2010). A research done in Australia emphasizes that after cardiac vascular

Figure 6. GNI per person in 2010, World Bank 2012
Source: World Bank, 2012

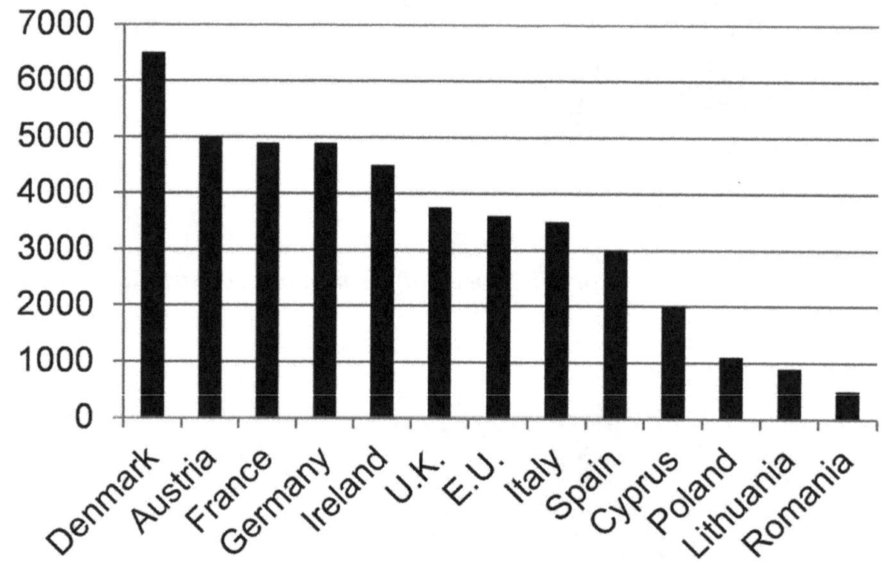

Figure 7. Health Expenditures per person in 2010, World Bank 2012
Source: World Bank, 2012

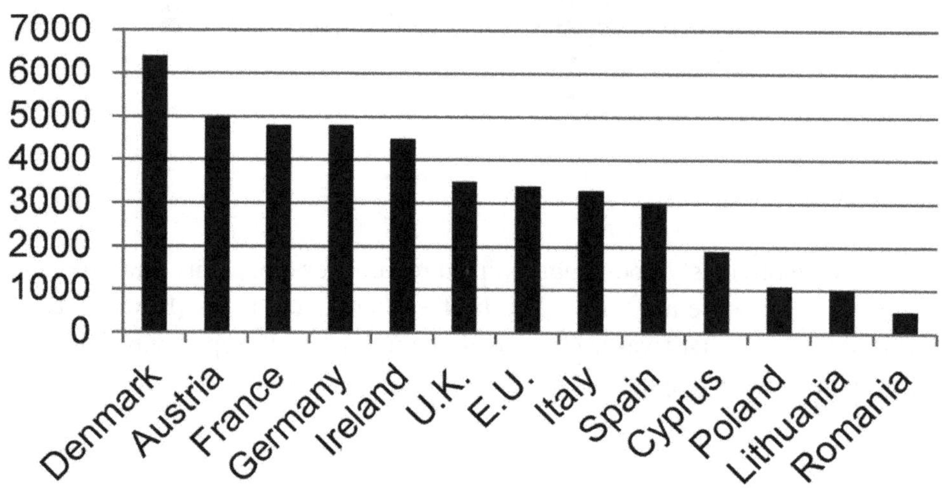

diseases, the second highest treatment cost occurs in oral diseases. In the same research it's shown that the cost of dental treatments is higher than the cost of cancer treatments (Australian Institute of Health and Welfare 2010). Other researches indicate that the more expensive treatment is dental treatment in industrialized countries (Schneider 1998, Bauer 2009).

In 2009, 5% of total health expenditures and 16% of private health expenditures are dental expenditures in OECD countries (OECD 2011).

In 2000, in the former European Union countries (15 countries), the total cost of services and treatments provided by dentists was 54 billion Euros (Widstrom & Eaton 2004). In the current EU, this number is about 79 billion Euros. This number is expected to be 93 billion Euros by 2020.

The regulations in patient contributions and dentists' tariff of fares directly impact the number and the cost of treatments. Since private dentists are more common in oral and dental health services, every regulation, treatment prices, payment plans and contributions of the state have a direct impact on dentists' and patients' needs for treatment.

Additionally, OECD reports show that people's own dental expenditures change upon the country's dental health system. In member countries, for example in Spain, oral health services are provided by private clinics and patients pay all the treatment costs. However, poor people have difficulties to pay for the service in such a system. In Denmark, the service is free for children under 18, however, adults pay for the treatment to the private clinics with the support of the state. In the other countries like France and Germany, preventive treatments are provided by health insurances and patients also contribute to the payments.

It's difficult to calculate the oral and dental health expenditures since people pay to the private clinics on their own. In most of the member countries like Greece and Italy, private expenditures can be calculated via the forms filled with patients, but this method doesn't reflect the exact data.

Dental diseases and its impacts are very costly for a person and for the society. In England, the cost of keeping the tooth in the mouth increases more and more (Steele Report 2009). Also, it should be kept in mind that oral diseases because the indirect costs like workforce loss. These problems emerge more and more with the aging population.

Preventive applications' importance of health economics are accepted in the literature. Lots of researches accepts that preventive applications, avoiding tooth decays are more profitable and useful than treating them (Oscarson 2007, Burt 1998). Also the usage of tooth paste including fluoride is one of the best methods considering its cost-effectiveness (Davies 2003, Yee 2004).

Sweden and Denmark managed to diminish the prevalence of oral diseases and the dental expenditures by concentrating on preventive applications (Wang, 1998).

Finally, a research analyzed the global situation as follows: "A system which primarily focuses on the treatment of a disease cannot be economically and socially supported by people and it's not ethically true. The most effective method is to concentrate on preventive applications" (Gooch 2009, Truman 2002, Tomar 2010).

Inequalities in the Treatment of Oral Diseases in Europe

The World Health Organization's 'Commission on Social Determinants of Health (CSDH)' states that: "The inequalities of health are mainly because of the inequalities of power, income and services" (CSDH, 2008).

European Parliament declared via "Resolution on Reducing Health Inequalities in the EU": "Among the countries that are member of EU, there's an increasing physical and mental health inequality (2011). In these countries, health inequalities generally occur between high and low income groups and also between highly educated and not-well educated groups.

In addition to economic, social and environmental factors, health is also affected by individuals' lifestyle and service providers. Lower socioeconomic groups have a tendency to unhealthy nutrition, smoke, drink alcohol. With combination of all these factors disease occurrence is inevitable.

Considering the socio-economic status, age, sex, general health status there is a serious inequality in oral health between EU countries. This inequality is more obvious at lower income levels of the society, such as

- People living in social deprivation areas (Marmot & Bell 2010)
- Those stays in psychiatric hospitals (Vigild, 1993)
- Elderly population (Griffin,2012)
- Convicts (Walsh, 2008)
- Homeless people (Depalma 2005)
- Refugees (Angelilo 1996)
- Immigrants (Heidmann 1985)
- Frequent traveler populations (Edwards 1997)
- Minority groups affected by social disadvantage (Christensen 2010)
- Adults with learning disabilities (Glassman 2003)

The groups listed above have extremely poor oral health and they have difficulties in accessing dental services. There groups usually apply to the medical institutions when it is an emergency.

Tooth Brushing Habits in Europe

In Europe, children around 12 years old who brush their teeth more than once a day tend to continue this behavior as a habit (Koivusilta, 2003).

A study about the 11 years old children's tooth brushing habits all across Europe shows that there is a direct relation between the family's income and brushing habits of children (HSBC 2010).

Another study conducted in Scotland about tooth brushing habits shows that familial factors have an important role in gaining tooth brushing habits (Levin & Currie 2010).

Access to Dental Services

Accessing to dental service units in an equal and fair way is a very important factor about to reduce the inequality in oral health. Reaching easily or not to the dental treatment services is the basic substructure of the system.

Government grant is needed for the kids and the deprived ones for the oral health system process. Considering the supply and the finance of the oral and dental health services it is possible to separate the EU Member States into various groups.

Cyprus: 80% of the population (all children of primary school age, low income individuals, civil servants, national security forces, and police) can take advantage of the free dental treatment services in State-owned clinics. Despite this, a large part of the population pay for the treatment in the private clinics.

Ireland: Children up to the age of 16 can receive a free service in the State-owned dental services. The others need to pay for the treatment in the private clinics.

Spain: All dental treatment services are provided by the private sector, all adult patients pay for expenses themselves. In some autonomous regions, taking advantage of the tax system, treatments of the children between the ages of 7-14 can be provided.

In Cyprus, Italy and Spain, state's contribution to the system is due to local taxes or in national revenue, but the given services are limited to only certain groups.

Denmark: Oral health services are being provided in schools and free until the age of 18. Free treatment service exists for the disadvantaged groups in the population (especially for old and poor individuals).

Italy: In theory, children under the age of 14 and disadvantaged groups may have free dental services, but in practice in most regions, only the emergency treatments are covered by the State.

England: Some groups' treatment expenses like the children under the age of 18, pregnant women and breastfeeding mothers, low income individuals and students under 19 who have part time school are covered by the State.

In countries such as Denmark, Italy, United Kingdom, in theory services exist for all citizens, while, in practice, treatment options can change and can be limited.

Countries providing health services with social insurance systems:

- **Germany:** A large majority of the population's treatment expenses is covered by the non-profit funds. There are State's dental clinics but they are just for the medical examination, medical diagnosis, and protecting implementations.
- **Austria:** Compulsory health insurance includes basic restorative and protecting dental treatments. Some protecting implementations are applied during education. Parents' health insurance covers their children's dental treatment expenses.
- **France:** Protecting implementations applied for the kids until 12 years old and also children between 6 and 18 can have free dental checkup at school. Other age groups have to cover their treatments under insurance on their own.
- **Lithuania:** State covers all oral treatments and dental treatments freely of the individuals up to 18 years. Adults between 18 and 65 can receive their treatments at the state-owned dental clinics with contribution payments.
- **Poland:** State has limitations about covering dental treatment expenses, only covers annual checkups. Young adults and pregnant may have enhanced treatments.
- **Romania:** Government health insurance also covers oral health care expenses. Dental treatments are free for those under the age of 18 and they have annual examinations. Despite unemployed, pregnant women, nursing mothers, military personnel, veterans and prisoners exempt from paying insurance, they are part of it.

Admission rates for dental health services are higher in developing member countries whose expenses met by the state than developed member countries which do not cover the dental health expenses. For example, in Catalonia there are no state support for oral and dental health services, having dental health service rates were, 32% of men, 38% of women in 2006 (Casals, 2007). In Belarus, state support is quite serious, 60% of the population went to the dentist in 2007 (Tserakheva, 2011). Before 1989, EU member Eastern European countries generally covered children's treatment expenses in schools. But today, because of increasing privatization of oral and dental health services, many public health programs has been stopped.

Each member country of the European Union supports the idea that each individual must be included in the state insurance or social insurance funds for the health care systems since it's a constitutional right.

Differences in Access to Dental Services

There are some recommended deadlines for regular dental examinations, the incidence of these periods varies between EU member countries.

Via the survey made by Eurobarometer, people have been asked that if they have visited a dentist in the last 12 months. Here are the results.

Compared with other regions in Europe, the values are higher in these countries. On the other hand, despite mandatory dentist controls are being held every 6 months and annually, these values are interestingly low (Eurobarometer 2010).

Visit rates in Eastern European Countries have lower values, Lithuania is % 46, Poland is %44, and Romania is % 34. Also Spain is % 43 and Portuguese is % 46 that can be counted in the same group. The rest of the countries have values like this, Austria is %56, Ireland is % 54, Cyprus is % 54, Italy is % 52, and France is % 52.

Differences in Dental Treatment

Differences do exist in the process of therapeutic and preventive treatment. In the countries such as Austria, France, Italy, operative treatment rates are higher. On the other hand countries such as Sweden, Denmark, Switzerland, and Netherlands have lower operative treatment rates than preventive treatment rates.

Table 4. Recommended Frequency in EU

Recommended Frequency	Member Country
Every six months	Poland
Once between nine and twelve months	Denmark
Yearly	Austria Cyprus France Germany Ireland İtaly Lithuania Romania
In case of need	England
Unclear	Spain

Figure 8. Dental treatment habits in EU

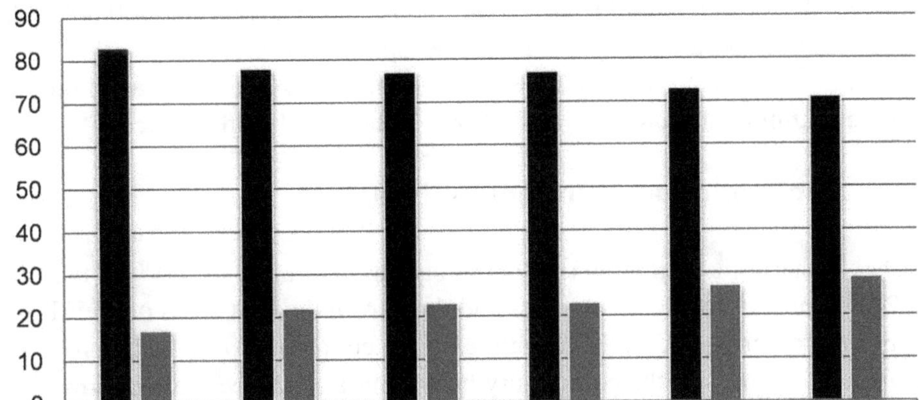

	Holland	Denmark	Germany	Luxemburg	Slovakia	Sweeden
■ YES	83	78	77	77	73	71
■ NO	17	22	23	23	27	29

THE STRATEGIES THAT CARRY ORAL AND DENTAL HEALTH SERVICES TO A BETTER LEVEL AND THE EVALUATION IN TERMS OF COST EFFECTIVENESS

In Turkey, there is an insufficient source in terms of the expenditures that is made in the oral and dental health services. We may compare some examples from foreign sources to understand the size of spending over oral and dental health services. In the United States with a population of 308.000.000, 108 billion dollars were spent for dental services in 2010. In Canada with a population of 33.000.000, 12.6 billion dollars were spent for dental services in 2009. Oral and dental health-related problems also create a loss such as the loss of a work/school day that we cannot explain financially. In Canada, 2.26 million school days, 4.15 million work days became loss due to the dental treatments or dental problems in 2010.

In Turkey, among all health expenditures, the part allocated to dental health is between 5-6%. In our country, almost all of the oral and dental health services which are given by the public sector consist of therapeutic services, namely 2nd step treatment services. According to the data of Social Security Institution for 2008-2009, dental treatment constitutes 33,8% of the dental applications. The proportion is 70% in West European countries. 60% of the oral and dental health services which is a large proportion, is provided by the private clinic and polyclinics where the services are mostly therapeutical. The cost of the first step, in other words, preventive health services' costs are much lower. The rosthodontic and restorative applications are mostly seen in the individuals who are not performed Preventive Dentistry applications and the financial burden to the Government is quite high. It is declared by the World Health Organization (WHO) that the DMFT (average number of teeth with decays-filling per individual and average number of lost teeth due to decay per individual) is the highest in the countries which have the dentistry services based on restorative applications, and again these countries at the same time, have the highest number of "toothless young age" individual. It is determined that the DMTF begins decreasing structurally in the countries that constitute their systems based on preventive philosophy and preventive applications. To explain with an example, the number of fillings that is needed in our country is 247.000.000 that has been revealed by the table 3 from the previous page. In the price list which has been determined by the Turkish Dental Association for 2012, the price of the filling for a tooth is 80 TL, the required amount of the all necessary fillings is 19.760.000.000 TL and this is the amount that is required for just one treatment method. The amount allocated to the Ministry of Health is 17.000.000.000 TL for 2011.

Although the tooth decays are one of the most widespread chronic diseases, they can be prevented. The cost may become lower with the some preventive measures. Here are some of the preventive measures that we'll be examining to lower the cost of oral and dental health services:

Fluor Varnish Application and Projection Example

Studies have shown that 80% of the dentistry applications is limited by 20% of the population. This proportion of 20% expresses as high risk caries and they, from the first years of their lives, tend to have continuous exposure to dental decay. Systematic early detection and prevention program of these risk groups is significant for not only the community health but also the economic terms. Early childhood decay (ECD) means that there is decay on the at least one surface of the teeth in children with up to the month of 71. ECD refers to permanent decay in the medium and long term; in other words, the children with ECD are the high risk groups of the future. Because of this reason, ECD related numbers are very important for making estimated tooth decay projections and correspondingly potential cost analysis. A projection work related to this subject has been made by D.Doğan and his friends. In this study, between the years of 2009-2010, in two different city centers, between 5-60 months old 499 children have been evaluated in terms of ECD prevalence and there have been evaluated the amount of decays, necessity treatments and the costs.

According to the studies, it is set that milk tooth of the 94% of the children with the tooth decay in their permanent tooth have also decay. It is declared that 83% of the children with no decay in their milk tooth have also no decay when they become 12 years old. It is seen that in comparison with the children who have no decay in their milk tooth, the children with decay in their milk tooth have 3 times more decay in their permanent teeth. In the projection based on of this study, 499 children have been examined and it is foreseen that 255 children out of 303 children who have decay will have a decay in their permanent tooth when they become 12 years old; however 33 children out of 196 children without any decay will have hardly a decay in their permanent tooth. The following is a table of the medium-term prediction decay and treatment cost:

The result of the study shows that even though it is expected that 58% of the 499 children have tooth decay when become 12 years old, thanks to fluor varnish application the amount may be decreased to 23%. In terms of cost, again with the fluor varnish application, the total cost may decrease from 42.486 TL to 17.082 TL. These results are noteworthy in terms of the country's economy and oral and dental

Table 5. Dental costs for treatment types

Treatment Types	Total Number	Unit Cost (TL)	Total Cost (TL)
Surface Covering	40	32	1280
Filling to one surface	999	73	72.927
Filling to two or more surface	169	77	13.013
Extracting	9	54	486
Crown	105	224	23.520
Total			**111.226 TL**

Table 6. Medium-term prediction decay and treatment cost

The Number of Decayed Tooth	The Number of Children	%85 Predictive Value/ The Number of Children who have Possibly Tooth Decay at 12 Years Old	Average Treatment Cost DMTF=2 (TL)	After Flour Varnish Application the Number of Children who have Possibly Tooth Decay at 12 Years Old	Average Treatment Cost (TL)
Without decay	196	33	33x146=4818	3	3x146=438
1-2 decays	106	93	93x146=13.578	28	28x146=4.088
3-4 decays	79	67	67x146=9.872	27	27x146=3.942
5 and more decays	115	98	98x46=14.308	59	59x146=8.164
Total	499	291	42.486	117	17.082

health and it is stated with the simple but continuous applications such as flour varnish which could be applied to the children between the ages of 0-3, significant results could be achieved with regards to medium-long term decay prevalence and treatment cost (see Table 6).

Fluoridation of Drinking Water

In drinking water, there has been fluoride naturally; on the other hand, this quantity is not at the optimal value. The optimal value that protects teeth from decay is 0.7- 1.2 ppm. All over the world, more than 40 countries and more than 300 million people consume their drinking water with fluorally. Only in USA 145 million people consume water which has been processed fluorally. In comparison with the other preventive applications, fluoridation has the lowest cost. Although it differs according to the population it is provided, the average cost of drinking water fluoridation annual per capita is between 20-50 cents. According to studies published by the CDC, the settlement which has a population of about 20.000 people or more, in response to every allocated 1 dollar for fluoridation, there occurs 38 dollars gain. Explaining with an example, in California average filling price is 14 dollars, fluoridation cost per capita is 50 cents, so it corresponds to 2 dollars for a family of four persons.

SOME SUCCESFUL COST-EFFECTIVE PROJECTS APPLIED IN EU TO PREVENT DENTAL DISEASES

- **Fluoridation of Water:** It's the process of the fluoridation of city water. It's safe, cheap and effective. In Europe England, Ireland, Spain and Poland are among the countries using this system.
- **Usage of Fluoridated Salt:** It's useful for the healthy development of children's permanent tooth. (Yeung, 2011). This program has been applied in Switzerland, Germany, Czech Republic and Slovakia.
- **Usage of Fluoridated Milk:** A method used in Bulgaria and England for children (The Borrow Foundation 2012, CED 2009). It's appropriate for regions in which fluoride cannot be provided via salt or water.

- **Childsmile Program, Scotland:** It's applied in regions in which the city water is not fluoridated. Oral health educations has been realized in all elementary and nursery schools, free tooth brushes and pastes have been distributed, families have been educated, fluoride polish applications have been made (CHILDSMILE 2012). DMFT scores of children participated to this program dropped from 1,86 in 2008 to 1,52 in 2010 (NDIP 2010).
- **Denmark's Preventive Oral Health Model:** In 1974, oral and dental health clinics were established under every municipality. Every person under 18 was obliged to be educated in these clinics. They were examined and benefited from preventive treatment.
- **Programs in Community Centers:** It's based on informing especially the migrated families in community centers in Sweden. This program contains the education of families, brushing and hygiene educations, nutrition advices and prescribing fluoride tablets for children (Wenhall 2008).
- **Oral Health Education Provided by Students:** This method is being used in some poor regions of Germany and Ireland. In Germany, the 4th grade students who took before an extensive oral hygiene education educated 1st grade students. A similar program applied also in Ireland.
- **The Addition of Oral Examinations to General Health Controls for Old People:** This is a method used in England.
- **Raise Awareness for Oral Hygiene Habits:** This is a method applied in Sweden. First, an education is given to the participants, then they gain the ability to diagnose bacterial plaque. During the program, there's an education every two months and dental controls every 3-12 months.
- **Cancer Screenings for high Risk Groups:** It started as a pilot application in Hungary. Media has been used to inform people. People have been invited to dental check-up and free examinations made for high-risk groups.
- **National Preventive Program Realized in Order to Rise the Frequency of Dental Visits of People in Adolescence Period:** Applied in 1997 in France. Within this program, free check-up right was given to people who were between 15-18 years old.
- **Supporting the Sugar-Free Products:** With lots of researches, it is proven that the sweetening (xylitol, sorbitol, mannitol etc.) avoid tooth decays (Deshponde 2008, Ly 2008). The sales of sugar-free products are encouraged in countries like Germany and Switzerland.
- **Imposing Restrictions on the Sales of Sugared Products / Encouraging the Labelling of Some Products:** This is made for giving more detailed information about the product contents. Some restrictions can also be imposed in order to reduce the sugar content of some products.

CONCLUSION

In the developing countries, the increasing cost of oral and dental health treatment compels the social security institutions. In this respect, it is quite substantial to identify the risky individuals from the early periods, launch applications for protection, provide training for the parents and to determine the prevalence of this type of individuals in the community and to make medium and long term cost projections.

Tooth decay, which are the most widespread and the most harmful among the oral illnesses, are periodontal diseases and oral cancers. Decays have been started being restrained with preventive programs which have been executed by various countries. On the other hand, it still poses a serious problem for the poor or deprived groups. The periodontal diseases have become more destructive by affecting more than 50% of the European population. The situation has seemed more desperate, the highest incidence of oral cancer is in Europe after South Asia.

It is obvious that the preventive applications are much more effective and cheaper than the therapeutic applications. In contrast, it is not clear that which applications are the most effective and necessary methods. The methods for enhancing and encouraging the health of the mouth are required to identify and explain in a good way. The determination of the best preventive applications will enable researchers to advance in that way and it will decrease the amount of money and time that are spent for the ineffective methods.

REFERENCES

Abuhanoğlu, H. C., & Ayanoğlu, Y. (2011). Mezuniyet Oncesi Tıp Egitimi Maliyetlerinin Belirlenmesi: Tıp Fakültesinde Bir Uygulama. *Sağlıkta Performans ve Kalite Dergisi, 4*.

Amariei, C., & Eaton, K. A. (2009). Systems for the provision of oral health care in the Black Sea countries part 1: Romania. *Oral Health and Dental Management in the Black Sea Countries*, *8*, 3–6.

Angelillo, I. F., Nobile, C. G., & Pavia, M. (1996). Oral health status and treatment needs in immigrants and refugees in Italy. *European Journal of Epidemiology*, *12*(4), 359–365. doi:10.1007/BF00145298 PMID:8891539

Araujo, M. W., Dermen, K., & Connors, G. (2004). 0ral and dental health among inpatients in treatment for alcohol use disorders: A pilot study. *Journal of the International Academy of Periodontology*, *6*, 125–130. PMID:15553979

Australian Institute of Health and Welfare. (2010). *Australia's health in 2010: Twelth biennial health report of the Australian Institute of Health and Welfare*. Retrieved from: www.aihw.gov.au/W0rkArea/DownloadAsset.aspx?id=6442452962 on O1/07/2012

Bauer J., Neumann T. & Saekel R. (2009). *Zahnmedizinische Versorgung in Deutschland*. Verlag: Hans Huber.

Blot, W. J., McLaughlin, J. K., Winn, D. M., Austin, D. F., Greenberg, R. S., & Preston-Martin, S. (1998). Smoking and drinking in rela-tion to oral and pharyngeal cancer. *Cancer Research*, *4*(23282), 7.

Borrow Foundation. (n.d.). Retrieved from: http://wwwborrowfoundation.org/why-fluoridate-milk

Boyle, P., & Levin, B. (2008). *World cancer report*. Lyon: International Agency for Research on Cancer.

Çalışkan, Z. (2009). Saglık Hizmetlerinde Önceliklerin Belirlenmesinde Ekonomik Degerlendirme Yontemi Olarak Maliyet-Etkililik Analizi. *Süleyman Demirel Üniversitesi İktisadi ve İdari Bilimler Fakültesi Dergisi*, *14*, 311–332.

Childsmile. (n.d.). Retrieved from: http://www.chiId-smile.org.uk

Christensen, L., Twetman, S., & Sundby, A. (2010). Oral health in children and adolescents with different socio-cultural and socio-economic backgrounds. *Acta Odontologica Scandinavica*, *68*(1), 34–42. doi:10.3109/00016350903301712 PMID:19878044

Chuang, S. C., Jenab, M., Heck, J. E., Bosetti, C., Talamini, R., Matsuo, K., & Hashibe, M. et al. (2012). Diet and the risk of head and neck cancer: A pooled analysis in the INHANCE consortium. *Cancer Causes & Control*, *23*(1), 69–88. doi:10.1007/s10552-011-9857-x PMID:22037906

Colak, H., Serdaroglu, L., & Dulgergil, C. (2010). Temel Agız Ve Dis Saglıgı Hizmetinde Restorasyon Uygulamalarının Yeri Önemi ve Sonucları. *Saglıkta Performans ve Kalite Dergisi,* (1).

Commission of the European Communities. (2009). *Reducing health inequalities in the EU. COM(2009) 567.* Retrieved from: http://ec.europa.eu/health/ph_determinants/socio_economics/documents/com2009_en.pdf

Corbet, E. (2007). Public health aspects of oral diseases and disorders — Periodontal diseases. In C. Pine & R. Harris (Eds.), *Community oral health* (2nd ed.). Surrey, UK: Quintessence.

Council of European Chief Dental Officers. (n.d.). *Database*. Retrivied from: http://www.cecdo.org/pages/database%20intro.html

Council of European Dentists. (2009). *EU manual of dental practice: Version 4.1.* Retrivied from: http://www.eudental.eu/index.php?lD=35918 on O2/04/2012

Council of European Dentists. (2011). *CED resolution 'for better oral health ofall EU citizens: Mutual integration of oral and general health.* Retrivied from: http://wwweudental.eu/inde><.php?lD=2741 on 25/O3/2012

Deshpande, A., & Jadad, A. R. (2008). The impact of polyol-containing chewing gums on dental caries: A systematic review of original randomized controlled trials and observational studies. *The Journal of the American Dental Association*, *139*(12), 1602–1614. doi:10.14219/jada.archive.2008.0102 PMID:19047666

Doğan, B. G. (2007). Toplum Agız ve Dis Saglıgı Göstergeleri. *Toplum Hekimligi Bulteni, 26*(2).

Droz, D., Guéguen, R., Bruncher, P., Gerhard, J. L., & Roland, E. (2006). Epidemiological study of oral dental health of 4-year-old children in french nursery schools. *Archives of Pediatrics & Adolescent Medicine*, *13*, 122Z–9. PMID:16860544

Eaton, K. A., Newman, H. N., & Bulman, J. S. (2003). National mean DMFF scores for Western European 12 year-olds — Are they Comparable? *Journal of Dental Research*, *82*(519), 334. PMID:12709497

Edwards, D. M., & Watt, R. G. (1997). Oral health care in the lives of Gypsy travellers in east Hertfordshire. *British Dental Journal*, *183*(252), 7. PMID:9364092

Ericsson, J. S., Abrahamsson, K. H., & Ostberg, A. L. (2009). Periodontal health status in Swedish adolescents: An epidemiological, cross-sectional study. *Swedish Dental Journal*, *33*, 131–139. PMID:19994563

Eurobaromoter 72.3 Oral Health. Special Eurobarometer 330. (2010). Retrivied from: http://eceuropa.eu/public_opinion/archives/ebs/ebs_330_en.pdf

Ferlay, J., Parkin, D. M., & Steliarova-Foucher, E. (2010). Estimates of cancer incidence and mortality in Europe in 2008. *European Journal of Cancer*, *46*(4), 765–781. doi:10.1016/j.ejca.2009.12.014 PMID:20116997

Glassman, P., & Miller, C. E. (2003). Preventing dental disease for people with special needs: The need for practical preventive protocols for use in community settings. *Special Care in Dentistry*, *23*(5), 165–167. doi:10.1111/j.1754-4505.2003.tb00305.x PMID:14965180

Gooch, B. F., Griffin, S. O., Gray, S. K., Kohn, W. G., Rozier, R. G., Siegal, M., & Zero, D. T. et al. (2009). Preventing dental caries through school-based sealant programs: Updated recommendations and reviews of evidence. *The Journal of the American Dental Association*, *140*(11), 1356–1365. doi:10.14219/jada.archive.2009.0070 PMID:19884392

Hashibe, M., Brennan, P., & Chuang, S. C. (2009). Interaction between tobacco and alcohol use and the risk of head and neck cancer: Pooled analysis in the INHANCE consortium. *Cancer Epidemiology, Biomarkers & Prevention*, *18*, 541–550. PMID:19190158

Işık, A., & Mutlu, A. (2011). *Saglık Ekonomisine Giris*. Ekin Basım Yayın.

Koivusilta, L., Honkala, S., Honkala, E., & Rimpela, A. (2003). Toothbrushing as part of the adolescent lifestyle predicts education level. *Journal of Dental Research*, *82*(5), 361–366. doi:10.1177/154405910308200507 PMID:12709502

Konig, J., Holtfreter, B., & Kocher, T. (2010). Periodontal health in Europe: Future trends based on treatment needs and the provision of periodontal services-position paper. *European Journal of Dental Education*, *1*, 4–24. doi:10.1111/j.1600-0579.2010.00620.x PMID:20415972

Levin, K. A., & Currie, C. (2010). Adolescent toothbrushing and the home environment: Sociodemographic factors, family relationships and mealtime routines and disorganisation. *Community Dentistry and Oral Epidemiology*, *38*(1), 10–18. doi:10.1111/j.1600-0528.2009.00509.x PMID:19845713

Ly, K. A., Milgrom, P., & Rothen, M. (2008). The potential of dental-protective chewing gum in oral health interventions. *The Journal of the American Dental Association*, *139*(5), 553–563. doi:10.14219/jada.archive.2008.0215 PMID:18451371

Marinho, V. C. C., Higgins, J. P. T., Logan, S., & Sheiham, A. (2003). Fluoride toothpastes for preventing dental caries in children and adolescents. *Cochrane Database of Systematic Reviews*, 1.

OECD Library. (2011). *HealthataGlance2011: OECD indicators*. Retrivied from http://www.oecd-ilibrary.org/sites/health_glance2011en/06/06/index.html;jsessionid=3dln9sdrovedm.delta?cOntentType=&itemld=/content/chapter/health_glance201157n&containerltemld=/content/serial/19991312&accessltemlds=/content/book/health_glance-2011-en&mimeType=text/html on 02/04/2012

Ozgen H., Tatar M. (2008). *Saglık Sektorunde Bir Verimlilik Degerlendirme Teknigi Olarak Maliyet-Etkililik Analizi ve Turkiye'de Durum.*

Pihlstrom, B. L., Michalowicz, B. S., & Johnson, N. W. (2005). Periodontal diseases. *Lancet*, *366*(9499), 1809–1820. doi:10.1016/S0140-6736(05)67728-8 PMID:16298220

Reinhardt, C. H., Lopker, N., Noack, M. J., Klein, K., & Rosen, E. (2009). Peer tutoring pilot program for the improvement of oral health behavior in underprivileged and immigrant children. *Pediatric Dentistry*, *31*, 481–485. PMID:20108738

Sabbah, W., Sheiham, A., & Bernabé, E. (2010). Income inequality and periodontal diseases in rich countries: An ecological cross-sectional study. *International Dental Journal*, *60*, 370–374. PMID:21141210

Sahinoz. T., Sahinoz. S. (2012). Demografik ve Bazı Saglık Gostergeleri Acısından Turkiye'nin Dunyadaki Durumu. *Gumushane Universitesi Saglık Bilimleri Dergisi, 1.*

Sahyoun, N. R., Lin, C. L., & Krall, E. (2003). Nutritional status of the older adult is associated with dentition status. *Journal of the American Dietetic Association*, *103*(1), 61–66. doi:10.1053/jada.2003.50003 PMID:12525795

Scully, C., & Bagan, J. (2009). Oral squamous cell carcinoma overview. *Oral Oncology*, *45*(4-5), 301–308. doi:10.1016/j.oraloncology.2009.01.004 PMID:19249237

Sheiham, A. (2006). Dental caries affects body weight, growth and quality of life in preschool children. *British Dental Journal*, *201*(910), 625–626. doi:10.1038/sj.bdj.4814259 PMID:17128231

Sheiham, A., & Nicolau, B. (2005). Evaluation of social and psychological factors in periodontal disease. *Periodontol*, *Z00039*(1), 118–131. doi:10.1111/j.1600-0757.2005.00115.x PMID:16135067

Shiau, H. J., & Reynolds, M. A. (2010). Sex differences n destructive periodontal disease: Exploring the biologic basis. *Journal of Periodontology*, *81*(11), 1505–1517. doi:10.1902/jop.2010.100045 PMID:20594052

Tserakhava T., Shakavets N., & Smirnoy A. (2011). Systems for the provision of oral health care in the black sea countries part 9: Belarus. *Oral Health and Dental Management, 10*, 115-118.

Turk Dishekimleri Birligi Dishekimlerinin Calısma Sekilleri. (n.d.). *Kurumlarda ve Ilcelerde.*

Vereecken, C. A. (2005). The Relative influence of individual and contextual socioeconomic status on consumption of fruit and soft drinks among adolescents in Europe. *European Journal of Public Health*, *15*(3), 224–232. doi:10.1093/eurpub/cki005 PMID:15905182

Watt, R., & Sheiham, A. (1999). Inequalities in oral health: A review of the evidence and recommendations for action. *British Dental Journal*, *187*, 6–12. PMID:10452185

Watt, R., & Sheiham, A. (2012). Integrating the common risk factor approach into a social determinants framework. *Community Dentistry and Oral Epidemiology*, *40*(4), 289–296. doi:10.1111/j.1600-0528.2012.00680.x PMID:22429083

Widstrom, E., & Eaton, K. A. (2004). Oral healthcare systems in the extended European Union. *Oral Health & Preventive Dentistry*, *2*, 155–194. PMID:15641621

World Bank. (n.d.). *World databank.* Retrivied from http://databank.worldbank.org

World Health Organisation. (2012a). *Oral health fact sheet N°318.* Retrivied from: http://www.who.int/media-centre/factsheets/fs318/en/index.html on 14/04/2012

World Health Organisation. (2012b). Oral health country/area profile programme. WHO Collaborating Centre, Malmo University, Sweden. Retrivied from: http://www.mah.se/CAPP/Country-Oral-Health-Profiles/EURO/

Yeung, C. A. (2011). Efficacy of salt fluoridation. *Evidence-Based Dentistry*, *12*(1), 17–18. doi:10.1038/sj.ebd.6400776 PMID:21436859

Yıldırım I., Dulgergil C., & Serdaroglu. (2010). Aile Hekimligi Uygulamalarında Erken Donem Koruyucu Dis Hekimligi Uygulamaları ve Önemi. *Saglıkta Performans ve Kalite Dergisi, 2.*

Zigon, G., Berrino, F., Gatta, G., Sanchez, M. J., Van Dijk, B., Van Eycken, E., & Francisci, S.EUROCARE Working Group. (2011). Prognoses for head and neck cancers in Europe diagnosed in 1995-1999: A population-based study. *Annals of Oncology*, *22*(1), 165–174. doi:10.1093/annonc/mdq306 PMID:20587510

KEY TERMS AND DEFINITIONS

Economics: Economics is the science which tries to give the most appropriate answer to the 'How to satisfy the unlimited wants with limited ressources?' question.

Gingival Diseases: Gingival diseases occur as a result of the infection of supportive tissues such as gingival and bones.

Health: According to the World Health Organization (WHO), "health is more than just the absence of illness or disability, but also is phsical, spiritual and social well-being." This definition explains all dimensions of health. Lately, "Living socially and economically a productive life" has been added to this definiton.

Health Economics: Health economics can be defined as the application of the rules of economics to the health services. It can also be defined as the efficient use of the ressources allocated to the health sector.

This work was previously published in Regional Economic Integration and the Global Financial System edited by Engin Sorhun, Ümit Hacıoğlu, and Hasan Dinçer, pages 110-129, copyright year 2015 by Business Science Reference (an imprint of IGI Global).

APPENDIX: MAIN RISK FACTORS FOR ORAL DISEASES

Oral diseases are generally preventable. Some harmful habits for general health increase the risk to catch oral diseases. These are:

- **Insufficient Nourishment/Malnutrition:** There's a close relation between insufficient nourishment/malnutrition and poor oral health (Nowjack-Raymer ve Sheiham 2003, Sahyoun ve Krall 2003).
- **Insufficient Oral Hygiene:** Brushing the theeth with toothpaste containing fluoride is effective in preventing the tooth decays and periodontal diseases (Marinho 2003, Wong 2011).
- **Cigarette/Tobacco Consumption:** Cigarette has been defined as an important risk factor for periodontal diseases (Johnson ve Guthmiller 2000). Cigarette is also one of the main causes of oral cancers.
- **Alcohol Consumption:** There's a well defined relation between excessive and wrong consumption of alcohol and oral diseases.
- **Oral Cancers:** Oral cancers are arising from tissues in and around the mouth such as tongue, lip, gingival and cheek.
- **Oral and Dental Health:** According to WHO, "Oral health is a state of being free from chronic mouth and facial pain, oral and throat cancer, oral sores, birth defects such as cleft lip and palate, periodontal (gum) disease, tooth decay and tooth loss, and other diseases and disorders that affect the oral cavity." Oral health can be divided into 3 groups: Tooth decays, periodontal diseases and oral cancers.
- **Tooth Decays:** Tooth decay is an illness which occurs with the resorption/perforation of tooth enamel.

Chapter 14
The Acceptability of Teleconsultations in Teledentistry:
A Case Study

Roxana Ologeanu-Taddei
Université Montpellier, France

Isabelle Bourdon
KEDGE Business School, France & Université Montpellier, France

Chris Kimble
KEDGE Business School, France & Université Montpellier, France

Nicolas Giraudeau
Université Montpellier, France

INTRODUCTION

Telemedicine and teledentistry are both relatively recent developments. Even telework, the field from which these specialties emerged, only dates back to the 1973-1974 oil crisis (Bailey & Kurland, 2002). Telework is often classified along three dimensions: organizational (working in the same or a different organization), spatial (working in the same or different physical space) and temporal (where communication with co-workers is either synchronous or asynchronous) (Kimble et al., 2000); as we shall see, these three basic divisions apply equally to telemedicine and teledentistry.

In its short history, various definitions have been put forward and various terms have been coined for telemedicine (Tulu, Chatterjee, & Laxminarayan, 2005). Perhaps the simplest is that proposed by Celler, Lovell, and Basilakis (2003, p. 242), telemedicine is "a system of healthcare delivery in which physicians examine patients through the use of telecommunications technology."

There have been a number of reviews of telemedicine (Roine, Ohinmaa, & Hailey, 2001; Hailey, Ohinmaa, & Roine, 2004) which put forward a wide range of potential benefits; nevertheless, despite the scope of the topic, certain themes appear consistently:

DOI: 10.4018/978-1-5225-1903-4.ch014

Figure 1. A classification scheme for teleworking
Kimble et al., 2000.

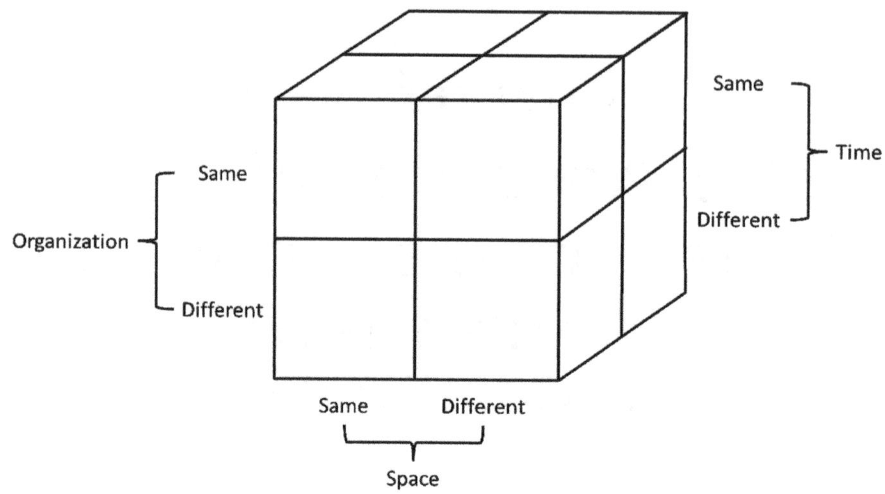

- Making specialist skills available in remote locations or to groups such as the elderly and disabled (Kimble et al., 2000; Asthana & Halliday, 2004; Noel, Vogel, Erdos, Cornwall, & Levin, 2004; Tulu et al., 2005).
- Improved adherence to standards and notions of best practice, particularly in the case of chronic conditions (Celler et al., 2003; Noel et al., 2004; Kimble, 2014).
- Reducing the cost of healthcare (Tulu et al., 2005; Bashshur, Shannon, Krupinski, & Grigsby, 2011; Kimble, 2014).

Although a number of activities can be placed under the heading of telemedicine, most involve some form of teleconsultation. Referring to Figure 1, a teleconsultation takes place when a physician in one location gives a consultation to a patient at some remote location (i.e. physician and patient are located in different spaces). The patient may, or may not, be supported by some other healthcare professional (i.e. a teleconsultation may involve a number of different organizations). The goal of the teleconsultation is for the patient and / or the healthcare professional to provide the physician with the information they need to make a diagnosis. Thus, finally, the communication between patient and physician, and the delivery of the diagnosis, may be either synchronous (e.g. via a live video link) or asynchronous (e.g. data is stored and accessed later).

Telemedicine is now well established in countries such as the United States and Australia (Celler et al., 2003) and there is growing interest in the topic in developing countries where problems of transport and access to healthcare facilities make telemedicine an attractive alternative to more traditional forms of healthcare provision (Chen, Cheng, & Mehta, 2013). Although various forms of telemedicine such as teleradiology, telepathology, teledermatology, and teleophthalmology are well established, teledentistry, the focus of this chapter, is relatively new.

According to Mihailovic, Miladinovic, and Vujicic (2011), the origins of Teledentistry can be traced back to the U.S. Army's Total Dental Access Project in 1994. They note that despite advances in the field of telemedicine, the field of teledentistry remains somewhat neglected. Although the situation is improving thanks to interest from transition and emerging economies such as Brazil (Torres-Pereira et al., 2008), Turkey (Ata & Ozkan, 2009) and India (Sukhabogi, Hameed, & Chandrashekar, 2014), teledentistry is still an emergent field. Below we briefly review some of potential benefits of teledentistry and some of the obstacles in the way of its further development.

TELEDENTISTRY: BENEFITS AND OBSTACLES

"Teledentistry is a combination of telecommunications and dentistry involving the exchange of clinical information and images over remote distances for dental consultation and treatment planning" (Jampani, Nutalapati, Dontula, & Boyapati, 2011). As indicated, this may include synchronous and asynchronous consultations on the same or different sites and the involvement of a variety of different professions.

Perhaps not surprisingly, many of the motivations for developing teledentistry are broadly the same as for telemedicine. It is claimed to improve access to and the delivery of oral healthcare whilst simultaneously decreasing costs (Golder & Brennan, 2000); to be particularly important in rural areas (Bhambal, Saxena, & Balsaraf, 2010) and for those who do not have easy access to dental healthcare, such as older people or prisoners (Sanchez Dils, Lefebvre, & Abeyta, 2004). Thus, for example, Berndt, Leone, and King (2008) report on an initiative to use teledentistry to provide services for socially disadvantaged children.

While noting that the evidence base for teledentistry is thin, Daniel and Kumar (2014) claim that teledentistry appears to have the potential to meet the triple aim of health care reforms in the United States: improved care quality, improved health outcomes, and reduced per-capita costs. However, they also note that despite this potential, a number of practical and organizational barriers remain; these include a lack of confidence from patients and health professionals, the modification of knowledge and skills required of health professionals, and organizational and bureaucratic difficulties concerning the reimbursement for telemedicine services.

Although Daniel and Kumar (2014) are specifically concerned with teledentistry in the US, many of the issues recur elsewhere. Below we briefly review some of these issues using the hierarchy produced by (Broens, Vollenbroek-Hutten, Hermens, van Halteren, & Nieuwenhuis, 2007), which identifies five factors (Table 1) that influence the implementation of telemedicine at different stages in a project's life cycle.

Table 1. Factors that influence the implementation of telemedicine

Factor	Stage in Life Cycle
Technology	Experimental Prototype
Acceptance	Pilot Project
Organization	Small-Scale Use
Finance	Large-Scale Use
Legal and Policy Issues	Operational Product

Broens et al., 2007.

Technology Issues

Once telemedicine projects move beyond the prototype stage, most of the technological issues relate to education and training. Prior experience or exposure to computer/health technology has been found to be crucial success factor (Or & Karsh, 2009). Giraudeau et al. (2014) also note the need for additional training on the side of nursing staff as a specific constraint for the growth of teledentistry.

Acceptance Issues

The idea of acceptance is related to perceived usefulness and ease of use (Davis, 1989). The attitude of medical staff has been found to be a significant determinant of technology adoption (Hu, Chau, & Sheng, 2002). Prior research has shown that, under certain circumstances, high levels of acceptance can overcome problems with the technology itself, even with a lack of adequate resourcing (Wade, Eliott, & Hiller, 2014).

Organizational Issues

The role of 'champion' (Chakrabarti, 1974) is a crucial factor in developing and continuing this type of project (Wade & Hamlyn, 2013). In effect, the champion promotes and builds legitimacy for the project through a network of relationships among the various stakeholders. Previous research (Vuononvirta et al., 2009), has identified ten different types of adopters in telehealth projects: enthusiastic user, positive user, critical user, hesitant user, positive participant, hesitant participant, critical participant, neutral participant, negative participant, and positive non-participant. Project staff and managers need to take into account all of these diverse attitudes as different people will require different actions to ensure the project is adopted.

Financing Issues

Chen et al. (2013) observe that although sustainable business models need to be developed in order to create value for a healthcare provider as well as for the patient, research on business models for telemedicine is limited. However, there are indications that viable business models exist. Kimble (2015) reviewed ten successful telemedicine projects and concluded that the IT component of such projects was often fairly basic, and the success of the project hinged on the way that networks of doctors, health workers, or counselors, were able to leverage existing resources; this was frequently facilitated by relatively minor changes to existing legal and medical codes.

Policy and Legislative Issues

As noted above, legal and policy issues are an important factor for the success of telemedicine, for example, from an Indian perspective, Sukhabogi et al. (2014) highlight legal issues and concerns about confidentiality as factors that inhibit telemedicine projects. Giraudeau et al. (2014) also list various legal and ethical constraints that prevent the establishment of a viable business model for teledentistry, including the reluctance of health insurance companies to pay for acts of telemedicine. Patel and Antonarakis (2013) cite similar concerns about the medico-legal aspects of service delivery.

Having delineated the field of teledentistry and highlighted some of the barriers to its further development, we now turn to the main topic of the chapter which is a case study of an ongoing teledentistry project in the south of France known as the e-DENT project. Below we describe the key problems and issues faced by the project and some of the potential solutions we have found. Based on this, we conclude by outlining some of the future research directions in the field of teledentistry.

THE e-DENT PROJECT

The e-DENT project is the first teledentistry project in France and probably the first official teledentistry project in Europe. The long-term goal of the project is to improve the provision of dental care for people who are not able to have regular consultations with a dentist, such as prisoners, the dependent elderly, or disabled people.

The project was initiated by a team from the faculty of Odontology in University of Montpellier who saw the lack of oral healthcare for elderly people as an important public health issue. It is based in the Languedoc-Roussillon area of southern France and is being carried out in collaboration with Montpellier public hospital and Oral-B, which is part of Procter & Gamble. The project is also supported by the regional public health agency of the Languedoc-Roussillon area who wish to know if teledentistry could be used as a tool to improve public dental health.

Currently, the project is in its pilot stage and involves 800 patients (100 prisoners, 100 frail people, and 600 elderly people) in twelve long-term care homes, three hospitals for frail people and a prison medical department (Giraudeau et al., 2014). In its present form, the project provides:

1. Information about oral health and the proper techniques for tooth brushing.
2. A teleconsultation to provide a diagnosis of the current state of the patient's oral health and, if appropriate, a recommendation for further treatment.

The teleconsultation process consists of three steps (Figure 2). To make it possible for the teleconsultations to be carried out, specific software (e-DENT® from e-DENTECH, Montpellier, France) needed to be developed.

Step 1: Nurses take pictures and videos of the patient's mouth and teeth using a specially developed intraoral camera, Soprocare®, which uses light of different wavelengths to highlight dental caries and gum inflammation without the need for dye solutions.

Step 2: When the filming and photography are complete, the data is sent to the server at the hospital where it is stored under secure conditions for review by a hospital dentist later.

Step 3: After reviewing the data, the hospital dentist makes a diagnosis and creates an appropriate plan for treatment, which may include the type of dentist and the intervention that is needed (e.g. regular or specialist dentist, general anesthesia, etc.)

Nurses follow a set protocol for the use of the camera with each patient, at the first evaluation, and after 4 to 6 months to observe any changes between consultations. Currently dental students from the Montpellier public hospital carry out the teleconsultations. Patients and medical staff are informed about any treatment that is needed, and organize any subsequent dental appointments.

Figure 2. Flow chart of a teleconsultation
Giraudeau et al., 2014.

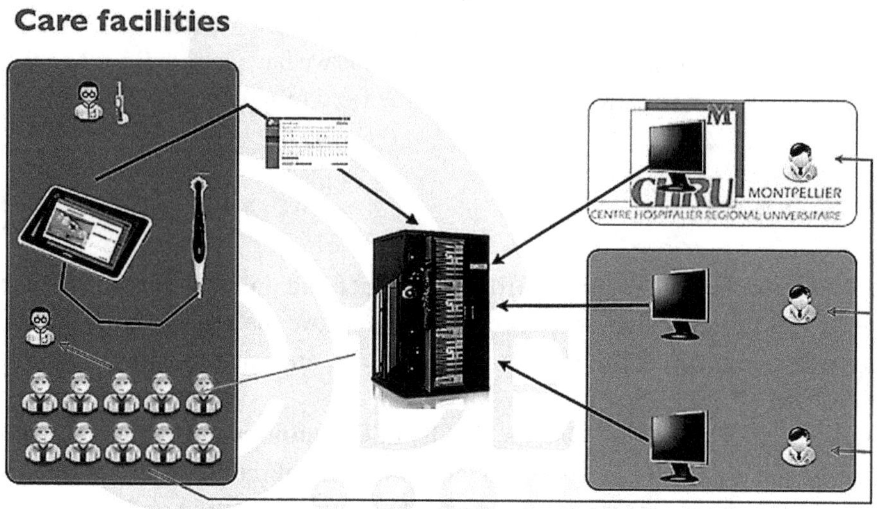

As this is a pilot project, one of the immediate concerns of the project is to evaluate how effective this teledentistry initiative is; as part of this, a qualitative survey has been carried out on the acceptability of the asynchronous teleconsultations to medical personnel. The results of this study, which highlight some of the problems faced in teledentistry, are reported, together with some potential solutions, below.

RESULTS AND DISCUSSION

As part of the e-DENT project, a qualitative study has been completed that involved interviews with nurses and managers of health facilities, dentists and the project manager. The study has highlighted some of the problems of acceptability associated with telemedicine in general and teledentistry in particular. The goal of the study is to gain a better understanding of the acceptability of the technique of teleconsultation from the key stakeholders (clinicians, nurses, patients, hospital managers). The approach is broadly inductive and may be described as an exploratory case study (Yin, 1994). The main data collection instrument was semi-structured interviews augmented with additional data from observations and documents. The results are presented using the hierarchy produced by (Broens et al., 2007) described earlier and highlight some of the issues we have found.

Technology Issues

As indicated above, many of the technology issues for this type of project relate to education and training. It appears that nurses' prior experience of computer technology will also be a crucial factor in the e-DENT project as some nurses lack the basic computer literacy skills needed to transfer the data to the server. In our case study, one nurse has abandoned the pilot project after 2 months because the technology was too threatening for her, even although she had completed all of the training required to operate the device. Thus, a lack of ongoing training, support, and education of nurses in the technology used in the project could become a barrier to its eventual success. In common with other teledentistry projects, users must be well trained and supported technically and professionally (Yellowlees, 2005).

Acceptance Issues

Although nurses' acceptance is seen as being particularly crucial for the success of the e-DENT project, we also need to deal with both the perceptions of patients and other health-care workers.

Nurses and Health-Care Workers

An essential aspect of the project concerns offering dental consultations in circumstances where access to such services would normally be limited. Although the benefits for the project as a whole are seen as things like increased access to dentistry services, increased communication between healthcare professionals, enhanced dentistry education opportunities and the identification of patients who require specific treatments, for nurses, the time that can be given to direct patient contact is viewed as an important potential benefit. The quality of communication with a nurse, who is known by the patient or is present when other clinicians are there, is crucial for certain aspects of teledentistry. The patient-nurse relationship is important as patients can have a fear of dentists and dental treatment. Nurses are able to reduce the anxiety of patients and enable them to remain in their own homes for consultations.

We believe that the acceptance for nurses is connected to their professional roles and status. Buccal teleconsultation is a new task for them; in addition to the technology, they have to accept providing this new service. The e-DENT project entails significant changes in nurses' work processes that affect the material conditions of their work and their relationships with other health care professionals (Nicolini, 2006); as a result, some modifications to their knowledge and skills are required. Consequently, acceptance of teledentistry is related both to technology and to the whole process that surrounds the provision of a teleconsultation.

These changes may be considered as a potential threat to a nurse's role and status; some nurses already consider their workload too high and for them the extra time and administration required for teleconsultation is not worth the investment.

Patients

The acceptance of patients is an important issue for the project; however, the evaluation of patient perceptions poses some problems. The normal techniques for measuring patient acceptance could not be used in the e-DENT project because of the particular characteristics of the patients. Many of the patients in the project have cognitive and/or intellectual disabilities and the Technology Acceptance Model (TAM) that is usually used to measure acceptance is based on uncovering the rationale for individual choices and behaviors. Consequently, we were inspired by approaches found in some medical papers to focus on patients' feelings and disposition. We are currently investigating the use of a modified PANAS grid (Watson, Clark, & Tellegen, 1988) using nurses' observations.

Organizational Issues

A big concern is the novel relationship between the clinical telehealth providers (i.e. the nurses and dentists) and the information technology (IT) providers that are needed to implement the tools used for the asynchronous consultation and diagnosis by dentists (Wade & Hamlyn, 2013). In the project, nurses capture images that are delivered and stored via an IT network to be consulted later by the dentist. The start of the project was delayed by 6 months because of problems related the internal IT departments of the hospital where the dentists were located. These problems included technical and organizational barriers to the installation of the equipment in the hospital's IT networks and a low priority given to the e-DENT project. In this relatively small-scale project, the e-DENT project leader effectively acted as the 'product champion', as it was he who initiated and promoted the project and it was he who had to resolve many of the low-level organizational problems.

Financing Issues

According to Broens et al. (2007), financing issues start to come to the fore as a project moves from a local, small-scale project to become more general and widespread. Although the e-DENT project is still local and relatively small-scale, some of the issues related to larger scale projects have already begun to appear.

The project is funded by the French Health Regulation Agency and by the Regional Union of Health-care Professionals, which provides support for the dentist's consultation fee. The Union provides an increased consultation fee to account for the additional time spent in the training of dentists for project. To grow, the project needs to find a way to continue without this specific form of financing. Any new arrangement needs to take into account the purchase of the device and its maintenance as well as the cost of the training for the dentist and nurses. Moreover, it has to construct an economic model with stakeholders that provide both a fee for the dentists who undertake the teleconsultations and a mechanism for reimbursing the time spent by nurses on preparing the data.

This is a particular problem in France because all consultations take place within a framework which is supported by the national Social Security system, which means dentists' fees are regulated and cannot exceed a certain amount. Consequently, even although the teleconsultation requires additional time, resources, and personnel, the dentists are unable to increase their fees. Similar problems arise when the nurse who collects the data is employed by a different organization to the doctor who consults the data.

Policy and Legislation Issues

Closely related to the problems of designing a viable business model for teledentistry are the changes to the law and to social policy that are needed to regularize the practice of telemedicine. In France, there is a specific law, introduced in 2010, that regulates telemedicine (sante.gouv, 2014). This law describes a judicial framework consisting of five different telemedicine acts, which are: tele-consultation; tele-expertise; tele-monitoring; tele-assistance and tele-regulation (see key terms and definitions below). The e-DENT project is related to teleconsultation (remote consultation with a patient) and tele-monitoring (where a remote physician interprets a patient's data). However, while this law provides legal recognition for acts of telemedicine in France it does so within a broader European framework of e-health, which covers areas such as electronic health records; consequently, there are many issues specific to teledentistry that are not covered. In the longer term, social policy and legislation issues will be crucial to the economic viability of teledentistry.

FUTURE RESEARCH DIRECTIONS

The e-DENT project raises numerous questions for future research. At this stage, which is essentially a pilot study, we have dealt with technology issues and issues related to the usability and quality of the system, as these needed to be analyzed before we could move forward. Concerning acceptance issues, it is clear that both patients' and professionals' attitudes toward teledentistry technology influence the success of the project. However, as we have indicated, the attitude of elderly patients needs to be better understood and metrics need to be developed to deal with their specificities (e.g. cognitive deficiencies).

In the pilot stages of the e-DENT project, the costs associated with the implementation and operation of teledentistry (including the initial investment, maintenance, and operational costs) have been funded by local and national initiatives. However, there is currently no structure for long-term financing, and a rigorous analysis of the cost-effectiveness of the process, which is needed for the development and financing of future projects, has not been undertaken.

In addition to this, the introduction of teledentistry will affect the (intramural) operation of individual organizations and require new (extramural) collaboration with other healthcare organizations. Those changes will in turn require modifications in the roles, rights, and responsibilities of stakeholders. This area has not been explored within the current literature on teledentistry.

However, the research area that is probably of the greatest importance currently concerns the need to create and/or redesign business models so that all of the participants can benefit from acts of teledentistry. The introduction of teledentistry influences the financial situation of various parties in the healthcare process, and leads to a redistribution of costs and revenues which is different to the financing of traditional (i.e. non-telemedicine) dental-care. In the longer term this will inevitably involve changes to and reform of the current legal framework that governs telemedicine.

Further legal research is needed to answer the numerous questions raised by teledentistry such as the issues raised by the transfer of medical data, the definition of acts of telemedicine and the legal restraints on cost sharing and remuneration between different medical specialties. Research in the field of public health policy could eventually lead to positive changes that would impact on teledentistry at both the level of public health and of patient care.

CONCLUSION

This project was driven by two key opportunities: the French law that created the legal framework for telemedicine and the financing provided by the French government for the experimental tele-medicine projects. Although the technology will continue to be developed, most of the major technological problems have now been solved. Issues of acceptance and organization, at least within the context of a small-scale implementation of teledentistry, are now being explored. The next major challenge is to find a suitable business model for teledentistry and to promote the more widespread acceptance of teleconsultations among dentists and nurses. In the longer term, this will require changes at national and/or European level.

REFERENCES

Asthana, S., & Halliday, J. (2004). What can rural agencies do to address the additional costs of rural services? A typology of rural service innovation. *Health & Social Care in the Community*, *12*(6), 457–465. doi:10.1111/j.1365-2524.2004.00518.x PMID:15717893

Ata, S. O., & Ozkan, S. (2009). *Information technology in oral health care: Attitudes of dental professionals on the use of teledentistry in Turkey*. Paper presented at the European and Mediterranean Conference on Information Systems.

Bailey, D. E., & Kurland, N. B. (2002). A review of telework research: Findings, new directions, and lessons for the study of modern work. *Journal of Organizational Behavior*, *23*(4), 383–400. doi:10.1002/job.144

Bashshur, R., Shannon, G., Krupinski, E., & Grigsby, J. (2011). The taxonomy of telemedicine. *Telemedicine Journal and e-Health*, *17*(6), 484–494. doi:10.1089/tmj.2011.0103 PMID:21718114

Berndt, J., Leone, P., & King, G. (2008). Using teledentistry to provide interceptive orthodontic services to disadvantaged children. *American Journal of Orthodontics and Dentofacial Orthopedics*, *134*(5), 700–706. doi:10.1016/j.ajodo.2007.12.023 PMID:18984404

Bhambal, A., Saxena, S., & Balsaraf, , S. V. (2010). Teledentistry: Potentials unexplored! *Journal of International Oral Health*, *2*(3), 1–6.

Broens, T. H., Vollenbroek-Hutten, M. M., Hermens, H. J., van Halteren, A. T., & Nieuwenhuis, , L. J. (2007). Determinants of successful telemedicine implementations: A literature study. *Journal of Telemedicine and Telecare*, *13*(6), 303–309. doi:10.1258/135763307781644951 PMID:17785027

Celler, B. G., Lovell, N. H., & Basilakis, J. (2003). Using information technology to improve the management of chronic disease. *The Medical Journal of Australia*, *179*(5), 242–246. PMID:12924970

Chakrabarti, A. K. (1974). The role of champion in product innovation. *California Management Review*, *17*(2), 58–62. doi:10.2307/41164561

Chen, S., Cheng, A., & Mehta, K. (2013). A review of telemedicine business models. *Telemedicine Journal and e-Health*, *19*(4), 287–297. doi:10.1089/tmj.2012.0172 PMID:23540278

Daniel, S. J., & Kumar, S. (2014). Teledentistry: A Key Component in Access to Care. *Journal of Evidence Based Dental Practice, 14,* 201-208.

Davis, , F. D. (1989). Perceived Usefulness, Perceived Ease of Use, and User Acceptance of Information Technology. *Management Information Systems Quarterly*, *13*(3), 319–340. doi:10.2307/249008

Giraudeau, N., Valcarcel, J., Tassery, H., Levallois, B., Cuisinier, F., Tramini, P., et al. (2014). Projet e-DENT: téléconsultation bucco-dentaire en EHPAD. *European Research in Telemedicine / La Recherche Européenne en Télémédecine, 3*(2), 51-56.

Golder, D. T., & Brennan, K. A. (2000). Practicing dentistry in the age of telemedicine. *Journal of the American Dental Association (1939), 131*(6), 734-744.

Hailey, D., Ohinmaa, A., & Roine, R. (2004). Study quality and evidence of benefit in recent assessments of telemedicine. *Journal of Telemedicine and Telecare*, *10*(6), 318–324. doi:10.1258/1357633042602053 PMID:15603628

Hu, P. J.-H., Chau, P. Y., & Sheng, O. R. L. (2002). Adoption of telemedicine technology by health care organizations: An exploratory study. *Journal of Organizational Computing and Electronic Commerce*, *12*(3), 197–221. doi:10.1207/S15327744JOCE1203_01

Jampani, , N. DNutalapati, R., Dontula, B. S. K., & Boyapati, R. (2011). Applications of teledentistry: A literature review and update. *Journal of International Society of Preventive & Community Dentistry*, *1*(2), 37–44. doi:10.4103/2231-0762.97695 PMID:24478952

Kimble, C. (2014). Electronic Health Records: Cure-All or Chronic Condition? *Global Business and Organizational Excellence*, *33*(4), 63–74. doi:10.1002/joe.21554

Kimble, C. (2015). Business Models for E-Health: Evidence From Ten Case Studies. *Global Business and Organizational Excellence*, *34*(4), 18–30. doi:10.1002/joe.21611

Kimble, C., & Bourdon, I. (2013). The Link among Information Technology, Business Models, and Strategic Breakthroughs: Examples from Amazon, Dell, and eBay. *Global Business and Organizational Excellence*, *33*(1), 58–68. doi:10.1002/joe.21523

Kimble, C., Li, F., & Barlow, A. (2000). *Effective Virtual Teams through Communities of Practice*. Strathclyde, UK: University of Strathclyde.

Mihailovic, B., Miladinovic, M., & Vujicic, B. (2011). Telemedicine in dentistry (teledentistry). In G. Graschew (Ed.), *Advances in telemedicine: applications in various medical disciplines and geographical area* (pp. 215–230). Rijeka, Croatia: InTech. doi:10.5772/14352

Nicolini, D. (2006). The work to make telemedicine work: A social and articulative view. *Social Science & Medicine*, *62*(11), 2754–2767. doi:10.1016/j.socscimed.2005.11.001 PMID:16343724

Noel, H. C., Vogel, D. C., Erdos, J. J., Cornwall, D., & Levin, F. (2004). Home telehealth reduces healthcare costs. *Telemedicine Journal and e-Health*, *10*(2), 170–183. doi:10.1089/tmj.2004.10.170 PMID:15319047

Or, C. K., & Karsh, B.-T. (2009). A systematic review of patient acceptance of consumer health information technology. *Journal of the American Medical Informatics Association*, *16*(4), 550–560. doi:10.1197/jamia.M2888 PMID:19390112

Patel, R. N., & Antonarakis, G. S. (2013). Factors influencing the adoption and implementation of teledentistry in the UK, with a focus on orthodontics. *Community Dentistry and Oral Epidemiology*, *41*(5), 424–431. PMID:23240902

Roine, R., Ohinmaa, A., & Hailey, D. (2001). Assessing telemedicine: A systematic review of the literature. *Canadian Medical Association Journal*, *165*(6), 765–771. PMID:11584564

Sanchez Dils, E., Lefebvre, C., & Abeyta, K. (2004). Teledentistry in the United States: A new horizon of dental care. *International Journal of Dental Hygiene*, *2*(4), 161–164. doi:10.1111/j.1601-5037.2004.00093.x PMID:16451490 sante.gouv. (2014). *Déploiement de la télémédecine: tout se joue maintenant*. Retrieved 17 Nov, 2014, from http://www.sante.gouv.fr/deploiement-de-la-telemedecine-tout-se-joue-maintenant.html

Sukhabogi, J., Hameed, I., & Chandrashekar, , B. (2014). Teledentistry: An essential need of the era. *Universal Research Journal of Dentistry*, *4*(2), 71–77. doi:10.4103/2249-9725.132965

Torres-Pereira, C., Possebon, R. S., Simões, A., Bortoluzzi, M. C., Leão, J. C., & Giovanini, , A. FPiazetta, C. M. (2008). Email for distance diagnosis of oral diseases: A preliminary study of teledentistry. *Journal of Telemedicine and Telecare*, *14*(8), 435–438. doi:10.1258/jtt.2008.080510 PMID:19047454

Tulu, B., Chatterjee, S., & Laxminarayan, S. (2005). A taxonomy of telemedicine efforts with respect to applications, infrastructure, delivery tools, type of setting and purpose.*Proceedings of the 38th Annual Hawaii International Conference on System Sciences*. doi:10.1109/HICSS.2005.56

Vuononvirta, , TTimonen, , MKeinänen-Kiukaanniemi, , STimonen, , OYlitalo, , KKanste, , OTaanila, , A. (2009). The attitudes of multiprofessional teams to telehealth adoption in northern Finland health centres. *Journal of Telemedicine and Telecare*, *15*(6), 290–296. doi:10.1258/jtt.2009.090108 PMID:19720766

Wade, V. A., Eliott, J. A., & Hiller, , J. E. (2014). Clinician Acceptance is the Key Factor for Sustainable Telehealth Services. *Qualitative Health Research*. PMID:24685708

Wade, V. A., & Hamlyn, J. S. (2013). The relationship between telehealth and information technology ranges from that of uneasy bedfellows to creative partnerships. *Journal of Telemedicine and Telecare*, *19*(7), 401–404. doi:10.1177/1357633X13506533 PMID:24218354

Watson, D., Clark, L. A., & Tellegen, , A. (1988). Development and validation of brief measures of positive and negative affect: The PANAS scales. *Journal of Personality and Social Psychology*, *54*(6), 1063–1070. doi:10.1037/0022-3514.54.6.1063 PMID:3397865

Yellowlees, P. M. (2005). Successfully developing a telemedicine system. *Journal of Telemedicine and Telecare*, *11*(7), 331–335. doi:10.1258/1357633305774472024 PMID:16238833

Yin, R. K. (1994). *Case Study Research, Design and Methods* (2nd ed.). Newbury Park, CA: Sage Publications.

KEY TERMS AND DEFINITIONS

Business Model: A unified conceptual description of the activities of value creation (the creation of a product that meets customers' needs), value capture (the marketing, support and sale of the product) and value architecture (the chain of activities that link customers and suppliers of a product) (Kimble & Bourdon, 2013).

Tele-Assistance: A doctor assists other health professionals at a distance in the performance of some medical act (sante.gouv, 2014).

Tele-Consultation: A doctor, based in one location, gives a consultation to a patient, who may or may not be supported by some other healthcare professional, at some other location. The patient and / or the healthcare professional provide the doctor with the data they need to make a diagnosis at a distance (sante.gouv, 2014).

Teledentistry: A combination of telecommunications technology and dentistry involving the exchange of data and images for the purposes of dental consultation and treatment planning (Jampani et al., 2011).

Tele-Expertise: A doctor seeking the opinion of one or more colleagues, at a distance, based on medical data related to the care of a patient (sante.gouv, 2014).

Tele-Monitoring: A doctor monitors and interprets medical parameters of a physically remote patient. The recording and transmission of data can be automated, performed by the patients themselves or by a health care professional (sante.gouv, 2014).

This work was previously published in the Encyclopedia of E-Health and Telemedicine edited by Maria Manuela Cruz-Cunha, Isabel Maria Miranda, Ricardo Martinho, and Rui Rijo, pages 1-12, copyright year 2016 by Medical Information Science Reference (an imprint of IGI Global).

Index

I

J

L

M

N

O

P

R

S

T

X

www.ingramcontent.com/pod-product-compliance
Lightning Source LLC
LaVergne TN
LVHW080621300926
849162LV00005B/1226